The Molecular Basis of Neurosurgical Disease

VOLUME 8: CONCEPTS IN NEUROSURGERY

The Molecular Basis of Neurosurgical Disease

VOLUME 8: CONCEPTS IN NEUROSURGERY

EDITORS

Corey Raffel, M.D., Ph.D.

Chief, Pediatric Neurosurgery
Mayo Eugenio Litta Children's Hospital
Associate Professor, Neurological Surgery
Mayo Medical School
Rochester, Minnesota

Griffith R. Harsh IV, M.D.

Associate Professor of Surgery
Harvard Medical School
Neurosurgical Service
Massachusetts General Hospital
Boston, Massachusetts

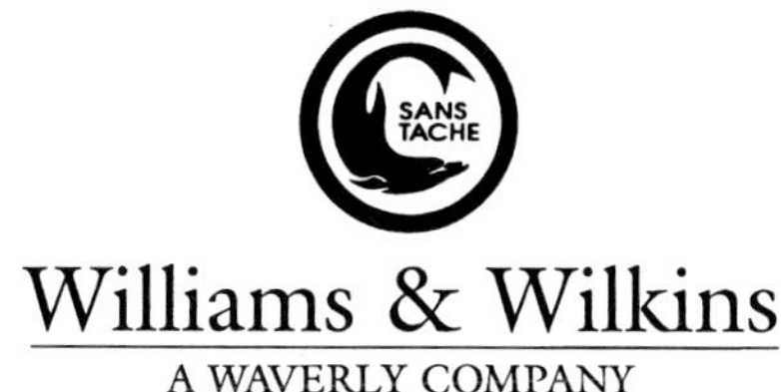

Williams & Wilkins

A WAVERLY COMPANY

BALTIMORE • PHILADELPHIA • LONDON • PARIS • BANGKOK
BUENOS AIRES • HONG KONG • MUNICH • SYDNEY • TOKYO • WROCLAW

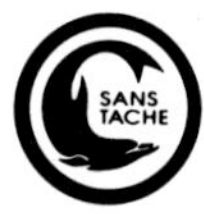

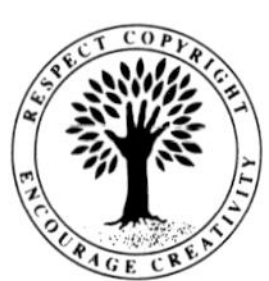

Accurate indications, adverse reactions, and dosage schedules for drugs are provided in this book, but it is possible that they may change. The reader is urged to review the package information data of the manufacturers of the medications mentioned.

Printed in the United States of America
(ISBN 0-683-18312-5)

96 97 98 99
1 2 3 4 5 6 7 8 9 10

Foreword

The revolution in molecular biology and genetics that is sweeping through the world of medicine holds great promise for the future. Diseases that heretofore have been untreatable and poorly understood may soon fall to the molecular scalpel. Much attention has been focused on diseases of the nervous system, often ones which neurosurgeons do not ordinarily treat. The importance of understanding the techniques, capabilities and current status of molecular biological approaches to nervous system disease is clear, and the neurosurgeon practicing 20 years from now will need to be familiar with this rapidly expanding area of medicine.

In continuing the CONCEPTS IN NEUROSURGERY series, the Congress of Neurological Surgeons looks forward, offering ways for the practicing neurosurgeon to remain up-to-date and to anticipate his or her educational needs for the future. Drs. Raffel and Harsh, both regularly working with molecular biological techniques, have gathered together knowledge about this subject relevant for neurosurgeons. We hope that this volume, provided as a service to members of the Congress, will help to prepare us all for the future of neurosurgery in the treatment of an increasing number of neurological diseases.

Stephen J. Haines, MD
Minneapolis, MN

Paul B. Nelson, MD
Indianapolis, IN

Preface

We are in the midst of a revolution in our understanding of the normal and aberrant functioning of an organism at the cellular, subcellular, and molecular levels. This is particularly true for brain and spinal cord function and for neurosurgical disease. As our understanding of the molecular alterations leading to disease increases, new strategies for treating disease by correcting these alterations are being developed.

This eighth volume in the *Concepts of Neurosurgery* series entitled, "The Molecular Basis of Neurosurgical Disease," reviews the new findings in molecular biology relevant to neurosurgery. Not surprisingly, given the wide range of diseases treated by neurosurgeons, there is a wealth of new relevant information. This volume is designed to pass from a discussion of the basic molecular biology of the central nervous system to the alterations of this biology in disease and then to potential treatments based on this molecular understanding of these processes. The first section includes two chapters discussing standard molecular biologic techniques and one discussing basic principles and strategies of gene therapy. An understanding of these techniques allows the neurosurgeon to review critically new information in molecular biology as it becomes available in neurosurgical and other journals. Following these basic chapters are chapters that discuss the normal function of the central nervous system—proliferation and differentiation of stem cells into mature central nervous system cells. The third section presents neuro-oncology from a molecular point of view. The gene alterations, the mechanisms by which they lead to various tumors, and the molecular mechanisms of various forms of therapy are discussed. The fourth section presents information regarding the molecular basis of cerebrovascular disease—specifically, stroke, vasospasm, and familial vascular malformations. Successive sections review the cellular and molecular mechanisms underlying the pathology and treatment of central nervous system trauma, epilepsy, pain, and deficiency diseases.

Some topics appear more than once in this volume. For example, the normal function of cell cycle proteins is presented in the chapter on proliferation, and their aberrant function is discussed more extensively in the neuro-oncology section. This repetition is intended to emphasize the importance of basic features, such as the cell cycle. In another example, calcium ion homeostasis is discussed in the chapters on both epilepsy and stroke. This repetition is intended to highlight the ways in which different cell processes share the same molecular mechanisms. It is our hope that this volume will be a reference for neurosurgeons seeking to expand their understanding of the molecular biology of the disease they treat and that they will be encouraged to take the lead in developing molecular neurosurgery.

Corey Raffel, M.D., Ph.D.
Rochester, MN

Griffith R. Harsh IV, M.D.
Boston, MA

Contributors

SERIES EDITORS

Stephen J. Haines, M.D., F.A.C.S.
Professor of Neurosurgery, Otolaryngology
  and Pediatrics
University of Minnesota
Minneapolis, Minnesota

Paul B. Nelson, M.D.
Professor and Chairman of Neurological Surgery
Indiana University School of Medicine
Indianapolis, Indiana

VOLUME EDITORS

Corey Raffel, M.D., Ph.D.
Chief, Pediatric Neurosurgery
Mayo Eugenio Litta Children's Hospital
Associate Professor, Neurological Surgery
Mayo Medical School
Rochester, Minnesota

Griffith R. Harsh IV, M.D.
Associate Professor of Surgery
Harvard Medical School
Neurosurgical Service
Massachusetts General Hospital
Boston, Massachusetts

CONTRIBUTORS

Joseph M. Alexander, Ph.D.
Assistant Professor of Medicine
Harvard Medical School
Assistant in Biochemistry, Neuroendocrine Unit
Massachusetts General Hospital
Boston, Massachusetts

Mitchel S. Berger, M.D.
Associate Professor
Department of Neurological Surgery
University of Washington
Seattle, Washington

D. H. Bhatt, M.D.
State University of New York
Stonybrook School of Medicine
Stonybrook, New York

Peter McL. Black, M.D., Ph.D.
Brain Tumor Center
Brigham and Women's Hospital
Children's Hospital
Dana Farber Cancer Institute
Joint Center for Radiation Therapy
Harvard Medical School
Boston, Massachusetts

Xandra O. Breakefield, Ph.D.
Harvard Medical School
Neurosurgical Service
Boston, Massachusetts

Adam Burkey, B.A.
Georgetown University Medical Center
Washington, DC

E. Antonio Chiocca, M.D., Ph.D.
Neurogenetics Center
Massachusetts General Hospital
Charlestown, Massachusetts

Dennis F. Deen, Ph.D.
Brain Tumor Research Center
Department of Neurological Surgery
University of California School of Medicine
San Francisco, California

Nicolas de Tribolet, M.D.
Division of Neurosurgery
Hôspital Cantonal Universitaire
Genève, Switzerland

Pierre-Yves Dietrich, M.D.
Laboratory of Tumor Immunology
Division of Oncology
Hôspital Cantonal Universitaire
Genève, Switzerland

Peter B. Dirks, M.D.
Brain Tumor Research Laboratory
Division of Neurosurgery
Hospital for Sick Children
Toronto, Canada

Martin A. Eglitis, Ph.D.
Laboratory of Cell Biology
National Institute of Mental Health
Bethesda, Maryland

Dan Fults, M.D.
Associate Professor Neurosurgery
University of Utah School of Medicine
Salt Lake City, Utah

John Golfinos, M.D.
Department of Neurosurgery
New York University Medical
New York, New York

B. A. Green, M.D.
Professor and Chairman
Department of Neurological Surgery
University of Miami School of Medicine
Chief of Neurosurgery Service
Jackson Memorial Hospital
Miami, Florida

Murat Gunel, M.D.
Section of Neurological Surgery
Yale University School of Medicine
Yale—New Haven Hospital
New Haven, Connecticut

Nalin Gupta, M.D.
Brain Tumor Research Center
Department of Neurological Surgery
University of California School of Medicine
San Francisco, California

Philip H. Gutin, M.D.
Brain Tumor Research Center
Department of Neurological Surgery
University of California School of Medicine
San Francisco, California

CONTRIBUTORS

Griffith R. Harsh IV, M.D.
Associate Professor of Surgery
Harvard Medical School
Neurosurgical Service
Massachusetts General Hospital
Boston, Massachusetts

Luc Jasmin, M.D., Ph.D.
Department of Neurosurgery
Georgetown University Medical Center
Washington, DC

Matthias Kirsch, M.D.
Brain Tumor Center, Brigham and Women's
    Hospital
Children's Hospital, Dana Farber Cancer
    Institute
Joint Center for Radiation Therapy, Harvard
    Medical School
Klinik fur Neurochirurgie
Carl-Gustav-Carus-Universitatsklinikum
Technische Universitat Dresden
Federal Republic of Germany

David N. Louis, M.D.
Molecular Neuro-Oncology Laboratory
Massachusetts General Hospital
Charlestown, Massachusetts

**R. Loch Macdonald, M.D., Ph.D.,
    F.R.C.S.(C)**
Assistant Professor
Section of Neurosurgery
University of Chicago Medical Center
Chicago, Illinois

Tim Mapstone, M.D.
Associate Professor of Neurosurgery
Division of Pediatric Neurosurgery
The University of Alabama at Birmingham
School of Medicine
Birmingham, Alabama

Linda S. Marton, Ph.D.
Research Associate
Section of Neurosurgery
University of Chicago Medical Center
Chicago, Illinois

Jeffrey McDonald, M.D., Ph.D.
Department of Neurological Surgery
University of Utah
Salt Lake City, Utah

Anil G. Menon, M.D.
Department of Molecular Genetics,
    Biochemistry and Microbiology
University of Cincinnati
Cincinnati, Ohio

Fredric B. Meyer, M.D.
Department of Neurosurgery
Mayo Clinic
Rochester, Minnesota

Hartmut P. H. Neumann, M.D.
Division of Nephrology and Hypertension
Department of Medicine
Albert-Ludwigs-University
Freiburg I. Br., Germany

Mark Noble, Ph.D.
Department of Oncological Sciences
University of Utah
Salt Lake City, Utah

Stephen H. Petersdorf, M.D.
Assistant Professor
Medical Oncology
University of Washington
Seattle, Washington

Corey Raffel, M.D., Ph.D.
Chief, Pediatric Neurosurgery
Mayo Eugenio Litta Children's Hospital
Associate Professor, Neurological Surgery
Mayo Medical School
Rochester, Minnesota

James T. Rutka, M.D., Ph.D.
Assistant Professor
Brain Tumor Research Laboratory,
    Division of Neurosurgery
The Hospital for Sick Children
Toronto, Canada

Thomas Santarius, M.D.
The Brain Tumor Center, Brigham
    and Women's Hospital
Children's Hospital
Dana Farber Cancer Institute
Joint Center for Radiation Therapy
Harvard Medical School
Boston, Massachusetts

CONTRIBUTORS

M. Priscilla Short, M.D.
Departments of Pediatric Neurology
 and Pathology
University of Chicago
Chicago, Illinois

Dennis D. Spencer, M.D.
Professor and Section Head
Section of Neurological Surgery
Yale University School of Medicine
Yale—New Haven Hospital
New Haven, Connecticut

Andreas Spuler, M.D.
Department of Neurosurgery
Mayo Clinic
Rochester, Minnesota

Brooke Swearingen, M.D.
Assistant Professor of Surgery,
 Harvard Medical School
Associate Visiting Neurosurgeon,
 Neurosurgical Service
Massachusetts General Hospital
Boston, Massachusetts

William K. M. Tan, Ph.D.
Department of Neurosurgery
Mayo Clinic
Rochester, Minnesota

Xiaoyu Wang, Ph.D.
Research Associate, Section of Neurosurgery
University of Chicago Medical School
Chicago, Illinois

Jack Wilberger, M.D., F.A.C.S.
Director of Neurotrauma, Professor of
 Neurosurgery
Allegheny General Hospital
Pittsburgh, Pennsylvania

Andreas von Deimling, M.D.
Institute for Neuropathology
University Hospital
Bonn, Germany

John S. Yu, M.D.
Harvard Medical School
Neurosurgical Service
Boston, Massachusetts

Joseph M. Zabramski, M.D.
Barrow Neurological Institute
Phoenix, Arizona

Berton Zbar, M.D.
Laboratory of Immunobiology
National Cancer Institute
National Institutes of Health
Frederick, Maryland

John Zhang, M.D.
Research Associate, Section of Neurosurgery
University of Chicago Medical Center
Chicago, Illinois

Contents

PART IV

Molecular Basis of Cerebrovascular Disease

PART V

Mechanisms and Treatment of Nervous System Trauma

PART VI

The Genetics and Subcellular Basis of Epilepsy

PART VII

Cellular and Subcellular Mechanisms of Pain

PART I

Molecular Strategies and Techniques

CHAPTER 1

Molecular Strategies and Techniques for Proteins

TIM MAPSTONE, M.D.

INTRODUCTION

This chapter provides a basic introduction to proteins: their structure, function, formation, decomposition, and experimental measurement by immunoprecipitation, HPLC, and Western blots. An understanding of techniques is critical to interpretation of data regarding aberrant or absent protein function because results can differ when different assays are used. The distinction between the presence of immuno-histochemically detectable protein and biochemically active protein is important. If, for example, a protein is dysfunctional because of post-transcriptional processing errors, an assay measuring its function will show a reduction, but one measuring its quantity immunohisto-chemically may show no change or even eleva-tion. The goal of this chapter is to review such basic principles of protein biochemistry so as to facilitate a critical reading of the current scien-tific literature.

STRUCTURE

Proteins are strings of amino acids. Gener-ally, if there are more than 50 amino acids in the string, the product is considered a protein; fewer than 50 amino acids constitutes a polypeptide. Since the basic structure and biochemistry are the same, the term protein will be used in this chapter to refer to both sizes.

Proteins have many roles in living organisms. They can be structural (*e.g.*, collagen or kera-tin); they can be enzymes that catalyze chemical reactions; they can transport ions and other el-ements essential to homeostasis; they are central to immune recognition and response; they can be both structural and functional (*e.g.*, myosin);

they can regulate DNA and RNA metabolism; and they can mediate many types of intracellu-lar signalling.

There are 20 common amino acids and a small number of derived amino acids formed from these common types. All amino acids are similar in structure. Each contains a central car-bon atom designated alpha. Covalently linked to this alpha carbon are four other entities: a single hydrogen atom, a carboxylic acid group (COO^-), an amino group (NH_3^+), and a side chain of varying complexity. The first three are common to all amino acids. The fourth is unique; it determines the physical and chemical characteristics of the amino acid and influences those of the proteins in which it is included. Furthermore, since amino acids are nonplanar, they can have mirror images, known as L-amino acid and D-amino acid, depending upon whether the amino group projects to the left or the right of the alpha carbon when viewed with the carboxyl group superior and the side chain inferior. Mammals contain only L-amino acids. The alpha carbon atom, the carboxylic acid group, and the amino group form what is re-ferred to as the protein backbone of carbon and nitrogen (*e.g.*, C-C-N-C-C-N).

Proteins are made by covalent linkage of one amino acid's carboxyl group to the adjacent amino acid's amino group. Once proteins are constructed, they assume unique three-dimen-sional conformations determined by the physi-cal and chemical properties of their constituent amino acids. This final configuration is de-scribed at four basic structural levels. Primary structure is simply the amino acid sequence of the protein. The secondary structure is the basic conformation of the carbon and nitrogen backbone of the protein (*e.g.*, an alpha-helix). The tertiary structure reflects the way the protein folds itself and places its side chains in three-dimensional space. This includes all covalent bonds between side chains, such as the disulfide bond between two cysteine residues (when this occurs in isolation—*i.e.*, two isolated cysteine amino acids forming a disulfide bond—it is known as the derived amino acid cystine). In this tertiary conformation, called the native conformation, the protein attains its lowest resting energy (*i.e.*, lowest Gibbs free energy state). The areas of the folded protein where the amino acids are tightly packed are called domains, and the areas between them are called interdomains. Interdomains are the most biochemically active parts of a protein. In enzymatic proteins, the domains are analogous to bumpers at a loading dock that help guide the trucks (*i.e.*, object to be worked upon) to the site where the work will be performed (*i.e.*, interdomain interface where substrate is bound). Many experimental techniques for assaying protein target the unique characteristics of tertiary structure. Quartenary structure connotes the association of multiple proteins into polymeric complexes.

SYNTHESIS

Proteins are made in an energy-requiring process called translation. This is separate from transcription, which is the process of making messenger RNA. Protein synthesis requires a decoding or translation of the messenger RNA sequence into the amino acid sequence. Each amino acid is specified by one or more RNA sequences of three nucleotides called codons. Each triplet codon specifies either a unique amino acid or a start or stop signal for translation. Transfer RNA is a nucleic acid that binds to both an amino acid and a trinucleotide sequence of messenger RNA. Each tRNA species has a specific pairing of trinucleotide sequence antisense to mRNA (the tRNA anticodon) and amino acid (specified by the mRNA codon). When a tRNA binds to mRNA at its appropriate site, it places the corresponding amino acid into the growing polypeptide chain.

Translation occurs at complexes of nucleic acid and protein called ribosomes. It begins with a group of incompletely defined proteins known as initiation factors. These factors bind to a special tRNA, known as methionyl initia-

tion tRNA, present only at initiation. This complex then binds to the 40s ribosome subunit, properly orientated by its own initiation factor. This complex of tRNA, 40s ribosome, and initiation factors then binds the mRNA in a fashion that allows it to be read or translated. The message (contained in the mRNA) is then scanned until the triplet AUG is identified. AUG is a unique and universal signal for starting translation. At this stage, the 60s ribosome subunit binds to the complex and protein synthesis begins. In an energy-requiring process utilizing GTP, the enzyme peptidyl transferase transfers the peptide from the preceding tRNA to the amino group of the tRNA next in line on the mRNA. This transfer involves a group of proteins known as elongation factors. Once the covalent bond between the amino group and carboxyl group of adjacent amino acids is formed, the mRNA and growing peptide must be repositioned by elongation factor 2 (translocase) to permit continued translation of the mRNA and elongation of the protein. Peptide bond formation always occurs between the amino group of the incoming tRNA amino acid and the carboxyl group at the end of the growing peptide chain. Once the protein has been translated, the ribosome-peptide complex encounters a codon which binds not a tRNA but rather a release factor that catalyzes a reaction freeing the protein and dissociating the ribosome and mRNA. Many proteins undergo post-translational modifications, such as the addition of sugars to form glycoproteins or the cleavage of a precursor protein (*e.g.*, proinsulin) into its active form (*e.g.*, insulin).

There are a number of places in this complex process where errors can yield defective proteins. The most common error is a point mutation where one nucleotide of the codon triplet is incorrect; this may result in an incorrect amino acid being inserted into the protein. A misplaced amino acid could alter the tertiary structure and thus the function of the protein. The protein may be completely useless or dysfunctional. For example, sickle cell disease occurs when a glutamic acid residue is replaced by lysine in the β chain of hemoglobin leading to the pathological precipitation of hemoglobin. This substitution also changes the physical properties of hemoglobin enough to permit separation of the aberrant protein from normal protein by gel electrophoresis or immunological techniques.

FUNCTION

Enzymes

Enzymes are catalytic proteins; they increase the rate at which a reaction reaches equilibrium and are not changed by the process. Some enzymes require co-factors for maximal catalysis. Most co-factors are a small molecule bound loosely to the enzyme (*e.g.*, copper or magnesium) or a prosthetic group that is bound more tightly to the enzyme. The compounds upon which the enzyme acts are called substrates.

Enzymes are grouped into six major classes: oxidoreductases, which catalyze oxidation-reduction reactions; transferases, which move functional groups from one place to another;

hydrolases, which are similar to transferase but only use water as the acceptor group; isomerases, which catalyze isomerizations; and ligases, which join two molecules in a reaction that requires energy usually supplied by ATP. Each of these classes is subdivided further according to substrate and energy source.

Enzyme function is usefully described kinetically in terms of quantity of product made per unit of time. Kinetic studies define a given enzyme's performance under specific physical conditions. By varying these conditions, one can quite accurately characterize an enzyme. This permits identification of an unknown enzyme and determination of whether an enzyme's function is altered by a mutation.

Enzymatic activity can be disrupted or regulated in a number of ways. Competitive inhibi-

Induction of TGFα mRNA in U-105MG Malignant Glioma Cells By Physiologic Concentrations of Epidermal Growth Factor

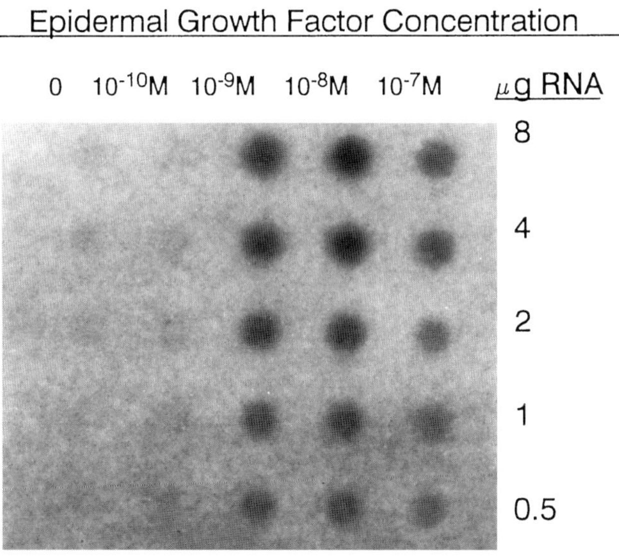

Figure 1.   Dot Blot analysis of Transforming Growth Factor-α mRNA expression in human glioma cell line U-105MG. Total RNA was extracted from post-log phase growth U-105MG cell cultures that had been exposed for 8 hours to varying concentrations of Epidermal Growth Factor (10^{-10} to 10^{-7} M) or saline. Serial dilutions of total RNA (0.5–8 μg) in 50 μl of Tris-EDTA buffer were blotted onto a nitrocellulose membrane clamped into a 96-well manifold vacuum device (Schleicher & Scheull), washed extensively, prehybridized and hybridized with a ^{32}[P]-labeled cDNA for TGFα (4). Autoradiographic exposure of the washed blot revealed hybridization of the cDNA probe to mRNA in a dose-dependent fashion with respect to the amount of EGF stimulation of TGFα mRNA expression. Unstimulated or sub-optimally stimulated U-105MG cells showed no detectable TGFα mRNA.

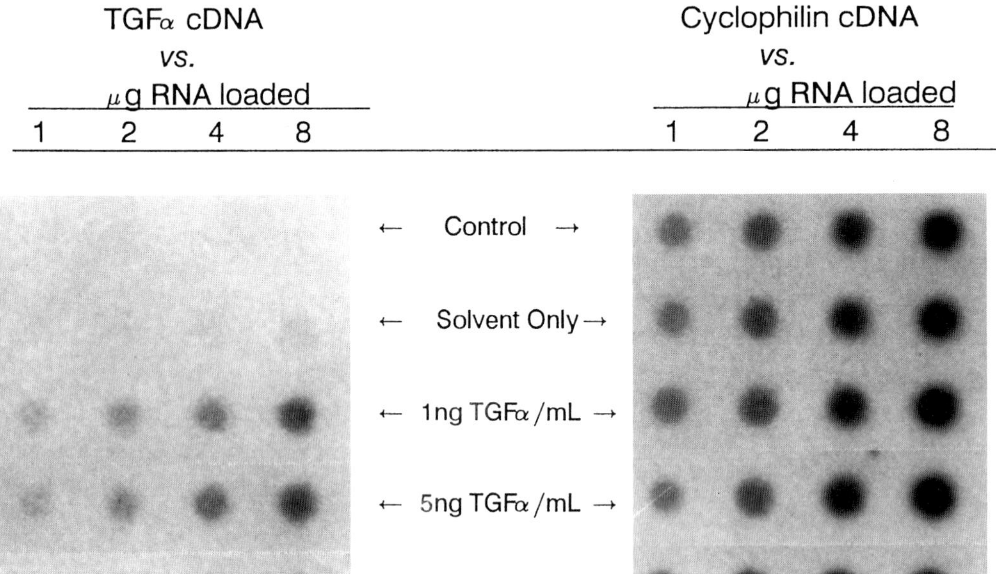

Figure 2. Dot Blot analysis of Transforming Growth Factor-α mRNA expression in human glioma cell line U-105MG. Total RNA was extracted from post-log phase growth U105MG cell cultures that had been exposed for 8 hours to varying concentrations of Transforming Growth Factor-α (1, 5 or 50 ng/ml) or saline. Serial dilutions of total RNA (1–8 μg) in 50 μl of Tris-EDTA buffer were blotted onto a nitrocellulose membrane clamped into a 96-well manifold vacuum device (Schleicher & Scheull), washed extensively, prehybridized and hybridized with a [32][P]-labeled cDNA for TGFα (4). Autoradiographic exposure of the washed blot revealed hybridization of the cDNA probe to mRNA, suggesting that TGFα is able to stimulate expression of its own mRNA. Unstimulated U-105MG cells showed no detectable TGFα mRNA. The blot was stripped and rehybridized with a [32][P]-labeled cDNA for cyclophilin (2) to demonstrate that equivalent amounts of mRNA were loaded for each of the variously treated cell cultures.

tors compete with substrate at the binding site. Methotrexate is a good example of a competitive inhibitor. It blocks access to the enzyme that makes thymidine monophosphate. After the drug is removed, however, the enzyme can function normally. Noncompetitive inhibitors bind elsewhere in a way that precludes enzymatic activity.

Enzymatic activity is affected by other features of the cellular environment. Most enzymes function as part of a metabolic pathway whose overall activity is determined at a rate-limiting step. The enzymatic activity at this rate-limiting step may be reduced by limiting the amount of substrate, adding cellular inhibitors of the enzyme (*e.g.*, feedback loops), limiting the amount of enzyme produced by the cell, or even increasing the rate of destruction of the enzyme. This intracellular manipulation of enzymatic activity is central to many experimental techniques for assessing whether an enzyme is normally present and active in a given setting.

Immunoglobulins

Immunoglobulins are vitally important proteins that identify and preserve self and destroy non-self structures in the organism. These very complex proteins were among the first to have their structure and synthesis elucidated by genetic techniques. It was originally thought that organisms encoded the myriad proteins required to recognize foreign substances in mobile DNA

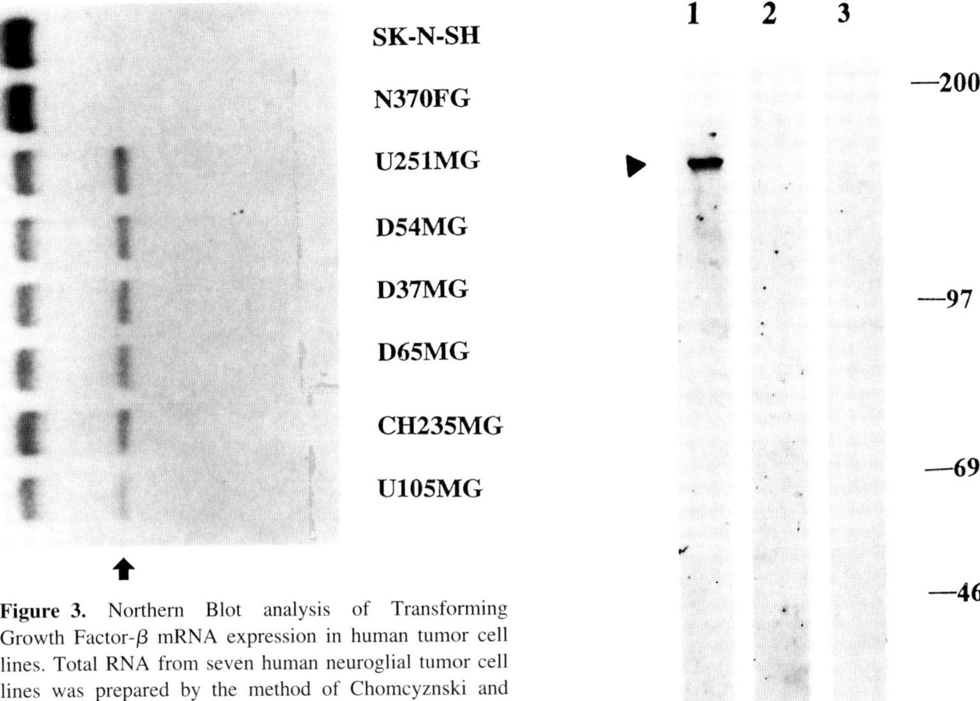

Figure 3. Northern Blot analysis of Transforming Growth Factor-β mRNA expression in human tumor cell lines. Total RNA from seven human neuroglial tumor cell lines was prepared by the method of Chomcyznski and Sacchi (xx) and 20 ng of each was loaded in each lane of a 1.2% agarose gel and resolved by electrophoresis for 60 minutes. RNA was blotted to Gene-Screen, the blot prehybridized and then hybridized at high stringency with a mixture of ^{32}[P]-labeled cDNA probes to TGFβ (pβas, 1.05 kbp insert (3)) and cyclophilin (p1B15, 743 bp insert (2)). After autoradiographic exposure of the hybridized blot, a 2.4-kb band, as expected for TGFβ mRNA, and a 1.0-kb band for cyclophilin mRNA were revealed. Cell lines that were negative for TGFβ expression were SK-H-SH (neuroblastoma) and N370FG (adenovirus-transformed fetal glial cell line); those positive for TGFβ expression included all five malignant glioma cell lines: U251MG, D54MG, D37MG, CH235MG and U105MG. cDNA probes for cyclophilin or other "house-keeping" genes that are relatively constantly expressed are employed routinely in northern or dot/slot blotting and to confirm that equivalent amounts of mRNAs were loaded.

Figure 4. Western Blot of a high-molecular weight TGFβ-like molecule using monoclonal antibody 12A12.D7. High molecular weight proteins ($>$100 kDa) secreted into the culture medium by human glioma cell line D54MG were prepared by gel filtration chromatography and resolved by electrophoresis in 1% SDS in 10% polyacrylamide gel (SDS-PAGE), blotted to nitrocellulose and the blot cut into strips. Each strip was reacted separately with (1) 12A12.D7 anti-TGFβ, (2) 15E2E2 anti-S100 protein antibody, or (3) saline. All three strips were incubated in biotinylated horse anti-mouse IgG antiglobulin and washed, and binding was visualized by sequential incubation in biotin-avidin a-conjugated alkaline phosphatase and NBT/BCIP. A 186-Da band was identified by monoclonal antibody 12A12.D7 to TGFβ Lower molecular weight species of TGFβ were not revealed.

segments whose movement within the gene generated novel DNA, and thus mRNA, sequences. Development of the concept of gene recombination and identification of the immunoglobulin genes has provided a better explanation. Immunoglobulins are comprised of two light chains derived from three distinct gene segments and two heavy chains derived from four distinct gene segments. Each chain is composed of variable segment and a constant segment. Rearranging and matching various genomic sequences provides near-limitless diversity. The heavy chain sequence defines the class of antibody as IgG, IgA, IgM, IgD, or IgE. The variable heavy chain gene segment and the variable light chain gene segments encode the portion of the protein that provides the antigen-binding capacity, and it is in these variable (and hypervariable) segments that the ability to bind so many diverse antigens arises. Each light chain binds to a portion of the heavy chain to create two antigen binding sites, and the con-

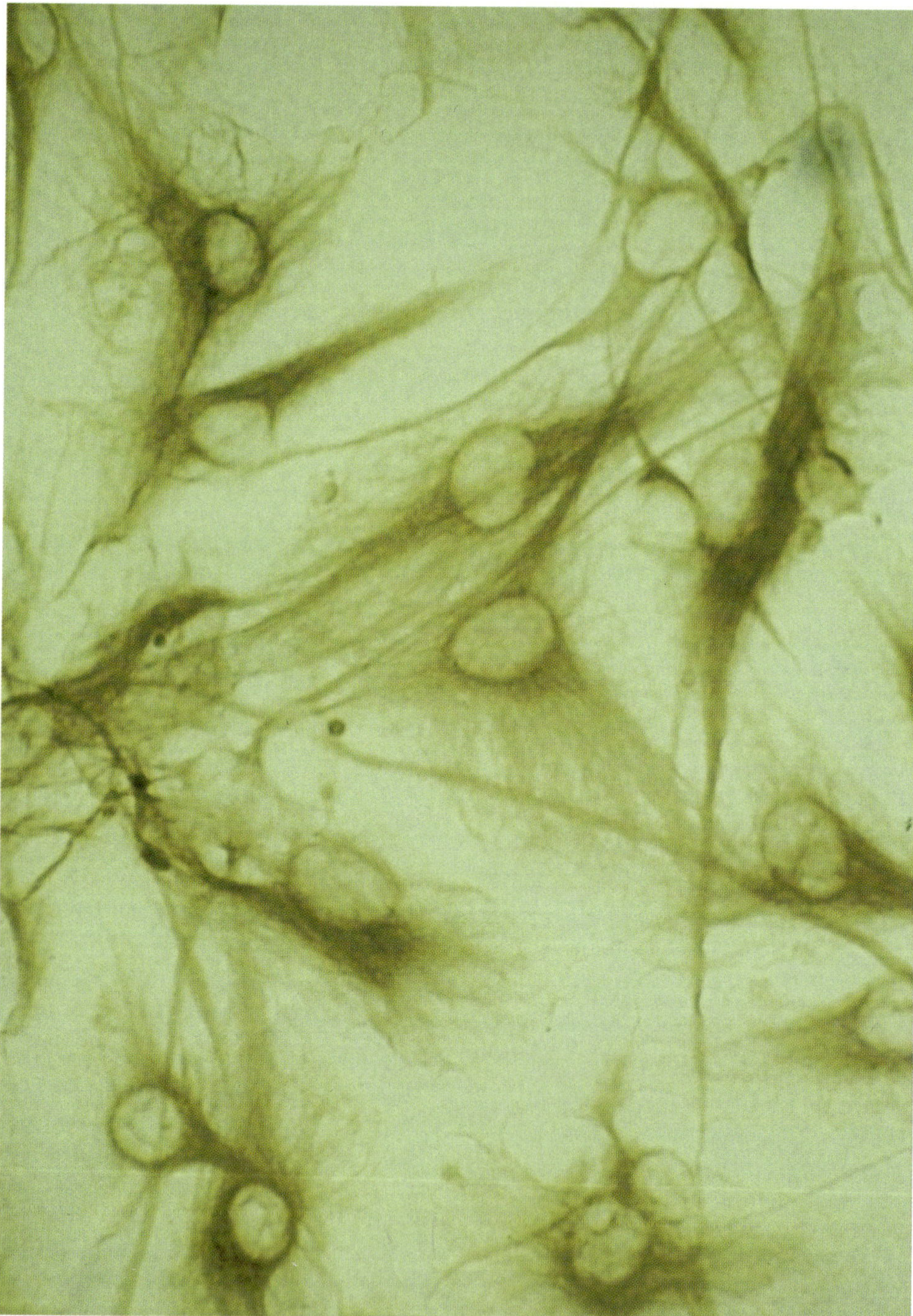

Figure 5.   Immunocytochemistry of malignant glioma cells. RT-3 rat glioma cells grown on coverslips were fixed with 4% paraformaldehyde, post-fixed in methanol-acetic acid and rehydrated in PBS. Cells were reacted with mouse monoclonal antibody 4A11.H9 to Glial Fibrillary Acidic Protein and biotinylated horse anti-mouse IgG antiglobulin. Binding of antibody was detected by avidin-biotin-conjugated horseradish peroxidase and diaminobenzidine. Note fine reticular staining of filaments within the cytoplasm of these cells.

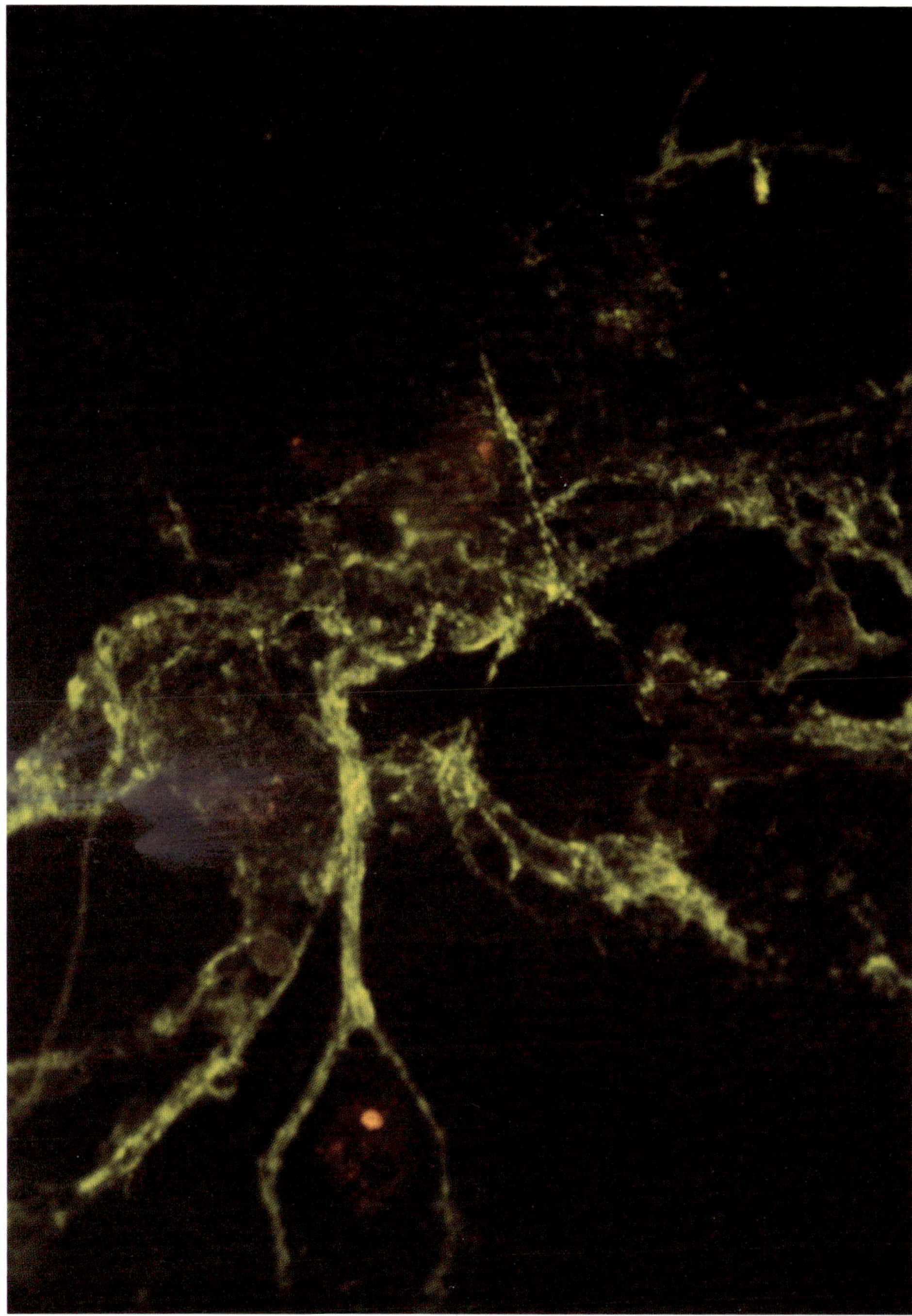

Figure 6. Immunofluorescence of malignant glioma cells. Freshly explanted tumor cells from a human malignant glioma were grown on coverslips, fixed with 2% paraformaldehyde and rinsed in PBS. Mouse monoclonal antibody L243 to human class II MHC antigen (HLA-DR) was reacted with cells followed by fluorescein isothiocyanate (FITC)-conjugated goat F(ab')2 anti-mouse IgG antiglobulin. Cells were visualized under mercury vapor UV light with an epi-illuminated fluorescence microscope equipped with a 475 nm excitation/515 nm barrier filter module. Note the fine punctate membrane-associated staining of some of the cells. Malignant glioma cells generally will express HLA-DR antigen immediately after culture but will lose this antigen expression with time in culture.

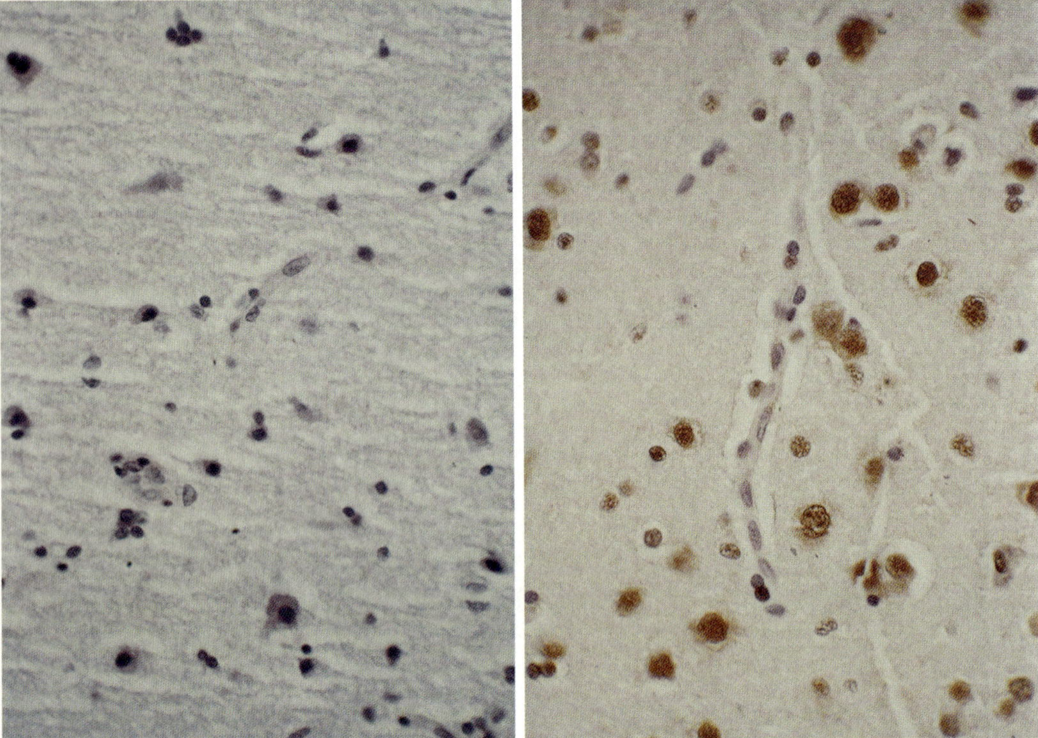

Figure 7.   Immunohistochemistry of human malignant glioma. Formalin-fixed, paraffin-embedded 10 μ thick sections of resected tissue from a malignant glioma and adjacent normal brain were mounted on TEPSA-coated slides, deparaffinized, rehydrated and reacted with monoclonal antibody 29.1.1 to the Epidermal Growth Factor Receptor. Sections were washed and antibody binding visualized by sequential incubation with biotinylated horse anti-mouse IgG antiglobulin, horseradish peroxidase-conjugated biotin-avidin and diaminobenzidine. Cytoplasmic and membrane staining of individual cells at the edge of the tumor bed identifies EGFR-positive, presumably malignant glial cells. No staining of cells in adjacent normal brain or of the capillary in the tumor section is apparent.

stant portions of the heavy chain bind together. The base of the resulting Y-shaped structure is the conjoined heavy chains, and each of the two arms is one light chain joined to one heavy chain. Each arm contains an antigen-binding site. The most distal portion contains the variable or hypervariable regions. Immunoglobulins, T-cell receptors, and the major histocompatibility proteins are closely related members of a group of proteins involved in cell-to-cell communication referred to as the immunoglobulin superfamily.

Immunoglobulins are formed when antigens are presented to the system via a complex mechanism requiring a number of different cells. A hapten is a molecule too small to be identified by an immune cell but, if attached to a large molecule, it is able to elicit an immune response. An epitope is that unique portion of the antigen that elicits the unique immunoglobulin. Since each antibody can bind two antigens (one at each end of the "Y"), cross-linking between antibody molecules to form a chain of antigen-antibody complexes is possible. These complexes can then be scavenged by appropriate cells. Specific binding of antigen is central to many assays of protein structure and function. Therapeutic potential lies with blocking antibodies that disrupt protein function. For example, an antibody that blocks a growth factor receptor might prove antineoplastic.

Signaling Systems

As our understanding of cellular biology increases, the dependence of cell homeostasis on signaling systems, comprised of enzymes, becomes abundantly clear. This section describes the neuronal calcium signaling system and its effect on multiple aspects of cellular metabolism as an example of cellular signaling systems in general.

Proteins maintain intracellular calcium homeostasis by pumping the ion into the endoplasmic reticulum or out to the extracellular space. Calcium may enter the cystosol by influx down a gradient, either through calcium channels within the cell membrane or from the internal endoplasmic reticulum stores. This flux is controlled precisely by multiple protein-based signaling systems. One avenue of entry of extracellular calcium is the NMDA-regulated calcium channel. This channel is blocked by a magnesium ion until a membrane-bound protein receptor is activated by binding glutamate. Binding changes the tertiary structure of the protein in a manner that releases the magnesium ion and allows influx of calcium. Receptor function is affected by other enzymes, such as protein kinase C (PKC), which phosphorylate the receptor. Phosphorylation alters the channel's physical characteristics, the ease of release of the magnesium ion, and, thus, channel function.

Intracellular calcium is released when protein receptors sensitive to inositol triphosphate or ryanodine are activated by their respective initiator. These initiators are released to the cytosol by a number of other transmembrane pathways activated by growth factors and neurotransmitters. The multiplicity of initiators and intersections of signaling pathways utilizing proteins affords abundant opportunity for modulation of signal amplitude and refinement of cellular responses.

Once the calcium-dependent signaling mechanism is initiated, the signal is transmitted to the nucleus. Although some intranuclear signaling is accomplished by calcium acting directly upon the nucleus, the Ras signaling pathway, which is activated by elevated calcium levels, is also involved. Ras protein, once it is activated by calcium, associates with and activates Raf (a serine-threonine kinase), which, in turn, activates a cascade of kinases including MEK1, MAP, and Rsks. These proteins then initiate activity in the nucleus. This cascade may alter the neuronal cytoskeleton and mediate the changes observed in the neuron after local changes in dendritic calcium. This cascade is used primarily to signal changes that require

new gene expression and consequent protein production.

Once calcium signals arrive in the nucleus, multiple pathways are available to effect activation or inhibition of gene activity. The first branch point occurs between the immediate early genes, which do not require new proteins for transcription, and the delayed response genes, which do require new protein synthesis. Delayed response genes are often also regulated by the proteins encoded by the immediate response genes. Delayed response genes generally code for proteins, such as nerve growth factor or apoptosis-inducing proteins, that directly affect cellular physiology.

This calcium-dependent signaling mechanism provides a paradigm for signaling systems within the cell and illustrates the exceedingly complex protein machinery involved. Calcium pathways that alter the cellular cytoskeleton may mediate vasospasm and its amelioration by calcium channel blockers. They may also be involved in the induction of apoptosis by overactivation of the NMDA receptor. Further understanding of these complex protein signaling systems should improve therapies of a variety of CNS diseases.

DNA Regulatory Proteins

Many cellular signaling systems impinge on the nucleus to activate DNA regulatory and cell cycle control proteins. These regulatory proteins, called DNA-binding proteins, control gene expression and are distinct from the histones (proteins), which help form chromatin structure. Soon after the structure of DNA was elucidated, transcription factors that control gene replication were identified. However, proteins controlling gene expression were not identified until sophisticated molecular biological techniques became available. Most DNA-binding proteins are facilitators or enhancers, rather than inhibitors, of transcription. By binding DNA, some prevent transcription initiation factors from binding to DNA and initiating mRNA production. There are four structural types: homeodomain, zinc finger, leucine zipper, and helix-loop-helix. Homeodomain proteins are comprised of multiple helical domains. Generally, one helical domain binds to the major groove of the DNA helix; other protein helical domains outside the DNA helix are available to bind transcriptional proteins. Zinc finger proteins enfold a zinc ion. The "finger" portion of the protein binds to DNA at a specific nucleotide sequence determined by the amino acid sequence of the "finger." An amino acid tail binds transcriptional proteins. Leucine zipper proteins have four or five leucine residues spaced to lie on the same side of the protein in a position to form a dimer with another similarly constructed protein. The side of the protein opposite the leucine residues binds to DNA. The immediate early nuclear genes *fos* and *jun* encode such proteins. Helix-loop-helix proteins, like the leucine zipper proteins, are dimers. These proteins have a major role in the control of cell growth and differentiation. Once these DNA-binding proteins have complexed with DNA, transcriptional factors attach to the other side of the protein to initiate mRNA production. The structure and function of these critically important proteins remain relatively unknown. Improved understanding of cellular control is contingent upon further elucidation of the function of this class of proteins.

TECHNIQUES OF PROTEIN IDENTIFICATION AND ISOLATION

Gel Electrophoresis

A protein in its natural state has particular physical and chemical properties that specify its unique characteristics. One-dimensional gels analyze the size and purity of a protein; two-dimensional electrophoresis also measures charge.

In one-dimensional gels, proteins run in only one direction. A solution of proteins is placed on a gel of polyacrylamide under a standard set of conditions. As an electrical field is applied across the gel, the proteins migrate through the gel with a velocity inversely proportional to molecular weight. A colorizing agent is then used to stain the proteins that appear as separate bands in the gel. The thinner and sharper the band, the purer the protein. A single band means only a single size of protein is present; multiple bands indicate that proteins of more than one size are present. This assay provides no information regarding function; it simply determines the presence or absence of protein at a given molecular weight.

Two-dimensional gel electrophoresis has two steps. The first separates proteins by charge; proteins in solution are allowed to migrate in an electric field to the point of isoelectric focusing. The second separates protein by size on a one-dimensional SDS polyacrylamide gel oriented 90° to the isoelectric focusing gel. Although a two-dimensional gel gives more information about the protein, it does not identify a specific protein or its function. Gel electrophoresis is basic to protein measurement, purification, and, when coupled with more specific techniques such as immunostaining, identification.

Chromatography—Conventional and High-Pressure Liquid Chromatography (HPLC)

Conventional chromatography separates proteins with respect to a chosen physical characteristic (such as size, charge, epitopes, shape, or size change based on pH). A solution of protein is passed through a column filled with a matrix that impedes the migration. The proteins are eluted sequentially by slowly modifying the parameter chosen for separation. The most basic chromatography technique, gel filtration, separates proteins by size. There are pores in the gel chromatography medium that trap small molecules as they pass through the gel. Larger molecules, which are not retarded by the pores, pass through rapidly and emerge from the column (elute) early. By sequentially collecting the eluent in small aliquots, sample proteins of decreasing molecular weight are obtained.

Ion exchange chromatography takes advantage of a protein's charge by running it through a gel with opposite charge. As the ionic strength of the elution buffer is increased, proteins are eluted through the column from least tightly bound to most tightly bound. Another technique uses antigen-antibody binding. Antibodies that recognize certain epitopes of the protein of interest are coupled to the matrix. The protein solution is poured over the column, and the protein of interest is bound to the gel as contaminants elute out. Changing the buffering solution dissociates the antigen-antibody complex, and the protein of interest is eluted. In affinity column techniques, essentially anything that can be bound to the matrix and slows the passage of the protein of interest can be used in the separation process. The parameters used for separation include size, charge (ion exchange), hydrophobic interaction, metal affinity, and bioaffinity.

HPLC uses rigid small-particle columns through which buffer is forced at high pressures (at times up to 400 Atm). HPLC permits rapid, precise purification of very small quantities of protein. Nonetheless, purification is still based on the physical structure not the function of the proteins.

Immunohistochemistry and Immunoprecipitation

The immune system provides a very powerful, precise method of identifying and quantifying proteins. Each protein has many antigenic sites against which multiple unique antibodies can be generated. Some antigenic sites are unique to a given protein configuration or activity state that presents distinctive amino acid sequences to the immune system.

Antibodies to a given protein can be generated by injecting the protein into an animal, usually a rabbit, that makes a full array of antibodies to the proteins. The serum from the immunized animal contains polyclonal antibodies—many different antibodies directed against the many antigenic sites on the protein. Many different subclasses of high-affinity antibodies that recognize many areas and conformations of the protein are generated. This is important for screening gene expression libraries and facilitates immunoprecipitation experiments. Making polyclonal antibodies is a technically difficult task that requires a highly purified immunogen. Because polyclonal antibodies recognize many different antigens on one protein, they are rarely used to study an individual domain (*e.g.*, to identify the deleted portion of the epidermal growth factor receptor in glial tumors).

Monoclonal antibodies are domain-specific. These are produced in a complex process that begins with immunizing the host animal to a given protein. B cells are isolated and fused, using hybridoma technology, to immortalized (myeloma) cells. Since an individual B cell encodes only one antibody, each hybridoma cell contains the specifications of only one antibody. One must then select the hybridoma cell that produces the antibody of interest. The monoclonal antibody it produces permits analysis of a specific domain. Monoclonal antibody is specific for a single epitope, not for the entire protein. If the epitope is found on more than one protein, then the monoclonal antibody is not protein-specific. The appropriate positive and negative controls must be used in experiments using monoclonal antibodies.

Once a protein of interest has been defined and the appropriate antibodies are available, many different assays can be performed. The most common technique is known as ELISA or enzyme-linked immunoabsorbent assay. In this technique, the immunoglobulin is covalently linked to a marker enzyme (often horseradish peroxidase) that facilitates recognition of the complex in such a fashion that the antigen-binding site and the active site of the enzyme remain functional. A frequently used and relatively sensitive type of ELISA, known as antibody sandwich, can detect less than 10 ng/ml of antigen. In this technique, antibodies are attached to the walls of microtiter plates, antigen is introduced and binds to the antibody, unbound antigen is washed away, and a different antibody fused to a marker enzyme is introduced to bind the fixed antigen. Enzyme-antibody-antigen-antibody complexes result. A substrate for the bound enzyme is added, and the amount of antigen present is quantified in terms of enzymatic product generated.

Immunohistochemistry can also be performed with a protein-specific antibody. Antibody is raised against a region of interest in a specific membrane bound or intracellular protein. A second antibody is then generated against the first antibody. This second antibody is covalently linked to the marker enzyme or molecule (*e.g.*, HRPO or radioactive label). As the first antibody is added to cells in suspension or fixed on a slide, the antibody binds to the protein of interest. Unbound antibody is rinsed away. The complex of second antibody and the marker is then added. This binds to the first antibody, thus attaching the marker enzyme to the protein of interest. An enzyme substrate is added, and the product is measured. This technique is powerful and sensitive. However, if great care is not taken, false positive results can arise from indiscriminate binding of antibody. Also, quantitation of product is often difficult, such that qualitative descriptions must be used.

Western blotting or immunoblotting is a rapid, sensitive technique that combines several of the techniques already discussed. First, proteins are electrophoretically separated by size on a polyacrylamide gel. Protein from this gel is then transferred to a membrane that binds the protein irreversibly, preserving the distribution by size from the gel. The membrane is then incubated with a solution containing protein-specific antibody: protein-bound antibody is then measured. This is a very sensitive test that needs controls to identify non-specific binding. Overly sensitive antibody probes can give false positive results. Immunoprecipitation experiments allow the isolation and identification of a specific protein. The protein mix is added to a solution of antibody directed against the protein of interest. The resultant antibody-protein complex can then be precipitated by various methods. This protein/antibody mixture then undergoes gel electrophoresis and assay as described for immunoblotting. None of these assays assesses protein function. They determine the presence or absence of a protein and, when radioactive densitometry is used, they may provide a quantitative estimate. Functional assays are required to verify specific protein activity.

Southwestern Blots

Our understanding of DNA regulatory proteins and their control of transcription has been greatly advanced by methods of identification and purification that utilize specific nucleotide-protein binding. DNA regulatory proteins bind to DNA with great specificity to form a DNA-protein complex. In a process analogous to immunoprecipitation, regulatory proteins can be separated from a crude protein mixture by binding the DNA regulatory sequence to a gel or column and adding the protein mixture. Regulatory proteins bind the appropriate DNA sites; unbound proteins pass through the column. The DNA-binding proteins are then eluted from the column by changing the elution buffer. When a gel is used, this technique is called Southwestern blotting or mobility shift gel electrophoresis. Since unbound DNA migrates more rapidly through a gel than the same DNA bound to its regulatory proteins, DNA-protein complexes can be separated from unbound DNA by gel electrophoresis of a solution of DNA admixed with crude protein extracts. These complexes will contain the regulatory protein. The affinity of the protein for the DNA can be assessed by

competitive inhibition. Addition of excess substrate—in this case, free DNA with various sites to which the protein can bind—establishes competition between the DNA sequence of interest and other DNA for the binding protein. By varying the amount of additional substrate and measuring the amount of protein binding to the DNA of interest, the affinity of the DNA regulatory protein for its target DNA sequence can be quantitated. Once a DNA sequence with high binding affinity is identified, it can be isolated and its base sequence determined.

SUMMARY

Understanding proteins is essential to understanding cell function. Numerous techniques have been developed to detect their presence and measure their function. Each has various strengths and weaknesses. Critical analysis of the literature of molecular neurosurgery demands close attention to experimental detail. One must be fully aware of the purpose, limitations, and potential errors of the techniques employed. This is particularly important for studies of proteins, as quantification of the presence of a particular species is too often assumed to demonstrate its function.

REFERENCES

1. Ausubel, F., Brent, R., Kingston, R., *et al. Current Protocols In Molecular Biology* 2. 1993.
2. Danielson, P. E., Forss-Petter, S., Brow, M. A., *et al.* p1B15: A cDNA clone of the rat mRNA encoding cyclophilin. DNA *7:*261–267, 1988.
3. Derynck, R., Jarrett, J. A., Chen, E. Y., *et al.* Human transforming growth factor-β complementary DNA sequence and expression in normal and transformed cells. Nature *316:*701–705, 1985.
4. Derynck, R., Roberts, A. B., Winkler, M. E., *et al.* Human transforming growth factor-α: Precursor structure and expression in *E. Coli.* Cell *38:*287–297, 1984.
5. Deutscher, M. *Guide to Protein Purification.* p. 182. 1990.
6. Devlin, T. *Textbook of Biochemistry with Clinical Correlations,* 3rd Ed. 1992.
7. Sambrook, J., Fritsch, E., and Maniatis, T. *Molecular Cloning,* 2nd Ed. 1989.
8. Watson, J., Gilman, M., Witkowski, J., and Zoller, M. *Recombinant DNA,* 2nd Ed. 1992.

CHAPTER 2

Nucleic Acids

JEFFREY McDONALD, M.D., Ph.D.

INTRODUCTION

Beginning with the first production of a biologically active recombinant DNA molecule containing genetic information from two species by Cohen and Boyer in 1973, progressing through the development of the polymerase chain reaction (PCR) by Saiki and coworkers in 1985, to the most recent advances in gene therapy and expression technologies, the revolution in biology known as "molecular biology" has been a revolution in techniques. The ingenuity and hard work of thousands of scientists in the field have produced a steady stream of new methods or adaptations of existing methods of studying biological macromolecules, each advance yielding new insights into the nature and control of life itself. This chapter will examine many of these techniques as prelude to the discussions of the genetic diseases discussed in other chapters of this textbook. For most of the techniques discussed in this chapter, there are published protocols; the individual steps of representative protocols will be summarized. The reader is referred to the original publications, as well as established laboratory manuals (1) for a more complete discussion of the various techniques, along with rationales for each.

GENE STRUCTURE AND REGULATION

Nucleic Acid Structure and Biochemistry

At its core, the field of molecular biology is the study of biological macromolecules called nucleic acids (deoxyribonucleic acid, or DNA, and ribonucleic acid, or RNA) and the cellular control mechanisms which have evolved to regulate their replication and expression. Nucleic acids are long polymers of individual subunits called nucleotides. A nucleotide is composed of a purine or pyrimidine base (indicating that at physiological pH they exist in the anionic form), and a cyclic pentose sugar attached to one or more phosphate groups (2). DNA contains four bases within its nucleotides: (A), thymine (T), guanine (G), and cytosine (C). RNA contains adenine, guanine, cytosine, and uracil (U).

The nucleotides of DNA and RNA are linked into very long linear molecules by their sugar moieties via phosphodiester covalent bonds. The sugar of the RNA polymeric backbone is ribose. The sugar of DNA is deoxyribose, in which the 2' hydroxyl group of the ribose ring is replaced by a proton. The phosphodiester bonds occur between the phosphate group attached to the 5' carbon of one sugar and the hydroxyl group attached to the 3' carbon of the adjacent sugar. By convention, the sequence of nucleotides is written in a 5' to 3' direction left to right on the printed page. Enzymes that act on DNA or RNA are frequently specific in their sequential direction of activity, moving in a 5'->3' or 3'->5' direction along the DNA or RNA strand.

DNA exists in the cell nucleus in a double-stranded form in which the nucleotide bases of one strand form hydrogen bonds with those of the other strand: A pairs with T, and G with C. This is the basis of semi-conservative replication of DNA in that each strand can serve as a template for duplication of the other strand prior to cell division. The double-stranded nature of DNA also allows for preservation of the integrity of the informational base of the genome, as repair of damage to one strand (mutation or loss of one or more nucleotides, as might occur by ionizing radiation or after exposure to chemical mutagens) is accomplished by pairing with the nucleotides of the second, undamaged strand. The two strands of DNA are thus termed complementary since the sequence of nucleotides of one always specifies that of the other (an A in one strand specifies a T in the other, etc.).

A single A/T or G/C pair within the double-stranded DNA molecule is termed a base pair. The length of a segment of DNA is given in terms of the number of base pairs (bp) of the two complementary strands contained within it. It is thus common to refer to DNA fragments as being, for example, 240 bp or 371 bp in length. Longer fragment sizes are given in terms of kilobase pairs (kbp), or thousands of base pairs. Genomic distance between two points on the DNA strand is given in terms of the number of kbp or even megabase pairs (millions of base pairs, Mbp), that separate them.

The two strands of nucleotides of the DNA molecule are aligned in 3-dimensional space in what is termed an antiparallel double helix. In this structure, first described by Watson and Crick in 1953, the $5'->3'$ orientation of each linear pentose phosphodiester backbone is aligned in opposite directions, and the corresponding bases of each nucleotide are within the interior of the helix, allowing for hydrogen bond formation between the A/T and G/C base pairs. The two strands of DNA are wound around each other such that there are approximately 10 nucleotides per turn of each helix; thereafter the structure repeats itself. Due to the geometry of the base pair interactions, the two pentose phosphodiester backbones of the DNA strands are not exactly 180 degrees apart, but rather are offset slightly. This creates what is termed a major and a minor groove in the DNA molecule. Access to the bases within the helix is greater on the major groove side, thus most known DNA sequence-specific interactions with proteins (as between upstream control elements of gene expression and transcriptional regulatory proteins) occur within this groove.

The structure of RNA differs from that of DNA in 3 principal ways. The two already discussed are the presence in RNA of ribose instead of $2'$-deoxyribose as the sugar in the pentose phosphodiester backbone, and uracil instead of thymine as the fourth base (along with G, C, and A). A third difference is that the RNA molecule is single-stranded, not double-stranded as is DNA. The single-strand structure allows for internal base-pairing within short stretches of the same RNA molecule, leading to the formation of unique hairpin, cruciate, and more complex tertiary structures. These tertiary structures are believed to play a significant functional role of many RNA moieties, particularly ribosomal and transfer RNAs.

Chromosome Structure

There are 46 chromosomes in human cells (2 sex chromosomes and 22 paired autosomes). Each chromosome is made up of a single long uninterrupted double helical strand of DNA from 50 million to 250 million bp in length. At a minimum, a piece of DNA requires three components to be a functional chromosome in a cell: a centromere, two telomeric ends, and specialized DNA sequences called origins of replication.

The centromere is the region near the mid-portion of the chromosome which attaches to the mitotic spindle during cell division to assure orderly segregation of one copy of the replicated chromosomes (i.e., one chromatid) into each progeny cell nucleus. Human centromeres are composed of unique DNA sequences in regions of highly repetitive DNA called alpha satellite DNA. The exact function of alpha satellite DNA is unknown, but the sequence of the repeat is specific for each chromosome centromere. This allows the distinction of one chromosome from another (e.g., chromosome 10 from chromosome 17) experimentally on direct inspection of a cell nucleus after hybridization to a specific alpha-satellite centromeric probe. A protein complex called the kinetochore attaches to the centromere of each chromosome, and at metaphase binds to and initiates outward movement along the kinetochore microtubule toward the spindle pole in the process of separation of the sister chromatids. Any replicating piece of DNA which contains a centromeric sequence within it will be reliably maintained in this manner through cell divisions. This is the basis for the cloning in yeast of large chromosome-sized pieces of human DNA called YACs in molecular biology research.

Telomeres are regions at the ends of chromosomes composed of stretches of highly repetitive DNA hundreds of nucleotides in length. Each tandemly arranged repeat unit within the telomere is quite short (in humans the sequence is GGGTTA). These repeats are synthesized during DNA replication not by using the adjacent complementary DNA strand as template, but rather by an enzyme called telomerase using an RNA template. The telomere maintains the length of the chromosome through many cell divisions despite the fact that initiation of DNA synthesis from the 5' end of the DNA strand always requires a short stretch of bases as leader sequence to allow for binding by the enzyme DNA polymerase before actual DNA synthesis then begins. Without the telomere regions, the 5' ends of the DNA strands would thus shorten by the length of the leader sequence with each round of DNA replication and cell division. The gradual decline in telomerase activity with advancing cell age may contribute to cell senecense and death by eventually allowing shortening and loss of telomeres in subsequent cell divisions.

During S phase of the cell cycle, the chromosomes are replicated to allow for subsequent chromosomal segregation into two daughter nuclei during mitosis. Chromosomal replication involves synthesis of a new DNA strand from each of the two strands of the original template double helix. Chromosomal *origins of replication* are specific sites on the DNA double helix at which the two strands focally separate, or denature, to allow a protein complex which includes the enzyme DNA polymerase to bind and begin DNA synthesis. In yeast, known replication origins consist of multiple copies of an 11 bp core sequence contained within a 100 bp region. A similar functional unit in the human genome almost certainly exist but is poorly characterized. In the eukaryotic genome, these sites appear to be clustered in groups of 20 to 80 replication origins, each separated by 30 to 300 kb of DNA. While the synthesis of one of the two new DNA strands (the leading strand) proceeds in a continuous linear manner in a $5'->3'$ direction, that of the other strand (the lagging strand) is discontinuous initially. On the lagging strand, short RNA primers are used to initiate synthesis of 100–200 base DNA fragments (called Okazaki fragments) homologous to the strand of the DNA region being replicated. The Okazaki fragments are subsequently joined together, or ligated, to form the continuous linear molecule of the DNA lagging strand.

The overall rate of DNA synthesis during replication of the human genome is 50 bp/sec, approximately 10 times slower than in bacteria. This slower rate reflects the fact that the DNA of eukaryotic chromosomes, unlike the bacterial genome, exists in the nucleus not as a bare double helix but rather in a highly protein-complexed state known as chromatin. Chroma-

tin serves several functions. First, it accomplishes compaction of a DNA chain that, if stretched out, would measure approximately a meter in length! Second, because of this great length, naked DNA is a fragile molecule prone to fragmentation due to shear forces. Associating it with the structural proteins of chromatin and compacting it protects the DNA and hence the genetic integrity of the cell. A third function of chromatin is to assist in the determination of cell phenotype by acting as one form of control of gene expression (3). More will be discussed in this regard in the following sections.

The principal proteins responsible for packaging the DNA into chromatin are the histones. The five known types of histones include H1, H2A, H2B, H3, and H4. Two copies each of H3 and H4 form a protein tetramer around which wraps 120 bp of DNA. One dimer of H2A–H2B is then added to either side of this tetramer-DNA complex, extending the length of DNA associated with each complex to 160 bp, to form the basic core unit of DNA packaging in the nucleus, called the nucleosome (4). An H1 molecule is then added as a linker between each adjacent DNA-octamer core, resulting in aggregation of the nucleosomes into an orderly array in a 30 nm thick chromatin fiber. Additional higher-order chromatin structures consisting of complex loops and even "loops of loops" of this 30 nm chromatin fiber account for the final condensed DNA structure known as chromosomes.

The exact state of compaction, or *condensation*, of chromatin varies from region to region in the genome, and indeed at times even within the same region during cell differentiation and lineage commitment. The most highly condensed state of chromatin is termed heterochromatin, which is in general more commonly observed in pericentromeric chromosomal locations. Genes present within regions of heterochromatin are generally inactive transcriptionally. Areas of chromatin containing transcriptionally active genes are in a less compact state, termed euchromatin, due to many factors including less tight H1 binding, modification of the acetylation and phosphorylation state of the nucleosomal core histones (particularly H4), and association with other non-nucleosomal proteins which are believed to partially unwind, or open up the chromatin structure focally. Euchromatin more readily permits the interaction of the DNA with gene regulatory proteins and proteins of the RNA transcriptional apparatus, interactions which are believed to require focal DNA-histone dissociation and nucleosome disruption. This open state of chromatin adjacent to actively transcribed genes can be experimentally observed by treating the chromatin with nucleases such as DNase I, which cleave the DNA in regions of open chromatin to which they have physical access. The modulation of the state of chromatin compaction is also a method of control of gene transcription.

Gene Structure

The specific sequence of nucleotides of the DNA is the basis for the biologic information contained therein. Genes are the units of inheritance which are encoded by this nucleotide sequence. In simplistic terms, a gene is a linear stretch of DNA nucleotides which encodes for the transcription of one RNA molecule that will then be translated by cytoplasmic ribosomes into the amino acids of one polypeptide protein chain. Eukaryotic RNA synthesis in reality is an extremely complex process. The recent development of in vitro systems to study the process has greatly facilitated our understanding. Although some of the details can be summarized here, for additional information the reader is referred to recent reviews on the subject (5, 6).

The three minimum components of a gene include (1) DNA sequences which identify for the RNA polymerase II enzyme complex where to start and where to stop transcribing RNA from the DNA template, called the transcription *start site* and *stop site*, (2) a stretch of DNA, which contains sequence information encoding for the polypeptide product of the gene, termed the *coding region* of a gene, and (3) short DNA sequences upstream of the transcription start site that serve as binding sites for the multiple regulatory proteins which influence how much transcript is made and at what time, in a region termed the *promotor* region. We will examine each these components of a gene in turn. Because the details of this process is worked out most clearly in yeast, the protein names given below are often for the yeast homologues. Human homologues are known for many of these proteins and the basic process is believed to be very similar for all eukaryotic organisms.

RNA transcription by the enzyme RNA polymerase II begins at a DNA sequence called the transcription start site (numbered +1 in the RNA transcript molecule). In the great majority of eukaryotic genes, this site is approximately 25 nucleotides downstream of a DNA sequence in the promotor region called the TATA *box*. This element is a stretch of approximately six A or T nucleotides (consensus sequence TATAAT) recognized by a specific DNA binding protein, called the TATA binding protein, or TBP. Binding of TBP to the TATA box is believed to be the first step in formation of the pre-initiation complex of proteins which will lead to RNA transcription (5). TBP is actually an intrinsic part of a large protein complex called TFIID, made up of TBP and 10 or more polypeptide TBP-associated factors, or TAFs (7). The functional enzymatic unit for RNA synthesis is the RNA polymerase II holoenzyme complex. This is composed of approximately 25 polypeptide subunits, including the RNA polymerase II enzyme, associated general transcription factors (with names such as Srb 2 to Srb 11, Gal11, Sin4, Rgr1, etc) and a complex of 10 proteins of the Swi/Swf group which are believed responsible for local opening up of chromatin structure by nucleosome disruption (7, 8).

Some genes do not have a TATA box sequence in their promotor region. This is principally observed in so-called *housekeeping* genes (such as those concerned with cell metabolic pathways) requiring steady basal levels of transcription in many or all cell types. Instead of a TATA box, these genes have a short DNA sequence at and immediately around the transcription start site called the *initiator element* (Inr). It appears that TBP and perhaps additional Inr-binding proteins, along with TFIID and the RNA Pol II holoenzyme complex, are required for efficient and accurate transcription initiation from at least some of these TATA-less genes (9).

After binding of the TBP/TFIID complex to the TATA box and the RNA polymerase II holoenzyme to the transcription start site, RNA transcription begins. While the TBP/TFIID complex remains at the promotor region, the RNA polymerase II holoenzyme initiates focal separation of the two strands of DNA in the coding region of the gene, using one (the so-called *negative* strand) as a template for the generation of the RNA transcript by catalyzing in a $5'->3'$ direction the addition of sequential complementary nucleotides. The non-template DNA strand (*positive* strand) corresponds in sequence to the RNA product, with the exception of course that the RNA transcript contains uracil bases in place of the thymine bases of the DNA sequence. By convention, the sequence of this non-template strand of DNA is given when the DNA sequence of a gene is specified.

The process of RNA transcript chain elongation proceeds at a synthesis rate of approximately 30 nucleotides per second. New transcripts are initiated prior to completion of the first RNA chain, and an RNA polymerase II holoenzyme density of one complex every 100 bp can be observed. The process of chain elongation continues until a stop, or termination, signal in the DNA is encountered by the RNA polymerase II holoenzyme. At the stop signal, RNA synthesis halts and the single strand RNA transcript and RNA polymerase II protein ensemble dissociate from the DNA double helix. The exact nature of the stop signal in eukaryotic genes remains poorly characterized.

Several modifications are made to the initial RNA transcript, including the addition of a 5' cap and a 3' poly(A) tail. The addition of a modified G residue (called the 7-methyl guanine cap) to the 5' end of the RNA transcript occurs almost immediately after initiation of synthesis of the RNA strand. The poly(A) tail is a long string (100–200 residues) of adenosine nucleotides added to a region near the 3' end of the RNA transcript, approximately 10–30 nucleotides downstream from the sequence AAUAAA by the enzyme poly(A)$^+$ polymerase. This poly(A) tail is believed to aid in the transport of the RNA molecule out of the nucleus and into the cytoplasm of the cell, where it then increases the stability and efficiency of translation of the mRNA into protein by ribosomes.

Eukaryotic genes differ from prokaryotic ones in many ways, one of the most important of which is the presence in eukaryotic genes of *introns* and *exons*. Introns are stretches of the DNA sequence of a gene which will be removed, or *spliced*, from the RNA molecule after initial transcription and modification by 5' capping and polyadenylation of the 3' end, and prior to translation into a protein product. Introns can range in size from a few scores of base pairs to a 100 kbp or more, and commonly comprise in length the majority of a gene sequence. Intron borders are defined by short consensus sequences called splice 5' donor site (consensus sequence . . . [C/A]AG:GU[A/G]-AGU . . ., where the colon specifies the exon:

intron border) and splice 3' acceptor site (consensus sequence . . . AG:[G/A] . . .). The DNA regions corresponding to RNA transcript segments retained after splicing and used for translation into a protein product are termed exons. In eukaryotic genes, there may be anywhere from one to dozens of exons. The RNA splicing process involves removal of the intron sequences by a large protein and RNA complex, called the spliceosome, and joining together of the two adjacent exon ends. Alternative splicing patterns of introns from a primary RNA transcript can lead to different protein products after translation. This is one process used by eukaryotic cells for regulation of gene expression.

Along with the promotor and coding regions of the gene, there are additional DNA sequence elements that bind other transcription control proteins. Binding of proteins to these elements can lead to increased or decreased expression of the corresponding RNA transcript. These transcriptional regulatory elements involved in control of gene expression will be discussed further in the next section.

Regulation of Gene Expression

The DNA content of the genome of nearly every cell of the body is identical. The fate of a particular cell is determined by which genes are transcribed within its nucleus. Genes encoding proteins involved in basic processes common to all cells (such as energy utilization and metabolic pathways, for example) are transcribed in every cell of the body. Other genes, however, are involved in cellular specialization and differentiation. A neuron differs from a hepatocyte, for example, due to the developmental program which it follows during differentiation, leading to a neuronal set of genes being actively transcribed in the former and a hepatic set transcribed in the latter. Some of the mechanisms which have evolved to regulate the choice of genes to be transcribed, in what form, when and to what level will be discussed in this section. These are issues of gene transcriptional regulation, which have in common the interaction of specific short (10–20 bp) DNA sequence stretches with regulatory proteins. Other mechanisms contributing to cellular differentiation, including control of gene expression by regulation of messenger RNA transport from the nucleus to the cytoplasm, RNA or protein stability, ribosomal control of RNA translation, and genetic imprinting are beyond the scope of this chapter.

The *promotor* region of a gene is the short sequence of DNA responsible for directing the binding of the proteins of the transcriptional apparatus to the proper start size for RNA synthesis by the RNA polymerase II holoenzyme complex. The promotor region contains the TATA box, which is the site of binding of transcription factors (including the TATA-binding protein, TBP, and the TFIID protein complex) located approximately 25 bp upstream of the start site of RNA transcription. Certain promotors are more efficient in binding this protein ensemble and thus are more likely to lead to higher rates of transcription and higher levels of transcript. These so-called strong promotors usually match more closely the consensus core sequence of the TATA box, TATAAT. Mutation of the TATA box to TACAAT, for example, tremendously decreases the strength of the promotor due to less efficient binding of the transcription initiation complex.

The amount of RNA transcribed from a gene, as well as the timing and tissue specificity of such transcription, is determined by the balance of positive and negative regulatory influences exerting control over the promotor region of the gene (6, 10). Studies of genes whose transcription is inducible by extracellular or metabolic factors have invariably identified multiple specific short sequences of DNA in the upstream region of the gene outside of the TATA box which serve as binding sites for transcriptional regulatory proteins. In response to an extracellular or intracellular signal, the nuclear concentration of one or more of these transcriptional regulatory proteins may increase, thereby leading to increased binding at these upstream binding sites. The result may be transcriptional activation or repression, depending on the specific function of the transcriptional regulatory protein.

We will next discuss several types of these upstream transcriptional regulatory elements, including enhancers, insulators, and transcriptional activators and repressors.

Enhancers are DNA sequences that are transcriptional control elements which differ from promotors in a number of important ways. First, there is no characteristic distance between the start site of RNA transcription and enhancer location. An enhancer may be many kilobases away and still be functionally active in modu-

lating gene transcription, and indeed can be located even within or downstream of a gene. Second, an enhancer sequence may be in either orientation relative to the direction of RNA transcription. Third, enhancers often convey tissue-specificity to transcription from an associated or even heterologous gene. For example, a gene may be transcriptionally active only in the nervous system, or only in the hepatic system (11) due to the proximity of the corresponding tissue-specific enhancer. This underlies the complex mechanism of tissue tropism observed in some viruses following infection in which, although the virus may be capable of infecting cells of many tissue types, productive or efficient infection arises in only a subset of tissues because of a tissue-specific enhancer within the viral genome.

An enhancer element is a short sequence of DNA containing multiple distinct binding sites for transcriptional activator proteins. These proteins bind, often synergistically, to the enhancer site via protein-DNA and protein-protein interactions to form a complex that has been termed an *enhanceosome* (12). The binding of this protein complex may either induce (13) or remove (12) local 3-dimensional bends in the DNA double helix in a manner that allows the formation of additional protein-protein interactions, leading to increased transcription from the associated gene. Enhancer elements stimulate transcription by inducing a loop in the DNA, bringing the enhancer/enhanceosome complex close to the promotor region (6). The enhanceosome complex in direct proximity to the promotor region then facilitates binding of the transcription initiation complex, TFIID and the RNA Pol II holoenzyme, leading to increased transcription of the gene. Alternatively (and perhaps not exclusively) the enhanceosome complex may track along the DNA helix from the enhancer site to the site of transcription initiation, where once again protein-protein interactions then induce transcriptional activation (14).

Enhancers are negatively regulated in the cell in one of several ways. The genomic region in which an enhancer lies may be maintained in a closed chromatin conformation, analogous to heterochromatin, in a process called silencing, discussed more blow. DNA sequence elements termed *insulators* may block the effect of an enhancer on its corresponding promotor in a reversible but location-dependent manner, only when the insulator is positioned in-between the enhancer and promotor. The distance between the enhancer and insulator elements, on the other hand, does not appear to be functionally important at distances up to 100 kb (15). The manner in which insulators function is under intense investigation; in at least one case, it establishes a DNA domain boundary which effectively sequesters the promotor from the effects of the enhancer, while not inactivating or directly blocking the enhancer itself (14, 16). The normal function of insulators may be to establish the boundaries of chromatin domains in which levels of gene transcription are regionally determined (3). Insulators, like enhancers, typically consist of multiple copies of short DNA sequences which serve as binding sites for the corresponding regulatory proteins.

Other upstream control elements function as transcriptional *activators* or *repressors* (13, 17). These sites are short stretches of DNA sequences located near the promotor region of a gene at which transcriptional regulatory proteins bind to the DNA helix. Transcriptional activator or repressor elements usually are close to the promotor (i.e., TATA box) region of a gene, and are under relatively tight constraints in regard to the distance and orientation of these elements from each other and from the promotor. This is the principal difference between these types of transcriptional regulatory elements and the enhancers and insulators previously discussed, which may be located in either orientation and at very great distances from the start site of transcription itself.

We have previously noted that changes in chromatin conformation may lead to alteration of gene transcription. Genes which are not actively transcribed within a particular cell (for example, globin genes in an oligodendrocyte) can be sequestered in a closed chromatin conformation, termed heterochromatin, inaccessible to the proteins of the transcriptional apparatus. These genes are frequently heavily methylated at the 5 position of cytosine residues in the CpG palindrome. DNA *methylation* of inactive genes is differentiation-related (18) and associated with closed chromatin environments that exclude access of regulatory sequences to transcription factors (19). Actively transcribed genes, on the other hand, (such as the same globin genes in a reticulocyte) are invariably in an open, or euchromatin, conformation. Spe-

cific developmentally-regulated DNA sequences exist in the human genome (for example, *locus control regions*, or LCRs) which serve to keep particular regions of the genome, and hence specific genes, in such an open chromatin conformation (20). If a locus control region is experimentally inserted into a particular region of a host genome (as in transgenic mice), open chromatin domains may be established. Genes within such open domains can be demonstrated to be more active transcriptionally as a result. This is believed to be one method of directing high level and tissue-specific expression of nearby genes, particularly important during development and differentiation of the host.

Nucleosome placement in chromatin is not random, but rather is, at least in part, sequence-dependent. The positioning of nucleosomes in the region of actively transcribed genes allows access of transcription factors to the regulatory sequences of promotor and other upstream regulatory areas (3). Conversely, chromatin silencers are specific DNA regulatory elements which appear to convey a closed chromatin environment to a region of the genome, silencing the effect of nearby enhancer elements. Silencers share several features with enhancer elements: they function in a manner that is orientation and position-independent, and they can act on other, unrelated genes located in their vicinity (21). One distinction between silencers and insulators is unidirectional effect of the establishment of domain bondarie, by insulators (16), rather than the regional, bi-directional effect of transcriptional down-regulation effected by silencers. Silencers and insulators share a common structural basis for their function, however, in conveying a closed chromatin environment when active.

Finally, most eukaryotic genes contain both introns and exons. Introns have arisen during eukaryotic evolution to provide another dimension of gene regulation-alternative splicing processes that produce different final protein products from the same region of DNA. In the splicing of a 5′ splice donor sequence to the 3′ splice acceptor sequence that removes the intervening intron, a choice of alternate 3′ splice acceptor sequences may exist in the same or adjacent intronic region. The use of a 3′ splice acceptor from the adjacent downstream intron, for example, will lead to the excision of the intervening exon sequences in the process of alternative splicing. The use of one 3′ splice acceptor rather than another will thus lead to a slightly different final mRNA sequence, and hence a different final protein product. The protein products of the various alternative splicing pathways may vary in their affinity for a specific ligand, or DNA binding sequence, for example. This process of alternative splicing can be under metabolic or developmental control.

GENE IDENTIFICATION, ISOLATION, AND EXPRESSION

In this section we will discuss several of the most commonly used techniques in molecular biology. The purification of nucleic acids is the fundamental starting point for many of the techniques which we will subsequently discuss. Upon initial purification, DNA and RNA solutions are extremely heterogeneous mixtures of sequences. The techniques described allow an investigator to visualize and clone (that is, isolate and amplify in pure form) individual DNA or RNA sequences from these complex mixtures.

Gels, Blots, and Hybridizations

DNA purification: DNA exists as chromatin in the cell nucleus. As discussed in the previous sections chromatin is composed of the double helix of DNA of the chromosomes wound into a compact and highly regulated three-dimensional structure by association with nuclear proteins. The process of purifying DNA or RNA involves lysing the cell and its nucleus, freeing the nucleic acids from these associated proteins, then finally isolating the DNA or RNA free from the other to collect one in pure form.

Cells from culture flasks (or dispersed cells from blood or tissue) are resuspended in a lysate and extraction buffer containing very low salt to induce cell swelling and lysis (1). High concentrations of ethylene diamine tetra-acetic acid (EDTA), sodium dodecyl sulfate (SDS), and ribonuclease (RNase) enzyme are also present in this buffer. The EDTA chelates calcium ions needed by many cellular enzymes (including deoxyribonuclease, or DNase) for activity. The SDS is a detergent which effectively dissolves cellular and nuclear membranes. It also contributes to the loss of protein secondary structure and thereby enhances the dissociation of DNA from chromatin-associated proteins. The RNase degrades cellular and nuclear RNA early in the DNA purification process, thus limiting its con-

taminating presence in later extraction steps. A protein-digesting enzyme such as proteinase K is then added to the solution, and during an incubation of several hours the cellular lysate proteins are degraded. Finally, an extraction step involving a mixed organic phase (usually a phenol/chloroform mixture, followed by chloroform alone to remove traces of the phenol) separates the relatively pure DNA (in the aqueous phase) from other cellular debris (in the organic phase or at the interphase). After collection of the aqueous phase, the DNA is precipated from the solution by addition of monovalent cations (NaCL to 0.2 M, sodium acetate to 0.3 M, or ammonium acetate to 2.5 M) and ice-cold alcohol (ethanol or isopropanol). Under these conditions, the solubility of DNA is greatly reduced, thus prompting its precipitation from the solution. It can then be collected by centrifugation and resuspended in a low-salt aqueous buffer such as TE (10 mM tris · HCl, 1 mM EDTA at ph 8.0).

Restriction Endonuclease Enzymes

Arguably the most significant advances in the field of molecular biology have arisen from the discovery of enzymes in eukaryotic and prokaryotic cells which can modify, cleave, join, synthesize, repair or replicate purified nucleic acids in a test tube. Indeed, it is these enzymes which are the fundamental "tools" of the molecular biologist. Part of the rapid progress in the field in recent years is attributable to the widespread availability of high-purity enzymes from commercial manufacturers at reasonable cost. The field has progressed greatly from the earlier days of 1970's when most of these enzymes had to be purified by the individual investigator at the investment of great expense and time.

One of the most basic and important classes of these enzymes is the so-called restriction endonucleases. These enzymes, isolated from bacterial cells, can create double-strand cleavages in DNA molecules. These enzymes cleave the DNA at specific sequences unique to each enzyme (so-called recognition sequences) of 4–8 nucleotides in length, and act in dimer pairs. This latter fact accounts for the typical dyadic symmetry of the recognition sequences on the two strands of DNA. Due to variation in the exact site of cleavage, some enzymes create single-strand termini of 2 or more nucleotides in length, while others create *blunt* non-overhanging DNA ends. Although the names of these enzymes appear quite strange on first glance, they derive from the convention of naming the enzyme based on the first letter of the genus followed by the first two letters of the species name of the bacteria from which the enzyme was isolated. If more than one such enzyme has been isolated from a given bacteria, then they are numbered in order of discovery (I, II, III, etc.). Thus, common enzymes include Hind III (the 3rd isolated enzyme from *Haemophilus Influenzae*, strain d) and Eco RI (the first isolated enzyme from *Escherischia coli*, strain R), etc.

The choice of which enzyme to use depends on the sequence of the DNA to be cleaved, and what is to be done with the DNA fragments generated. If the DNA is to be ligated with another molecule, then choosing an enzyme which leaves overhanging single-strand ends (usually only 2–4 nucleotides long) allows more efficient binding to and subsequent ligation with compatible overhanging ends of DNA (as in a similarly-cleaved plasmid for cloning) in the next step. Blunt-end ligation (joining together of 2 double-strand DNA ends without single-strand overhangs) is possible but is much slower and less efficient in the test tube. On the other hand, at times the goal of the digestion is to generate very large fragments of DNA, as in the generation of genomic libraries for position cloning. Enzymes whose recognition sites are rarely present in the genome, and hence separated by great distances, are preferred in this case. These so-called *rare-cutting restriction enzymes* usually have recognition sites of 8 or more bp in length.

The actual digestion of DNA by restriction endonucleases is straightforward. The purified DNA is incubated with the enzyme under appropriate buffer salt conditions for 1–2 hours at 37 °C (or, rarely, another specified temperature). The restriction enzyme can often then be inactivated by heat (usually 10 minutes at 65 °C), or extracted from the DNA solution with phenol and chloroform, or the DNA can simply be loaded onto a gel for separation by electrophoresis.

Agarose Gel Electrophoresis

The goal of the investigator frequently is to identify a particular piece of DNA or a specific transcript of RNA from the complex mixture of nucleic acid molecules present after nucleic acid purification. The first step in this process often involves fractionation of the nucleic acid molecules based on their size using the technique of gel electrophoresis. This technique is so fundamental to the field of molecular biology, in fact, that it has been said that a molecular biologist, is "one who runs gels", that is, performs gel electrophoresis.

DNA and RNA are densely charged molecules due to the phosphate backbone of their strands. These are fully ionized, and hence negatively charged, at physiological pH. Application of an electric field will consequentially induce migration of the nucleic acids due to the applied voltage. When the nucleic acid molecules are forced to migrate through a semisolid gel matrix such as agarose, which is a polymer of carbohydrates residues extracted from seaweed, the smaller molecules will migrate more freely through the gel. Larger molecules get hung up due to the "sieve-like" properties of the gel matrix, and hence migrate more slowly. Agarose of 0.3% to 1.2% concentration is typically used, the concentration being inversely proportional to the effective size range of nucleic acids which can be separated (i.e., a low agarose concentration is used for separation of large nucleic acid fragments, and vice versa). The gel is poured as a warm solution into a gel mold (typically horizontal due to fragility of the gel itself), then allowed to cook and solidify. Molecular weight *markers* of known size are loaded onto the gel in an adjacent lane to that which is carrying the nucleic acid mixture to be size-fractionated. After application of voltage (1–5 V/cm) for a sufficient period of time (typically 30 minutes to 12 hours), the gel is removed from the electrophoresis apparatus and is ready for transfer of the nucleic acids in the gel to a membrane for hybridization analysis, or one can directly visualize the nucleic acids in the gel by staining them with ethidium bromide. This compound intercalates between the bases of the nucleic acids, and on illumination of the gel with ultraviolet light induces fluorescence. In this way, a fragment of nucleic acid of particular size can be identified for subsequent isolation.

Both DNA and RNA can be size-fractionated in this manner. DNA is usually separated using a tris-borate-EDTA (TBE) buffer. RNA of course is single-stranded, and thus exists in solution in complex secondary and tertiary structures due to internal base-pairing. If these structures are not denatured, the RNA molecule will migrate through the gel in a manner faster than would be predicted based on its size due to its compact nature and its reduced tendency to be slowed down by the gel matrix. RNA agarose gels, then, are usually run under denaturing conditions in formaldehyde buffer (22), as described further below.

Southern Hybridization

In 1975 E. M. Southern described a technique (23) for visualization of particular DNA sequences of interest by gel electrophoresis and transfer of the DNA to a solid nitrocellulose filter. This technique eventually was named for its originator, and termed *Southern blotting*. By methods described below, hybridization of the DNA on the filter with a labeled known DNA fragment, or *probe*, can identify the location of DNA fragments on the filter homologous to the probe itself.

The technique of Southern hybridization (1) involves size-fractionation of DNA fragments generated by restriction endonuclease digestion of genomic or cloned DNA. After gel electrophoresis, a photograph is taken of the ethidium bromide-stained gel with molecular weight markers to document the distance of migration of DNA fragments of particular sizes. The gel is then transferred to a dish, where it is soaked in a series of solutions designed to denature the DNA so it will bind efficiently to the nitrocellulose filter or synthetic membrane upon transfer out of the gel. Alkaline conditions (0.5 M NaOH, 1.0 M NaCl) for 10 to 30 minutes accomplishes the denaturation. The exact conditions chosen for binding to the filter or membrane depend on the type of membrane chosen. Nitrocellulose (or nitrocellulose derivatives) filters, nylon membranes, or positively-charged cellullose derivatives with nylon backing are usually used for DNA immobilization after transfer from the agarose gel. After transfer to the membrane, the exact pattern of the original DNA migration in the gel is preserved. The DNA is bound on the membrane either non-covalently through hydrophobic interaction (as with nitrocellulose) or covalently (as with nylon or charged cellulose derivatives), or is linked to the membrane matrix irreversibly by exposure to ultraviolet irradiation. Because the DNA on the membrane is single-stranded (due to the denaturing step), it will readily bind to homologous sequences of single-strand DNA (or even RNA) labeled probes through base-pairing. In this manner, Southern hybridization accomplishes direct visualization of DNA sequences of interest on the membrane.

For Southern hybridization, the membrane following DNA transfer is placed in a small plastic bac and 5–20 cc of a hybridization solution is added. Following a preincubation of 1–2 hours for blocking of nonspecific binding sites, a labeled single-strand probe (usually radioactively labeled with ^{32}P) is added and the incubation continues, typically for an additional 12–24 hours. Thereafter the filter is removed and washed at high temperatures and low salt conditions for 30 minutes or more. The filter is then dried briefly, and placed in an autoradiography film holder with Xray film. The film is exposed for 15 minutes to a week or more (depending on the strength of the hybridization and the activity of the labeled probe) and then developed. The region where the probe hybridized to homologous sequences on the membrane is identified as a band, or focal area of exposure, on the Xray film. This can then be accurately traced back to a specific region of the gel, and hence sized accurately, by determination of migration distance of the band. Southern blotting is a very powerful technique to identify the specific size of a DNA fragment homologous to a known probe sequence after restriction endonuclease digestion of the original DNA mixture.

The Polymerase Chain Reaction

In the 12 years since its first description, the polymerase chain reaction, (PCR), has quickly become one of the standard procedures of molecular biology. It is an extremely powerful technique which has numerous applications, including amplification of a segment of DNA for cloning, sequencing, or mutation analysis; microsatellite analysis for loss of heterozygosity (LOH) determination of chromosomal deletions in cancer cells; and generation of mixtures of complementary DNA molecules (cDNA libraries) from mRNA extracted from cells. The principle of PCR is that of exponential amplification of DNA fragments as the products of one reaction cycle become the templates for the next cycle. The reaction cycles are defined by sequential temperature-driven denaturation and annealing steps of DNA fragments.

In essence, PCR requires three elements: *primers* which define the ends of the amplification product, a DNA or RNA fragment to be amplified (termed the *template*), and an enzyme to accomplish the synthesis of the DNA. The primers are two short oligomeric pieces of DNA of specific sequence. They are typically 15–20 nucleotides in length, and in sequence are homologous to complementary sequence stretches on the template. The template nucleic acid is mixed with the primers (present in great molar excess to the template) and enzyme under ideal salt conditions. The mixture is typically heated to 94 °C for denaturation of the nucleic acids (primers and template) to single-strand form, then allowed to cool to 55–60 °C during which the primer strands anneal to the single-strand template. Temperature elevation to 72 °C thereafter allows DNA synthesis by the enzyme to proceed at an efficient rate. DNA synthesis proceeds in a 5′ to 3′ direction, using the primer as a starting point for strand elongation. The enzyme used is usually *Taq* polymerase, isolated from the thermophilic bacterium *Thermus aquaticus*. This DNA polymerase is tolerant of very high temperatures, which would heat-inactivate most other enzymes. After the synthesis of DNA complementary to the template, the entire cycle is repeated beginning with a 94 °C denaturation step. The thermal cycling reactions are fast, and each cycle takes approximately 10 minutes or less.

For the second PCR cycle, both the original template and the newly-synthesized product become sites of primer annealing, and hence subsequent DNA synthesis as the amplification process begins. This cycle results in the production of two new complementary product molecules. The next cycle produces 4 product molecules, the following 8, etc. Twenty to forty cycles of PCR may be performed, resulting in the exponential increase in product DNA. Up to 1 microgram of product DNA can be produced from one nanogram of template DNA after 30–35 cycles of amplification (1). The amplification product of routine PCR is typically 2–500 bp in length. Longer products (up to 10 kbp or more) are possible under rigorous conditions termed LR-PCR (long-range PCR).

Whether several hundred base pairs in length or 10kbp or more, the amplified products are suitable for many subsequent applications. The products may be directly characterized for DNA sequence and mutation analysis, separated by gel electrophoresis for size fractionation, labeled radioactively for probe preparation, or subcloned into a plasmid DNA molecule for cDNA library construction or clone purification. Additional discussion regarding the preparation of amplified DNA products from a mRNA starting mixture (reverse transcriptase-PCR, or RT-PCR) is presented below.

Molecular Cloning

Cloning is the production of multiple copies of a DNA fragment of interest (termed the *insert*) by insertion of the fragment into a self-replicating piece of DNA (the *plasmid*, or *vector*), then introduction of the DNA construct into a host cell (usually a bacterium). Each replication cycle of the plasmid in the bacterial cells also replicates the insert DNA. This, along with the division of the bacteria during a period of exponential growth, leads to the production of many millions of copies of the original construct in a short period of time.

Many methods exist for DNA cloning (1). In general, however, the DNA fragment to be cloned is typically produced by restriction endonuclease digestion of genomic DNA, or production of cDNA from an RNA template. Single-strand overhanging ends of the insert DNA, when incubated in solution with compatible ends on the plasmid molecule (generated by digestion with the same or compatible restriction endonuclease) anneal to form a closed circular molecule. The two pieces of DNA (plasmid and insert) are then covalently linked by incubation with the enzyme DNA ligase. The DNA construct molecule may then be efficiently introduced into a host bacterial strain that has been rendered *competent* for DNA transfection (i.e., the cells are permissive for the entry of foreign molecules of DNA). The generation of such competent bacteria involved the rapid placement of exponentially growing cells into an ice-cold solution of $CaCl_2$, then briefly warming the cells in the presence of the exogenous DNA. For reasons that are poorly understood, the cells transiently take up the exogenous DNA, which then replicates inside the host bacteria. The presence of the plasmid DNA inside the host cell is maintained by choice of a vector which contains an antibiotic resistance gene, followed by growth of the bacteria in media containing the antibiotic. Plasmid molecules can be purified from the bacterial cells free of the host DNA genome due to the size difference between the much smaller plasmid and the larger bacterial genome. So-called *rapid plasmid preps* permit the isolation of large quantities of relatively pure plasmid DNA (each containing a copy of the insert fragment) in a matter of hours.

A *library* may be constructed in an identical manner if the original insert DNA is actually a heterogeneous mixture of DNA fragments. If the source of the insert fragments is genomic DNA digested with a restriction endonuclease, then the resulting mixture of transformed bacterial cells, each one carrying a unique plasmid construct containing a different inserted genomic fragment, is called a genomic library. Because of the great number of genomic insert fragments which would be required to span the entire genome, large inserts are desirable in the construction of genomic libraries so as to reduce the total number of clones required to entirely span the genome. Specialized vectors derived from viruses which infect bacterial cells have been developed to accept such large insert DNA fragments. Cosmids are vectors derived from lambda bacteriophage which will accept inserts in the 15–35 kb range. P1 bacteriophage vectors have been constructed which will accept inserts up to 100 kb in size. Genomic libraries composed of such vectors are useful for chromosomal mapping and gene cloning projects termed *position cloning*. Other bacterial plasmids and viruses are typically chosen to accept the smaller inserts of a cDNA library, discussed below.

Measurement of Gene Expression

RNA purification: RNA is present only transiently in the cell nucleus transcripts. Most of it is present in the cell cytoplasm as ribosomal complexes with associated ribonuclear proteins. The RNA initially isolated from cells is a heterogeneous mixture composed of 80–85% ribosomal RNA, 15–20% small nuclear RNA and transfer RNA moieties, and 1–5% messenger RNA. The principal difference in the isolation of RNA versus DNA stems from the extreme sensitivity of RNA to the presence of seemingly ubiquitous RNase enzymes in the cellular lysates, as well as in the environment, including on investigators' skin. Tissue from which RNA is to be isolated must be directly flash-frozen into liquid nitrogen ($-400\,^{\circ}$C) or

used immediately when fresh in order to avoid RNA degradation. Glassware and solutions used in RNA isolation must also be specially treated with RNase-inactivating chemicals prior to use. Such handling constraints are not necessary for isolation of the much more stable DNA molecule. To maintain the integrity of the RNA during isolation, cells are typically lysed directly into a solution containing strong protein-denaturing compounds to inactivate these RNases. Later steps in RNA isolation also frequently include protein RNase inhibitors in the solutions for similar reasons.

A common method of RNA isolation (24, 25) involves placing living cells or flash-frozen tissue directly into guanidinium isothiocyanate solution. The cellular lysate is viscous due to the release of high-molecular weight DNA. Following homogenization of the mixture to shear this DNA and addition of detergent and EDTA, the mixture is layered over a dense cesium chloride cushion and centrifuged. Careful choice of cesium chloride density and centrifugation conditions leads to the selective pelleting of only the RNA molecules in a relatively pure form. This RNA pellet is resuspended in TE buffer (pH 7.6). This pH is lower than for DNA purification due to the base-sensitivity of the RNA molecule. The RNA is then precipitated once again out of solution by addition of monovalent cations and ethanol. This final RNA pellet is then resuspended once again in Te (pH 7.6) buffer).

Often it is the messenger RNA (mRNA) which is of interest to an investigator, as these are the molecules which encode sequences to be translated by the ribosomal apparatus in the cell into proteins. The mRNA must be separated from the much more common ribosomal and transfer RNA molecules present in the isolated mixture of *total* RNA. Almost all mammalian messenger RNA molecules contain a string of adenosine residues 100–200 long on the 3′ end, and are thus called poly(A)$^{+}$ RNA collectively. The presence of the poly(A) tails is exploited in the purification of mRNA from the other RNA moieties in the mixture. Most methods use affinity chromatography to accomplish this using cellulose microparticles to which strings of deoxythymidine (oligo-dT) nucleotides have been covalently linked. When the RNA mixture isolated from the cells is passed over a column of oligo-(dT)-cellulose beads in a buffer of high salt concentration (0.5 M NaCL), the mRNA species bind non-covalently to the cellulose beads via interaction of the poly(A) tails and the oligo-(dT)-strings. Other RNA molecules pass through the column. The mRNA is then eluted from the column by addition of a low-salt buffer in which the affinity of the poly(A) tail and oligo-(dT) string is greatly decreased.

Northern Hybridization

The method of Southern (23) for detection of specific DNA fragments in a complex mixture of sequences was quickly adapted (26) for identification of RNA fragments following RNA gel electrophoresis. In an intentional pun on the name of the DNA technique, this method of RNA transfer to a filter followed by hybridization to a labeled probe was quickly known by investigators in the field as *northern blotting*. (Indeed, a similar technique was also developed for proteins and termed *western blotting*. To date, an "Eastern blot" has not been described!).

Detection of specific RNA sequences after gel electrophoresis is nearly identical in principle to Southern blotting described earlier, varying only in the details of the solutions and conditions employed. The total or poly(A)$^+$ RNA is electrophoresed through a horizontal agarose gel to separate the molecules by size. Smaller RNA molecules pass through the sieve of the agarose more readily, and thus migrate further in the gel during the period of voltage application (typically 3–6 hours). In order to denature the secondary and tertiary structure of the RNA, which is extensive due to internal base-pairing of the single-strand molecules, the gel is formed and run with formaldehyde in the solutions, and the RNA before loading onto the gel is heated in a solution containing formaldehyde and formamide (22). Depending on the abundance of the transcript being detected by northern analysis, typical amounts of RNA loaded per gel lane are 10 micrograms of total RNA or 1–2 micrograms of poly(A)$^+$ RNA. After electrophoresis, the gel is rinsed to decrease the formaldehyde concentration, then the RNA is transferred to a nitrocellulose or nylon membrane by capillary action as described for transfer of DNA by Southern blotting. The conditions for prehybridization, hybridization with a labeled probe, and washing are likewise essentially identical to Southern analysis. Autoradiography for exposure of Xray film to the membrane after hybridization and washing re-veals the size of the transcript homologous to the probe employed, as well as its relative abundance. A transcript which is present in the original RNA solution at twice the relative abundance, for example, will yield a band on autoradiography that is twice as intense on scanning for the Xray film after exposure.

Complementary DNA

A messenger RNA molecule is a linear single strand of nucleotides covalently linked via a phosphodiester backbone in a 5′–>3′ direction. The terminal several hundred nucleotides at the 3′ end of the messenger RNA molecule is a string of adenosine nucleotides composing the poly(A) tail. For several reasons, it is often desirable to convert this single-stranded RNA molecule into a *complementary* DNA (abbreviated cDNA) double-stranded form, one strand of the double helix of which is homologous to the original messenger RNA sequence, and the other strand of which is identical to the RNA sequence (except of course for the substitution of thymidine residues in the DNA in place of uridine in the RNA). Reasons for the conversion of a messenger RNA molecule into a cDNA form include the ability thereafter to clone the DNA and determine the sequence of nucleotides comprising it using the technique of DNA sequencing and the greater stability of the DNA during routine handling and long-term storage.

The conversion of mRNA into cDNA takes place in two basic stages. The first, termed *first strand synthesis*, involves synthesis of a single strand of DNA homologous to the RNA strand utilizing an enzyme called *reverse transcriptase*. There are several specific reverse transcriptases currently available; each is a RNA-dependent DNA polymerase isolated from RNA viruses which infect mammalian cells. The function of the enzyme in the virus life cycle is to convert the viral RNA genome into a DNA form after infection of the host cell. A commonly used enzyme for cDNA synthesis is from the Moloney murine leukemia virus (MMLV). The reverse transcriptase requires a primer of DNA to initiate the synthesis process, thus an oligo-(dT) strand 10–20 nucleotides in length is annealed to the poly(A) tail of the mRNA first, followed by addition of nucleotides and MMLV reverse transcriptase to accomplish the first DNA strand synthesis.

The second stage is termed *second strand synthesis*, and entails several steps. First, the original mRNA strand of the new RNA:DNA hybrid molecule is removed, usually enzymatically using an enzyme called RNase H which specifically degrades the RNA part of any RNA:DNA hybrid molecule. Second, an enzyme called terminal transferase is used to add a *homopolymeric tail* of residues (usually cytosine) to the 3′ end of the first-strand DNA molecule, creating a poly-(dC) tail. Third, a primer of G residues is annealed to this newly-synthesized poly-(dC) tail. This oligo-(dG) primer is used to initiate DNA synthesis of the second strand of the cDNA molecule using a DNA polymerase enzyme (DNA-dependent DNA polymerase) such as E. coli DNA polymerase I. The end result of this process is a double strand DNA molecule homologous in sequence to the original mRNA transcript, with a tail at one end of oligo-(dT):poly(A) residues and a tail at the other end of oligo-(dC):oligo-(dG) residues.

There are a great many technical variations on the theme of conversion of mRNA into cDNA. One of the most commonly used, termed homopolymeric tailing is that discussed above (27). In practice today, this is usually carried out via modification of the method devised by Okayama and Berg in 1982 (28) in which the initial oligo-(dT) primer of first strand synthesis is part of a plasmid vector capable of replication in a bacterial cell. After completion of second strand synthesis, the vector with newly-synthesized double strand cDNA attached is circularized and joined using the enzyme DNA ligase. In this form, the cDNA inserted into the plasmid vector is ready for direct introduction into bacteria for molecular cloning. This methodology has subsequently been further modified to include *linkers* adjacent to the oligo-(dT) and oligo-(dG) primers used in first and second strand synthesis, respectively. These linkers are short 10–20 nucleotide stretches of DNA which correspond in sequence to the recognition sites of one or more restriction enzymes (29). This allows the efficient manipulation of the cDNA insert into and out of the vector molecule during the process of cloning of the cDNA, and is included in almost all currently-employed protocols for cDNA synthesis.

RT-PCR

The powerful amplification ability of the polymerase chain reaction has been applied to the process of generation of complementary DNA molecules from a purified or heterogeneous mixture of RNA molecules. This process, termed reverse transcriptase polymerase chain reaction, or RT-PCR, allows the detection of extremely rare (low-abundance) messenger RNA molecules in a mixture of total RNA prepared directly from cells or tissues. With a few additional steps, the direct cloning of these amplified molecules is also achievable. Further, the prior isolation of poly(A)$^+$ RNA as a starting material is not necessary, greatly simplifying and speeding up the process of transcript detection and cloning.

The process of RT-PCR (30) involves the generation and amplification of cDNA molecules corresponding to specific mRNA transcripts. The first step is the synthesis of the first strand DNA complementary to the original mRNA using an RNA-dependent DNA polymerase enzyme (typically MMLV reverse transcriptase) and an oligo-(dT) primer which binds to the poly(A) tails of the messenger RNA molecules. Unlike the subsequent DNA synthesis steps utilizing *Taq* polymerase, this reaction takes place at 37 °C since the reverse transcriptase enzyme is not heat-stable. The second strand of DNA synthesis and all subsequent PCR cycles proceed as described previously for routine PCR amplification of a DNA template using *Taq* polymerase, elevated temperature cycling, and two unique primers. The primers are chosen to each correspond to a 10–20 nucleotide stretch of the sequence of the specific transcript which is to be amplified. The region of transcript in between the two primer sites is amplified using standard PCR methodology. For additional sensitivity in detecting rare transcripts, the PCR products may be transferred via the Southern blot technique to a membrane, then probed with a labeled clone of the transcript of interest to demonstrate expression. (Fig 1.) Quantitation of level of expression of a particular transcript is also possible using so-called quantitative RT-PCR. This is essentially the same methodology as described for routine RT-PCR with additional internal controls to ascertain that the amplification process is performed under conditions which maintain a lin-

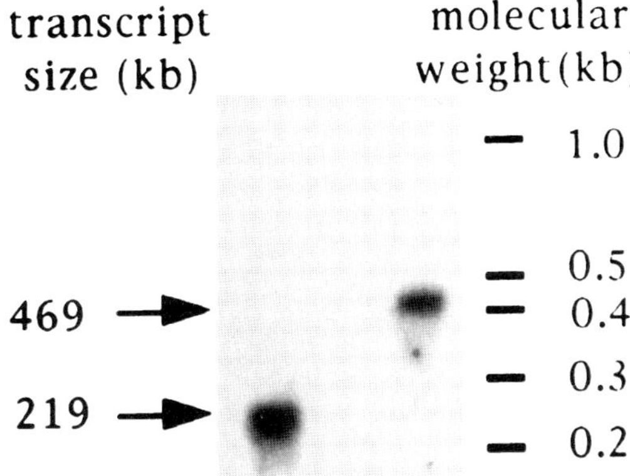

Figure 1. Reverse-transcriptase PCR (RT-PCR) analysis demonstrating expression of a gene called ABR in normal human brain. Total RNA was isolated from normal brain, then amplified with primer pairs corresponding to the ABR gene segments for Mber-region exons 1–3 (219 bp) and 1–5 (469 bp). The amplification products are visible after Southern hybridization to a radiolabaeled ABR probe and autoradiography for 12 hours.

ear relationship between amount of product and amount of starting material (31).

If a mix of random primers is chosen in the amplification steps of RT-PCR, then a representative array of amplified cDNA products may be generated from a starting heterogeneous mixture of mRNA or total RNA. A cDNA library may thus be generated by subcloning these cDNA products into a plasmid vector. The resulting mix of transformed bacterial colonies may be screened for a specific product of interest using colony hybridization techniques (1). This combination of reverse transcription (synthesizing a complementary DNA strand from a mRNA template) and the powerful amplification capabilities of PCR allows the construction of a cDNA library from a very small amount of starting mRNA.

GENETIC MUTATIONS AND ANALYSIS

One of the principal goals of the molecular biologist frequently is to identify genes whose mutation is responsible for a disease state. In the next several sections we will discuss modes of analysis to accomplish this important task.

Types of Mutations

The maintenance of the integrity of the nuclear genome and its sequence, as well as its fidelity during replication, is obviously of vital importance to the organism. A *mutation* is a change in DNA sequence that becomes permanent by passage to future cell progeny during the process of genome replication and cell division. It has been estimated that the likelihood of a mutation arising in the genome is on the order of one base pair change per 10^9 bp replicated in a cell division (32), which corresponds to roughly one base change in an average gene per 10^6 cell generations. The cell has thus evolved proofreading and repair mechanisms dedicated to identifying and correcting errors in replication, and to repair damage to the DNA of its genome. When a mutation arises which escapes these repair and proofreading mechanisms, a mutation may be inherited by that cell's progeny. Types of mutations include *point mutations*, in which a single base pair in a gene is changed (for example, G/C base pair changed to A/T). An *inversion* is the excision, 180 degree flipping, and then reinsertion of a DNA segment in the genome. A *deletion* is the simple loss of a region of a chromosome or gene, while a *translocation* is the movement of a segment of a chromosome from its original location, and reattachment to another chromosomal location.

The great majority of mutations are likely to be deleterious to the function of the gene product. Point mutations or small deletions and inversions may lead to a substitution of one amino acid for another in the protein encoded for by that gene, or truncation of the gene product by early termination of transcription. The effect of the mutation may be classified in several ways, including null, gain- or loss-of-function, or dominant-negative. A *null* mutation leads to total loss of function of the protein encoded by that gene. This is usually recessive in that the function of the gene product of the other, nonmutated allele is unaltered. A *gain-of-function* mutation, on the other hand, is usually dominant in that the mutated gene product acquires new activities or substrate spectra, or maintains its normal activity in a non-regulated and overactive manner. A *loss-of-function* mutation is similar to the null mutation, except that instead of complete abolishment of activity of the gene product, the activity is instead either diminished or abolished. This is usually a recessive mutation. A loss-of-function mutation which is dominant even in the presence of a normal gene product is termed *dominant negative*. This is observed when the mutated gene product interferes with the activity of the normal protein, and is frequently seen in instances when the gene product acts in a dimeric or multimeric form.

Linkage Analysis

Linkage analysis is the study of the transmission of genetic markers, genes, and phenotypes through generations of a study population. It is a powerful technique which permits the identification of genetic markers mapping to specific regions of the genome, and the identification of regions of the genome and specific genes whose mutation may give rise to disease. Linkage analysis is based on two principles: first, chromosomes are long molecules of DNA composed of genetic loci linked end-to-end in linear array. Second, homologous chromosomes (for example, each of the two copies of chromosome 17) at time of meiosis prophase I align at the spindle and undergo exchange of genetic information in the crossing-over process of genetic recombination. On average, two or three cross-over events occur between each pair of homologous chromosomes during this process. The term genetic linkage refers to the tendency of two loci which are physically located close to each other on a chromosome prior to meiotic crossing-over to remain together (i.e., linked) afterwards.

Linkage analysis is useful in predicting the physical distance between two genetic loci on a chromosome from the fact that the probability that a recombination event will occur between the loci reflects the distance separating them. In terms of genetic units, one Morgan is defined as the distance over which there occurs, on average, one crossing-over event per meiosis. One centiMorgan (abbreviated cM, for 1/100th Morgan) corresponds on average to approximately one million base pairs in physical distance.

The study of inheritance of genetic markers (disease states and DNA sequence polymorphisms, for example) among extended families reveals the segregation of specific loci within the pedigree. Two statistical methods were developed in the 1940s and 1950s for estimating the likelihood of genetic linkage. A detailed discussion of the statistical calculations is beyond the scope of this chapter, although the reader is referred to recent reviews on the subject (33, 34). The *method of maximum likelihood* evaluates the hypothesis that the two loci are linked versus the competing hypothesis that they segregate independently at meiosis, against the observed marker segregation patterns in the study population. The log-odds, or *LOD score*, is a related statistical calculation which is more widely reported. A LOD score of 3.0 or greater is generally accepted as strong evidence for linkage (1000:1 odds for linkage) while a score of -2.0 is considered strong evidence against linkage (100:1 odds against linkage).

The compilation of recombination frequencies for genetic loci in large study populations has permitted over the years the construction of genetic linkage maps (35). These maps assign predicted chromosomal location and order to the studies markers. With this information, the power of the genetic linkage analysis technique is revealed in the subsequent ability to predict the location of unknown disease genes based on the study of inheritance patterns of nearby (linked) known markers in affected populations. That is, when a specific pattern of inheritance of known genetic markers in a region of the genome is identified in individuals afflicted with the disease state, one may predict through LOD score analysis the linkage of the unknown disease gene to one or more of the mapped genetic markers. Thus the location of the unknown disease gene may be inferred, permitting its further characterization and molecular cloning using physical molecular genetic techniques such as position cloning.

Loss of Heterozygosity Analysis

Another method of identifying regions of the genome which may contain genes whose deletion or mutation may be associated with disease pathogenesis (particularly tumor etiology or progression) is through analysis of loss of heterozygosity (LOH). LOH analysis relies on the discovery in the 1980's that there are between individuals many sites of DNA sequence variability in the human genome known as DNA polymorphisms. These polymorphisms are located in non-coding regions within genes or in regions in between genes. These were identified (36, 37) as regions containing short DNA sequence repeat elements ranging in length from dinucleotide length elements (usually cytidine: adenosine, or CA repeats) to tandem arrays of imperfect repeats of 100–200 nucleotide elements (termed variable number of tandem repeat, or VNTR). Although thousands of these repeats exist in the human genome, they have no known genetic function. They have proved extremely useful, however, for genetic mapping studies since they are highly polymorphic in the general population, and are usually stably inherited. Thus, it is common for an individual to inherit a marker allele of a certain specific length from the maternal chromosomal complement, and an allele of a different length from the paternal complement. In this event, the marker is said to be *informative* for that study individual. Useful markers for LOH analysis are highly informative, typically revealing length polymorphisms in 70–90% of individuals.

VNTR repeats are responsible for creating restriction fragment length polymorphisms (RFLP) when genomic DNA is digested with a restriction enzyme with recognition sites spanning the repeat element itself. RFLP analysis consists of digesting genomic DNA with the suitable flanking restriction endonuclease, followed by gel electrophoresis, Southern transfer to a membrane, and hybridization to a labeled DNA probe homologous to the VNTR sequence (Fig. 2). Sites of variable dinucleotide or tetranucleotide repeat elements are studied by microsatellite analysis. Its principal advantage relative to RFLP analysis is the ease and speed of the study, as well as the minimal amount of genomic DNA consumed in this PCR-based analysis. Oligomeric primer pairs corresponding in specific sequence to the repeat being analyzed are annealed to genomic DNA, then the repeat element is amplified using PCR methodology. Radioactive label is incorporated in the amplified product, then the reaction mix is size-separated by polyacrylamide gel electrophoresis, which is performed at higher voltage, with greater resolution than agarose electrophoresis (Fig. 3).

If markers on RFLP or microsatellite analysis reveal unique allele lengths for maternal and paternal chromosome to which the marker mapped, then the loss of one of the two alleles is observable through LOH analysis. When such loss of genetic information is reproducibly associated with a disease state, particularly tumorigenesis, the presence of a gene important in preventing the disease state on the region of loss is inferred. This is the basis of the use of LOH analysis to identify regions containing tumor suppressor genes (see chapter 4).

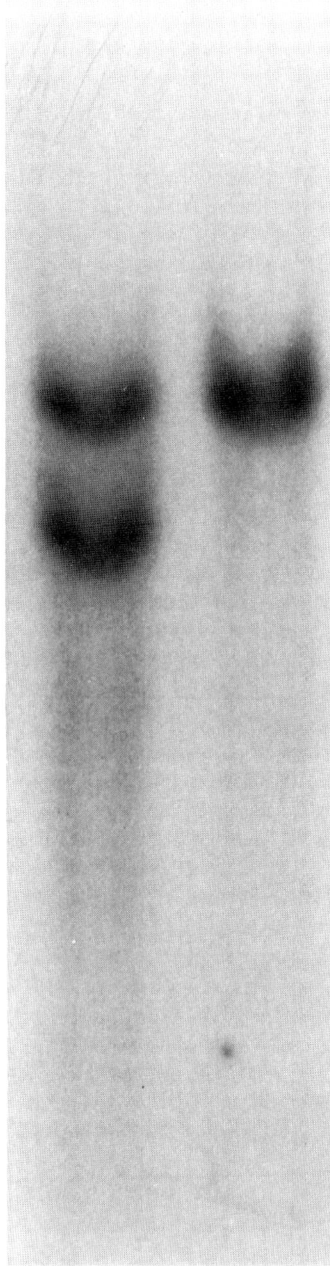

Figure 2. Loss of heterozygosity demonstrated by RFLP analysis using a VNTR probe in the p53 gene located on chromosome 17p13.1 The loft lane demonstrates two alleles after restriction endonuclease digestion of 10 micrograms of DNA isolated from the patient's peropheral leuko cytes, and Southern hybridization to rhe labeled VNTR prove. This maker is thus informative in this patient. The right lane demonstrates loss of heterozygosity by deletion of the smaller allele in DNA isolated from the patient's medulloblastoma tumor.

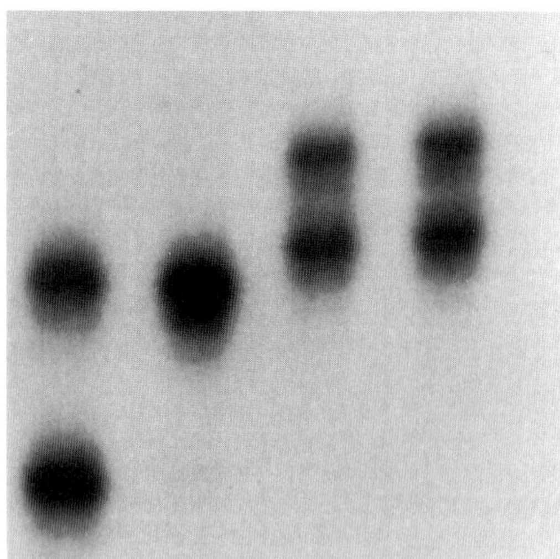

Figure 3. Microsatellite analysis in tumor specimens from two medulloblastoma patients. Primers for the microsatellite marker UT49 located on chromosome 17p were used to amplify DNA from each patieni's peripheral blood leukcytes and medulloblastona tumors. Lane 1 demonstrates marker informativeness in DNA isolated from patient #39, and loss of heterozygosity in the tumorgenome (lane 2). Lanes 3 and 4 demonstrate marker informativeness and retention of heterozygosity in DNA isolated from patient #41 leukocyto and tumor DNA, respectively.

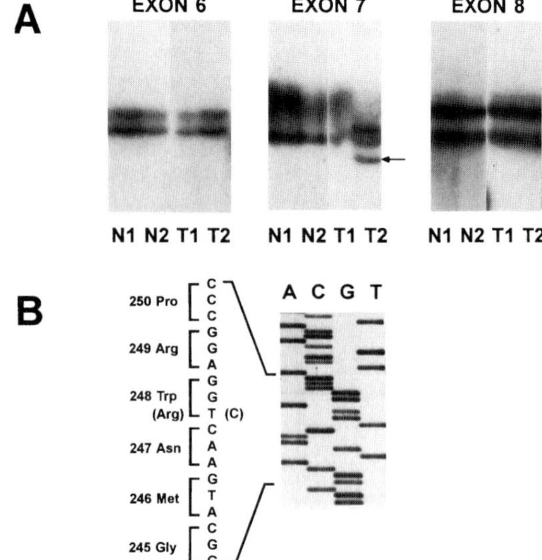

Figure 4. Single strand sequence polymorphism analysis (A) of exons 6, 7, and 8 from the p53 gene in 2 patients with astrocytoma demonstrationg a point mutation in the tumor genome of patient 2 in exon 7 (lane T2, arrow). No mutation is evident in the tumor of patient 1 (T1), nor the leukocyto DNA of either patient (N1, N2). The point mutation was xonfirmed by direct DNA sequence analysis (B), showing a C->T mutation in the T2 genome, leading to an Arg->Trp amino acid substitution. (Kindly provided by Dan Fults, M.D.).

Point Mutation Analysis

The detection of a single base pair mutation within a genome of 3 billion base pairs would seem a daunting task. Searching for such a mutation by DNA sequencing of even small parts of the genome, is impractical. In 1989, however, Orita and coworkers (38) reported an extremely rapid and sensitive technique which has made it possible to screen a large number of individuals or tumor specimens, for example, for point mutations in defined regions of a gene of interest. This technique, called *single strand conformation polymorphism* (SSCP) analysis, is more rapid than direct DNA sequencing, and is preferred for projects involving large-scale screening of multiple genomic specimens.

In SSCP analysis, genomic DNA is annealed to specific oligomeric primers designed to encompass the region of interest (typically approximately 200 bp long). This region is amplified using standard PCR methodology, then electrophoresed on a non-denaturing polyacrylamide gel. Under these conditions, the electrophoretic mobility of the two DNA strands of the PCR product is dependent not only on the length of the strand but also on the nature and extent of intra-strand base-pairing creating tertiary structural (i.e., conformational) changes in the DNA. Since these conformational changes are dependent on the DNA sequence of the strand, the electrophoretic mobility is sequence- as well as size-dependent. Point mutations are thus detected as gel band shifts (Fig. 4). The identification of a gel shift on SSCP analysis suggests a point mutation, which is then confirmed in individual specimens by direct DNA sequencing of the PCR product.

REFERENCES

1. Sambrook, J., Fritsch, E. F., Maniatis, T. Molecular Cloning: a laboratory manual. 2nd ed. Plain View: Cold Spring Harbor Laboratory Press, 1989.
2. Alberts, B., Bray, D., Lewis, J., Raff, M., Roberts, K., and Watson, J. D. Molecular biology of the cell. 3rd ed. New York/London: Garland Publishing, Inc. 1994.
3. Wolffe, A. P. Transcription: in tune with the histones. Cell. 77:13–16, 1994.
4. Hayes, J. J., Clark, D. J., and Wolffe, A. P. Histone

contributions to the structure of DNA in the nucleosome. Biochemistry. *88:*6829–6833, 1991.

5. Buratowski, S. The basics of basal transcription by RNA polymerase II. Cell. *77:*1–3, 1994.

6. Tjian, R. and Maniatis, T. Transcriptional activation: a complex puzzle with a few easy pieces. Cell. *77:*5–8, 1994.

7. Struhl, K. Chromatin structure and RNA polymerase II connection: implication for transcription. Cell. *84:* 179–182, 1996.

8. Wilson, C. J., Chao, D. M., Imbalzano, A. N., Schnitzler, G. R., Kingston, R. E., and Young, R. A. RNA polymerase II holoenzyme contains SWI/SNF regulators involved in chromatin remodeling. Cell. *84:* 235–244, 1996.

9. Weis, L., and Reinberg, D. Transcription by RNA polymerase II. initiator-director formation of transcription-competent complexes. FASEB J. *6:*3299–3309, 1992.

10. Robertson, L. M., Kerppola, T. K., and Vendrell, M., et al. Regulation of c-fos expression in transgenic mice requires multiple interdependent transcription control elements. Neuron. *14:*241–252, 1995.

11. Allan, C. M., Walker, D., and Taylor, J. M. Evolutionary duplication of a hepatic control region in the human apolipoprotein E gene locus. J Biol Chem. *270:*26278–26281, 1995.

12. Thanos, D. and Maniatis, T. Virus induction of human IFNβ gene expression requires the assembly of an enhanceosome. Cell. *83:*1091–1100, 1995.

13. Van der Vliet, P. C., and Verrijzer, C. P. Bending of DNA by transcription factors. Bioessays. *15:*25–32, 1993.

14. Scott, K. S. and Geyer, P. K. Effects of the su(Hw) insulator protein on the expression of the divergently transcribed drosophila yolk protein genes. EMBO J. *14:*6258–6279, 1995.

15. Dorsett, D. Distance-independent inactivation of an enhancer by the suppresser of hairy-wing DNA-binding protein of drosophila. Genetics. *134:*1135–1144, 1993.

16. Gerasimova, T. I., Gdula, D. A., Gerasimov, D. V., Simonova, O., and Corces, V. G. A drosophila protein that imparts directionality on a chromatin insulator is an enhancer of position-effect variegation. Cell. *82:* 587–597, 1995.

17. Jackson, M. E. Negative regulation of eukaryotic transcription. J Cell Science. *100:*1–7, 1991.

18. Grubinska, B., Laszkeiwicz, I., Royland, J., Wiggins, R. C., and Konat, G. W. Differentiation-specific demethylation of myelin associated glycoprotein gene in cultured oligodendrocytes. J Neurosci Res. *39:*233–242, 1994.

19. Costello, J. F., Futscher, B. W., Kroes, R. A., and Pieper, R. O. Methylation-related chromatin structure is associated with exclusion of transcription factors from and suppressed expression of the 0–6-methylguanine DNA methyltransferase gene in human glioma cell lines. Mol Cell Biol. *14:*6515–6521, 1994.

20. Festenstein, R., Tolaini, M., Corbella, P., et al. Locus control region function and heterochromatin-induced position effect variegation. Science. *271:*1123–1125, 1996.

21. Laurenson, P. and Rine, J. Silencers, silencing, and heritable transcriptional states. Microbiol Rev. *56:* 543–560, 1992.

22. Lehrach, H., Diamond, D., Wozney, J. M., and Boedtker, H. RNA molecular weight determinations by gel electrophoresis under denaturing conditions, a critical reexamination. Biochemistry. *16:*4743–4751, 1977.

23. Southern, E. M. Detection of specific sequences among DNA fragments separated by gel electrophoresis. J Mol Biol. *98:*503–517, 1975.

24. Glisin, V., Crkvenjakov, R., and Byus, C. Ribonucleic acid isolated by cesium chloride centrifugation. Biochemistry. *13:*2633–2637, 1974.

25. Ullrich, A., Shine, J., and Chirgwin, J., et al. Rat insulin genes: construction of plasmids containing the coding sequences. Science. *196:*1313–1319, 1977.

26. Alwine, J. C., Kemp, D. J., and Stark, G. R. Method for detection of specific RNAs in agarose gels by transfer to diazobenzyloxymethyl-paper and hybridization with DNA probes. Proc Natl Acad Sci. *74:*5350–5354, 1977.

27. Wensink, P. C., Finnegan, D. J., Donelson, J. E., and Hogness, D. S. A system for mapping DNA sequences in the chromosomes of drosophila melanogaster. Cell. *3:*315–325, 1974.

28. Okayama, H., and Berg, P. High-efficiency cloning of full-length cDNA. Mol Cell Biol. *2:*161–170, 1982.

29. Coleclough, C., and Erlitz, F. Use of primer-restriction-end adapters in a novel cDNA cloning strategy. Gene. *34:*305–314, 1985.

30. Frohman, M. A., Dush, M. K., and Martin, G. R. Rapid production of full-length cDNAs from rare transcripts: amplification using a single gene-specific oligonucleotide primer. Proc Natl Acad Sci USA. *85:*8998–9002, 1988.

31. Gause, W. C., and Adamovicz, J. The use of the PCR to quantitate gene expression. PCR Methods Appl. *3:*S123–S135, 1994.

32. Drake, J. W. Comparative rates of spontaneous mutation. Nature. *221:*1132, 1969.

33. Lalouel, J. and White, R. Analysis of genetic linkage. In: Emery, A. E. H., Rimoin, D., eds. Principles and practice of medical genetics. New York: Churchill Livingstone, 149–164, 1990.

34. Meyers, D. A. Genetic approaches to familial aggregation. In: Khoury, M. J., Beaty, T. H., Cohen, B. H., eds. Fundamentals of genetic epidemiology. New York/Oxford: Oxford University Press. 284–311, 1993.

35. Collins, F. S. Positional cloning moves from perditional to traditional. Nature Genet. *9:*347–350, 1995.

36. Nakamura, Y., Leppert, M., O'Connell, P., et al. Variable number of tandem repeat (VNTR) markers for human gene mapping. Science. *235:*1616–1622, 1987.

37. Weber, J. L. Informativeness of human $(dC-dA)_n \cdot (dG-dT)_n$ polymorphisms. Genomics. *7:*524–530, 1990.

38. Orita, M., Suzuki, Y., Sekiya, T., and Hayashi, K. Rapid and sensitive detection of point mutations and DNA polymorphisms using the polymerase chain reaction. Genomics. *5:*874–879, 1989.

CHAPTER 3

Basic Concepts of Gene Therapy

JOHN S. YU, M.D., GRIFFITH R. HARSH IV, M.D.,
XANDRA O. BREAKEFIELD, Ph.D.

INTRODUCTION

Potential Utility of Gene Therapy

As recombinant DNA techniques reveal the genetic etiology of neurologic diseases, gene therapy is being explored as a means to treat diseases at the genetic level. The identification of genes causing diseases of the nervous system has highlighted the paucity of effective therapies for many of them. Originally, gene therapy was envisioned as a cure for hereditary diseases at the gene level to be achieved by replacing a deleted gene or correcting a mutant gene in tissues dependent on the normal gene. Such gene therapy is particularly attractive for inherited diseases of the nervous system, as many are attributable to defects in a single gene. This therapy directed at the primary lesion would obviate the need to reverse the secondary effects of gene loss or dysfunctional gene products. Replacing a deleted gene is more feasible than correcting a mutated one. Correction of a mutant gene would require site-directed recombination into the host cell genome. Although this is feasible in culture, its relative inefficiency in vivo limits its clinical utility.

Currently, gene therapy is being developed for both hereditary and nonhereditary conditions. It attempts either to augment expression of a deleted or insufficiently expressed gene or to express genes that might prevent pathologic manifestations of the aberrant gene. The first strategy could provide the normal gene product in monogenic recessive and X-linked diseases in which a gene is deleted or expressed at insufficient levels. The second strategy may selectively reduce expression of the diseased gene or counteract the effects of its products in dominantly inherited diseases with aberrantly functioning gene products. Gene therapy may also be useful for disorders not attributable to a single inherited genetic defect. For diseases of the central nervous system (CNS), such as Parkinsonism and neoplasia, this might involve delivering genes whose products promote neuronal survival or inhibit tumor growth, respectively (48, 84, 91). This chapter reviews the targeting of somatic, rather than germ cells, by both strategies of gene therapy for CNS disease (25).

Progress in the development of viral vectors and in the understanding of the pathophysiology of neurologic diseases has brought gene therapy to the threshold of clinical use. The excitement regarding this powerful technology is tempered by clinical concerns about the safety and the difficulty of delivering genes to the nervous system. Diseases of the nervous system pose special challenges to gene delivery: 1) the skull and blood-brain barrier hinder access to diseased tissue, 2) specialization of function within the brain requires precise delivery to a particular neuroanatomical region, and 3) delivery-related toxicity is more likely to produce clinically significant injury in the brain whose cells are postmitotic and highly specialized. The complexity of neural anatomy, the intricate interrelationships of neurons and glia, and our limited understanding of brain function and pathophysiology increase the difficulty of applying gene therapy to neurologic disease. These challenges are being addressed by study of different modes of packaging genes for delivery—such as naked nucleic acid and DNA in liposomes, dextran conjugates and viral vectors, or in cells genetically modified to produce either a desired gene product or a viral vector carrying the therapeutic gene. Different routes of gene delivery to the brain—through the parenchyma, the vascular system, and the cerebrospinal fluid—are also being explored.

The Two Paradigms of Gene Therapy

Gene therapy approaches employ one of two basic paradigms in which transduction of the therapeutic gene into cells occurs either in vivo or ex vivo. In the in vivo paradigm, the patient's cells are transduced in situ. Complexes of nucleic acids, viral vectors, or cells modified to produce viral vectors containing the therapeutic gene are delivered to the brain, where transduction of the targeted cell population occurs. Advantages of in vivo transduction include the relative ease of delivering small particles (except when vector-producing cells [VPC] are used) and, when replication-competent vectors are involved, the possibility of increasing the range of gene delivery by engendering secondary waves of transduction. Disadvantages include a low rate of transduction and toxicity. In the ex vivo paradigm, cells from established cell lines or primary cells harvested from patients are genetically modified in tissue culture and then delivered to the brain. This method is suitable for the delivery of genes producing diffusible compounds, such as biosynthetic enzymes for neurotransmitters (50), trophic factors (79), lysosomal enzymes (115, 151), cytokines (41), and enzymes activating antineoplastic prodrugs (29, 45). Advantages of ex vivo transduction are its efficiency and the opportunity to expand stocks of transduced cells by allowing them to proliferate before use. Disadvantages include the need to deliver cells rather than vectors or nucleic-acid complexes and the inability to engender secondary transduction within the patient.

Vectors for Gene Therapy of CNS Disease

Viral vectors have been the mainstay of gene therapy to the nervous system because of the high efficiency with which they can deliver genes to cells in culture and in vivo. Viral vectors are viruses modified so as to retain viral genetic elements that allow efficient transduction of the target cell but to disrupt the elements responsible for replication and toxicity. Several classes of viral vectors have been developed for use in the central nervous system (150, 169). The type of virus used depends in part on the disease being treated, as each has advantages and disadvantages that vary with the nature of the disease and the type of cell being targeted. For instance, in degenerative disease of the nervous system, neurons and glia are the common targets of gene therapy. In the postnatal CNS, these cells are predominantly postmitotic. This population of nondividing cells can be infected by DNA virus vectors but not transduced by retroviral vectors. This precludes direct retroviral in vivo gene transfer in deficiency diseases but is an advantage for retroviral gene therapy of tumors (152). Proliferating tumor cells are vulnerable, but quiescent neurons and glia are not. Viral vectors carry the inherent disadvantage that they elicit an immune response to viral antigens which, in turn, limits gene delivery, especially in secondary applications, and may lead to rejection of target cells expressing viral antigens and the transgenes.

Nonviral vectors are an alternative means of delivering therapeutic genes to the CNS. Use of nonviral vectors has thus far been limited by their low efficiency of gene transduction. However, their safety is a powerful attraction. Chimeric vectors that combine viral elements for enhanced gene transfer efficiency with nonviral elements that ensure safety may provide a nontoxic, efficient means of delivering therapeutic genes to the central nervous system.

PRINCIPLES OF GENE DELIVERY

The goal of gene therapy methods is expression of the transgene(s) in target cells in vivo. There are a number of steps needed to achieve this; critical issues are the choice of delivery vehicle or vector, the mode of entry of the vector into cells, the state of the transgene within cells, and regulation of transgene expression (Fig. 1). Most current modes of vector entry into cells are not specific to cell types. Certain cell populations can be targeted, however, by the choice of delivery route. Vector entry into the nervous system can be achieved by focal, stereotactic injection into the parenchyma; uptake from nerve terminals in the periphery with retrograde transport to neuronal

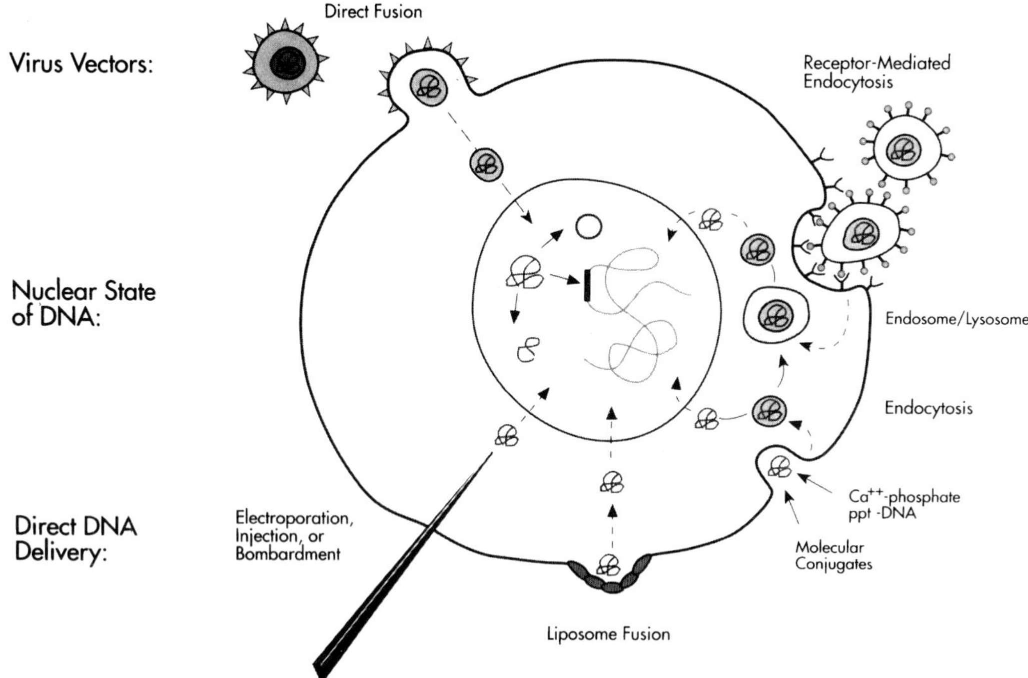

Figure 1. Entry and state of foreign DNA in cells. DNA can be introduced into cells in a number of ways. Some viruses, like herpes and retrovirus, have a membrane envelope that fuses to the cell surface, depositing the virions directly into the cytoplasm. Liposomes bearing elements that fuse at neutral pH can also be taken up in this direct manner. Other viruses, like adenovirus and AAV, are taken up by receptor-mediated endocytosis and then use acid-triggered fusigenic proteins to escape from the endosomes and avoid degradation in lysosomes. Receptor mediated endocytosis is also used by Ca^{++} phosphate DNA precipitates and molecular conjugates. DNA can also be delivered through the membrane by temporary disruption using electroporation, injection or particle bombardment. Models of transit through the cytoplasm to the nucleus are less well defined although some viruses travel on actin and microtubular elements. Some viruses, like HIV, have nuclear localization signals on viral proteins to target the nucleus. DNA can pass into the nucleus through nuclear pores. Retrovirus entry requires dissolution of the nuclear membrane at mitosis. Within the nucleus DNA elements can integrate into the cellular genome, or exist as replicating or non-replicating extrachromosomal DNA elements.

cell bodies within the nervous system; or introduction into the vasculature or intrathecal space. There are two basic modes of transgene delivery, mechanical and viral.

Vehicles for Transgene Delivery

In the case of mechanical delivery, DNA is usually packaged to neutralize its negative charge and to reduce shear forces on it, thus decreasing degradation and facilitating delivery (13, 178). DNA can be precipitated with calcium phosphate, bound to gold particles, encapsulated in artificial membranes, termed liposomes, and/or complexed with positively charged proteins, termed molecular conjugates. Particles can be delivered by electroporation or bombardment, in which case they pass directly through the cell membrane, temporarily disrupting it. Liposomes can fuse to the membrane, thus releasing their contents directly into the cytoplasm. Conjugates can be taken up by endocytosis or pinocytosis; they end up within membrane vesicles in the cytoplasm and must exit from those vesicles before they enter the degradative endosomal-lysosomal pathway. Mechanical means of gene delivery can be very inefficient because of a low level of cellular uptake, degradation within cells, and poor access to the nucleus. Alteration of the transgene by incorporating specific viral proteins or DNA sequences, sometimes from several different viruses, creates synthetic vectors with facile mechanical delivery, stable DNA, and efficient transgene expression.

In the case of viral delivery, the transgene is integrated within viral sequences so it is packaged with viral nucleic acid in virus capsids. The transgene in the resultant viral vector enters cells by the mode characteristic of that particular virus. For virus vectors in current use, cellular recognition molecules are present on most cells and thus entry is not cell specific, although there may be differences in the relative efficiency of infection among cell types and species for particular viruses. Viruses commonly used for gene delivery do so by two mechanisms; herpes virus (usually derived from herpes simplex virus type 1, HSV1) and retrovirus (usually derived from Moloney murine leukemia virus, MoMLV) enter by direct fusion of the viral envelope to the cell membrane, such that the capsid is released into the cytoplasm while adenovirus and adenoassociated virus (AAV) vectors are taken up by receptor-mediated endocytosis.

Site of Transgene Expression

Most transgenes are designed to be expressed within the cell nucleus. The route of vectors from the cytoplasm into the nucleus is not well understood. Transgenes introduced by most vectors can access the nucleus even in non-mitotic cells. In general, however, breakdown of the nuclear membrane facilitates nuclear entry of the vector, as well as replication of the host's DNA. It also promotes integration of the foreign DNA and expression of the transgene. Some virus vectors, such as retrovirus, can only access nuclear space when the nuclear membrane breaks down during mitosis; others, such as AAV and HIV, can enter the nucleus and integrate into the genome of dividing, as well as non-dividing cells. "Free" DNA in the nucleus can be transcriptionally active for some time, but is eventually degraded or lost during mitosis. Some viruses, *e.g.*, HSV and Epstein Barr virus (EBV), can maintain their genome as a stable extra-chromosomal (episomal) element in the host cell nucleus. Latent HSV establishes a nucleosomal configuration in some postmitotic cells, *e.g.*, sensory neurons, while EBV maintains itself as replicative element, replicating in phase with host lymphoid cells. Incorporation of the EBV origin of DNA replication, oriP, and the gene encoding the viral DNA

binding proteins, EBNA1, into an expression plasmid can permit retention and expression of transgenes over a number of cell generations. Theoretically, incorporation of mammalian origins of replication into such expression plasmids would be similarly useful. Most of the mammalian origins described to date are quite large, >12 kb, and require larger cloning vehicles. However, several groups have shown extended retention of plasmids with smaller mammalian origins of DNA replication (66). Within the nucleus, the transgene can also integrate into the host cell genome, usually at random sites, but, in the case of AAV, preferentially on human chromosome 19q. Although integration of nonviral DNA sequences is a very inefficient process, some viruses have developed means to promote this process, *e.g.*, retrovirus, AAV, and elements from these viruses can be used to promote transgene integration.

Other vectors can express transgenes in the cytoplasm without requiring nuclear import. These include those derived from vaccinia, Sindbis, and bacculovirus viruses (16). Self-promoting DNA transcription cassettes express genes in the cytoplasm without the need for nuclear access. They encode prokaryotic RNA polymerases which express the transgenes from the appropriate prokaryotic promoter. Messages generated in the cytoplasm must be able to function without the post-transcriptional modifications that normally occur in the nucleus, including capping the 5′ terminal, splicing of introns, and polyadenylation.

Control of Transgene Expression

One of the unresolved problems regarding control of transgene expression is the choice of appropriate promoters. Expression of transgenes tends to be extinguished over time in vivo, even when the DNA is still present in cells. Several factors contributing to this problem have been identified. In general, viral promoters are recognized as "foreign" in eukaryotic cells and shut-down, primarily through DNA methylation. Thus, for example, the cytomegalo-virus (CMV) promoter, which can give extremely strong transient transgene expression, is eventually shut off in most mammalian cells. In general, if the DNA bearing the transgene is replicating, and thus in an "open" configuration, expression continues (161). Depending on the site of transgene integration into the host cell genome, condensation of the DNA into a nucleosomal configuration can also decrease transgene expression. The identification of a movable locus control region (LCR), which flanks the globin gene and "holds the DNA open" to transcription, has been a promising finding (1). However, this region is specific for erthyroid cells and similar regions have yet to be identified for other cell types.

Mammalian promoters can achieve transgene expression for longer periods in vivo, even months, but again are strongly influenced by neighboring DNA elements. The phosphoglycerate kinase (PGK) promoter (a strong housekeeping promoter) mediates strong transgene expression in a number of cell types in vivo (115). Combinations of enhancer elements and promoters also maintain transgene expression in vivo—e.g., the muscle-specific creatinine kinase enhancer element linked to the CMV promoter for differentiated muscle cells (34). For neural cells, a number of different promoters, defined in transgenic mice, may prove useful. These include the promoter for the glial fibrillary acidic protein (GFAP) for astrocytes (20); the neurofilament heavy chain promoter for neurons (145); the PO promoter for Schwann cells (2); and the myelin basic protein promoter for oligodendrocytes (113). More specific neural promoter elements may produce transgene expression limited to particular types of neurons (83)—e.g., the sodium channel promoters for certain neurons (104) or the tyrosine hydroxylase promoter for catecholaminergic neurons (122).

Self-promoting and inducible promoters are also being developed. For example the T7-T7 cytoplasmic expression cassette bears T7 polymerase and the transgene each under a separate T7 promoter (97). Placement of an internal ribosomal entry sequence 5' to the translation initiation codon results in capless messages being transcribed via these promoters (54). Introducing T7 RNA polymerase, or the RNA encoding it, into the cytoplasm along with the transgene primes the cassette, which then generates more polymerase and transgene.

Another self-priming vector system is the GAL4:VP16 transactivating fusion protein combined with multiple copies of the GAL4 binding site (140). The GAL4 protein (derived from yeast) binds to the GAL4 DNA site, and VP16 (derived from HSV) serves as a potent transactivator of transcription. The fusion protein can drive synthesis of its own message as well as that of a transgene (57). This system has been made drug-inducible by adding a truncated form of the hormone binding domain of the progesterone receptor to the GAL4:VP16 transactivator; this truncated portion no longer binds progesterone, but does bind a steroid analog drug, which can activate the transactivator (167).

Among other inducible promoters (61), the prokaryotic-derived tetracycline (tet) regulatable promoter system appears to be the most effective. It incorporates a tet repressor: VP16 transactivator protein and the tet operator linked to the CMV promoter. This comes in both a tet-on (63) and tet-off form (62). The latter has been incorporated in a self-contained retrovirus vector (125). This construct is able to tightly control transgene expression even within rodent brain. Still the ability to reproducibly achieve long term (>6 month) regulatable expression in cells in the nervous system has remained elusive. The use of promoter elements for the latency associated transcripts (LATs) produced by some neurons (e.g., sensory neurons) during the latent phase of infection by HSV vectors appears most promising currently (39, 57, 177).

The field of gene therapy is still very much in an exploratory phase. Although many techniques are being tried, only a few have been directly compared. Over the next few years, coalescence of more sophisticated promoter technology, improved mechanical and viral gene delivery, and the availability of synthetic vectors which retain viral elements required for efficient delivery and eliminate those that cause toxicity should make gene therapy a viable treatment option.

VIRAL VECTORS

Retrovirus

Structure and Life Cycle of Retroviruses

Retroviruses are single-stranded RNA viruses with a 9 kb long genome bearing longitudinal repeat (LTR) sequences at both ends. Virions contain two copies of the RNA genome, as well as reverse transcriptase, integrase, and other viral proteins within an icosahedral capsid surrounded by a lipoprotein envelope.

Most retroviruses used as vectors are derived from the Moloney murine leukemia virus (MoMLV), which has a broad host range (117). New vectors derived by modification of the MoMCV genome and from endogenous retroviral genomes in mice (163) may have the advantage of more sustained gene expression in vivo. Retroviruses require the target cell to be dividing for proviral integration into the host genome to occur (81, 146). Stable integration into the genome of mitotic cells and passage to cell progeny, extensive characterization, and a record of safety make retroviral vectors the vectors of choice for most experimental and clinical studies thus far (31).

Packaging Cell Lines

The establishment of packaging cell lines which produce replication-defective vectors, free of wild-type retrovirus virus, is the most significant advance in the safe use of retroviruses as gene vectors (Fig. 2) (35, 110, 126). Packaging cell lines are stably transfected cell lines that release retrovirus vectors containing the gene of interest. Most packaging cell lines are derived from the murine fibroblast line, 3T3, and can produce either ecotropic virus, which efficiently infects murine cells, or amphotropic virus, which infects cells from a broad range of species. The species specificity of infection depends on the envelope (env) protein the packaging line expresses.

Packaging lines are generated by stably transfecting cells with mutated retrovirus sequences. In its simplest form, the gag, pol, and env sequences are preserved, but the packaging sequence, psi, contains an inactivating mutation. This allows all proteins involved in viral replication and packaging to be expressed but prevents retrovirus RNA encoding them to be packaged into viral particles. Therefore, until a plasmid with retroviral sequences bearing the psi signal is transfected into the packaging line, it releases particles that either are empty or contain only RNA derived from defective retrovirus sequences endogenous to the host genome. New versions of packaging cell lines bear fragmented retrovirus sequences with multiple mutations that further reduce the possibility of generating wild-type virus by recombination between vectors and retrovirus sequences in the host genome (35, 110, 126).

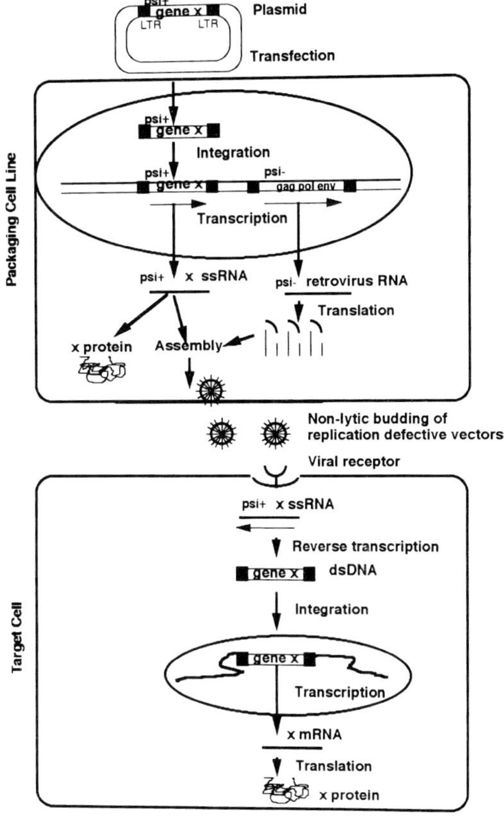

Figure 2. Generation of and infection by retrovirus vectors. The packaging cell line contains wild type retroviral sequences, including gag, pol, and env, integrated into the host cell genome, but lacks the packaging signal, psi, for incorporation of viral encoded RNA into the virions. A plasmid containing the gene of interest and the psi packaging signal between the retroviral LTR sequences is transfected into the packaging cell line. After genomic integration, the gene of interest is transcribed into single stranded RNA (ssRNA) that can be packaged into assembling virions. Nonlytic budding occurs and retrovirus vectors from the supernatant are used to infect cells. Alternatively, packaging cell lines can be transplanted in vivo for on site vector generation and infection. The retrovirus infects the cells by fusion of the virion envelope with the plasma membrane of the cell. The retroviral RNA undergoes reverse transcription to form double stranded DNA (dsDNA) and integrates at random sites in the genome of actively dividing cells. The integrated gene is transcribed and translated into the protein of interest.

Vector plasmids contain the retrovirus LTRs and psi sequence; the rest of the genome is replaced by transgene sequences (Fig. 3). Following transfection of packaging cells with the

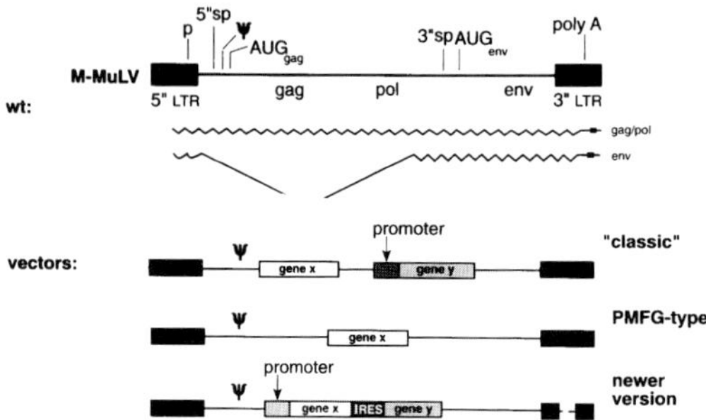

Figure 3. Retrovirus vectors. The wild type (wt) MoMLV genome generates two types of transcripts (wavy lines): unspliced (gag/pol) and spliced (env) RNA, both under regulation of the 5′ LTR (left black box): p = promoter, sp = RNA splice sites, psi (ψ) = packaging signal, AUG = start site of translation, polyA = polyA addition site in the 3′ LTR. (Reprinted with permission from Gilboa *et al.*, 1986.) Some vector formulations are also shown: in the classic type, one transgene, X, is placed under the 5′ LTR promoter and another transgene, Y, is placed under another promoter inserted within the construct. The pMFG vector design (Mulligan, 1993) carries only a single transgene but gives high titers by virtue of an extended gag sequence 3′ to the psi sequence. In newer vectors, transgenes are placed in tandem, separated by an IRES sequence to allow translation to initiate at start sites on the same messenger RNA. A promoter is placed internally to the 5′ LTR and a deletion in the 3′ LTR removes its ability to act as a promoter when it becomes the 5′ LTR following genomic integration, thus preserving the integrity of the internal promoter (reprinted with permission from Sena-Esteves *et al.*, 1995).

vector plasmid, the RNA corresponding to the viral vector and transgene(s) is encapsidated and infectious viral particles bud off from the surface of the packaging cell line. Conditioned medium from these cells is filtered and used as viral stock. The number of infectious particles per milliliter is usually titered by colony-forming units under selection when the vector includes a drug selection gene, such as the neomycin gene or by histochemistry for lacZ.

Entry into the Cell

Glycoproteins of the viral envelope mediate binding to the cell surface and hence cell specificity (4, 111). The envelope fuses with the cell membrane releasing the virion contents into the cytoplasm. The RNA genome is copied into a double-stranded genome by reverse transcriptase and forms a pre-integration complex with other viral proteins. The preintegration complex of MoMLV retrovirus accesses the cell

nucleus during mitosis and integration into the host genome is mediated by integrase.

The generation of vectors with different envelope proteins is a major technical advance in retroviral gene delivery. Pseudotyped viruses are engineered either by generation of recombinant env proteins or by concurrent infection of cells with different strains of retroviruses. This produces vectors with novel env proteins or with env proteins from different taxonomic groups on their coats. Such modifications alter the host specificity of the virus (176). In addition to broadening the host range, pseudotyping can also increase the stability of viral particles. This allows them to be concentrated up to 300-fold to titers of 10^9 infectious units/ml (23, 183).

Specificity of the envelope protein has also been altered in other ways—for example, chemical modification with lactose. This produces artificial asialoglycoproteins that can target particles to asialoglycoprotein receptors on human hepatocytes (120). Strepavidin-biotin-strepavidin ridged antibodies, which are bispecific for the virus particle and cell surface epitopes (*e.g.*, MHC class I and II molecules and EGF and insulin receptors) have also been utilized to infect target cells albeit with low efficiency (44, 108, 138). Chimeric env proteins have been created with recombinant DNA techniques (*e.g.*, erythropoietin sequence added in frame at the *N*-terminal of the ecotropic env sequence) to achieve cell type specificity in human cells (85). Expanding the host range of vectors permits their use in a wider range of experimental models. Targeting vectors to specific cell types would greatly increase the precision of gene delivery at the cellular level.

Access to the cell genome depends on mitosis for the breakdown of nuclear membrane (132). Further, the low titers and instability of retroviral vectors limit their use for direct delivery in vivo, even to dividing cells. Some of these limitations may be overcome with pseudotyping, which involves incorporation of more stable envelope elements from other viruses into the virion particles (85). For diseases of the CNS, retrovirus vectors are used either in an ex vivo approach, in which vectors are used to deliver genes efficiently to dividing cells in culture, which are subsequently grafted intraparenchymally to deliver therapeutic gene products to brain cells, or an in vivo approach by grafting of packaging cells into tumors for on-site selective gene delivery to dividing tumor cells (148, 160).

Intracellular Processing of a Retroviral Vector

Following entry into the host cell, the retroviral RNA genome is copied into a linear double-stranded cDNA form by reverse transcriptase, a product of the pol gene. The double-stranded DNA is circularized via the long terminal repeats (LTRs) and enters the nuclear space as a nucleosome complex when the nuclear membrane is disassembled at mitosis. Integration into the host genome is mediated by integrase, the product of the viral gene, int. The site of integration is relatively random although transcriptionally active regions may be preferred (147).

Expression of the Transgene

When integrated into the host cell genome, the vector is typically transcribed from the viral 5′ LTR promoter. Depending on the site of integration, there is the potential for cis-activation of host cell gene expression, which can trigger transformation and neoplasia. Dysregulation of transgene expression by components of the surrounding host genome may also "shut down" the LTR promoter. Downregulation of the LTR promoter frequently, but not always, occurs in vivo (124). Transgene expression can be maintained by using a strong mammalian promoter to drive transgene expression in the targeted cells. For example, the phosphoglycerate kinase (PGK) promoter remains active over months in fibroblast grafts in vivo (115); and a combination of the muscle-specific creatinine kinase enhancer and the cytomegalovirus (CMV) promoter allows continued expression in differentiated muscle cells in vivo (34).

Multiple gene products can be expressed if the genes encoding them total less than 8 kb (Fig. 3). For example, a reporter gene such as lacZ and a drug resistance gene, such as neoR, can be expressed from the 5′ LTR promoter and an internal promoter, respectively, or from the same promoter with an internal ribosome entry site (IRES). The IRES allows translation to initiate from the middle, as well as from the beginning, of the transcript (2, 54). Internal promoters utilized in retroviral vectors include promoter/enhancer elements from (CMV), Rous sarcoma virus (RSV), and SV40. To prevent the

relatively strong LTR promoter from "overriding" internal promoters, a small deletion can be made in the 3′ LTR, which becomes the 5′ LTR after integration. This inactivates LTR promoter function and reduces the chance of cis activation of a cellular proto-oncogene (184).

Adenovirus

Structure and Life Cycle of Adenovirus

Adenovirus virions are 80–90 nm in diameter and consist of a non-enveloped capsid. Virions bind to an, as yet, unidentified receptor on the cell surface through a fiber protein extending from the capsid (166). There is little cell specificity of infection by wild-type particles, but modifications of the fiber protein may allow cell targeting (109). Virions are engulfed by receptor-mediated endocytosis. As endosomes acidify, the penton-base capsid protein undergoes a conformation change which allows fusion to the endosome membrane and release of the virion into the cytoplasm. Transport of the viral DNA into the nucleus is an ATP-dependent process mediated by nuclear targeting signals in the capsid. Replication of the virus leads to cell death. Although adenovirus does not integrate into the host cell genome and does not have a stable episomal state, replication-defective adenovirus genomes can persist in an extrachromosomal state for months in vivo.

Cell Entry and Intracellular Processing

The adenovirus genome is linear, double-stranded DNA approximately 36 kb in length. It encodes at least 30 mRNA species. The genome is divided into several regions with different roles and times of expression during replication (Fig. 4). Each end of the viral chromosome has a 100–140 bp redundant sequence, the inverted terminal repeat (ITR), which is necessary for viral replication. The packaging signal sequence is localized next to the 5′ ITR and mediates encapsidation of viral DNA into preassembled capsids. The transcriptional units are classified according to their time of expression during virus propagation. The E1 region is active immediately after the virus enters the host cell nucleus. It encodes transactivators of early gene transcription and proteins that shut off cellular RNA translation. The E2 region encodes proteins needed for viral DNA replication and RNA splicing. The proteins encoded in the E3

RECOMBINANT ADENOVIRUS VECTOR

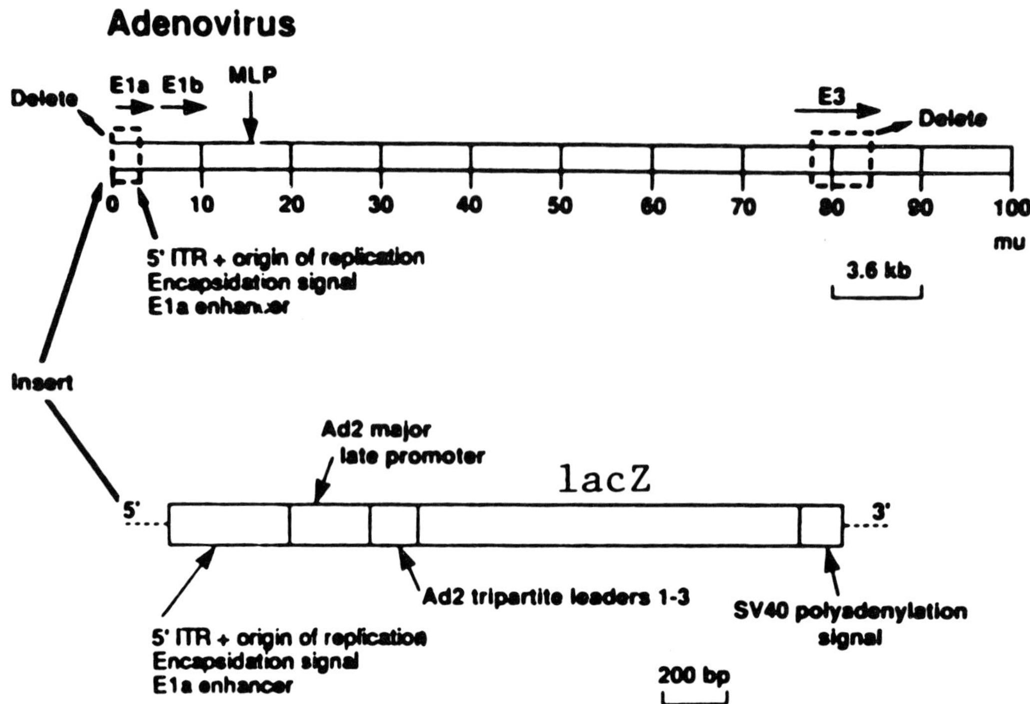

Figure 4.   Adenovirus vector. Wild-type adenovirus type 5 genome showing the E1a, E1b, and E3 regions and the major late promoter (MLP). The recombinant vector, Ad-alpha1 lacZ, was constructed by deleting the majority of the E3 region and 2.6 mu from the left end of the virus and inserting a lacZ expression cassette consisting of the 5′ inverted terminal repeat (ITR), the E1a enhancer and MLP promoter regulating expression of lacZ (reprinted with permission from Rosenfeld *et al.*, 1991).

region help the vector-infected cell evade immune surveillance. One of these, the 19 kDa glycoprotein localized in the endoplasmic reticulum, blocks transport of major histocompatibility complex (MHC) class I proteins to the cell surface and thereby cytotoxic T lymphocyte-mediated killing of the adenovirus-infected cell. The E4 region encodes transcriptional regulators of viral genes and inhibitors of cellular gene expression. The major late region codes for most of the polypeptides that comprise the capsid.

Adenovirus vectors are used in many experimental animal models and clinical studies (3, 173). They can be grown to high titer, infect a wide variety of cell types, and efficiently deliver genes to both mitotic and nonmitotic cells. Adenoviruses cause mild upper respiratory tract infections but are not oncogenic in humans. They have been used as vaccines clinically and hence have an established record of safety.

Creation of Adenoviral Vectors

Adenovirus vectors are derived by deleting a portion of the genome and replacing it with transgenes. They can be constructed by ligation of plasmids bearing modified adenoviral genes into adenoviral DNA in vitro or by transfection of cells with plasmids and virion DNA. In this latter case, viral DNA is either linear or contained in a circular plasmid and homologous recombination occurs within cells. The first-generation vectors had deletions in the E1 and E3 regions, which provided space for about 7.5 kb of foreign sequences. Since E1 functions are critical for generation of virions, these vectors

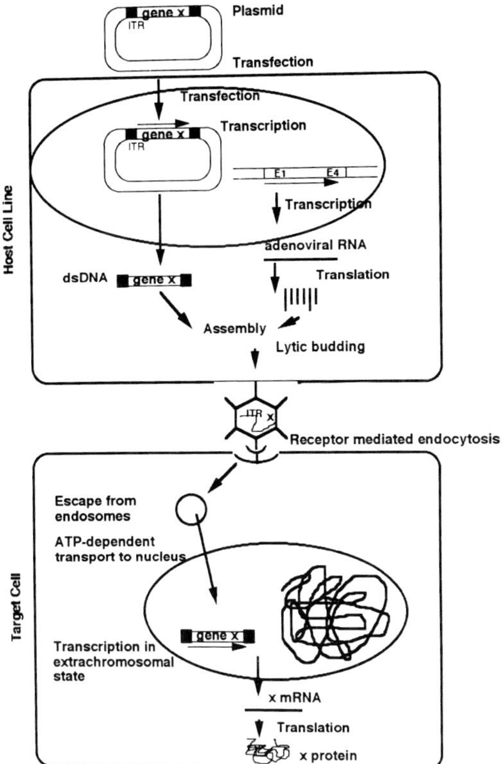

Figure 5. Generation and infection by adenovirus vectors. The host cell line typically contains the adenoviral E1 and/or E4 regions needed for viral replication. A plasmid containing a packaging signal, other adenovirus genes, and the transgene is transfected into host cells. The gene of interest is packaged as double stranded DNA in virions, and virions are released by lytic budding. The adenovirus particles containing the gene of interest enter the target cells by receptor mediated endocytosis. The virions are released from endosomes into the cytoplasm and are transported to the nucleus where DNA enters through nuclear pores in an ATP-dependent process. The replication defective adenoviral genome persists in an extrachromosomal element for some time in the nucleus, but does not have a stable episomal state.

are produced in cells, human embryonic kidney 293 cells, previously transfected with the E1 gene (Fig. 5). These vectors are replication-defective in most other cells, but some cells, including some tumor cell lines, can provide the missing viral functions in trans. Also, recombination is possible between the E1 region in the 293 cellular genome and the mutant virus to generate wild-type virus. Loss of the E3 region increases the transgene capacity of the vector

without compromising replication of the virus. However, this deletion reduces the ability of viral antigens to avoid immune detection. The relatively brief transgene expression observed with these early E3-deleted vectors results from immune rejection of infected cells expressing viral antigens (94).

Vectors with deletions of E1 and parts of E4 have been developed. These are propagated in cells transfected with intact E1 and E4 sequences (127). Since the ITRs and the adjacent packaging sequence are the only cis-acting signals required for virus replication and packaging, these vectors can potentially accommodate transgenes up to 30 kb even while retaining the E3 region. They should prove useful once adenovirus packaging cell lines or schemes become available. Since such minimal vectors would not induce expression of viral antigens, infected cells should not be rejected by the immune system. Nonetheless, the immune response to the virion inoculum could limit the efficiency of infection, especially with repeated use of the vector.

Adenovirus Vectors in the Brain

In several studies, direction inoculation of adenovirus vectors into the brain parenchyma has produced strong transgene expression in neurons, astrocytes, microglia, oligodendrocytes, and ependymal cells (3, 9, 36, 93). Adenovirus vectors can be delivered across the blood-brain barrier following its osmotic disruption (121); in these studies, a preference for infection of astrocytes, rather than neurons, was noted (116). The adenovirus virions are transported retrogradely from nerve terminals to neuronal cell bodies, *e.g.*, inoculation of skeletal muscle labels motor neurons in the spinal cord.

The number of cells expressing the transgene declines over months. Downregulation of promoters, degradation of vector DNA, and immune rejection of infected cells may all contribute to this extinction. Larger inoculums of vector are toxic to the brain, possibly because they induce a strong host immune response. The adenovirus virions are transported retrogradely from nerve terminals to neuronal cell bodies; *e.g.*, inoculation of skeletal muscle labels motor neurons in the spinal cord.

The robust, relatively brief gene expression mediated by adenovirus vectors is well suited to treating brain tumors. A number of studies have shown repression of experimental brain tumors by direct intratumoral injection of adenovirus vectors bearing the HSV-TK gene followed by systemic ganciclovir treatment (26, 137). Delivery through the vasculature combined with barrier disruption preferentially targets tumors in the brain whose neovasculature has a poorly developed barrier. Under these conditions, however, replication-defective adenovirus vectors deliver less transgene than do replication-conditional HSV vectors (14, 121).

Adenoassociated Virus

Structure and Life Cycle

Adenoassociated virus (AAV) is a 4.7-kb ssDNA virus that infects cells of all mammalian species. Co-infection with adenovirus or herpes virus is required for the production of AAV virus (6, 11). In the absence of helper virus, the AAV genome integrates into the host cell genome. In human cells this occurs preferentially at a specific nonessential locus, termed AAVS1, on chromosome 19 but can also occur at other sites in the genome of human and rodent cells (56, 87). AAV is typically found in respiratory infections in association with other viruses and alone is not pathologic. It enters cells by receptor-mediated endocytosis, using an as yet unidentified receptor. The viral genome is flanked by 145 bp inverted terminal repeats (ITRs) which have promoter activity and are critical to viral replication, encapsidation, integration, and rescue. The viral genome encodes the Rep and Cap proteins. Rep proteins are involved in replication, gene expression, and integration into the genome. Two of the four isoforms of Rep bind to an homologous repeat element, which is present in both the virus ITRs and the human AAVS1 locus. The helicase and recombinase activities of the rep protein mediate integration into the host cell genome. Cap proteins make up the virions, which are physically different from those of the helper virus.

AAV Vectors

AAV vectors are an important new tool for gene delivery because of their ability to integrate into the cellular genome in both mitotic and postmitotic cells (11, 119). Site-specific integration into a noncoding locus avoids disruption of cellular genes and potentially provides a platform for exploring controlled pro-

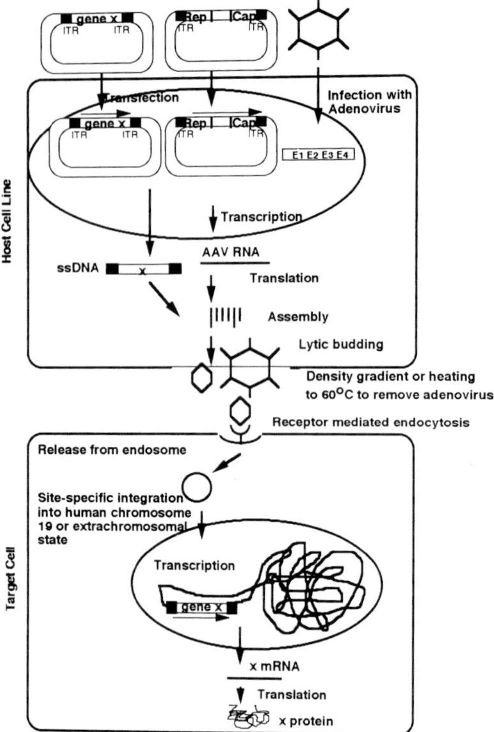

Figure 6. Generation and infection by adeno-associated viral vectors. The host cell line is infected with helper adenovirus and co-transfected with a plasmid containing the gene of interest between the AAV ITRs and a plasmid containing rep and cap genes between the adenovirus ITRs. Rep and Cap proteins are translated and allow replication of the ITR-bearing transgene cassette and packaging into viral particles. The helper virus renders the cell permissive to AAV propagation. Recombinant AAV and adenovirus particles are released by lytic budding. Density gradient centrifugation or heating at 60°C is performed to remove or inactivate adenovirus, respectively. Recombinant AAV particles are taken up by receptor mediated endocytosis into the target cells. ITR-flanked transgenes can integrate randomly or into a specific site in human chromosome 19. They can also be maintained in a relatively stable extrachromosomal state.

moter/enhancer elements. Current AAV vectors are generated from plasmids containing cis acting ITRs, between which the transgene of interest and its regulatory sequences are inserted (Fig. 6). Because of the limits on size posed by the virion, AAV vectors can only package an insert between 4.0 and 4.7 kb. If the Rep gene is included in the vector, the insert size is reduced to approximately 2 kb.

When plasmid DNA containing the transgene and ITRs is transfected into permissive cells in the presence of adenovirus and a helper AAV plasmid, the ITRs and the sequences between them are rescued from the plasmid and packaged in AAV virions (Fig. 6). The helper plasmid contains adenovirus ITRs, which cannot be packaged in this context and supplies complementing gene products, Rep and Cap, for AAV replication and capsid production. Both AAV vectors and adenovirus are released from cells. Adenovirus can be removed by density gradient centrifugation or inactivated by heating the preparation at 60°C for 30 minutes. This system allows production of AAV vector stocks which are free of infectious wild-type AAV and helper virus (141). Typical titers obtained for AAV vectors are 10^5–10^6 transducing units/ml although these can be concentrated by density gradient centrifugation. The relatively low titers of AAV vectors are attributed in part to limiting amounts of the rep and cap gene products. The establishment of cell lines with high levels of expression of Rep and Cap proteins has been problematic due in part to the cytotoxicity of Rep. Flotte *et al.* (47) have recently described an increase in titer of 50-fold over previous packaging methods by transfecting cell lines that have integrated an ITR-flanked transgene with plasmids that express large amounts of Rep from the HIV promoter. After density-gradient centrifugation and concentration, titers of approximately 10^{10} transducing units/ml were reported.

ITR-flanked transgenes can integrate into the host cell genome at random sites or in human cells, at a specific site on chromosome (19, 142). Preferential sites in rodent cells have not been identified. During this time, multiple copies of the viral genome are maintained in a relatively stable extrachromosomal state in the cell nucleus. Resistance to exonucleases is conferred by the hair-pin structures formed by the ITRs. AAV integrate into the genome of nondividing, as well as dividing, cells although DNA synthesis increases the efficiency of integration and dividing cells are transduced 200-fold more efficiently than nondividing cells (139). Stimulation of DNA repair can facilitate integration of AAV sequences in nondividing cells (5). Russell *et al.* (139) have shown that the AAV genome can replicate and persist in an extrachromosomal state for up to 12 days in nondividing cells and any time throughout this period can integrate or be passed onto progeny in a nonintegrated state if cells are stimulated to divide.

AAV Vectors in the Brain

Only a few studies have used AAVs to transduce neural cells. In the presence of helper virus, wild-type AAV can replicate in human astrocytoma and oligodendroglioma cell lines, indicating that the receptor for AAV is present on these cells (162). Stereotaxic injection of AAVs into rat brain yielded long-term (three-month) expression of a tyrosine hydroxylase transgene driven by the CMV promoter (82). The ratio of infectious vector particles to transduced cells was about 10:1 as assessed by transgene expression two days following injection. Subsequently the number of positive cells declined, presumably because the AAV genome was degraded and/or the promoter was downregulated. Immunocytochemical analyses of brain sections reveal that most transduced cells were neurons and glia. Thus, AAV vectors can be used for transgene delivery in the CNS, but it is not yet clear whether they can integrate into the genome of these cells or how stable gene expression will be.

Herpes Simplex Virus

Structure and Life Cycle

Among the over 80 types of herpes viruses, three are common pathogens in humans: Herpes simplex virus type 1 (HSV1) and type 2 (HSV2) and varicella zoster (72). Vectors derived from HSV1 have been used experimentally to deliver genes to a number of tissues in vivo and are particularly well suited for delivery to neurons (18, 57, 80) and brain tumors (17, 75). HSV1 is a large DNA virus with a genome of 150 kb containing 75 genes (105). The virus particle (150 nm in diameter) consists of an icosahedral capsid surrounded by tegument proteins and a membranous envelope (135).

HSV in the Cell

Although cells differ in the efficiency of viral entry, HSV1 virus can infect essentially all cell types in a wide range of species, the virus enters cells following binding of glycoproteins in its envelope to heparin sulfate and other, as yet unidentified, components of the cell membrane.

Binding is followed by fusion of the envelope and cell membrane with release of the virus capsid and associated tegument proteins directly into the cytoplasm. Once inside the cell, the virus capsid is delivered to the nucleus by association between viral tegument proteins and microtubules and retrograde transport. The capsid opens outside the nucleus, and viral DNA with associated tegument proteins enters through the nuclear pores (101). Within the nucleus, the viral DNA can either proceed to productive infection or enter into latency (133). In productive infection, there is a sequence of expression of viral genes that progresses from immediate early (IE, alpha) genes, which code primarily for transactivating factors, to early (E, beta) genes, coding for enzymes involved in viral DNA synthesis, to late (L, gamma) genes, which produce structural virion proteins. Two important features of productive infection are activation of IE viral genes by the tegument protein, VP16, and interference with host cell macromolecular synthesis by tegument protein, vhs. Productive infection leads to generation and release of thousands of virions. The host cell dies within 24 hours.

Alternately, in some cells, such as neurons, the virus can enter a state of latency where there is virtually no expression of viral genes. In latency, the viral genome assumes a stable extrachromosomal state in the cell nucleus. Only one type of viral transcript, a nuclear RNA species of unknown function, termed the latency associated transcript(s) (LATs), has been detected (156). The viral DNA has a nucleosomal configuration and can exist in this state for years with no apparent alteration of neuronal physiology. Changes in the cell state in response to temperature, hormones, or stress can reactivate the viral genome leading to viral production. Less virus is produced following reactivation from latency than by productive infection, and the host cell does not necessarily die.

HSV Vectors

HSV is well-suited for gene delivery to the nervous system (18). First, it is potentially safe in humans. HSV1 is a common pathogen in humans and only rarely causes serious complications although productive infection in the brain can rapidly engender lethal encephalitis (30, 96, 174). HSV1 may access the brain to assume a state of latency with no clinical man-

ifestations in many people (10). A number of antiherpetic drugs are also available which can effectively block virus replication (135). Second, the virus particles are stable and can be generated at high titers, up to 10^{12}/ml. These high titers are compatible with the small volumes of inoculum tolerated in the CNS and allow multiple routes of administration. Third, the state of latency is virtually benign to neurons and allows the potential for long-term expression of the transgenes (155). Fourth, anterograde and retrograde transport of the virus allows traverse from the periphery into and throughout the CNS along neuronal pathways (165). Fifth, the virus can be mutated to insert >30 kb of transgene sequence and to reduce toxicity (57, 134).

The HSV1 appears to be particularly well suited for use in brain tumor therapy (103). Mutation of several of the viral genes involved in DNA replication—UTPase, thymidine kinase (TK), and ribonucleotide reductase (RR)—render the virus replication-defective in normal postmitotic cells, like neurons, but replication-competent in dividing cells, which can complement the defect (28, 59). In addition, the HSV-tk gene product can convert ganciclovir, acyclovir, and other drugs to nucleotide analogues which block both viral and cellular replication, thereby selectively killing dividing tumor cells (8).

Critical considerations in the potential clinical application of these vectors include their inherent toxicity, the possible reactivation of latent wild-type virus, and the immune responses engendered (17). A number of viral proteins are toxic to cells: IE gene products, ICP4, ICP0, and ICP27; the virion host shut off function (vhs) and associated UL13 gene products; the VP16 virion component; and products of genes associated with neurovirulence, gamma 34.5 and UL5 (27, 90). Most of these potentially harmful genes can be mutated in vectors; the resultant vectors can be propagated in cultured cells transfected with complementing, essential viral genes. Such mutant viruses should be virtually nontoxic to normal cells in vivo.

Herpes virus vectors are very versatile agents of genetic manipulation. Two types, recombinant virus vectors and amplicon vectors, can be generated as independent entities or propagated in tandem. Recombinant virus vectors contain

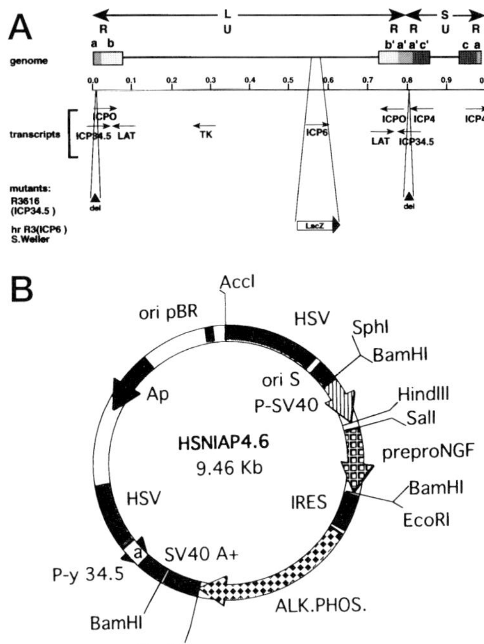

Figure 7. HSV1 recombinant virus and amplicon vectors. (A) Recombinant virus vector. The 151-kb HSV 1 genome is shown at the top. U = unique regions, L = long, and S = short. R = repeat elements ab and b′a′ flanking UL, a′c′ and ca flanking Us. Some transcripts are indicated as arrows in the direction of transcription. A typical vector, here MGH1, was derived by homologous recombination of a plasmid bearing a lacZ marker insertion in the ICP6 (ribonucleotide reductase) gene (Goldstein and Weller, 1988) in a gamma34.5 mutant virus (Roizman, 1993) (Dr. Christof Kramm, Dr. Antonio Chiocca and Maureen Chase, unpublished data). It is similar to the one described by Mineta *et al.*, 1995. Mutation in ICP6 renders the vector replication competent only in dividing cells; mutation in gamma34.5 reduces neurovirulence; and the lacZ gene allows detection of viral infection. (B) Amplicon plasmid. This 9.46-kb plasmid contains three kinds of genetic elements: 1) sequences that allow propagation in E. coli—the ampillicin resistance gene (Ap) and the E. coli origin of DNA replication (ori pBR); 2) sequences that support propagation and packaging of plasmid DNA by a helper HSV 1 virus—an HSV1 origin of DNA replication (Oris) and a packaging site within the repeat element; and 3) a transcription unit including the SV40 promoter and the mouse prepro-NGF cDNA, an IRES translational read-through, the human alkaline phosphatase marker gene, and the SV40 poly-adenylation site (designed by Dr. Peter Perchan) (reprinted from Breakefield *et al.*, 1995, with permission)

full-length herpes genomes in which various viral genes have been mutated and replaced by transgenes (Fig. 7A). Amplicons are plasmids bearing only an HSV origin of replication and packaging signal (Fig. 7B). Deletion mutations in viral genes maximize space for transgenes and reduce the chance of recombination or mutational reversion to wild type. For packaging in the HSV virion, it is necessary to retain packaging signals, DNA origin(s) of replication, and structural components of the viral particle and to maintain a genome size within 8 kb of the normal 152 kb HSV1 genome. For recombinant virus vectors, these functions are encoded in the vector itself; for amplicon vectors, they are supplied by an HSV1 helper virus.

Viral genes are classified as nonessential or essential. The nonessential genes, over 40 in number, are not required for growth of the virus in permissive cells; *e.g.*, Vero cells in culture (57). In four regions of the viral genome, the nonessential genes occur in tandem, thus allowing insertion of up to 10 kb of transgene sequence at four different sites. Mutations in some of the genes needed for viral DNA replication render the virus replication-competent only in dividing cells that can supply a complementary cellular function in trans. Essential genes are needed for viral propagation in any type of cell. Many essential gene products can be provided in trans by transfecting packaging cells with the essential viral gene(s). Vectors defective in essential genes are replication-defective in all cells except those transfected with the missing viral gene(s). Newer vectors contain mutations in multiple toxic genes—*e.g.*, ICP4-minus and a mutant form of VP16 (171); ICP4-minus, ICP27-minus, vhs-minus, and RR-minus (179); and gamma 34.5-minus and RR-minus (88, 112).

Recombinant Vectors

Recombinant virus vectors are being developed for two main purposes, stable gene delivery to neurons and gene therapy for brain tumors. For gene delivery to neurons, the key features are low toxicity, entrance into latency, and long-term gene expression. Mutations in multiple viral genes can be used to virtually eliminate the toxicity of HSV vectors, although many of these mutations also reduce virus titers. It is also possible that infection with the vector could lead to reactivation of wild-type virus in neurons harboring latent HSV1. Theoretically, antiherpetic drugs which block viral replication could reduce the toxicity of such wild-type virus without interfering with gene delivery by replication-defective vectors. Other factors can promote entrance into and maintenance of latency in neurons: NGF (123, 175), certain isoforms of Oct2 (99), and low multiplicity of infection (MOI). Still, it is unclear which types of neurons and whether any glia harbor the virus in latency. Recent studies on HSV infection in the CNS and in sensory neurons indicate that neurons maintain multiple copies of the HSV1 genome in a latent state (131). Maintaining transgene expression from latent viral DNA in neurons is difficult, although transgene expression for at least three months has been noted with modified LAT promoters (39, 57, 177) and the neuronal specific enolase promoter (7). Gene expression in latency may be limited by the tightly packaged configuration of the viral DNA in this state, as well as the absence of appropriate transactivating factors.

For gene therapy of brain tumors, some viral toxicity can be tolerated, and transient transgene expression can be effective. Investigators have taken advantage of replication-conditional vectors which selectively propagate in, and thereby kill, dividing tumor cells but are replication-defective in neurons and other postmitotic cells (12). Toxicity to tumor cells can be increased by incorporating transgenes with antioncogenic activity into the vectors. For example, the viral tk gene can convert nucleoside analogues, like ganciclovir, to toxic nucleotide analogues which disrupt DNA replication, kill dividing cells, and block further virus replication. Toxicity to normal cells can be decreased by mutating nonessential toxic or neurovirulent viral genes.

Recombinant virus vectors are typically generated by homologous recombination in a two-step process. First, a portion of the viral genome, cloned in a plasmid, is modified by deletion replacements. Most of the viral gene is deleted and replaced by transgene sequence, leaving at least 500 bp of viral sequence on either side of the transgene. Second, this plasmid is transfected into permissive cells which are then either transfected with infectious virus DNA or infected with virus. Homologous recombination occurs between the viral sequences in the plasmid and the corresponding locus in the viral genome such that some proportion of the virus progeny (typically 1/1000) will be recombinants. The progeny can then be

screened for these recombinants in several ways: by selecting for loss or restoration of tk activity through propagation in acyclovir or HAT medium, respectively (134); by histochemical staining for loss or gain of a marker gene—*e.g.*, lacZ (69); for growth following rescue of an essential viral gene linked to a transgene ("marker rescue") (38), or by in situ hybridization of infected cells with transgene sequences (71). Recent cloning of infectious viral DNA into a set of cosmids (33) and introduction of lox sequences (51), which allow recombination in vitro, should simplify generation of recombinant virus vectors in the future.

HSV Amplicon Vectors

HSV amplicon vectors were initially developed by Spaete and Frenkel (153) to shuttle vectors between mammalian and bacterial cells. The amplicon plasmids contain an *E. coli* origin of DNA replication and a gene for antibiotic resistance to allow propagation and selection in bacteria, as well as an origin of DNA replication (oriS) and packaging signal (pac) from HSV1 to permit their replication and packaging into HSV particles during active HSV1 infection of mammalian cells (70) (Fig. 8). The resulting amplicon vectors typically contain ten tandem copies of a 10 kb plasmid sequence per virion particle and are coproduced with the helper HSV1 virus in a <1:1 ratio (89). The helper virus and amplicon vector are identical particles which cannot be physically separated from each other. Typically, the helper virus is replication-defective and can be a recombinant virus vector in its own right (100). In the future, it may be possible to package amplicon vectors without generating helper virus (53). This would be ideal for long-term nontoxic delivery, as there would be no viral gene expression by infected cells. Amplicon vectors are very easy to generate and promoter activity, at least short-term, may be more reliable provided enhancer elements in the incorporated HSV1 sequences can be minimized. These amplicon concentrates can apparently exist in a "free" state in the cell nucleus and are stable for weeks to months, at least in nondividing cells. They have been used for gene delivery to a number of cell types, including neurons in vivo, and shown to produce functional changes (43, 46, 92). Amplicon vectors should prove useful for gene therapy of brain tumors, as they can potentially be generated in

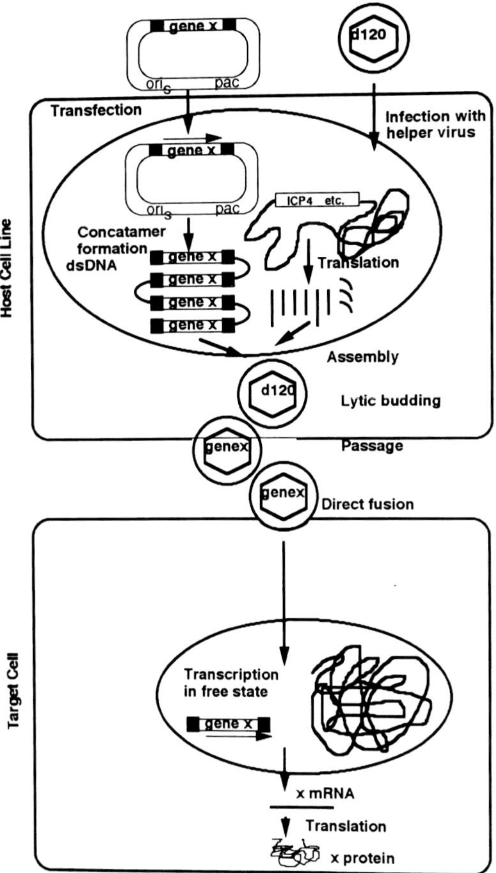

Figure 8. Generation of HSV amplicon vectors. The host cell line contains an HSV1 immediate-early gene essential for viral replication, typically the IE3 gene encoding ICP4. Amplicon plasmids containing a HSV origin of DNA replication (Oris) and packaging signal (pac), as well as the transgene (gen x), are transfected into the host cells with subsequent infection with a mutant HSV helper virus, which contains a deletion in the same immediate-early gene, e.g. d120 (DeLuca *et al.* 1985). The plasmid replicates as a rolling circle, and a concatenate of the amplicon plasmid is packaged into virions in parallel with helper virus particles. Lytic budding occurs and serial passages are performed to increase viral titers and the ratio of amplicon vectors to helper virus.

vivo and coupled to a recombinant (helper) virus vector, such that replication of the virus depends on an essential function encoded by the amplicon.

Other Virus Vectors

A number of other virus vectors are being developed to expand the range of cell targets and the potential uses for gene delivery. In particular, it would be helpful to have vectors that were maintained as extrachromosomal nuclear elements (episomes) in dividing and nondividing cells and others that could replicate and express genes in the cytoplasm without having to enter the cell nucleus. An episomal vector which can be maintained in dividing cells has been derived from Epstein-Barr virus (EBV) (67, 182). This human herpes virus has a trophism for B lymphocytes and pharyngeal epithelial cells. This limited host cell range could prove useful in targeting delivery to lymphoid and epithclial cells. Its 172 kb genome is maintained in a latent state as a circular DNA element which replicates in cycle with proliferating lymphoid cells (172). The EBV-encoded protein, EBNA-1, is a DNA binding protein which, together with cellular factors, initiates EBV DNA replication at EBV oriP sequences. The oriP, which contains multiple EBNA-1 binding sites, functions not only as an origin of DNA replication, but also as a transcriptional enhancer and chromosomal retention factor.

Autonomously replicating DNA vectors can be generated by incorporating the EBNA-1 gene and oriP into plasmids, usually with a drug resistance gene to select for retention of the plasmid over successive cell generations (42, 182). Such vectors can be transfected into a number of different cell types and can carry up to 330 kb of foreign DNA. An EBV vector-expressing antisense RNA for IGF1 appeared to change the phenotype of rat glioblastoma cells, thereby enhancing immune recognition of tumor antigens (164). It may also be possible to achieve autonomous, episomal replication of vectors using mammalian origins of DNA replication; these, however, are not well defined and usually cover large zones (>10 kb) of DNA sequence (22). Given the size limitation of most vectors it would be worthwhile to test smaller elements with some replication potential—*e.g.*, a 4.8-kb sequence downstream of the amplifiable dihydrofolate reductase gene in CHO cells (24, 186); "ors" sequences isolated as DNA "bubbles" in S phase (102); and a 3.5-kb domain 5′ to the amplifiable c-myc proto-oncogene (106).

Given the difficulties in transit of vectors from the plasma membrane to the cell nucleus, it is also useful to have vectors which can express genes in the cytoplasm. Both DNA (vaccinia) and RNA (Sindbis) vectors with this ability have been described. Vaccinia is a dsDNA pox virus which is enveloped and enters cells by direct membrane fusion. The 191 kb genome has been sequenced and contains terminal ITRs and over 200 open reading frames (ORFs), most of unknown function. The transcriptional machinery is packaged in the virus core and includes DNA-dependent RNA polymerase, transcription factors, RNA capping and methylating enzymes, termination factor, and poly (A) polymerase (114). Expression of transgenes via vaccinia vectors is usually short-term and must be under the control of vaccinia promoters. Replicative infection can be toxic to cells, but highly attenuated vectors with deletions in 18 ORFs have been developed that allow cell survival (95). Typically high level gene expression can be achieved with these vectors. Sindbis virus is a ssRNA virus containing sense RNA (12 kb) that is capped and polyadenylated (128). It enters the cell by endocytosis and can be translated directly as a sense message, or replicated through an antisense intermediate to yield amplification of the sense message. These vectors can give transient high-level expression, but can also be toxic to cells.

SYNTHETIC VECTORS

The inherited toxicity of virus vectors has prompted development of synthetic vectors. Synthetic vectors have a combination of physiochemical properties and molecular genetic features that facilitate packaging of the DNA, delivery into the cytoplasm, usually into the cell nucleus, and transgene expression. Although these synthetic vectors are currently less stable and less efficient at gene delivery than most virus vectors, major advances in this field can be expected in the near future. Two basic modes of DNA packaging have been used—molecular conjugates and liposomes. Molecular conjugates are DNA (negatively charged) condensed through electrostatic, noncovalent interaction with polycationic amines, usually poly (L) lysine (positive charged). Liposomes are composed of a variety of different lipids which spontaneously form vesicles of variable size and encapsulate the DNA with varying efficiency (149, 168). It is difficult to package DNA in anionic liposomes, but cationic liposomes can achieve 100% encapsulation. Recently Dr. Leaf

Huang and colleagues combined anionic and cationic lipids with DNA-polylysine conjugates to produce stable particles the size of virions (80 nm in diameter) (52). Other molecules can be bound to the conjugates or the liposomes to target them to specific cells and to promote their cellular entry. Typical targeting molecules are ligands for cell surface receptors, such as transferrin, which binds to the transferrin receptor prevalent on hematopoietic and proliferative cells (154); antibodies to proteins on the cell membrane, which allow some specificity for targeting (185); or virion components, such as inactivated adenovirus particles or capsid proteins (109). Inclusion of viral proteins into conjugates or liposomes, however, potentially increases their antigenicity; the resultant host immune response can inhibit gene delivery and evoke toxic inflammatory responses.

Liposomes deliver genes directly into the cytoplasm by fusing with the cell membrane. Liposomes can be made fusigenic at neutral pH by virtue of their lipid composition (74) or by the incorporation of fusigenic proteins from viruses. A number of enveloped viruses, including influenza virus (Sendai virus), hemagglutinating virus of Japan (HVJ), and HIV, have envelope proteins that change conformation upon binding to the cell membrane. This exposes a hydrophobic domain in the virion that mediates fusion of the viral envelope and the host cell membrane (40, 74, 98). Liposomes incorporating such viral proteins are termed "virosomes." More typically, synthetic vectors are taken up by receptor-mediated endocytosis. This is a relatively efficient uptake process, but the DNA then becomes trapped in endosomes where it can be degraded through the lysosomal pathway. Virus capsid proteins, which are fusigenic at the acidic pH of the endosomes, can be incorporated into vectors to promote the release of vector DNA into the cytoplasm. These include the vesicular stomatitis virus glycoprotein (VSV-G) (74), the hemagglutinin peptide of HVJ (170), and the adenovirus penton protein (64).

Transfer of DNA from the cytoplasm to the nucleus remains an inefficient process. Modifications attempting to improve transfer, such as inclusion of proteins like the HIV matrix protein that contain nuclear localization signals (157), and incorporation of high mobility group proteins normally associated with nuclear DNA, have had limited benefit. As with certain viruses, it is also possible to achieve cytoplasmic expression of transgenes with synthetic vectors. For example, "T7-T7" vectors use the phage T7 promoter to drive expression of both the gene encoding the phage RNA polymerase and the transgene (10, 97). Such vectors need to be primed with RNA polymerase but then are self-sustaining, with the caveat that overexpression of T7 RNA polymerase can be toxic to some cells. The necessity for capping of mRNA is avoided by including sequences for internal ribosomal entry prior to the AUG codon for translation initiation. For vectors that are transported into the nucleus, it is possible to include sequences—*e.g.*, ITRs and Rep from AAV (56), or lox sequences, and the gene for CRE recombinase (143)—that will promote integration into the cellular genome. The AAV ITRs can also stabilize DNA as an extrachromosomal element by forming hairpin structures at the ends which render the DNA resistant to exonucleases (119). Vectors can also contain viral elements—*e.g.*, EBV oriP or EBNA-1 or mammalian origins of replication (see above) that will allow them to replicate along with the host cell genome. Other elements—*e.g.*, NTS from the 5′ flanking end of mammalian rRNA genes (68) or sequences near the dihydrofolate reductase (24) and N-myc genes (144)—can promote amplification of DNA elements within the nucleus.

MODES OF DELIVERY

Principles of Vector Delivery

The choice of method of targeting genes to treat neurological diseases must consider the specific anatomical defects of the disease. The affected region in the nervous system can be localized, as in the substantia nigra and striatum in Parkinson's disease, or global, as in lysosomal storage disorders or infiltrative brain tumors. Localized disorders may prove well suited for viral gene delivery via stereotactic injection. The postmitotic and vulnerable state of neurons in the brain requires that toxicity be avoided while controlled transgene delivery is achieved. The extent of gene delivery depends on the titer and stability of the vector, its diffusibility through the parenchyma, and the efficiency with which it infects different cell types. The parenchymal injury by the vector depends on its inherent toxicity, the presence and acti-

vation of other viruses, the immunogenicity of the vector and encoded proteins, and the volume of injection. Only a few microliters can be injected in rodent brain without causing injury. Convection-enhanced infusion of macromolecules can achieve high concentrations of compounds with a more uniform distribution in white matter and gray matter; this technique may prove useful for gene transfer when more global gene delivery is needed.

Viral vectors have been explored most extensively as agents of gene delivery to the nervous system because of the high titers and efficient infectivity that can be achicved, especially with adenovirus and herpes vectors. Different vectors have relative advantages and disadvantages. Adenovirus vectors can be isolated at titers higher than those of other viral vectors and appear to have some selectivity for astrocytes in the CNS (116). They can sustain expression of transgenes for months, although immunogenicity caused by expression of viral antigens by infected cells limits long-term expression and causes some toxicity. HSV vectors can also be produced at high titers and have a preference for infecting neurons in the CNS (116). High transgene expression can be obtained, but its duration in the CNS with current vectors is limited to less than a few months except in a few neurons. Gene delivery is more efficient and stable in peripheral sensory neurons. AAV vectors can potentially integrate into the host cell genome and provide long-term expression, but they are currently limited by low titers and small transgene capacity. Retrovirus vectors are relatively inefficient at direct gene delivery in the postnatal brain because of their low titers. their instability, and the paucity of dividing cells in normal brain. Relatively efficient gene delivery to experimental brain tumors can be achieved, however, by grafting retrovirus packaging lines into the tumor mass (32, 148). In immunocompetent animals, retrovirus is released over an extended period (one to two weeks) until the packaging cells are rejected. In logarithmically growing brain tumors, a transgene can be delivered to up to 50% of tumor cells (130, 161) by dircct infection and subsequent transmission to tumor cell progeny. A new generation of hybrid retrovirus vectors, incorporating vesicular somatitis virus envelope protein for increased virion stability and HIV matrix and associated proteins for gene delivery to postmitotic cells, may provide a means of transgene integration into neurons.

Methods of Disseminated Delivery

Three methods have been used to disseminate viral vectors through large volumes of brain in rodents: on-site vector propagation, vascular delivery, and intrathecal delivery (Fig. 9).

On-Site Vector Propagation

Limited propagation of vectors within brain tumors has been achieved with both retrovirus vectors and herpes vectors and can potentially be achieved with most other vectors. Retrovirus vectors can be generated on site by grafting of packaging cells or by injection of packaging cells infected with wild-type retrovirus. In the latter case, tumor cells infected with both retrovirus vector and wild-type, replication-competent virus become packaging cells for retrovirus vectors in their own right (159). Replication-competent retrovirus vectors, with a limited transgene capacity, which can propagate by themselves in dividing cells, have also been

developed (158). In a similar manner, AAV vectors could be generated in mitotic, or postmitotic, cells by co-infection with AAV and adenovirus or herpes virus. Cells infected with adenovirus vectors lacking the essential E1A gene can generate more vectors following cotransfection with a molecular conjugate encoding the E1A gene (58). Both amplicon and recombinant virus herpes vectors can also be propaged in vivo. Recombinant vectors, which are replication-compromised, for example, by defects in the immediate early ICPO gene, can produce a "smoldering" infection in the brain without apparent compromise of animal health for some time (73). Mutations in some of the viral genes needed for DNA synthesis—*e.g.*, UTPase, TK, and RR—render the virus replication competent only in dividing cells. Thus, in experimental brain tumors, the virus propagates selectively in dividing tumor cells, killing them as it spreads from the site of inoculation along infiltrating strands of tumor while sparing normal brain tissue (15). The on-site generation of

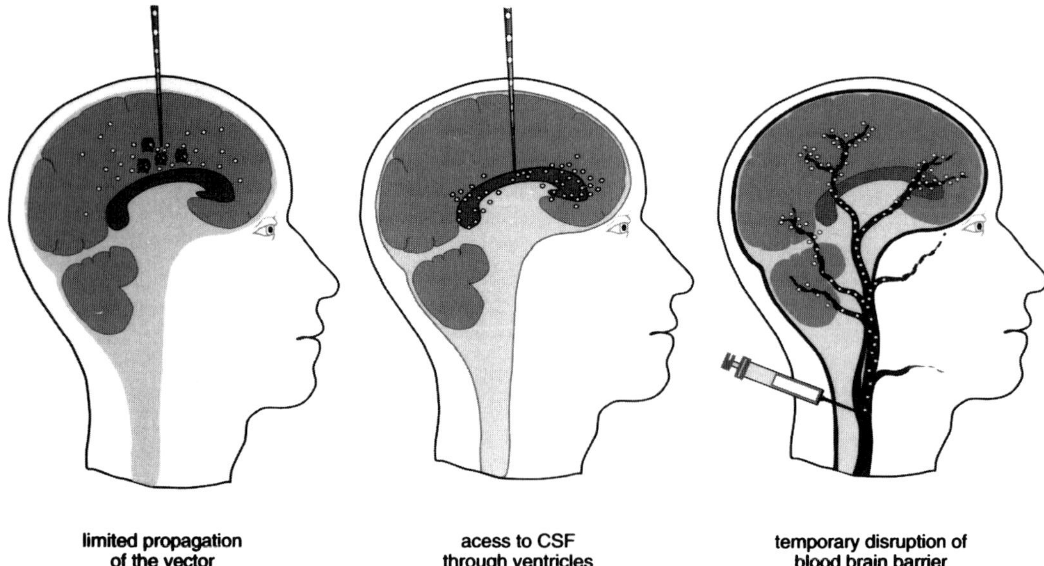

Figure 9.   Disseminated gene delivery to the brain. Stable, high-titer vectors, such as HSV1, can theoretically be delivered to brain tumors through three routes (from left to right). (*A*) Replication-conditional vectors injected into the tumor spread out to infiltrating tumor cells by on-site propagation in dividing tumor cells, diffusion and secondary infection. (*B*) Vectors injected into the ventricles spread throughout the CSF and can reach tumor cells throughout this space. In some regions the virus can pass across into the brain parenchyma. (*C*) Virus injected into the carotid artery in combination with pharmacologic agents, such as bradykinin, or with osmotic disruption, which temporarily increase access across the blood vessels, can reach tumor cells selectively because the neovasculature in the tumor has a weaker blood-tumor barrier, as compared with the blood-brain barrier in normal brain (reprinted from Breakefield *et al.*, with permission)

amplicon vectors in the brain should also be possible through coupling to a replication-conditional helper virus—*e.g.*, in the piggyback system. Clearly, unchecked virus propagation in brain could be toxic because of viral functions and the immune response to the infection, but vector replication can be blocked with antiherpetic drugs if necessary.

Transarterial Delivery

By virtue of their high titers and stability, adenovirus and HSV can be delivered across the blood-brain barrier in conjunction with temporary disruption by osmotic shock or pharmacologic agents. Thousands of normal neural cells, both astrocytes and neurons, are transfected in the ipsilateral hemisphere following injection into the carotid artery during osmotic disruption (116). When an experimental tumor is present intracranially, the bulk of gene delivery is to the tumor bed (121). Pharmacologic agents, such as bradykinin and RMP-7, which increase access across the blood-brain barrier (77, 78) yield significant and selective gene delivery by virus vectors to tumors, with very little or no access to normal brain (129). Access to brain tumors is facilitated by neovasculature which has a less complete blood-brain barrier. In fact, intra-arterial vector delivery during osmotic or pharmacologic barrier modification preferentially yields gene delivery to the periphery of the tumors, which are regions of the most active neovascularization (121, 129). How these large viral particles, 50–100 nm in diameter, cross the blood vessel endothelium is unclear. Presumably, they pass between endothelial cells, although in the case of replication-conditional herpes vectors, they may propagate in dividing endothelial cells, thereby killing them and releasing virus to the surrounding tissue.

Intrathecal Delivery

Virus vectors can also access neural cells through the CSF. Adenovirus, herpes virus, and retrovirus packaging cells have been injected into the lateral ventricles or cisterna magna of rodents. Adenovirus and herpes virus spread rapidly throughout the intrathecal space by CSF flow and infects ependymal cells throughout the brain (9, 36, 88). In the case of HSV vectors, there is also uptake into neuronal processes extending near the ventricles. Intracisternal injection of retrovirus packaging cells and herpes

vectors can also infect glioma cells which have spread throughout the subarachnoid space. In the case of replication-conditional HSV vectors, intraventricular delivery is more toxic than intravascular or intraparenchymal delivery, possibly because of damage to the ependyma and/or the inflammatory immune response to the virus.

CONCLUSION AND FUTURE DIRECTION

Gene therapy, although having almost limitless potential for the amelioration of disease, will require another generation of scientific study before it becomes a major component of clinical care. Initial clinical trials have reported discouraging results in treating cystic fibrosis, muscular dystrophy, and hypercholesteremia (49, 65, 86, 107). The exuberance with which the advocates of gene therapy have projected cures has been tempered by the reality of the infancy of this technology. Fundamental issues of gene delivery and expression need to be addressed before viral vectors can be used effectively for the treatment of diseases at the molecular level.

The characteristics that make a vector highly desirable for gene therapy are the same for any vector system although the priorities may vary with the application: 1) the vector should contain the transgene(s) of interest and be produced in pure stock at high titers; 2) the vector should be highly selective and efficient for gene delivery to target cells; 3) the expression of the transgene should be appropriate to achieve disease correction in a tissue-specific regulatable and/or sustained manner; 4) if desirable, the transgenes should be stably retained by cells and chromosomal integration should be site-specific; and 5) vectors and transgenes should be resistant to immunologic rejection by the host to reduce toxicity and allow repeated treatments.

Although these goals are within reach for some of the current vectors, each component requires critical evaluation and comparison with other methods. Perhaps the ultimate solution will require combinations of the useful components of various viral systems. Adenovirus-mediated gene delivery has produced efficient gene expression, and the development of third-generation vectors with disruption of additional viral genes may permit longer transgene expression (180). With tissue-engineering techniques and immunomodulation, it may be possible to prevent immune rejection of vectors by hosts that recognize them as foreign agents and thus allow repeated treatment (60, 180, 181). Herpes vectors are also efficient for gene delivery to the nervous system and have the added characteristics of neuronal tropism and latency. The development of multiple deletion mutants should reduce the toxicity of these vectors and alleviate safety concerns about the risk of reversion to wild-type (112). Alteration of retroviral env proteins to achieve cell selectivity based on receptor recognition can be incorporated into other vectors and should allow targeted gene expression along with the use of tissue-specific promoters and drug-inducible promoters to allow greater control of gene expression. Integration of transgenes into postmitotic cells may be achieved using HIV components (157). The site-specific integration by adenoassociated virus is especially desirable as it would prevent cis activation of genomic sequences and site-specific variation in viral promoter activity. Attempts at incorporating human immunodeficiency virus components into retrovirus vectors have shown that cellular transcription factors coupled to the preintegration complex may also allow site-specific integration of transgene sequences. As another means of achieving long-term, tissue-specific gene expression, mammalian artificial chromosome vectors are being developed that can carry large pieces of DNA and replicate and segregate as independent artificial chromosomes in dividing cells (21, 76). Ultimately, the successful clinical application of gene transfer techniques will rely on the convergence of vector technologies, as well as a deeper understanding of the cell biology of gene delivery and the immunology of viral infection.

REFERENCES

1. Ace, C. I., McKee, T. A., Ryan, J. M., *et al.* Construction and characterization of a herpes simplex virus type 1 mutant unable to transinduce immediate-early gene expression. J. Virol. *63:*2260–2269, 1989.
2. Adam, M. A., Ramesh, N., Miller, A. D., and Osborne, W. R. Internal initiation of translation in retroviral vectors carrying picronavirus 5′ nontranslated regions. J. Virol. *65:*4985–4990, 1991.
3. Akli, S., Caillaud, C., Vigne, E., *et al.* Transfer of a foreign gene into the brain using adenovirus vectors. Nat. Genet. *3:*224–228, 1993.
4. Albritton, L. M., Tseng, I., Scaddan, D., and Cunning-ham, J. M. A putative murine ecotropic retrovirus receptor gene encodes a multiple membrane-spanning protein and confers susceptibility to virus infection. Cell *37:*659–666, 1989.
5. Alexander, I. E., Russell, D. W., and Miller, A. D. DNA-damaging agents greatly increase the transduction of nondividing cells by adeno-associated virus vectors. J. Virol. *68:*8282–8287, 1994.
6. Ali, M., Lemoine, N. R., and Ring, C. J. A. The use of DNA viruses as vectors for gene therapy. Gene Ther. *1:*367–384, 1994.
7. Andersen, J. K., Barber, D. A., Meaney, C. A., and Breakefield, X. O. Gene transfer into mammalian CNS using herpes virus vectors: long-term expression of bacterial lacZ in neurons using the neuron-specific enolase promoter. Hum. Gene Ther. *3:*487–499, 1992.
8. Andrei, G., Snoeck, R., and De Clercq, E. Susceptibilities of several drug-resistant herpes simplex virus type 1 strains to alternative antiviral compounds. Antimicrob. Agents Chemother. *39:*1632–1635, 1995.
9. Bajocchi, G., Feldman, S. H., Crystal, R. G., and Mastrangeli, A. Direct in vivo gene transfer to ependymal cells in the central nervous system using recombinant adenovirus vectors. Nat. Genet. *3:*229–234, 1993.
10. Baringer, J. R., and Pisani, P. Herpes simplex virus genomes in human nervous system tissue analyzed by polymerase chain reaction. Ann. Neurol. *36:* 823–829, 1994.
11. Bartlett, J. S., Quattrocchi, K. B., and Samulski, R. J. The development of adeno-associated virus as a vector for cancer gene therapy. In: *The Internet Book of Gene Therapy: Cancer Therapeutics,* edited by R. E. Sobol, and K. J. Scanlon, pp. 27–39, Appleton and Large, Stamford, CT, 1995.
12. Bolovan, C. A., Sawtell, N. M., and Thompson, R. L. ICP34.5 mutants of herpes simplex virus type 1 strain 17syn+ are attenuated for neurovirulence in mice and for replication in confluent primary mouse embryo cell cultures. J. Virol. *68:*48–55, 1994.
13. Bottger, M., Vogel, F., Platzer, M., Kiessling, U., Grade, K., and Strauss, M. Condensation of vector DNA by the chromosomal protein HMG1 results in efficient transfection. Biochem. Biophys. Acta *950:* 221–228, 1988.
14. Boviatsis, E. J., Chase, M., Wei, M. X., *et al.* Gene transfer into experimental brain tumors mediated by adenovirus, herpes simples virus (HSV), and retrovirus vectors. Hum. Gene Ther. *5:*183–191, 1994a.
15. Boviatsis, E. J., Scharf, J. M., Chase, M., Harrington, K., and Breakefield, X. O., Chiocca, E. A. Antitumor activity and reporter gene transfer into rat brain neoplasms inoculated with herpes simplex virus vectors defective in thymidine kinase or ribonucleotide reductase. Gene Ther. *1:*323–331, 1994b.
16. Boyce, F. M., and Bucher, N. L. R. Baculovirus-mediated gene transfer into mammalian cells. Proc. Natl. Acad. Sci. U.S.A., in press.
17. Breakefield, X. O., Kramm, C. M., Chiocca, E. A., and Pechan, P. A. Herpes simplex virus vectors for tumor therapy. In: *The Internet Book of Gene Therapy: Cancer Therapeutics,* edited by R. E. Sobol

and K. J. Scanlon, pp. 41–56, Appleton and Large, Stamford, CT, 1995.

18. Breakefield, X. O., and DeLuca, N. A. Herpes simplex virus for gene delivery to neurons. New Biol. *3:*203–218, 1991.

19. Bredenbeek, P. J., Frolov, I., Rice, C. M., and Schlesinger, S. Sindbis virus expression vectors: packaging of RNA replicons by using defective helper RNAs. J. Virol. *67:*6439–6446, 1993.

20. Brenner, M., Kisseberth, W. C., Su, Y., Besnard, F., and Messing, A. GFAP promoter directs astrocyte-specific expression in transgenic mice. J. Neurosci. *14:*1030–1037, 1994.

21. Brown, W. R. A. Mammalian artificial chromosomes. Curr. Opin. Genet. Dev. *2:*479–486, 1992.

22. Burnhans, W. C., and Huberman, J. A. DNA replication origins in animal cells: a question of context. Science *263:*639–640, 1994.

23. Burns, J. C., Friedmann, T., Driever, W., *et al.* Vesicular stomatitis virus G glycoprotein pseudotyped retroviral vectors: concentration to very high titer and efficient gene transfer into mammalian and nonmammalian cells. Proc. Natl. Acad. Sci. U.S.A. *90:*8033–8037, 1993.

24. Caddle, M. S., and Calos, M. P. Analysis of the autonomous replication behavior in human cells of the dihydrofolate reductase putative chromosomal origin of replication. Nucleic Acids Res. *20:*5971–5978, 1992.

25. Chang, P. L. (ed.). *Somatic Gene Therapy.* CRC Press, 1995.

26. Chen, S. H., Shine, H. D., Goodman, J. C., Grossman, R. G., and Woo, S. L. Gene therapy for brain tumors: regression of experimental gliomas by adenovirus-mediated gene transfer in vivo. Proc. Natl. Acad. Sci. U.S.A. *91:*3054–3057, 1994.

27. Chou, J., Kern, E. R., Whitley, R. J., *et al.* Mapping of herpes simplex virus-I neurovirulence to gamma 34.5, a gene nonessential for growth in culture. Science *250:*1262–1266, 1990.

28. Coen, D. M., Kosz-Vnenchak, M., Jacobsen, J. G., *et al.* Thymidine kinase-negative herpes simplex virus mutants establish latency in mouse trigeminal ganglia but do not reactivate. Proc. Natl. Acad. Sci. U.S.A. *86:*4736–4740, 1989.

29. Connors, T. A. The choice of prodrugs for gene directed enzyme prodrug therapy of cancer. Gene Ther. *2:*702–709, 1995.

30. Corey, L., and Spear, P. G. Infections with herpes simplex viruses. N. Engl. J. Med. *314:*749–757, 1986.

31. Cornetta, K., Moen, R. C., Culver, K., *et al.* Amphotropic murine leukemia retrovirus is not an acute pathogen for primates. Hum. Gene Ther. *1:*15–30, 1990.

32. Culver, K. W., Ram, X., Waebridge, S., Ishii, H., Oldfield, E. H., and Blaese, R. M. In vivo gene transfer with retroviral vector-producer cells for treatment of experimental brain tumors. Science *256:*1550–1552, 1992.

33. Cunningham, C., and Davison, A. J. A cosmid-based system for constructing mutants of herpes simplex virus type 1. Virology *197:*116–124, 1993.

34. Dai, Y., Roman, M., Naviaux, R. K., and Verma, I. M. Gene therapy via primary myoblasts: long-term expression of factor IX protein following transplantation in vivo. Proc. Natl. Acad. Sci. U.S.A. *89:*10892–10895, 1992.

35. Danos, O., and Mulligan, R. C. Safe and efficient generation of recombinant retroviruses with amphotropic and ectropic host ranges. Proc. Natl. Acad. Sci. U.S.A. *85:*6460–6464, 1988.

36. Davidson, B. L., Allen, E. D., Kozarsky, K. F., Wilson, J. M., and Roessler, B. J. A model system for in vivo gene transfer into the central nervous system using an adenoviral vector. Nat. Genet. *3:*219–223, 1993.

37. DeLuca, N. A., McCarthy, A., and Schaffer, P. A. Isolation and characterization of deletion mutants of herpes simplex virus type 1 in the genes encoding immediate-early regulatory protein. ICP4. J. Virol. *56:*558–570, 1985.

38. Desai, P., Homa, F. L., Person, S., *et al.* A genetic selection method for transfer of HSV-1 glycoprotein B mutations from the plasmid to the viral genome. Virology *204:*312–322, 1994.

39. Dobson, A. T., Margolis, T. P., Sedarati, F., *et al.* A latent, nonpathogenic HSV-1 derived vector stably expresses beta-galactosidase in mouse neurons. Neuron *5:*353–360, 1990.

40. Doms, R. W. Protein conformational changes in virus-cell fusion. Methods Enzymol. *221:*61–72, 1993.

41. Dranoff, G., Jaffee, E., Lazenby, A., *et al.* Vaccination with irradiated tumor cells engineered to secrete murine granulocyte-macrophage colony-stimulating factor stimulates potent, specific, and long-lasting anti-tumor immunity. Proc. Natl. Acad. Sci. U.S.A. *90:*3539–3543, 1993.

42. DuBridge, R. B., Tang, P., Hsia, H. C., *et al.* Analysis of mutation in human cells by using an Epstein-Barr virus shuttle system. Mol. Cell Biol. *7:*379–387, 1987.

43. During, M. J., Naegele, J. R., O'Malley, K. L., and Geller, A. I. Long-term behavioral recovery in parkinsonian rats by an HSV vector expressing tyrosine hydroxylase. Science *266:*1399–1403, 1994.

44. Etienne-Julan, M., Roux, P., Carillo, S., *et al.* The efficiency of cell targeting by recombinant retroviruses depends on the nature of the receptor and the composition of the artificial cell-virus linker. J. Gen. Virol. *74:*3251–3255, 1992.

45. Ezzeddine, Z. D., Martuza, R. L., Short, M. P., Platika, D., Malick, A., Choi, B., and Breakefield, X. O.: Selective killing of glioma cells in culture and in vivo following retrovirus transfer of the herpes simplex virus thymidine kinase gene. New Biol. *3:*1–7, 1991.

46. Federoff, H. J., Geschwind, M. D., Geller, A. I., and Kessler, J. A. Expression of nerve growth factor in vivo from a defective herpes simplex virus 1 vector prevents effects of axotomy on sympathetic ganglia. Proc. Natl. Acad. Sci. U.S.A. *89:*1636–1640, 1992.

47. Flotte, T. R., Barraza-Ortiz, X., Solow, R., Afione, S. A., Carter, G. J., and Guggino, W. B. An improved system for packaging recombinant adeno-associated virus vectors capable of in vivo transduction. Gene Ther. *2:*29–37, 1995.

48. Friedmann, T. Gene therapy for neurological disorders. Trends Genet. *10:*210–214, 1994.

49. Friedmann, T. Human gene therapy—an immature genie, but certainly out of the bottle. Nature Med. *2:*144–147, 1996.

50. Gage, F. H., and Fisher, L. J. Intracerebral grafting: a tool for the neurobiologist. Neuron *6:*1–12, 1991.

51. Gage, P. J., Sauer, B., Levine, M., *et al.* A cell-free recombination system for site-specific integration of multigenic shuttle plasmids into the herpes simplex virus type 1 genome. J. Virol. *66:*5509–5515, 1992.

52. Gao, X., Jaffurs, D., Robbins, P. D., and Huang, L. A sustained, cytoplasmic transgene expression system delivered by cationic liposomes. Biochem. Biophys. Res. Commun. *200:*1201–1206, 1994.

53. Geller, A., Song, S., Lim, F., *et al.* A helper virus-free packaging system for HSV-1 plasmid vectors that supports efficient gene transfer in the rat brain. Soc. Neurosci. Abst. *20:*Abst 79.18, 1994.

54. Ghattas, I. R., Sanes, J. R., and Majors, J. E. The encephalomyocarditis virus internal ribosome entry site allows efficient coexpression of two genes from a recombinant provirus in cultured cells and in embryos. Mol. Cell Biol. *11:*5848–5859, 1991.

55. Gilboa, E., Eglitis, M. A., Kantoff, P. W., and Anderson, W. F. Transfer and expression of cloned genes using retroviral vectors. Biotechnology *4:*504–512, 1994.

56. Giraud, C., Winocur, E., and Berns, K. I. Site specific integration by adeno-associated virus is directed by a cellular DNA sequence. Proc. Natl. Acad. Sci. U.S.A. *91:*10039–10043, 1994.

57. Glorioso, J. C., Bender, M. A., Goins, W. F., *et al.* Herpes simplex virus as a gene-delivery vector for the central nervous system. In: *Viral Vectors*, pp. 1–23, Academic Press, 1995.

58. Goldsmith, K. T., Curiel, D. T., Engler, J. A., *et al.* Trans complementation of an E1A-deleted adenovirus with codelivered E1A sequences to make recombinant adenoviral producer cells. Hum. Genet. Therap. *5:*1341–1348, 1994.

59. Goldstein, D. J., and Weller, S. K. An ICP6:lacZ insertional mutagen is used to demonstrate that the UL52 gene of herpes simplex virus type 1 is required for virus growth and DNA synthesis. J. Virol. *62:*2970–2977, 1988.

60. Golumbek, P. T., Azhari, R., Jaffee, E. M., *et al.* Controlled release, biodegradable cytokine depots: a new approach in cancer vaccine design. Cancer Res. *53:*5841–5844, 1993.

61. Gossen, M., Bonin, A. L., and Bujard, H. Control of gene activity in higher eukaryotic cells by prokaryotic regulatory elements. Trends Biochem. Sci. *18:*471–475, 1993.

62. Gossen, M., and Bujard, H. Tight control of gene expression in mammalian cells by tetracycline-responsive promoters. Proc. Natl. Acad. Sci. U.S.A. *89:*5547–5551, 1992.

63. Gossen, M., Freundlieb, S., Bender, G., Muller, G., Hillen, W., and Bujard, H. Transcriptional activation by tetracyclines in mammalian cells. Science *268:*1766–1769, 1995.

64. Greber, U. F., Willetts, M., Webster, P., and Helenius, A. Stepwise dismantling of adenovirus 2 during entry into cells. Cell *75:*477–486, 1993.

65. Grossman, M., Rader, D. J., and Muller, D. W. M. Ex vivo gene therapy of familial hypercholesterolaemia. Human Gene Ther. *3:*179–222, 1992.

66. Hamlin, J. L. Mammalian origins of replication. Bioessays *14:*651–659, 1992.

67. Hammerschmidt, W., and Sugden, B. Genetic analysis of immortalizing functions of Epstein-Barr virus in human fl lymphocytes. Nature *340:*393–397, 1989.

68. Hemann, C., Gartner, E., Weidle, U. H., and Grummt, F. High-copy expression vector based on amplification-promoting sequences. DNA Cell Biol. *13:*437–445, 1994.

69. Ho, D. Y., and Mocarski, E. D. Beta-galactosidase as a marker in the peripheral and neural tissues of the herpes simplex virus-infected mouse. Virology *167:*279–283, 1988.

70. Ho, D. Y. Amplicon-based herpes simplex virus vectors. Methods Cell Biol. *43:*191–210, 1994.

71. Homa, F. L., Otal, T. M., Glorioso, J. C., *et al.* Transcriptional control signals of herpes simplex virus type 1 late (gamma 2) gene lie within bases −34 to +124 relative to the 5′ terminus of the mRNA. Mol. Cell. Biol. *6:*3652–3666, 1986.

72. Honess, R. W. Herpes simplex and "the herpes complex": diverse observations and unifying hypothesis. J. Gen. Virol. *65:*2077–2107, 1984.

73. Huang, Q., Vonsattel, J.-P., Schaffer, P. A., Martuza, R. L., Breakefield, X. O., and DiFiglia, M. Introduction of a foreign gene (lacZ of E. Coli) into rat neostriatal neurons using herpes simplex virus mutants: a light and electron microscopic study. Exp. Neurol. *115:*303–316, 1992.

74. Hug, P., and Sleight, R. G. Fusogenic virosomes prepared by partitioning of vesicular stomatitis virus G protein into preformed vesicles. J. Biol. Chem. *269:*4050–4056, 1994.

75. Hunter, W., Rabkin, S., and Martuza, R. Brain tumor therapy using genetically engineered replication-competent virus. In: *Viral Vectors*, pp. 259–274, Academic Press, 1995.

76. Huxley, C. Mammalian artificial chromosomes: a new tool for gene therapy. Gene Ther. *12:*, 1994.

77. Inamura, T., and Black, K. L. Bradykinin selectively opens blood-tumor barrier in experimental brain tumors. J. Cereb. Blood Flow. Metab. *14:*862–870, 1994.

78. Inamura, T., Nomura, T., Bartus, R. T., and Black, K. L. Intracarotid infusion of RMP-7, a bradykinin analog: a method for selective drug delivery to brain tumors. J. Neurosurg. *81:*752–758, 1994.

79. Isacson, O. On neuronal health. Trends Neurosci. *16:*306–308, 1993.

80. Johnson, P. A., and Friedmann, T. Replication-defective recombinant herpes simplex virus vectors. Methods Cell Biol. *43:*211–230, 1994.

81. Jolly, D. Viral vector systems for gene therapy. In: *The Internet Book of Gene Therapy: Cancer Therapeutics*, edited by R. E. Sobol and K. J. Scanlon, pp. 3–16, Appleton and Large, Stamford, CT, 1995.

82. Kaplitt, M. G., Leone, P., Samulski, R. J., Xiao, X., Pfaff, D. W., O'Malley, K. L., and During, M. J. Long-term gene expression and phenotypic correc-

tion using adeno-associated virus vectors in the mammalian brain. Nat. Genet. *8:*148–154, 1994.

83. Kaplitt, M. G., Kwong, A. D., Kleopoulos, S. P., Mobbs, C. V., Rabkin. S. D., and Pfaff, D. W. Preproenkephalin promoter yields region-specific and long-term expression in adult brain after direct in vivo gene transfer via a defective herpes simplex viral vector. Proc. Natl. Acad. Sci. U.S.A. *91:*8979–8983, 1994b.

84. Kaplitt, M. G., and Loewy, A. D. Gene therapy and neuroscience applications. In: *Viral Vectors.* Academic Press, 1995.

85. Kasahara, N., Dozy, A. M., and Kan, Y. W. Tissue-specific targeting of retroviral vectors through ligand-receptor interactions. Science 1373–1376, 1994.

86. Knowles, M. R., Hohneker, K. W., Zhou, Z., *et al.* A controlled study of adenoviral-vector-mediated gene transfer in the nasal epithelium of patients with cystic fibrosis. N. Engl. J. Med. *333:*823–831, 1995.

87. Kotin, R. M., Menninger, J. C., Ward, D. C., *et al.* Mapping and direct visualization of a region-specific viral DNA integration site on chromosome 19q13-qter. Genomics *10:*831–834, 1991.

88. Kramm, C. M., Sena-Esteves, M., Barnett, F. H., *et al.* Gene therapy for brain tumors. Brain Pathol. *5:*345–381, 1995.

89. Kwong, A. D., and Frenkel, N. Biology of herpes simplex virus (HSV) defective viruses and development of the amplicon system. In: *Viral Vectors,* edited by M. G. Kaplitt, and A. D. Loewy, pp. 25–42, Academic Press, 1995.

90. Kwong, A. D., and Frenkel, N. The herpes simplex virus virion host shut off function. J. Virol. *63:* 4834–4839, 1989.

91. Latchman, D. S. Genetic *Manipulation of the Nervous System.* Academic Press, 1996.

92. Lawrence, M. S., Ho, D. Y., Dash, R., and Sapolsky, R. M. Herpes simplex virus vectors overexpressing the glucose transporter gene protect against seizure-induced neuron loss. Proc. Natl. Acad. Sci. U.S.A. *92:*7247–7251, 1995.

93. Le Gal La Salle, G., Robert, J. J., Bernard, S., *et al.* An adenovirus vector for gene transfer into neurons and glia in the brain. Science *259:*988–990, 1993.

94. Lee, M. G., Abina, M. A., Haddada, H., and Perricaudet, M. The constitutive expression of the immunomodulatory gp 19k protein in E1-, E3-adenoviral vectors strongly reduces the host cytotoxic T cell response against the vector. Gene Ther. *2:*356–363, 1995.

95. Lee, S. S., Eisenlohr, L. C., McCue, P. A., Mastrangelo, M. J., and Lattime, E. C. Intravesical gene therapy: in vivo gene transfer using recombinant vaccinia virus vectors. Cancer Res. *54:*3325–3328, 1994.

96. Leib, D. A., and Olivo, P. D. Gene delivery to neurons: is herpes simplex virus the right tool for the job? BioEssays *15:*547–554, 1993.

97. Lieber, A., Andig, W., Sommer, S., *et al.* Stable high-level gene expression in mammalian cells by T7 phage RNA polymerase. Methods Enzymol. *217:* 47–66, 1993.

98. Lifson, J. D. Fusion of human immunodeficiency virus-infected cells with uninfected cells. Methods Enzymol. *221:*3–12, 1993.

99. Lillycrop, K. A., Howard, M. K., Estridge, J. K., *et al.* Inhibition of herpes simplex virus infection by ectopic expression of neuronal spice variants of the Oct-2 transcription factor. Nucleic Acids Res. *22:* 825–830, 1994.

100. Lowenstein, P. R., Fournel, S., Bain, D., *et al.* Simultaneous detection of amplicon and HSV-1 helper encoded proteins reveals that neurons and astrocytoma cells do express amplicon-borne transgenes in the absence of synthesis of virus immediate early proteins. Mol. Brain Res. *30:*169–175, 1995.

101. Lycke, E., Hamark, B., Johansson, M., *et al.* Herpes simplex virus infection of the human sensory neuron. An electron microscopy study. Arch. Virol. *101:*87–104, 1988.

102. Mah, D. C. W., Kijkel, P. A., Todd, A., Klein, V., Price, G. B., and Zannis-Hadjopoulos, M. Ors12, a mammalian autonomously replicating DNA sequence, associates with the nuclear matrix in a cell cycle-dependent manner. J. Cell. Sci. *105:*807–818, 1993.

103. Martuza, R. L., Malick, A., Markert, J. M., *et al.* Experimental therapy of human glioma by means of a genetically engineered virus mutant. Science *252:* 854–856, 1991.

104. Maue, R. A., Kraner, S. D., Goodman, R. H., and Mandel, G. Neuron-specific expression of the rat brain type II sodium channel gene is directed by upstream regulatory elements. Neuron *4:*223–231, 1990.

105. McGeoch, D. J., Dalrymple, M. A., Davison, A. J., *et al.* The complete DNA sequence of the long unique region in the genome of herpes simplex virus type 1. J. Gen. Virol. *69:*1531–1574, 1988.

106. McWhinney, C., and Leffak, M. Autonomous replication of a DNA fragment containing the chromosomal replication origin of the human c-myc gene. Nucleic Acids Res. *18:*1233–1242, 1990.

107. Mendell, J. R., Kissel, J. T., Amato, A. A., *et al.* Myoblast transfer in the treatment of Duchenne's muscular dystrophy. N. Engl. J. Med. *333:*832–838, 1995.

108. Michael, S. I., and Curiel, D. T. Strategies to achieve targeted gene delivery via the receptor-mediated endocytosis pathway. Gene Ther. *1:*223–232, 1994.

109. Michael, S. I., Hong, J. S., Curiel, D. T., and Engler, J. A. Addition of a short peptide ligand to the adenovirus fiber protein. Gene Ther. *2:*660–668, 1995.

110. Miller, A. D. Retrovirus packaging cells. Hum. Gene Ther. *1:*5–14, 1990.

111. Miller, D. B., Edwards, R. M., and Miller, A. D. Cloning of the cellular receptor for amphotropic murine retroviruses reveals homology to that for gibbon ape leukemia virus. Proc. Natl. Acad. Sci. U.S.A. *91:*78, 1994.

112. Mineta, T., Rabkin, S. D., and Martuza, R. L. Attenuated multimutated herpes simplex virus-1 for the treatment of malignant gliomas. Nat. Med. *1:*938, 1995.

113. Miyao, Y., Shimizu, K., Moriuchi, S., *et al.* Selective expression of foreign genes in glioma cells: use of

the mouse myelin basic protein gene promoter to direct toxic gene expression. J. Neurosci. Res. *36:* 472–479, 1993.

114. Moss, B. Vaccinia virus: a tool for research and vaccine development. Science *252:*1662–1667, 1991.

115. Moullier, P., Bohl, D., Heard, J.-M., *et al.* Correction of lysosomal storage in the liver and spleen of MPS VII mice by implantation of genetically modified skin fibroblasts. Nat. Genet. *4:*154–159, 1993.

116. Muldoon, L. L., Nilaver, G., Kroll, R. A., Pagel, M. A., Breakefield, X. O., Chiocca, E. A., Davidson, B. L., Weissleder, R., and Neuwelt, E. A. Comparison of intracerebral inoculation and osmotic blood brain barrier disruption for delivery of adenovirus, herpesvirus and iron oxide particles to normal rat brain. Am. J. Pathol. *147:*1840–1851, 1995.

117. Mulligan, R. C., and Berg, P. Selection for animal cells that express the Escherichia coli gene coding for xanthineguanine phosphoribosyltransferase. Proc. Natl. Acad. Sci. U.S.A. *78:*2072–2076, 1981.

118. Mulligan, R. C. The basic science of gene therapy. Science *260:*926–932, 1993.

119. Muzyczka, N. Use of adeno-associated virus as a general transduction vector for mammalian cells. Curr. Topics Microbiol. Immunol. *158:*97–129, 1992.

120. Neda, H., Wu, C. H., and Wu, G. Y. Chemical modification of an ecotropic murine leukemia virus results in redirection of its target cell specificity. J. Biol. Chem. *266:*14143, 1991.

121. Nilaver, G., Muldoon, L. L., Kroll, R. A., Pagel, M. A., Breakefield, X. O., Davidson, B. L., and Neuwelt, E. Delivery of herpesvirus and adenovirus to nude rat intracerebral tumors following osmotic blood-brain barrier disruption. Proc. Natl. Acad. Sci. U.S.A. *92:*9829–9833.

122. Oh, Y. J., Moffat, M., Wong, S., Ullrey, D., Geller, A. I., and O'Malley, K. L. A herpes simplex virus-1 vector containing the rat tyrosine hydroxylase promoter directs cell type-specific expression of beta-galactosidase in cultured rat peripheral neurons. Mol. Brain Res. *35:*337–236, 1996.

123. Pakzaban, P., Geller, A. I., and Isacson, O. Effect of exogenous nerve growth factor on neurotoxicity of and neuronal gene delivery by a herpes simplex amplicon vector in the rat brain. Hum. Gene Ther. *5:*987–995, 1994.

124. Palmer, T. D., Rosman, G. J., Osborne, W. R., Miller, A. D. Genetically modified skin fibroblasts persist long after transplantation but gradually inactivate introduced genes. Proc. Natl. Acad. Sci. U.S.A. *88:*1330–1334, 1990.

125. Paulus, W., Baur, I., Boyce, F. M., Breakefield, X. O., and Reeves, S. A. Self-contained, tetracycline-regulated retroviral vector system for gene delivery to mammalian cells. J. Virol. *70:*62–67, 1996.

126. Pear, W. S., Nolan, G. P., Scott, M. L., and Baltimore, D. Production of high-titer helper-free retroviruses by transient transfection. Proc. Natl. Acad. Sci. U.S.A. *90:*8392–8396, 1993.

127. Perricaudet, M. Towards the development of a new generation of adenoviral vectors. Intl. Conf. Gene. Ther. CNS Disord. 1995.

128. Piper, R. C., Slot, J. W., Li, G., Stahl, P. D., and James, D. E. Recombinant sindbis virus as an expression system for cell biology. Methods Cell Biol. *43:*55–78, 1994.

129. Rainov, N. G., Zimmer, C., Chase, M., *et al.* Selective uptake of viral and monocrystalline particles delivered intraarterially to experimental brain neoplasms. Hum. Gene Ther. *6:*1543–1552, 1995.

130. Ram, Z., Culver, K. W., Walbridge, S., Blaese, R. M., and Oldfield, E. H. In situ retroviral-mediated gene transfer for the treatment of brain tumors in rats. Cancer Res. *53:*83–88, 1993.

131. Ramakrishnan, R., Levine, M., and Fink, D. J. PCR-based analysis of herpes simplex virus type 1 latency in the rat trigeminal ganglion established with a ribonucleotide reductase-deficient mutant. J. Virol. *68:*7083–7091, 1994.

132. Roe, T., Reynolds, T. C., Yu, G., and Brown, P. O. Integration of murine leukemia virus DNA depends on mitosis. EMBO J. *12:*2099–2108, 1993.

133. Roizman, B., and Batterson, W. Herpes viruses and their replication. In: *Virology*, edited by B. N. Fields, pp. 497–526, New York, Raven Press; 1991.

134. Roizman, B., and Jenkins, F. J. Genetic engineering of novel genomes of large DNA viruses. Science *229:* 1208–1214, 1985.

135. Roizman, B., and Sears, A. E. Herpes simplex viruses and their replication. In: *The Human Herpesviruses*, edited by B. Roizman, R. J. Whitely, and C. Lopez, pp. 11–68, New York, Raven Press, 1993.

136. Rosenfeld, M. A., Siegfried, W., Yoshimura, K., Yoneyama, K., Fukayama, M., Stier, L. E., Paakko, P. K., Gilardi, P., Stratford-Perricaudet, L. D., Perricaudet, M., Jallat, S., Pavirani, A., Lecocq, J.-P., and Crystal, R. G. Adenovirus-mediated transfer of a recombinant alpha1-antitrypsin gene to the lung epithelium in vivo. Science *252:*431–434, 1991.

137. Ross, B. D., Kim, B., and Davidson, B. L. Assessment of ganciclovir toxicity to experimental intracranial gliomas following recombinant adenoviral-mediated transfer of the herpes simplex virus thymidine kinase gene by magnetic resonance imaging and proton magnetic resonance spectroscopy. Clin. Cancer Res. *1:*651–657, 1995.

138. Roux, P., Jeanteaur, P., and Piechaczyk, M. A versatile and potentially general approach to the targeting of specific cell types by retroviruses: application to the infection of human cells by means of major histocompatibility complex class I and class II antigens by mouse ecotropic murine leukemia virus-derived viruses. Proc. Natl. Acad. Sci. U.S.A. *86:* 9079–9083, 1989.

139. Russell, D. W., Miller, A. D., and Alexander, I. E. Adeno-associated virus vectors preferentially transduce cells in S phase. Proc. Natl. Acad. Sci. U.S.A. *91:*8915–8919, 1994.

140. Sadowski, I., Ma, J., Triczenberg, S., and Ptashne, M. GAL4-VP16 is an unusually potent transcriptional activator. Nature –335:563–564, 1988.

141. Samulski, R. J., Chang, L. S., and Shenk, T. Helper-free stocks of recombinant adeno-associated viruses: normal integration does not require viral gene expression. J. Virol. *63:*3822–3828, 1989.

142. Samulski, R. J. Adeno-associated virus: integration at

a specific chromosomal locus. Curr. Opin. Genet. Dev. *3:*74–80, 1993.

143. Sauer, B., and Henderson, N. Site-specific DNA recombination in mammalian cells by the Cre recombinase of bacteriophage P1. Proc. Natl. Acad. Sci. U.S.A. *85:*5166, 1988.

144. Schwab, M., Corvi, R., and Amler, L. N-MYC oncogene amplification: a consequence of genomic instability in human neuroblastoma. Neuroscientist *1:*277–285, 1995.

145. Schwartz, M. L., Katagi, C., Bruce, J., and Schlaepfer, W. W. Brain-specific enhancement of the mouse neurofilament heavy gene promoter in vitro. J. Biol. Chem. *269:*13444–14450, 1994.

146. Sena-Esteves, M., Aghi, M., Pechan, P. A., Kaye, E. M., and Breakefield, X. O. Gene delivery to the nervous system using retroviral vectors. In: *Genetic Manipulation of the Nervous System*, edited by D. Latchman, pp. 149, Academic Press, 1996.

147. Shih, C.-C., Stoye, J. P., and Coffin, J. M. Highly preferred targets for retrovirus integration. Cell *53:* 531–537, 1988.

148. Short, M. P., Chio, B., Lee, J., *et al.* Gene delivery to glioma cells in rat brain by grafting of a retrovirus packaging cell line. J. Neurosci. Res., *127:*427–439, 1990.

149. Singhal, A., and Huang, L. Gene transfer in mammalian cells using liposomes as carriers. In: *Gene Therapeutics: Methods and Applications of Direct Gene Transfer*, edited by J. A. Wolff, pp. 118–142, Birkhauser, Boston, 1994.

150. Smith, F., Jacoby, D., and Breakefield, X. O. Virus vectors for gene delivery to the nervous system. Res. Neurol. Neurosci. *8:*21–34, 1995.

151. Snyder, E. Y., Taylor, R. M., and Wolfe, J. H. Neural progenitor cell engraftment corrects lysosomal storage throughout the MPS VII mouse brain. Nature *374:*367–370, 1995.

152. Sobol, R. E., and Scanlon, K. J. Cancer Therapeutics. In: *The Internet Book of Gene Therapy*. Appleton and Lance, Stamford, CT, 1995.

153. Spaete, R., and Frenkel, N. The herpes virus amplicon: a new encaryotic defective-virus cloning-amplifly-ing vector. Cell *30:*295–304, 1982.

154. Stavridis, J. C., Deliconstantinos, G., Psallidopoulos, M. C., Armenakas, N. A., Hadjiminas, D. J., and Hadmininas, J. Construction of transferrin-coated liposomes for in vivo transport of exogenous DNA to bone marrow erythroblasts in rabbits. Exp. Cell Res. *164:*568–572, 1986.

155. Stevens, J. G., Wagner, E. K., Devi-Rao, G. B., *et al.* RNA complementary to a herpesvirus gene mRNA is prominent in latently infected neurons. Science *253:*1056–1059, 1987.

156. Stevens, J. G. Human herpesviruses: a consideration of the latent state. Microbiol. Rev. *53:*318–332, 1989.

157. Stevenson, M. Portals of entry: uncovering HIV nuclear transport pathways. Trends Cell Biol. *6:*9–15, 1996.

158. Stuhlmann, H., Jaenisch, R., and Mulligan, R. C. Construction and properties of replication-competent murine retroviral vectors encoding methotrexate resistance. Mol. Cell biol. *9:*100–108, 1989.

159. Takamiya, Y., Short, M. P., Ezzeddine, Z. D., Moolten, F. L., Breakefield, X. O., and Martuza, R. L. Gene therapy of malignant brain tumors: a rat glioma line bearing the herpes simplex virus type 1-thymidine kinase gene and wild type retrovirus kills other tumor cells. J. Neurosci. Res. *33:*394–503, 1991.

160. Takamiya, Y., Short, M. P., Ezzeddine, Z. D., Moolten, F. L., Breakefield, X. O., and Martuza, R. L. Gene therapy of malignant brain tumors: a rat glioma line bearing the herpes simplex virus type 1-thymidine kinase gene and wild type retrovirus kills other tumor cells. J. Neurosci. Res. *33:*493–503, 1992.

161. Tamiya, T., Wei, M. X., Chase, M., *et al.* Transgene inheritance and retroviral infection contribute to the efficiency of gene expression in solid tumors inoculated with retroviral vector producer cells. Gene Ther. *2:*531–538, 1995.

162. Tenenbaum, L., Darling, J. L., and Hooghe-Peters, E. Adeno-associated virus (AAV) as a vector for gene transfer into glial cells of the human central nervous system. Gene Ther. *1:*580, 1994.

163. Torrent, C., Gabus, C., and Darlix, J. L. A small and efficient dimerization/packaging signal of rat VL30 RNA and its use in murine leukemia virus-VL30-derived vectors for gene transfer. J. Virol. *68:*661–667, 1994.

164. Trojan, J., Johnson, T. R., Rudio, S. D., Ilan, J., Tykoolnski, M. L., and Ilen, J. Treatment and prevention of rat glioblastoma by immunogenic C6 cells expression antisense insulin-like growth factor 1 RNA. Science *259:*94–97, 1993.

165. Ugolini, G., Kuyers, H. G., and Strick, P. L. Trans-neuronal transfer of herpes virus from peripheral nerves to cortex and brainstem. Science *243:*89–91, 1989.

166. Varga, M. J., Weibull, C., and Everitt, E. Infectious entry pathway of adenovirus type 2. J. Virol. *65:* 6061–6070, 1991.

167. Vegeto, E., Allan, G. F., Schrader, W. T., *et al.* The mechanism of RU486 antagonism is dependent on the conformation of the carboxy-terminal tail of the human progesterone receptor. Cell *69:*703–713, 1992.

168. Vieweg, J., Boczkowski, D., Roberson, K. M., *et al.* Efficient gene transfer with adeno-associated virus-based plasmids complexed to cationic liposomes for gene therapy of human prostate cancer. Cancer Res. *55:*2366–2372, 1995.

169. Vos, J.-M. H. *Viruses in Human Gene Therapy*. Carolina Academic Press, Durham, NC, 1995.

170. Wagner, E., Plank, C., Zatloukal, K., *et al.* Influenza virus haemagglutinin HA-2 N-terminal fusogenic peptides augment gene transfer by transferrin-polylysine-DNA complexes: towards a synthetic virus-like gene transfer vehicle. Proc. Natl. Acad. Sci. U.S.A. *89:*7934–7938, 1992.

171. Wang, J. J., Friedmann, T., and Johnson, P. A. Differentiation of PC12 cells by infection with an HSV-1 vector expressing nerve growth factor. Gene Ther. *2:*323–335, 1995.

172. Weisz, O. A., and Machamer, C. E. Use of recombinant vaccinia virus vectors for cell biology. Methods Cell Biol. *43:*137–159, 1994.

173. Weitzman, M. D., Wilson, J. M., and Eck, S. L. Adenovirus vectors in cancer gene therapy. In: *The Internet Book of Gene Therapy: Cancer Therapeutics*, edited by R. E. Sobol, and K. J. Scanlon, pp. 17–23, Appleton and Large, Stamford, CT, 1995.

174. Whitley, R. J. Herpes simplex virus. In: *Virology*, edited by B. N. Fields, D. M. Knipe, *et al.*, p. 1843, 2nd ed. New York, Raven Press, 1990.

175. Wilcox, C. L., Smith, R. L., Freed, C. R., and Johnson, E. M., Jr. Nerve growth factor-dependence of herpes simplex virus latency in peripheral sympathetic and sensory neurons in vitro. J. Neurosci. *10:*1268–1275, 1990.

176. Wilson, C., Reitz, M. S., Okayama, H., *et al.* Formation of infectious hybrid virions with gibbon ape leukemia virus and huma T-cell leukemia virus retroviral envelope glycoproteins and the gag and pol proteins of Moloney murine leukemia virus. J. Virol. *63:*2374–2378, 1989.

177. Wolfe, J. H., Deshman, S. L., and Fraser, N. W. Herpes virus vector gene transfer and expression of beta-glucuronidase in the central nervous system of MPS VII mice. Nat. Genet. *1:*379–384, 1992.

178. Wolff, J. A. Methods and applications of direct gene transfer. In:*Gene Therapeutics*. Birkhauser, 1994.

179. Wu, N., Glorioso, J., and DeLuca, N. A. Multiple mutants of HSV as vectors for gene transfer, Abst # 204. 19th International Herpes Virus Conference 1994.

180. Yang, Y., Li, Q., Ertl, H. E., *et al.* Cellular and humoral immune responses to viral antigens create barriers to lung-directed gene therapy with recombinant adenoviruses. J. Virol. *69:*2004–2015, 1995a.

181. Yang, Y., Xiang, Z., Ertl, H. C., *et al.* Upregulation of class I major histocompatibility complex antigens by interferon gamma is necessary for T-cell-mediated elimination of recombinant adenovirus-infected hepatocytes in vivo. Proc. Natl. Acad. Sci. U.S.A. *92:*7257–7261, 1995b.

182. Yates, J. L., Warren, M., and Sugden, B. Stable replication of plasmids derived from Epstein-Barr virus in various mammalian cells. Nature (London) *313:*812–815, 1985.

183. Yee, J.-K., Miyanohara, A., LaPorte, P., *et al.* A general method for the generation of high-titer, pantropic retroviral vectors: highly efficient infection of primary hepatocyte. Proc. Natl. Acad. Sci. U.S.A. *91:*9564–9568, 1994.

184. Yee, J. K., Moores, J. C., Jolly, D. J., *et al.* Gene expression from transcriptionally disabled retroviral vectors. Proc. Natl. Acad. Sci. U.S.A. *84:*5197–5201, 1987.

185. Yoshida, J., and Mizzuno, M. Simple method to prepare cationic multilamellar liposomes for efficient transfection of human interferon-B to human glioma cells. J. Neurooncol. *19:*269–274, 1994.

186. Zannis-Hadjopoulos, M., Nielsen, T. O., Todd, A., and Price, G. B. Autonomous replication in vivo and in vitro of clones spanning the region of the DHFR origin of bidirectional replication. Gene *151:* 273–277, 1994.

PART II

Molecular Neurobiology

Recent Advances in Cell Proliferation: The Cell Cycle—Its Drivers, Engines, and Brakes

PETER B. DIRKS, M.D., JAMES T. RUTKA, M.D., Ph.D.

INTRODUCTION

The past decade has witnessed major advances in understanding the factors controlling cell proliferation. These include identification of cyclins and cyclin-dependent kinases as the molecules regulating cell cycle progression, delineation of the interaction of these molecules with products of tumor suppressor genes in the control of normal and neoplastic cell proliferation, and the discovery of apoptosis. Cyclins and cyclin-dependent kinases govern cell cycle progression. Their activities are regulated by phosphorylation and dephosphorylation. Inactivating mutations of tumor suppressor genes may lead to uncontrolled cell proliferation and tumor formation. Cell number reflects not only the rate of cell division as determined by positive and negative influences on the rate of cell cycling, but also the rate of cell loss. One means of cell loss is apoptosis or programmed cell death. Several of the biochemical pathways subserving apoptosis have now been well defined. Imbalances in these apoptotic pathways may contribute to the development and progression of cancer.

Just as prior study of cell kinetics and the biochemistry of cell proliferation led to understanding of tumor growth and the design of antineoplastic agents, recent analysis of the cell cycle with the techniques of molecular biology has identified the molecular mechanisms of tumorigenesis and new strategies for reducing tumor cell proliferation. These new strategies specifically target the cell cycle proteins driving neoplastic proliferation. In a different setting, molecular manipulation of the cell cycle might enhance the proliferative potential of normal tissues in repair or replacement of injured tissues.

In this chapter, current knowledge of the cell cycle and its distinct phases is described. The mechanisms by which the cell cycle is controlled by cyclins, cyclin-dependent kinases, and cyclin-dependent kinase inhibitors are detailed. The impact of growth factors on cell signalling and cell cycle pathways is discussed. Finally, the role of tumor suppressor genes in controlling cell proliferation and the process of programmed cell death is reviewed.

THE CELL CYCLE

A proliferating cell passes through an orderly sequence of phases which comprise the cell cycle (Fig. 1). Following mitosis, a cell enters an interphase consisting of three parts. Differentiated cells exit the cell cycle after mitosis to enter a state of quiescence called G0. The proliferating cell progresses into the first phase of interphase called gap 1 (G1), which is characterized by cell growth and synthesis of components necessary for DNA synthesis. S phase follows G1 and is the period in which chromosomal DNA is replicated. The next phase, called gap 2 (G2), is shorter than G1 and precedes mitosis. During this phase, DNA replication must be completed before the cell begins mitosis. In the mitotic phase, equal amounts of chromosomal material migrate to opposite poles of

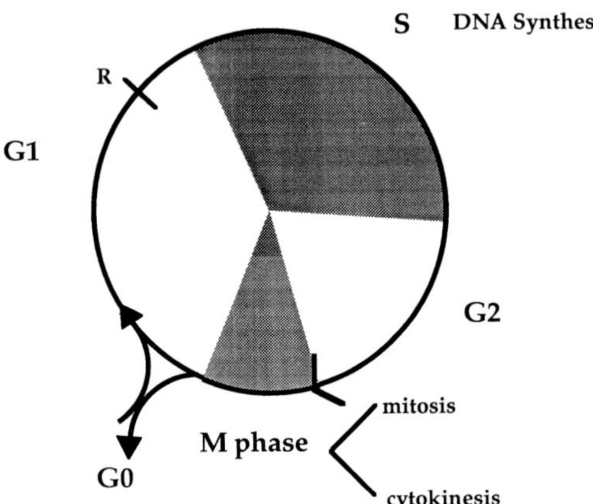

Figure 1. The cell cycle is an orderly sequence of phases that are tightly regulated. Timely execution of events during all phases is essential to obtaining two normal daughter cells. Following completion of mitosis, a cell can exit the cell cycle and enter a state of quiescence known as G0 phase. Cells undergoing terminal differentiation reside in G0. If a cell is destined to continue to proliferate, it enters G1 phase which is characterized by cell growth and preparation for DNA synthesis. During this phase the cell is sensitive to conditions in its environment. If these conditions are unfavorable, the cell can arrest in G1. There is a point, called restriction point (*R*), beyond which a cell is committed to complete mitosis regardless of the conditions of the environment. S phase brings DNA synthesis. In G2 phase DNA replication is assessed for errors before mitosis begins. In mitotic phase, the duplicated DNA material is equally distributed to two daughter cells containing equal amounts of cytoplasm.

the cell. The subsequent division of the cytoplasm, cytokinesis, results in two identical but separate daughter cells. In a rapidly dividing human cell, the entire cell cycle lasts about 24 hours. G1 lasts 12 hours; S phase, 6 hours; G2, 6 hours; and mitosis, 30 minutes (118). The critical genetic and enzymatic events controlling the normal cell cycle have recently been characterized (for reviews see Nurse (124), Sherr (158), Heichman and Roberts (57), and King 1994). An understanding of these is critical to understanding both normal cell proliferation and its aberration in tumors, such as glioblastoma multiforme.

FOUR MAIN PHASES OF THE CELL CYCLE

G1 Phase

During the G1 phase of the cell cycle, the cell prepares for S phase by enlarging and by pro-

ducing proteins and other macromolecules necessary for DNA synthesis. G1 is an appropriate phase for regulating cell cycle progression because it immediately precedes DNA synthesis and mitosis (132). Extracellular influences such as growth factors may affect whether a quiescent cell remains quiescent or enters the cell cycle to proliferate (G0 to G1) and whether a proliferating cell continues to proliferate or exits the cell cycle to become quiescent (G1 to G0) (132). For example, a proliferating cell may become quiescent if the extracellular environment lacks growth factors. There is a point late in G1, however, beyond which a cell is committed to divide even without growth factor signals. In mammalian cells, this point is called the restriction point. At the restriction point, the decision regarding cell cycle progression is made. It precedes S phase by 1–3 hours (132). The molecular event critical for G1 progression is inactivation of the retinoblastoma tumor suppressor protein (pRb) by phosphorylation by D-cyclin/CDK4 or CDK6 complexes (see below). As a general rule, progression within G1 is controlled predominantly by extracellular factors, whereas events in S phase, G2, and M are controlled by intracellular factors (132).

S Phase

During S phase, the complete DNA complement of the nucleus is replicated in a number of hours. Bidirectional DNA replication is initiated at many sites along chromosomes. The chromosomal protein scaffolding is also replicated so that the entire complex chromosomal structure is ready for segregation in mitosis (84). Entry into S phase is precipitated by the association of cyclin E with CDK2. Cyclin A-CDK2 complexes are also involved in both entry into and progression through S phase (see below) (57). Very stringent control of DNA replication ensures that the chromosomal material is only replicated once prior to the next cell division. Cell fusion experiments demonstrated that replicated nuclei are unable to reenter S phase until they have completed mitosis (84). Disturbance of S phase is disastrous for the cell's progeny. Mitosis will not begin until DNA replication is complete.

G2 Phase

During G2 phase, DNA replication is completed, and the replicated DNA is screened for damage (118). The identification of DNA damage arrests the cell cycle at particular checkpoints within G2. As an example, if radiation during G2 causes DNA strand breaks, the cell does not enter mitosis until DNA has been repaired (198).

Mitosis

During mitosis, the replicated chromosomes and the cytoplasm are segregated equally into two daughter cells. Mitosis consists of an orderly sequence of distinct phases (for reviews see McIntosh and Koonce (105), Koshland (82), and Murray and Hunt (118)). In prophase, the chromosomes condense to a state suitable for transport. Condensation allows the chromosomes not only to move without getting entangled, but also to withstand the mechanical forces exerted by the mitotic spindle (118). Chromosome condensation probably begins as early as the end of S phase (118). DNA is wound around histone proteins, and histones are phosphorylated during mitosis by cyclin-dependent kinases (see below). This may be an important control point. The cytoskeleton of the cell disassembles and reorganizes, and the nuclear envelope dissolves. The breakdown of the nuclear envelope involves phosphorylation of lamins, intermediate filament proteins beneath the inner nuclear membrane (118). Complexes of cyclin B and the cyclin-dependent kinase CDK1 (also called CDC2) phosphorylate lamins (see below). Breakdown of the nuclear envelope permits separation of DNA in mitosis. To effect DNA segregation, the centrosome, which is composed of two specialized microtubular structures called centrioles, duplicates to yield two pairs of centrioles. The centrioles migrate to opposite ends of the cell to form spindle poles which then form the spindle apparatus (118). The Golgi apparatus and the endoplasmic reticulum fragment into tiny vesicles dispersed throughout the cytoplasm. Pineocytosis ceases, RNA synthesis stops, and protein synthesis declines dramatically. In metaphase, the chromosomes move to the cell's midplane and align such that sister chromatids face opposite ends of the cell. Microtubules, which form the spindle apparatus, arise from a microtubular organizing center at opposite poles of the cell and attach to each side of the centromere of each chromosome via specialized DNA binding proteins called kinetochores. The microtubules

of the spindle apparatus are dynamic, constantly elongating and shrinking by the addition and removal of tubulin subunits. Cyclin B/CDK1 phosphorylation of protein microtubules facilitates formation of the spindle apparatus. At anaphase, the sister chromatids separate along the axis of the spindle apparatus and migrate to a spindle pole at opposite ends of the cell. This separation of sister chromatids permits daughter nuclei to form (118). It is associated with degradation of cyclin proteins. During telophase, chromosomes expand when they reach the spindle poles, the nuclear envelope reforms, and lamins entering the nucleus through nuclear pores repolymerize to support the nuclear membrane (105, 118). Following nuclear division, cytoplasmic division occurs by cytokinesis. A contraction ring of microfilaments pinches off the cytoplasmic material to produce two daughter cells. Cytokinesis also requires inactivation of the cyclin B/CDK1 complex (118).

DETERMINATION OF CELL CYCLE PROGRESSION BY CYCLINS AND CYCLIN-DEPENDENT KINASES

Progression through the cell cycle is governed by the orderly activation of cyclin-dependent kinases (CDKs) as they associate with their regulatory subunits, the cyclins. CDKs are protein kinases whose phosphorylation of specific substrates effects particular cell cycle events. Three examples are notable: 1) During mitotic phase, cyclin B1/CDK1 complexes phosphorylate H1 histones, which in turn participate in chromosome condensation in prophase; 2) Phosphorylation of nuclear lamins by cyclin B1/CDK1 complexes allows dissolution of the nuclear envelope, facilitating formation of the mitotic spindle (56, 137, 183); and 3) During G1 phase, phosphorylation of the retinoblastoma susceptibility protein, pRb, by D-cyclins and CDK4/CDK6 permits entry into S phase (104, 107, 158). CDK enzymatic activity varies in a tightly regulated manner throughout the cell cycle, but CDK protein levels remain constant.

CYCLINS AS THE REGULATORY SUBUNITS OF CDKS

Cyclins are a group of structurally similar proteins that share homology of a conserved 100-amino acid domain known as the cyclin box (112). This region is essential for CDK binding and CDK activation. Cyclin-CDK interactions are promiscuous: specific CDKs can interact with a number of different cyclins, and a given cyclin can interact with different CDKs (112) (Fig. 2). CDK activity is partly determined by cyclin levels, which oscillate in a cell cycle-dependent manner (Fig. 3). Cyclins were originally discovered in sea urchin embryos, in which levels of a set of proteins oscillate sharply during the transition from G2 to M phase (36). The determinants of cyclin levels are not well understood in mammalian cells and likely differ for different types of cyclins. The substrate, subcellular localization, and temporal pattern of activation of a cyclin determine these parameters of activity for the CDKs with which it associates (112).

There are two main families of cyclins, the mitotic cyclins and the G1 cyclins. Mitotic cyclins consist of cyclin B and cyclin A. Cyclin A also has a second role in S phase of the cell cycle. The G1 cyclins are cyclins C, D1–3, and E.

Mitotic Cyclins

Cyclin B: Association with Mitosis

The union of studies in yeast, *Xenopus oocytes*, and sea urchin embryos led to the discovery that a common protein kinase, called M phase-promoting factor (MPF), is involved in the transition from G2 to M phase in all eukaryotic cells. MPF has two subunits: cyclin B, the regulatory subunit, and CDC2 (CDK1), a pro-

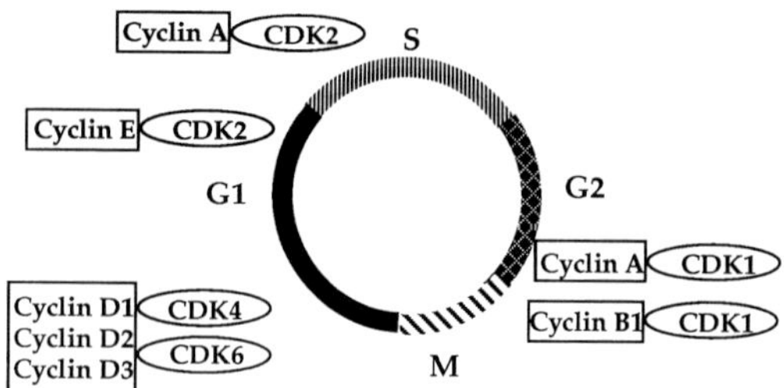

Figure 3. Cyclins are the regulatory subunits of CDKs. Cyclins associate with different CDKs at various stages of the cell cycle. A CDK can associate with more than one cyclin, and a cyclin can interact with more than one CDK. Cyclins target CDKs to their substrates and determine the timing of CDK activity. In this figure, cyclin/CDK pairs are shown for different phases of the cell cycle.

tein kinase. The rate of synthesis of cyclin B during metaphase-anaphase transition at mitosis varies little throughout the cell cycle; the decline in cyclin B reflects its rapid degradation. For the cell to exit mitosis, Cyclin B must be degraded by the ubiquitin-dependent proteolytic pathway (45). Cyclin B associates only with CDK1; the kinase activity of this complex rises sharply at the start of mitosis. Cyclin B-CDK1 complexes reside in the cytoplasm until the start of mitosis, at which time they are transported to the nucleus (138).

Cyclin A: Association with S phase Progression and G2-M Phase

Cyclin A expression begins early in S phase; levels of cyclin A peak during the G2-M transition. Just as the level of expression of cyclin A varies with different phases of the cell cycle, so does the particular CDK, depending on what it associates with. Cyclin A can bind and activate CDK2 during S phase, and CDK1 during G2-M. Cyclin A expression is essential for S phase progression (131). Cyclin A's localization to sites of DNA replication in S phase nuclei suggests a direct role in the assembly or activation of DNA replication complexes (13). Its importance in S phase is highlighted by the demonstration that microinjection of cyclin A antibodies prevents cells from entering S phase (44, 131). Its presence in S and M phases suggests that cyclin A helps orchestrate the cell's progression through these two phases. Cyclin A may also be the target of adhesion-dependent signals that control cell cycle progression. In fact, overexpression of cyclin A results in an-

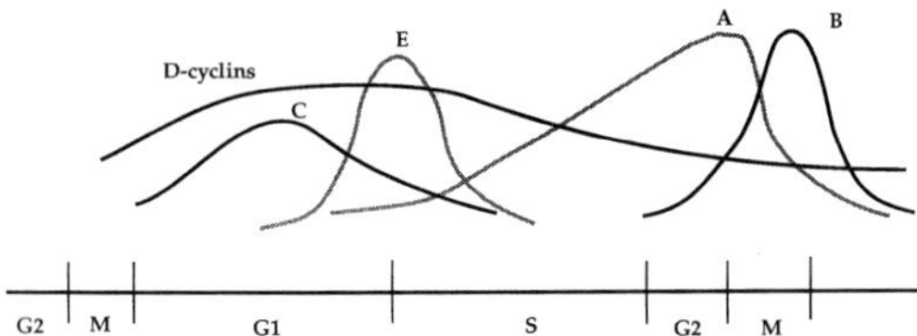

Figure 2. Expression pattern of cyclins in the cell cycle. When cells, stimulated by serum, emerge from quiescence, D-type cyclins (cyclins D1–3) are expressed early in G1 phase and do not fluctuate much if cells are allowed to cycle continuously. Expression of D cyclin in particular is influenced by growth factor stimulation. Cyclin E levels rise and fall sharply at the start of S phase; its expression is critical for the onset of DNA synthesis. Cyclin A levels begin to arise early in S phase; expression is essential for progression through S phase. Cyclin A is also expressed at high levels early in mitotic phase. Cyclin B1 expression is associated with the start of mitosis; its degradation during anaphase is essential for exit from mitosis.

chorage-independent cell growth—a hallmark of cancer cells (48).

Cyclins in G1

D Cyclins: Growth Factor Sensors Essential for G1 Progression

The D cyclins (cyclin D1, D2, and D3) are delayed early-response genes whose expression is induced by growth factors (190). Following the addition of serum to serum-deprived cells, expression of D cyclin rises in early- to mid-G1 phase and gradually declines over the remainder of the cell cycle. If growth factors are withdrawn, D cyclin levels decrease slowly (190). Cells that are continuously cycling have little variation in levels of D cyclin. Therefore, D cyclins link growth factor-induced signals to cell cycle regulators. Interestingly, cyclin D1 overexpression occurs in cells containing activated *ras*, and the cyclin D1 promoter is inducible by *c-jun*, an immediate early growth factor-induced gene (39, 59, 90). These results suggest that growth factor signalling pathways stimulate proliferation by inducing cyclin D1 expression (39, 59).

The different D cyclins are expressed in a cell type-specific manner. Most cells express cyclin D3 and either cyclin D1 or D2 (65, 157). Human D cyclins restore G1 progression to yeast cells devoid of D cyclins. Cyclin D1 may be involved in tumorigenesis: 1) cyclin D1 is possibly oncogenic in parathyroid adenomas in which a chromosomal translocation places the cyclin D1 gene (*PRAD1*) next to the parathyroid hormone gene enhancer (115); 2) expression of antisense cyclin D1 mRNA in an esophageal cell line with amplified cyclin D1 diminishes cell proliferation and tumorigenicity; and 3) overexpression of cyclin D1 results in neoplastic transformation (61, 70, 203).

D cyclins associate routinely with CDK4, but with CDK6 only in serum. They selectively phosphorylate pRB (104). D cyclins contain an LXCXE amino acid sequence that binds the small pocket region of pRb to catalyze phosphorylation of pRb (37, 75).

Cyclin D1 has been extensively studied. Overexpression of cyclin D1 in fibroblasts shortens G1 phase. Injection of anticyclin D1 antibodies into G1 phase cells prevents their entry into S phase (94). In cells lacking cyclin D1, overexpression of cyclin D2 or D3 shortens

G1 phase. Interestingly, cyclin D1 is unnecessary for G1 progression if the cell lacks functional pRb (5, 93). Levels of cyclin D1 are very low in pRb-deficient cells. pRb may regulate expression of cyclin D1 as pRb stimulates the cyclin D1 promoter (117).

The biological effects of increasing cyclin D1 expression are quite complex. As an example, overexpression of cyclin D1 causes inhibition rather than stimulation of cell proliferation of some types of cells. In a mammary epithelial cell line with low levels of endogenous cyclin D1, stable overexpression of cyclin D1 protein decreases its growth and tumorigenicity (51).

Expression of Cyclin E at G1-S Transition— Essential for Entry into S phase

Cyclin E is expressed in late G1 phase with a sharp peak at the G1-S transition. Cyclin E's kinase partner is CDK2. The kinase activity of this complex is also maximal at the G1-S transition (30, 81). Cyclin E expression precedes cyclin A expression and the onset of DNA synthesis. Microinjection of anticyclin E antibodies in G1 phase inhibits entry into S phase, suggesting that cyclin E expression is essential to the G1-S transition (126). Microinjection of anticyclin E antibodies in S phase has no effect on cell cycle progression (126). Microinjection of anticyclin E antibodies in G0 does not block entry into S phase, but microinjection of cyclin D1 antibodies does. Perhaps these two different cyclins act at different points in G1 phase. Overexpression of cyclin E accelerates G1 progression and decreases the amount of serum required for growth (125). Cyclin E-CDK2 complexes may be important to maintenance of pRb phosphorylation (185).

ACTIVATION OF CDKS BY CAKS (CYCLIN-ACTIVATING KINASES)

Activation of CDKs involves a series of phosphorylations by kinases and dephosphorylations by phosphatases (Fig. 4) (40, 47, 112). Phosphorylation may be either inhibitory or activating, depending on which residue is phosphorylated. Regulation of CDK activity is best understood for cyclin B/CDK1 complexes in yeast. Cyclin B binding to CDK1 occurs in S phase when cyclin B begins to reach significant levels. Binding of a cyclin to a CDK is essential for CDK activation. As cyclin B binds to

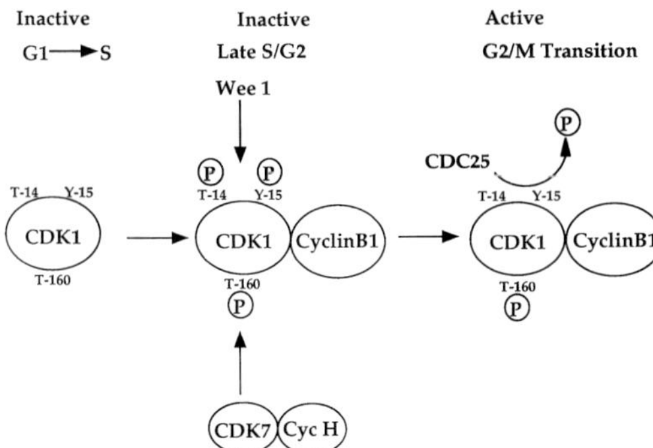

Figure 4. CDK activity is regulated by a complex series of phosphorylations at different sites. Binding of a cyclin is necessary for activation of a CDK by a CAK through phosphorylation at a threonine residue at position 160. In the case of cyclin B1/CDK1 complexes, phosphorylations at other sites, threonine-14 and tyrosine-15, restrain the activity of the enzyme complex. The CDK is then rapidly activated at the beginning of mitosis as the inhibitory phosphates are removed by the CDC25 phosphatase.

CDK1, CDK1 is phosphorylated at a threonine 161 by CAK. CAK contains two subunits, one catalytic and one regulatory (40). CAK's catalytic subunit is structurally similar to CDK's and has been called CDK7. CDK7 has a threonine residue homologous to that of CDK, suggesting that it too is regulated by phosphorylation. The regulatory subunit is also a cyclin, cyclin H. This CAK-cyclin H/CDK7 complex can activate multiple CDKs, including CDK1, CDK2, and CDK4. Cyclin binding to CDK likely triggers activation of CDK by the CAK. Cyclin binding induces a conformational change in the CDK that changes the orientation of a bound ATP binding site and exposes the enzymes substrate (68).

As phosphorylation at threonine 161, important for eventual CDK1 activation occurs, removal of inhibitory phosphates on CDK1, Tyr14 and Tyr15 is also accomplished. A kinase called wee1, originally discovered in yeast, catalyzes these inhibitory phosphorylations. Wee1 kinase activity diminishes during mitosis, and this facilitates activation of CDK1. Removal of these inhibitory phosphates at Thr 14 and Tyr 15 is performed by phosphatase CDC25. When CDC25 is phosphorylated by CDK1, its phosphatase activity is increased, and a positive feedback activation of CDK1 occurs as its inhibitory phosphates are removed. This coordinated balance of phosphorylation and dephosphorylation activates cyclin B/CDK1 at the start of mitosis. Cyclin B/CDK1 is then able to phosphorylate substrates in both the cytoplasm and the nucleus which effect nuclear and cytoplasmic division (56).

CYCLIN-DEPENDENT KINASE INHIBITORS AS BRAKES ON THE CELL CYCLE

Cell proliferation is regulated by the balance between expression of genes stimulating growth and expression of those inhibiting growth. Positive growth regulators, such as cyclins and CDKs, are opposed by cyclin-dependent kinase inhibitors (CDKIs) (for reviews see Elledge and Harper (35), Sherr and Roberts (159), and Hunter and Pines (65) (Fig. 5). These inhibit cyclin-CDK complexes. Because they inhibit cell cycle progression, they could be tumor suppressor genes.

Most cyclins and CDKs do not exist as mere binary complexes. Rather, they form quaternary protein complexes consisting of a cyclin, CDK, proliferating cell nuclear antigen (PCNA), and a CDKI. The CDKIs retard cell proliferation. In addition, CDKIs may be involved in such diverse processes as terminal cell differentiation, DNA replication, DNA repair, induction of apoptosis, and cellular senescence (159). Loss of expression of a CDKI may have disastrous consequences for the cell. For example, loss of the CDKI, p16, has been linked to many human cancers. There are two main classes of inhibitors, those that inhibit multiple cyclin-CDK complexes such as p21, $p27^{KIP1}$, and $p57^{KIP2}$ and those that inhibit the G1 D-type cyclin and CDK4/CDK6 complexes: $p16^{INK4A}$, $p15^{INK4B}$, $p18^{INK4C}$, and $p19^{INK4D}$.

p21 As a Universal Inhibitor of CDKs

p21 was first identified as a component of the quaternary complexes of multiple cyclins, CDKs, and PCNA, a protein involved in DNA replication and repair in normal cells. However, p21 is notably absent in transformed cells (193, 194). In transformed cells the typical quaternary complex is reduced to a binary cyclin/CDK complex, suggesting that the presence of p21 in quaternary complexes is important for restraining cell growth (194). Interestingly, p21 is also absent from cyclin/CDK complexes in spontaneously immortalized Li-Fraumeni fibroblasts

A)

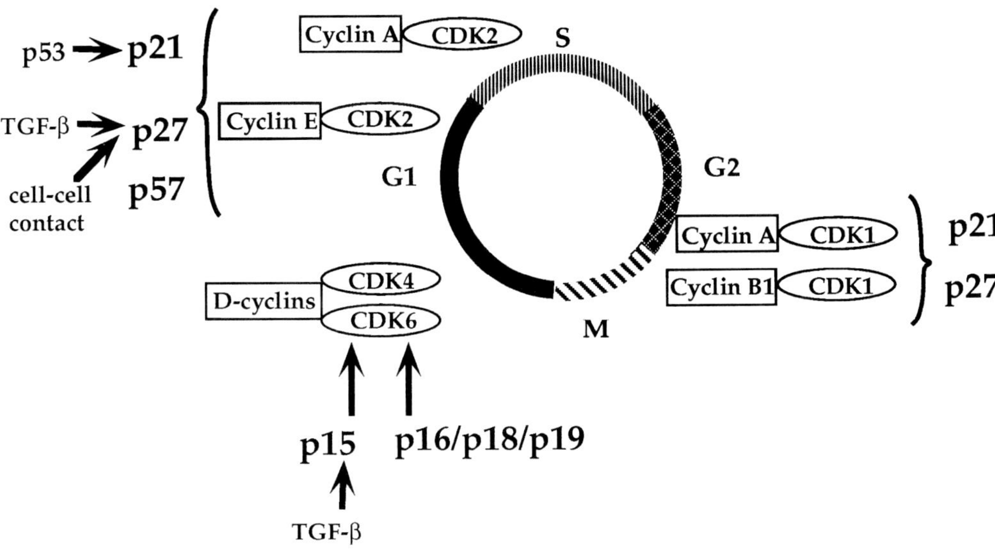

B)

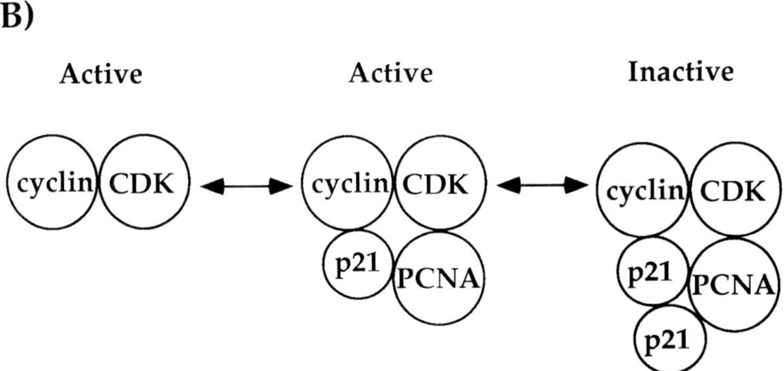

Figure 5. (*A*) Cyclin/CDK activity is inhibited by a number of specific inhibitors. Two main families are defined by similarities in structure and inhibitory action. The p21/p27/p57 family inhibits multiple cyclin/CDK complexes, whereas the p16/p15/p18/p19 family specifically inhibits CDK4/CDK6-associated complexes. The G1 arrest by certain stimuli is mediated by these inhibitors. As examples, radiation-induced G1 arrest is mediated by p53 induction of p21; and TGF-β1-mediated G1 arrest is mediated by p15 and p27. (*B*) Cyclin/CDK complexes are binary complexes that associate with other proteins. A critical stoichiometric relationship is required for inhibition of kinase activity by a CDK inhibitor. In normal fibroblasts, cyclins and CDKs exist in a quaternary complex with proliferating cell nuclear antigen (*PCNA*) and the CDK inhibitor p21. Binary cyclin/CDK complexes have kinase activity as do those complexes with a single p21 molecule. If the complex associates with another p21 molecule, the complex is no longer active. p27 likely inhibits cyclin/CDKs by a similar mechanism. p16 can prevent CDK binding to D-cyclins and can inhibit already active D-cyclin-CDK complexes. (Adapted from Zhang, H., Hannon, G. J., and Beach, D. p21 containing cyclin kinases exist in both active and inactive states. Genes Dev. 8:1750–1758, 1994; see also Sherr and Roberts (159)).

which have lost the function of both p53 alleles (194). Expression of the p21 gene is induced by p52, an inhibitor of CDKs abundant in senescent cells. The p21 gene is also expressed in differentiated melanoma cells.

p21 lowers cyclin/CDK activity (194). It plays an important role in p53-mediated G1 cell cycle arrest induced by DNA damage. p21 inhibits activation of cyclin/CDK by binding to the catalytically active site of the quaternary complex (201). Saturation of cyclin/CDK complexes with p21 sterically blocks CAK's ability to phosphorylate the threonine-161 residue of CDK (201). In addition to decreasing the activity of cyclin/CDK complexes, p21 also blocks the ability of PCNA to activate DNA polymerase-δ, the main enzyme for DNA replication (180). Interestingly, p21 inhibits PCNA-dependent DNA replication but does not affect PCNA-associated DNA repair (88). The carboxy terminus is involved in CDK inhibition (95). Although p21 is involved in p53-mediated G1 arrest, it does not appear to be involved in p53-mediated apoptosis (181). p21 expression can also occur independent of p53 induction. In cultured cells that do not express functional p53, p21 expression is induced in early G1 by serum stimulation (108).

p16^{INK4A} As a Specific CDK4/CDK6 Inhibitor and a Tumor Suppressor Gene

Another CDK inhibitor, p16^{INK4A} (inhibitor of CDK4, also called multiple tumor suppressor 1, MTS1, and CDKN2) is a potentially important tumor suppressor gene. This gene was originally cloned from yeast as a protein which could interact with CDK4 (154). p16^{INK4A} binds to CDK4 in binary fashion and inhibits the kinase activity of cyclin D-CDK4 complexes. p16^{INK4A} disrupts the cyclin/CDK association by binding to the CDK. It also prevents activation of CDKs by blocking CAK phosphorylation (3). p16^{INK4A} is also a specific inhibitor of CDK5, the other important kinase partner of D-cyclins. This inhibition is likely important in the regulation of cyclin D-CDK4/CDK6 phosphorylation of pRb, an important step in the initiation of S phase. Kamb et al. identified p16 as a tumor suppressor gene located on chromosome 9p21, a locus commonly deleted in malignant melanomas (73). In their study, p16^{INK4A} was homozygously deleted in a large proportion of human tumor cell lines (73).

Although the frequency of homozygous deletions is much lower in primary tumors, this gene probably plays an important role in familial melanoma, primary pancreatic adenocarcinoma, and glioblastoma multiforme (11, 66, 69, 74, 116, 122).

Interestingly, the expression of *p16^{INK4A}* in tumor cells seems inversely related to the expression of pRb (89, 127, 129, 133). In tumor cells with normal pRb there is often little p16^{INK4A} expression; if pRb is functionally inactivated, p16^{INK4A} is expressed. This suggests that these proteins act along the same pathway to restrain cell growth and that pRb is downstream from p16^{INK4A}. Inactivation of either pRb or p16^{INK4A} may allow a cell to enter S phase unchecked (127, 154). pRb restraint on cell growth can thus be inactivated either by a pRb mutation that results in a nonfunctional or absent pRb or by absence of p16^{INK4A} which leads to hyperphosphorylation of pRb by CDK4/CDK6. This hypothesis is supported by an experiment in which transfection of wild-type p16^{INK4A} into osteosarcoma cells lacking functional pRb (SAOS-2 cell line) did not cause G1 cell cycle arrest, but its transfection into osteosarcoma cells bearing wild-type pRB (U-2-OS cells) did (93). In normal cells, pRb transcriptionally represses p16^{INK4A} (89). This suggests that a feedback loop may exist such that when pRb is inactivated by phosphorylation, p16 transcription increases to inhibit CDK4/CDK6 activity (89).

Other inhibitors of CDK4/CDK6 complexes, such as p15^{INK4B}, p18^{INK4C}, and p19^{INK4D}, (15, 49, 52, 62) have structural homology to p16^{INK4A} and form binary inhibitory complexes with CDK. p15^{INK4B} also occurs at the 9p21 chromosomal locus (30 kilobases away), and it is usually codeleted with p16^{INK4A} in glioblastomas (52, 69, 143). p15^{INK4B} expression in keratinocytes increases 30-fold following G1 cell cycle arrest induced by transforming growth factor-β1 (TGF-β1). p15^{INK4B} is normally expressed in a wider range of normal tissues than *p16^{INK4A}*, suggesting that there may be tissue-specific functions for CDKIs (69, 143).

Mediation of Cell Cycle Arrest from Cell-Cell Contact of TGF-β Treatment by p27

p27^{KIP1} (kinase inhibitory protein) is a CDK inhibitor with structural homology to p21 (140).

Similar to p21, $p27^{KIP1}$ inhibits multiple cyclin/ CDK complexes. This CDKI is involved in G1 cell cycle arrest produced by extracellular signals such as TGF-β or contact inhibition (139, 140, 174). $p27^{KIP1}$ cooperates with $p15^{INK4B}$ to produce cell cycle arrest in response to TGF-β (146). $p27^{KIP1}$ binds stoichiometrically to cyclin/CDK complexes, thus interfering with CAK activation of CDK (76, 140, 174). Unlike p21, $p27^{KIP1}$ does not bind PCNA. A newly cloned p27-like CDKI, $p57^{KIP2}$ appears to have more tissue-specific expression (86, 103).

REGULATION OF THE CELL CYCLE BY RETINOBLASTOMA PROTEIN AND E2F TRANSCRIPTION FACTORS

pRb is an important substrate for cyclin D-CDK4, cyclin D-, CDK6, and cyclin E-CDK2. pRB phosphorylation is critical to control cell cycle progression in G1 (for review see Weinberg (185) and Ewen (37) (Fig. 6)). pRb is phosphorylated in a cell cycle-dependent manner (9, 25A). Levels of pRb protein do not vary during the cell cycle, but the extent of its phosphorylation does. It is hypophosphorylated during cell quiescence. Phosphorylation begins in mid-G1 phase and peaks in S phase. pRb then reverts to the hypophosphorylated state by the beginning of the next G1 phase. This pattern of phosphorylation suggests that pRb is a substrate for cyclin/CDKs. Which cyclin/CDK complex is most important for phosphorylating pRb is unknown. D-cyclin-CDK4/CDK6 kinase complexes are very important in early to mid-G1 phase; cyclin E/CDK2 complexes are important at the G1-S transition, and cyclin A/CDK2 complexes help maintain pRb phosphorylation in S phase. There are two pRb-related proteins, p107 and p130, which are also phosphorylated in a cell cycle-dependent manner by cyclin/CDK complexes. When overexpressed, p107 and p130 can induce cell cycle arrest. However, to date, no mutations in these genes have been found in human cancers. Therefore, they do not qualify as classic tumor suppressor genes like pRb.

Following phosphorylation of pRb (or p107 or p130), E2F transcription factors are released. E2Fs bind only to the hypophosphorylated active form of pRb. An extremely important function of pRb is restraint of the E2F activity (185). A number of E2F proteins (E2Fs 1–5) bind with different affinities to various members of the pRb family. E2Fs are DNA-binding proteins which initiate transcription of multiple genes

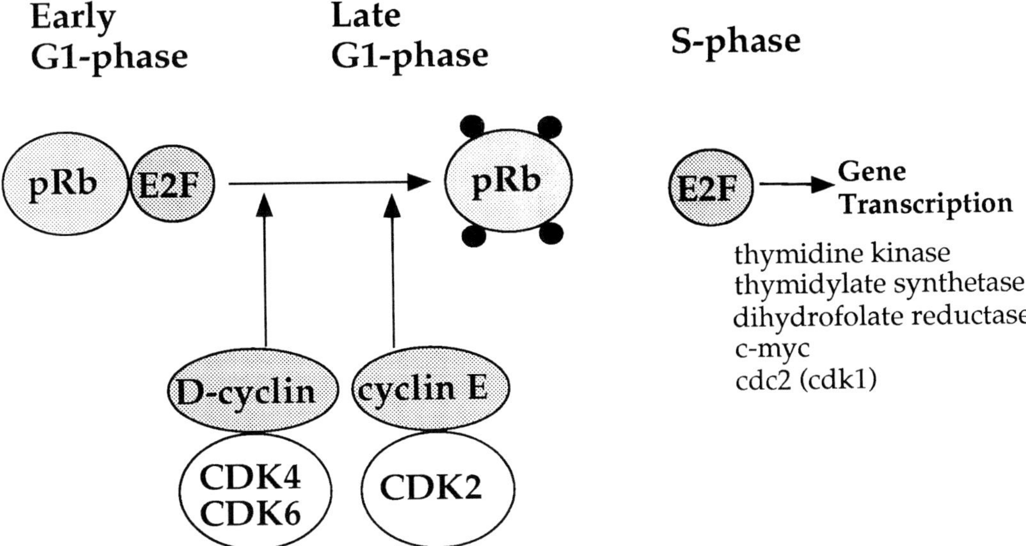

Figure 6. Progression through the cell cycle is controlled by sequential activation of cyclins and CDKs. In G1 phase, one target of CDKs is the retinoblastoma protein (*pRb*). Phosphorylation of pRb by cyclin-CDK complexes releases E2F transcription factor. E2F is then free to bind to DNA to activate transcription of genes important to cell cycle progression. Which particular cyclin-CDK complexes are critical to pRb modification is unknown, although the ones shown are the most likely candidates. Retinoblastoma proteins and E2F transcription factors are also involved.

important to cell cycle progression (38, 121). The genes activated by E2F contain E2F-binding consensus sites in their promoters and include dihydrofolate reductase, thymidine kinase, DNA polymerase-α, thymidylate synthetase, B-*myb*, CDK1, and c-*myc*. All these genes are important to entry into or progression through the cell cycle (38). E2F can both induce S phase entry and effect neoplastic transformation in the absence of serum. This suggests that E2Fs can act as oncogenes (72, 156, 164, 195). Restraint of E2F activity is not pRb's only function. In its hypophosphorylated state, pRb also represses the E2F transcription state. It is unclear whether pRb acts alone in this regard or whether DNA binding of E2F also contributes (8, 187).

This pRb-E2F pathway is extremely complex and central to the control of proliferation. Disruption of this pathway contributes to the development of many different human tumors.

GROWTH FACTORS

Growth factors are critical to cell proliferation and tumorigenesis. Oncogenes are dominant mutant forms of normal cellular genes (proto-oncogenes). Many oncogenes encode for proteins involved in the growth factor signaling cascade (12). Growth factors are soluble secreted proteins that exert biological effects on target cells by binding to a specific transmembrane receptor. Activation of a growth factor receptor initiates an intracellular signaling cascade of complex protein-protein interactions and changes in phosphorylation that ultimately alters expression of genes important for cell proliferation (Fig. 7). Many different growth factors have their signals transduced by a common pathway, the Ras-Raf-mitogen-activated kinase pathway. Abnormalities in a number of molecules, both activating molecules and their negative regulators, along this pathway contribute to uncontrolled cell proliferation. As an example, mutations in the ras proto-oncogene that produce a constitutively activated ras protein and signaling pathway contribute to the development of a number of human cancers. Conversely, abnormalities in proteins that decrease ras expression or activation may also produce uncontrolled proliferation. The neurofibromin protein, which is defective in neurofibromatosis type I, normally converts ras from an active to an inactive state. Loss of this important regulator of ras activity is tumorigenic. The tumorigenicity of derangements in this pathway manifest its importance in regulating cell proliferation. In this section, the mechanism of signal transduction by growth factors will be outlined. Platelet-derived growth factor will be discussed as an example of growth factor-mediated control of cell proliferation.

In addition to regulating cell proliferation, growth factors also affect cell differentiation, the cytoskeleton, and membrane-bound vesicle transport (23, 101). The effect of a growth factor depends on the cell's type, its state of differentiation, the local concentration of the growth factor, the duration of cell activation by a growth factor, and simultaneous binding of other growth factors to their specific receptors. Since multiple types of growth factors act simultaneously, signals from multiple types of factors are integrated in intracellular signaling pathways. Other factors such as the adhesion of the cell to the extracellular matrix may influence the effect of a growth factor-induced signal. The signal transduction pathway from growth factor receptor to the nucleus is extremely complex, and the following discussion is simplified for the purposes of this chapter.

In order to proliferate, cells must be stimulated by growth factors. For example, to maintain the growth of fibroblasts in culture, growth factors must be present in the growth media. Removal of growth factors from the culture media may cause cell cycle arrest or apoptosis (see apoptosis section). Platelet-derived growth factor (PDGF) accounts for 50% of the platelet-derived mitogenic activity of serum; epidermal growth factor and TGF-β contribute to the other half (150). *In vivo*, PDGF released by platelets when they aggregate stimulates division of fibroblasts and smooth muscle cells in wound repair. Growth factors do not enter the cell but rather exert their effects by binding to receptors which are tyrosine kinases. A growth factor receptor is a transmembrane protein with three domains. There is an extracellular domain which binds the growth factor, a small transmembrane domain which anchors the receptor in the plasma membrane, and a larger intracellular (cytoplasmic) domain containing tyrosine kinase activity which initiates the intracellular signaling cascade.

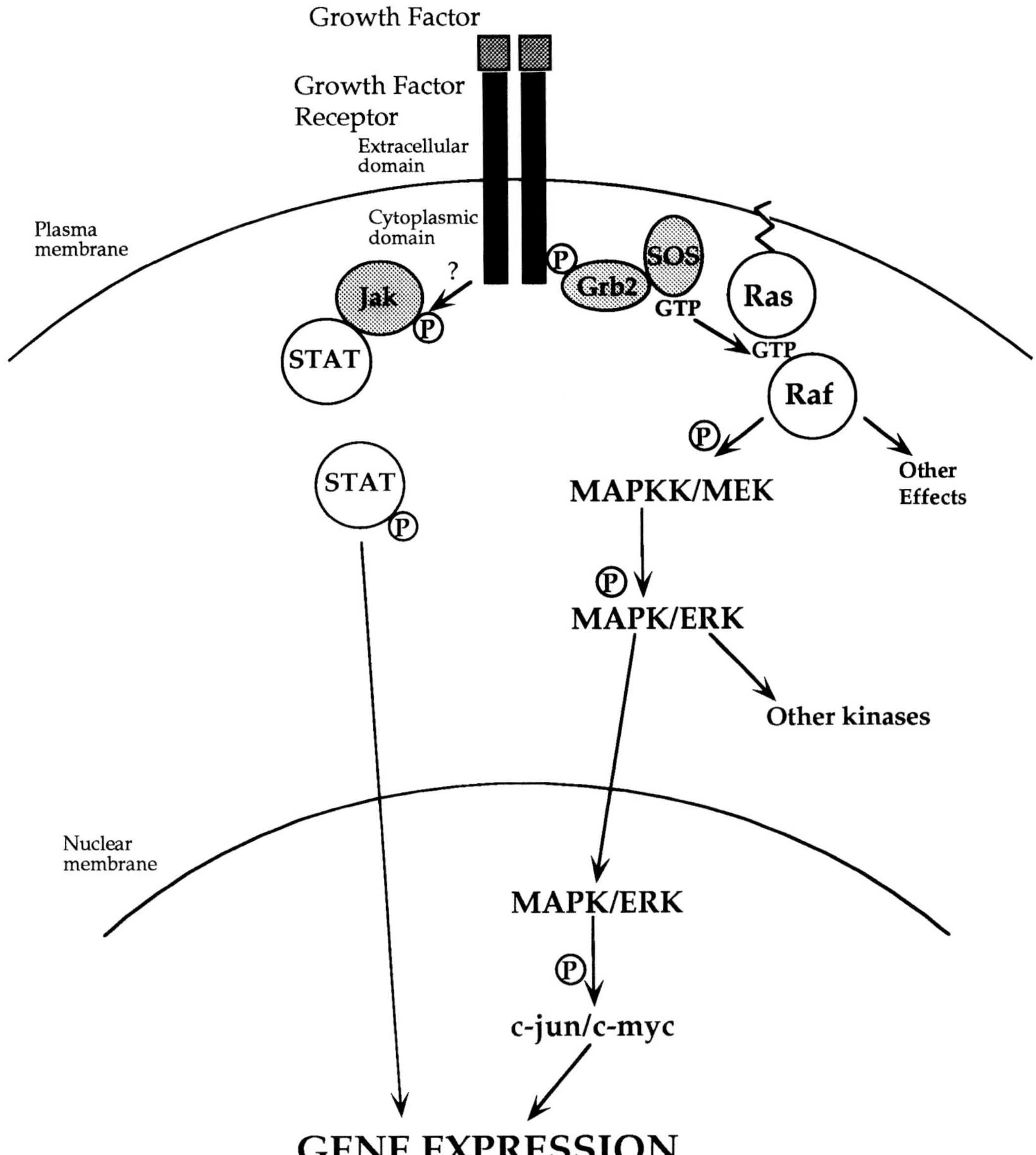

Figure 7. Growth factor signaling via the Ras-MAP kinase pathway. Binding of a growth factor to a specific receptor results in an intracellular signaling cascade characterized by activation of proteins through phosphorylation. Ultimately, this pathway stimulates transcription factor binding to DNA and induces expression of genes important for cell proliferation or differentiation. Another pathway, Jak-STAT may also mediate growth factor signaling, particularly the response of immune cells to cytokines. Activation of a cell surface receptor recruits a Jak kinase which phosphorylates a STAT protein. Once phosphorylated the STAT is directly translocated from the membrane to the nucleus to bind to DNA and cause a change in gene expression.

PDGFs and Receptors: Prototypes

PDGF, the first growth factor characterized, is a dimer of two polypeptide chains joined by disulphide bonds. Two polypeptides, A and B, form homodimers (PDGF-AA or PDGF-BB) or heterodimers (PDGF-AB) (150, 153). PDGF-B is the normal cellular homologue of v-*sis*, the oncogene of simian sarcoma virus (150). PDGF is secreted by platelets, mononuclear phagocytes, endothelial cells, vascular smooth muscle (VSM) cells, embryonic cells, and a variety of transformed cells. PGDF has pleiotrophil effects on cells with PDGF receptors; it stimulates proliferation of fibroblasts, VSM cells, glial cells, and chondrocytes (150). It can also indirectly enhance the proliferation of some cells lacking PDGF receptors (150).

PDGF binds to a receptor composed of two different subunits, α and β, joined noncovalently. The α-subunit can bind either PDGF-A or PDGF-B, but the β subunit binds only PDGF-B (153). Thus, PDGF-BB can bind to all receptor isoforms, PDGF-AB binds to platelet-derived growth factor receptor (PDGFR)-$\alpha\alpha$ or PDGFR-$\alpha\beta$, and PDGFR-$\beta\beta$ binds only to PDGF-BB. PDGF-$\alpha\alpha$ functions as the universal PDGFR. The PDGFR isoforms are present in varying amounts on different cell types, and as a result, the effect of PDGF stimulation depends on the type of PDGF dimer (which varies according to the source cell) and the type of receptor present on the target cell. This permits the response to PDGF to vary with a cell's physiological state as manifested by the types of PDGFR expressed (153). Mapping of the patterns of expression of different growth factor isoforms and receptor isoforms in the nervous system of mice shows that PDGF-B and PDGFR-β are not expressed in astrocytes, but PDGF-B is expressed in neurons and PDGFR-β in brain capillary endothelial cells (151). Neuronal injury could lead to glial chemotaxis and proliferation by releasing PDGF-B which binds PDGFR on astrocytes (151). PDGF-A is expressed at high levels by glial cells and neurons throughout the nervous system (197). The genes for the PDGF chains and PDGFR subunits are located on different chromosomes, and their expressions are independently regulated (153).

Autocrine stimulation is possible when a cell both produces PDGF and expresses the appropriate PDGFR subunits. PDGF binds the cell's PDGFRs to stimulate proliferation. Autocrine stimulation could promote uncontrolled cell proliferation; this may occur in sarcomas, lung carcinomas, and malignant astrocytomas (23, 155). This autocrine loop frees the cell from dependence on its environment.

Mutation in growth factor receptor tyrosine kinases can also produce uncontrolled cell pro-

liferation. Mutations in the extracellular domain may release the cytoplasmic domain from the normal restraints of the extracellular domain or may alter the conformation of the protein to yield dimerization and activation in the absence of ligand binding (175). Mutations in the transmembrane domain may cause dimerization and activation, and mutations of the cytoplasmic domain may constitutively activate tyrosine kinase activity.

Numerous other growth factor and receptor systems affect the proliferation and differentiation of multiple cell types. These include the fibroblast growth factors, epidermal growth factors, transforming growth factors-α, insulin-like growth factors, and vascular endothelial growth factors (VEGFs). Some of these growth factor systems have been implicated in the pathogenesis of human neoplasia, including brain neoplasms (186, 199). In particular, amplification and rearrangement of epidermal growth factor receptors occur in approximately 40% of glioblastomas (31, 32, 113, 119, 165). VEGF stimulates endothelial cell growth and tumor angiogenesis, particularly in glioblastomas (119).

The Intracellular Growth Factor Signaling Cascade

Typically, binding of a growth factor to a receptor induces dimerization of two individual receptors. Receptor dimerization results as binding of ligand to the extracellular domain induces a conformational change that facilitates interaction between the bound receptor and a nearby receptor (175). The aggregation of growth factor receptors following ligand binding induces autophosphorylation of the intracellular domains. Each receptor phosphorylates the other usually on a tyrosine residue in a kinase domain (175). Autophosphorylation removes an internal constraint on the intracellular domain such that the receptor can attain a conformation able to phosphorylate protein substrates. Phosphorylation of tyrosine residues opens binding sites for a specific 100-amino acid domain of a number of other proteins. This domain is called the src homology 2 region (SH2) (135, 136). Src is a nonreceptor protein tyrosine kinase involved in signal transduction. The homologous protein, v-src, is the transforming protein of the Rous sarcoma virus. The SH2 region and a 50-amino acid domain called SH3 mediate protein-protein interactions involved in many intracellular signaling pathways. Growth factor receptors lack SH2 and SH3 domains. After a growth factor binds to a receptor and intracellular signals are initiated, the receptor-ligand complex is rapidly internalized and degraded.

The autophosphorylated intracellular growth factor receptor domains bind other proteins with SH2 domains. The specificity of binding of an SH2 domain is determined by the amino acids surrounding a phosphorylated tyrosine residue (19, 135). For example, activation of the epidermal growth factor receptor (EGFR) or PDGFR by tyrosine phosphorylation creates a binding site for the SH2 domain of an adaptor protein, Grb2 (92). Grb2 is normally present in the cytoplasm bound to a guanine nucleotide exchange factor called SOS. Activation of the intracellular domain of the growth factor receptor permits interaction of the Grb2 SH2 domain with the phosphorylated tyrosine residue on the growth factor receptor (6, 19). This interaction juxtaposes Grb2 and SOS and Ras. Ras is activated as SOS exchanges the GDP on Ras for GTP. Ras, when bound to GTP, is activated and initiates further intracellular signaling. Thus, Ras functions as a binary switch, cycling between an inactive GDP-bound state and an active GTP-bound state (50). Ras itself has intrinsic GTPase activity; as it slowly hydrolyses bound GTP back to GDP, ras is inactivated (79). GTPase-activating proteins (GAPs), such as neurofibromin, hasten termination of Ras activity. The impaired GTPase activity of some mutant Ras proteins reflects insensitivity to GAPs; constitutive activation of Ras and uninterrupted stimulation of cell proliferation can result (43).

Ras proteins are involved in a wide variety of intracellular processes such as cell proliferation, cell differentiation, control of the cell cytoskeleton, and regulation of traffic between membranous intracellular compartments (6). Ras mutations occur in many human cancers. Ras mutations are found in approximately 30% of many types of human tumors, such as lung, thyroid, colon, and pancreatic cancers (79).

Ras activation by growth factors activates a series of serine/threonine kinases called the mitogen-activated protein (MAP) kinase cascade or extracellular signal-related kinases, ERKs/ cascade. This ultimately activates nuclear transcription factors c-jun and c-myc by phosphorylation (60, 101). These transcription factors bind to DNA to induce expression of genes important in cell proliferation. Many signaling pathways converge on Ras as a common route to the nucleus.

Activation of Ras to the GTP-bound form shifts cytosolic Raf to the cell membrane (87, 168, 179). Raf, like Ras, is a proto-oncogene (144). To activate the carboxy terminus of Raf, Ras must receive a farnesyl group (lipid moiety) which then links Ras to the plasma membrane (14, 43). Inhibition of farnesyl transferases, the enzymes that catalyze farnesylation of Ras, is a new strategy for cancer treatment (43). When bound to the plasma membrane and to GTP, Ras associates with the amino terminus of Raf. This association leads to tyrosine phosphorylation of Raf and activation of its serine/threonine kinase activity (99). Once activated, Raf dissociates from Ras but remains bound to the cytoskeleton at the plasma membrane. The integrity of the cytoskeletal anchoring molecules is critical to this signaling pathway as they serve to compartmentalize the various signaling molecules to their sites of action (111). Raf (also called MAP kinase kinase kinase) then activates MAP kinase kinase (MAPKK, also called Mek) by phosphorylation, which in turn activates MAP kinase (MAPK) (22, 60, 101). Mek is a point of integration for the Ras-Raf pathway and several other intracellular signaling pathways. G-proteins signal through Mek. Cell adhesion signals mediated by integrin cell surface molecules also send a proliferative stimulus through MAPK (17).

The MAPK pathway is the common path to the nucleus of a number of signaling systems. MAPKs (including extracellular signal-related kinases ERK-1 and ERK-2) activate a large number of substrates, both cytoplasmic and nuclear transcription factors (25, 101). MAPKs translocate into the nucleus to activate transcription factors such as c-myc and c-jun by phosphorylation. Ras activates other pathways in addition to the MAPK pathway. Ras may activate other similar GTP-binding proteins, such as Rho and Rac, which are involved in modulating the cell cytoskeleton (147, 148). Ras activation of Rac may be essential to cell transformation by oncogenic Ras (142).

The Jak-STAT signal transduction pathway also mediates growth factor signaling. Ligand binding stimulates a receptor tyrosine kinase to phosphorylate. The activated receptor activates by phosphorylation a Janus (JAK) kinase associated with the cytoplasmic domain of the receptor. The JAK kinases in turn phosphorylate a group of cytoplasmic proteins called STATs (signal transducers and activators of transcription). Interaction between Jaks and STATs are mediated by SH2 domains on STATs (58). Phosphorylated STATs translocate to the nucleus where they dimerize, bind to specific sequences on DNA, and activate transcription (24).

TUMOR SUPPRESSOR GENES

Cancer can arise from inactivation of both copies of a gene whose product restrains cell growth. Such genes are termed tumor suppressor genes. Cancer caused by homozygous inactivation of tumor suppressor genes is thus a recessive process. This contrasts with the dominant effect of mutations of proto-oncogenes that produce a gain of function; alteration of one allele is sufficient for tumorigenesis. Tumor suppressor genes include genes whose product inhibits progression through the cell cycle, such as Rb, p53, p15, and p16 or downregulates Ras activity, such as NF1 and organic membrane proteins, such as NF2. Other candidate tumor suppressor genes identified by their homozygous deletion in tumors do not yet have their function identified. These genes include DCC which is deleted in colon cancer, the Wilm's tumor suppressor gene WT1, the adenomatous polyposis coli gene APC, and BRCA1 (a putative suppressor of breast cancer). The following discusses the Rb gene as a model of tumor suppressor genes. The p53 tumor suppressor gene will also be discussed. The tumor suppressor gene that inhibits CDKs, p16^{INK4A}, has been discussed in the cell cycle section. The tumor suppressor genes NF1 and NF2 will be discussed in the sections on phakomatoses.

RETINOBLASTOMA AS A MODEL

Study of familial cancer syndromes led to the important discovery of tumor suppressor genes. The existence of these genes was predicted from statistical analysis of patients with retinoblastoma (80). The hypothesis that retinoblastoma is caused by two mutational events has been confirmed by the demonstration that a mutation occurs in each copy of the retinoblastoma susceptibility gene (Rb), a tumor suppressor gene. In the hereditary form of retinoblastoma tumors result from inheritance of a mutated Rb allele from a parent and acquisition of mutation in a

remaining normal Rb allele in a somatic cell. The second mutation leads to either a complete lack of pRb expression or the production of a functionally inactive protein. Tumors in the nonhereditary form arise from two sporadic mutations in the same somatic cell. Patients with the hereditary form often have bilateral retinoblastomas, earlier appearance of the disease, and an increased incidence of tumors in other tissues. Because every somatic cell in the affected individual contains a single mutation in Rb, only one inactivating mutation in the remaining normal Rb allele of any cell is required for neoplastic transformation of that cell. The frequency of somatic mutation is sufficiently high that a second mutation in Rb is highly likely to occur. The phenotype of retinoblastomas thus appears to be dominantly inherited. The likelihood of an inactivating somatic mutation in each allele of a gene in the same cell is extremely low. Therefore, nonhereditary, sporadic retinoblastomas are typically unilateral, appear later in life, and affected individuals do not have an increased incidence of other tumors.

Rb was the first tumor suppressor gene discovered. The cloning of the Rb gene followed by 10 years detection of deletions in chromosome 13q14 in sporadic and hereditary forms of retinoblastoma (100). Rb can be inactivated by a variety of genetic lesions, including large deletions, splice mutations that lose an exon, and microdeletions in the promoter region (100). The higher frequency of germline R6 mutations during spermatogenesis suggests that genomic imprinting may affect which allele is mutated (100). The tumor suppressor role of Rb is supported by the suppression of growth and neoplastic phenotype by wild type Rb introduced into osteosarcoma cells (SAOS-2) that lack Rb (64). Expression of the exogenous Rb in these cells resulted in reversal of the transformed phenotype. Conversely blocking production of pRb in human fibroblast cells by injecting oligonucleotides antisense to Rb, increases the rate of mitosis (169).

Rb mutations also occur in human cancers other that retinoblastomas and osteosarcomas that can be hereditary. Loss of heterozygosity for Rb has been found in 44% of a small group of studies on glioblastoma multiforme (176). Sporadic sarcomas, small cell lung carcinomas, bladder carcinomas, and breast carcinomas also have Rb mutations, but many other tumor types do not (184). It is unclear why only a few types of tumors contain mutations in Rb, a gene expressed in all tissues. However, it is not uncommon that a ubiquitously expressed gene such as Rb is altered in only a minority of cancers. Perhaps this reflects the variety of cancers and of genetic alterations that can be oncogenic. Interestingly, in small cell lung carcinomas, levels of pRb and $p16^{INK4A}$ vary inversely (129).

Studies of transgenic mice lacking one or both Rb alleles confirm Rb as a tumor suppressor gene and an important regulator of cell proliferation. Mice heterozygous for a mutation in Rb were created by disrupting one Rb allele through homologous recombination in mouse embryonic stem cells grown *in vitro* (67, 85). Heterozygous offspring were then mated to produce homozygous progeny. Mice with a single mutant Rb allele are susceptible to pituitary tumors but, paradoxically, not retinoblastomas. The pituitary tumor's expression of the remaining wild-type Rb allele lacks a "second hit." Loss of this second allele manifests a lack of DNA injury and confirms the importance of Rb in the genesis of these tumors. It is unclear why these mice do not develop retinoblastomas. Most homozygous mice appear normal at day 11 of gestation but die by day 15; this implies that expression of pRb is essential for normal development. In these mice, there is a profound defect in erythropoiesis and widespread neuronal death.

p53 Tumor Suppressor Gene

p53 is a nuclear and sequence-specific binding protein involved in the regulation of transcription (26, 141, 177). It is central to important cellular processes such as cell cycle arrest in response to DNA damage and the induction of apoptosis. Loss of the p53-mediated G1 cell cycle checkpoint may produce genomic instability, as DNA aberrations occur following prolonged culture of cells containing mutant p53. Genomic instability is a hallmark of transformed cells (200). Indeed, because of its role in cell cycle arrest following DNA damage and its role in DNA repair, p53 has been called a "guardian of the genome."

p53 is the most frequently mutated gene in sporadic human cancer. p53 mutations occur in tumors of the colon, lung, esophagus, breast, liver, brain, and hemopoietic tissues (63). The spectrum of p53 mutations varies with tumor type; for example, a mutation in codon 273 predominates in brain tumors (141). Mutations in p53 tend to occur at one of four hot spots where they preclude binding of p53 to DNA and its activation gene transcription (177). Other mutations alter conformation of the protein, such that it both inactivates and interferes with wild-type molecules. In this blocking of the function of wild-type protein p53, mutants act in a "dominant negative" fashion (177). p53 is also inactivated by DNA viral oncoproteins (SV40 large T-antigen, adenovirus E1B, and human papilloma virus E6) that bind p53, inhibit its activity, and engender transformation. p53 can also be inhibited by binding the MDM2 protein, whose gene is amplified in some sarcomas (177).

The importance of p53 as a tumor suppressor gene is highlighted in Li Fraumeni syndrome (96, 97). Individuals affected by this rare familial cancer syndrome develop a wide variety of neoplasms, most commonly breast carcinomas and soft tissue sarcomas, but also brain tumors, osteosarcomas, lung carcinomas, adrenocortical carcinomas, and leukemias. The pattern of inheritance is autosomal dominant. Tumors occur at young ages, and multiple primary tumors are common. By age 30 the risk of cancer is 50%, compared to 1% in the general population (96). Affected individuals have a germ line mutation in one p53 allele, and their tumors have lost the remaining wild-type allele (97).

Transgenic mice with loss of one or both alleles appear developmentally normal but are prone to develop tumors (27). Tumor formation is rare in heterozygous animals but almost universal in homozygous animals. Approximately 75% of homozygous mice have tumors at 6 months of age, most commonly malignant lymphomas and sarcomas.

CELL SENESCENCE

Tumor cells *in vitro* are commonly able to divide indefinitely as long as they are provided with adequate nutrients and growth factors. Such tumor cells are said to be immortal. On the other hand, normal diploid cells in culture usually proliferate only for a limited number of cell divisions before they lose the ability to synthesize DNA and undergo mitosis. Then they are unable to divide despite growth factors in the medium and competent growth factor receptors on their cell surface (134). A normal cell in this state is said to be senescent. Escape from senescence may be tumorigenic. Cell senescence is important to both normal and neoplastic control of cell proliferation as well as to human degenerative disorders in which it may be prematurely activated.

Most studies of cellular senescence use fibroblast cells in culture. Normal diploid fibroblasts can proliferate in culture for approximately 50 population doublings before they acquire the senescent phenotype (54). Senescent fibroblast cells are larger, less motile, and grow at a lower saturation density than young fibroblasts (46). These cells have more RNA, proteins, glycogen, and lipids, although most have a normal amount of DNA (46). Senescent cells acquire chromosomal aberrations possibly related to loss of telomeric DNA (see below). In a population of senescent cells, fewer cells cycle, and those that do have increased cell cycle length. Senescent cells are unable to progress through the cell cycle and synthesize DNA in response to growth factor stimulation (178). Senescent cells unable to divide are arrested in the G1 phase of the cell cycle (152, 160). Senescent cells can be distinguished from quiescent cells, which are also growth arrested in G0 phase by their larger size (160). The time to senescence is an innate biological property of the cell. It correlates with the number of previous cell divisions and not the actual chronological age of the cell (54). As an example, if a culture of cells is growth arrested by serum starvation or contact inhibition, the length of time spent at growth arrest does not affect the total number of cell divisions that a cell can achieve (54, 178).

In fibroblast cells, the senescent phenotype is dominant. Fusion of young and old cells prevents the young nucleus from synthesizing DNA. This suggests that a cytoplasmic factor in the old cells prevents initiation of DNA synthesis (46). Senescence resembles a state of cellular differentiation characterized by an altered specific profile of gene expression (46, 178). At the end of a cell's proliferative life span, a pattern of gene expression is activated that leads to growth arrest and morphological change. At the same time, the expression of genes stimulating growth may be downregulated. The transcription of the proto-oncogene c-fos is suppressed in senescent cells (46). Some of the genes, including senescence genes, may actually be tumor suppressor genes.

Senescent cells predominantly express the hypophosphorylated or growth inhibitory form of the retinoblastoma protein, although the total amount of pRb is unaltered (42, 178). Senescent cells have decreased mRnA for CDK1, cyclin A, and cyclin B1 (1, 166) and decreased CDK2 protein (28). However, the interaction among cyclins, CDKs, and pRb in senescence is extremely complex. Induction of CDK expression in senescent cells does not restore proliferative ability. Although increased levels of cyclin D1 and cyclin E occur in senescent fibroblasts (28), these proteins are hypophosphorylated and are likely trapped in inactivated protein complexes (28).

Expression of the sdil (senescent cell-derived inhibitor) inhibits DNA synthesis. It was cloned from senescent fibroblasts which expressed it at levels 10- to 20-fold higher than do young cells (123). Sdil encodes the previously described p21 involved in inhibition of p53-regulated CDK. p21 is thus likely important to cell cycle arrest and inhibition of DNA synthesis in senescent cells (178). p21 expression increases in senescent cells (171). Other CDKIs such as p16^{INK4} may also be involved in cellular senescence. Escape from senescence by Li-Fraumeni fibroblasts is associated with loss of the remaining p53 allele and loss of p16^{INK4} expression (149). Other candidate senescence genes may reside on chromosome 1. Human-hamster cell fusions that escape cell senescence lack both copies of chromosome 1 (170). Reintroduction of chromosome 1 into these cells restore cell senescence (170).

In cells that become senescent the telomeres, the ends of the chromosomes, progressively shorten as the cell ages (21). Telomeres consist of repetitive DNA sequences (TTAGGG) and protein. Because DNA polymerases are unable to completely replicate linear DNA molecules, DNA of the telomere region must be replicated without DNA template guidance by enzymes called telomerases (21). Telomerases reverse transcribe their own RNA to produce the repeat DNA (163). Telomeres protect the ends of the chromosomes against illegitimate recombination and may be involved in chromosomal attachment to the nuclear envelope (21). Loss of telomeres leads to chromosome instability and deletions which may arrest cell proliferation.

The length of telomeres in fibroblasts, cells with a limited life span *in vitro*, correlates with the remaining number of cell divisions which can occur before they senesce (163). Normal cells with unlimited proliferative potential, such as unicellular organisms and germ cells, have stable telomeres and active telomerases (21, 163). Immortal cells and tumor cells also preserve telomere length. Reactivation of telomerases in these cells may allow addition of repetitive DNA to the ends of the chromosomes and preservation of proliferative ability. Reactivation of telomerases is likely a late step in tumor formation, as cells of many tumors have shortened telomeres. However, in a model of neoplastic transformation of normal mammalian cells by viral oncoproteins, cells initially develop shorter telomeres, but those cells that become immortal preserve telomere length and express telomerases (21). Telomerase activity is prevalent in biopsies of malignant tumor and germline tissues but is absent in normal tissues (178).

APOPTOSIS

Homeostasis in a multicellular organism involves sophisticated control of not only cell proliferation and differentiation but also cell death (167). Apoptosis is a type of cell death distinct from necrosis, defined by characteristic biochemical and morphological changes. Apoptotic cell death is unique in being gene directed; there is a growing repertoire of genes whose expression or lack thereof is linked to apoptosis. Cell death by apoptosis eliminates cells produced in excess, improperly developed cells, and damaged cells (173). In a number of circumstances, apoptosis can be considered "physiological" cell death as it is used to limit cell number in normal physiological processes, such as the regression of lactating breast tissue following weaning (77).

Apoptotic cell death is common during development. During maturation of a limb, death of cells in the interdigital spaces leads to the formation of fingers and toes (20). The terms "programmed cell death" and apoptosis have often been used interchangeably in the literature, and there is ongoing debate over the precise use of these terms. Apoptosis occurs in every organ and is widely conserved throughout evolution, from worms to fruit flies to mammals (20).

Although triggered by a diverse array of signals, apoptosis is probably executed through a common pathway (173) (Fig. 8). Apoptotic cell death can follow with intrinsic or extrinsic influences on the cell (167). Apoptotic cell death during development likely represents timely execution of a cell death pathway whose activation is innate to the developing cell. However, extrinsic factors can be difficult to separate from intrinsic factors. The actual choice of which particular cell dies during apoptosis may be determined by the local concentration of growth factors, the absence of cell to cell contact, or the absence of cell contact with the extracellular matrix (189). Other extrinsic stimuli leading to apoptosis include ionizing radiation, reactive oxygen species, chemotherapeutic drugs, and viral infection (167).

Disordered apoptosis has been implicated in numerous important human diseases: degenerative neurological disease such as Alzheimer's disease, autoimmune disease such as systemic lupus erythematosis, and cancer. A chromosomal arrangement characteristic of follicular lymphoma results in excessive expression of bcl-2 gene that prevents apoptosis. Loss of cells in the reperfused zone of an ischemic stroke occurs by apoptosis. As apoptosis is better understood, new therapeutic strategies may target imbalances in apoptotic pathways.

The Morphology and Biochemistry of Apoptosis

The term apoptosis was first used to describe the death of cells associated with atrophy of the liver induced by ligating a large branch of the portal vein (78). It is characterized by shrinkage of cells and fragmentation of chromatin. A characteristic pattern of DNA fragmentation appears as a ladder on electrophoresis (98, 191).

Apoptosis is characterized by cell shrinkage and compaction of chromatin against the nuclear membrane (for review see Kerr (77) and Manjo (98)). The nucleus may fragment, and the cell frequently develops cytoplasmic processes that envelope these pyknotic nuclear fragments. The processes may separate from the cell as apoptotic bodies which are then phagocytosed by macrophages. Swelling of organelles or mitochondria does not occur. An important feature of apoptosis is that the dying cell is contained within the plasma membrane. Because none of the cell's contents leak into the

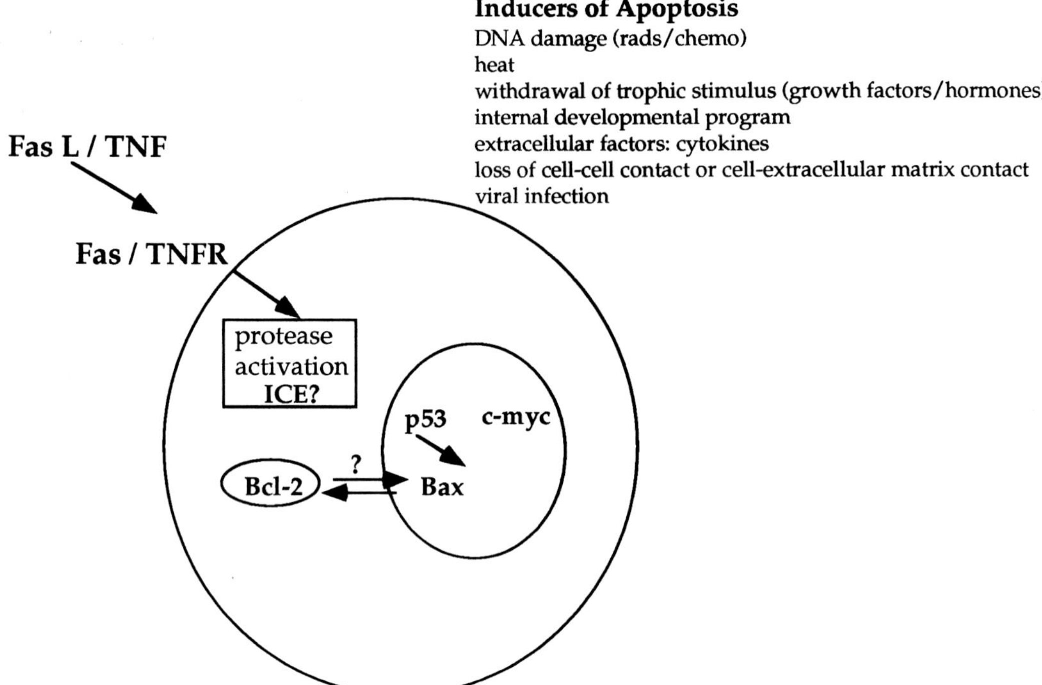

Figure 8. Understanding of the mechanisms of programmed cell death is limited. A few of the genes associated with apoptosis have been discovered, but the mechanisms by which they cause cell death are still largely unknown. This figure lists some precipitants of cell death and some of the gene products involved. In lymphocytes, activation of cell surface receptors, Fas or TNFR, leads to cell death by an undescribed pathway. DNA damage can induce p53 expression, and p53 may induce expression of Bax which is associated with apoptosis. Bcl-2 prevents cell death, and in some experimental systems, the relative amounts of Bax and Bcl-2 determines whether a cell dies or lives. C-myc may also trigger apoptosis in the event of conflicting cellular signals. For example, protease activation by ICE in lymphocytes may be a common effector mechanism for initiating the cellular changes of apoptosis.

extracellular environment, there is no inflammatory reaction. The ladder pattern of DNA fragmentation results from DNA cleavage between nucleosomes. This produces fragments that are multiples of 180 base pairs (a nucleosome is the basic subunit of the chromosome consisting of 180 bp of DNA wrapped around histone proteins).

Necrotic cell death, such as that following arterial infarction, is very different from apoptotic cell death. During necrosis, mitochondrial dysfunction reduces the energy required to maintain function of membrane ion channels and cells swell (20). Cell rupture releases intracellular contents that induce an inflammatory reaction. The nuclei undergo condensation followed by clumping into irregularly defined masses. Organelles initially swell and then disintegrate. In necrosis contiguous cells are usually affected, whereas in apoptosis the cells involved are dispersed (77). Necrosis is always pathological.

Bcl-2 and Protection from Apoptosis

The genetics of apoptosis has been studied in the roundworm, *Caenorhabditis elegans* (for review see Steller (167)). In this simple organism of only 1000 somatic cells, 131 cell deaths occur as the worm matures. Two genes, ced-3 and ced-4, are absolutely required for death of the 131 cells. Mutations in either one of these genes permits survival of the 131 cells otherwise destined to die. One other gene, ced-9, is required to protect cells that should survive from apoptotic cell death; mutations in this gene cause widespread ectopic cell death (167). The regulators of apoptosis in *C. elegans* have homologues in mammalian cells. Ced-3 is homologous to the apoptosis effector protein inter-leukin-1β-converting enzyme (ICE) (see discussion below), and ced-9 is homologous to bcl-2 (B-cell lymphoma/leukemia-2 gene), a proto-oncogene frequently dysregulated in follicular lymphoma (145).

Bcl-2 expression is overexpressed in B-cell malignancies by virtue of a chromosomal translocation t(14;18) which places an immunoglobulin heavy chain enhancer adjacent to the bcl-2 gene (145). Bcl-2 expression promotes cell survival without increasing cell proliferation (145). Microinjection of a bcl-2 expression vector into neurons that are normally dependent on certain neurotrophic factors protects these neurons when the neurotrophic factors are withdrawn (2). Overexpression of bcl-2 can protect a variety of cells from apoptosis induced by stimuli, such as chemotherapeutic drugs, gamma or ultraviolet irradiation, and free radicals (145). Conversely, reductions in bcl-2 expression by antisense techniques accelerates cell death when growth factors are withdrawn (145). Bcl-2 also inhibits apoptosis mediated by the proto-oncogene c-myc and the tumor suppressor gene p53 (145). However, some stimuli can initiate apoptosis even when bcl-2 is overexpressed (145).

Most agents to which bcl-2 confers resistance against apoptosis cause DNA damage. Bcl-2 neither protects cells from the damage nor aids in their repair, but it does prevent damaged DNA from activating the apoptosis pathway. Unfortunately, little is known so far about the actual function of bcl-2. Immunohistochemical staining localizes the protein to the nuclear envelope, endoplasmic reticulum, and the mitochondrial membrane. This suggests that bcl-2 may be involved in nuclear transport, nuclear envelope maintenance, and intracellular calcium homeostasis (145). The cellular protective effects of bcl-2 involve interactions with other proteins that have structural homology to bcl-2 (128). Bcl-2 can form heterodimers with a protein called bax, and it must associate with bax to prevent cell death (128, 198). Overexpression of bax leads to cell death (128). The relative amounts of bcl-2 and bax may determine survival or cell death following apoptosis (128). If bax homodimers predominate, cell death ensues; if there is sufficient bcl-2 to bind the bax that is present, then cell death is prevented (198).

Other bcl-2-related genes are involved in apoptosis. The bcl-x gene encodes multiple bcl-x proteins through alternatively spliced mRNA. Bcl-xL, highly expressed in adult brain, inhibits apoptosis whereas Bcl-xS, highly expressed in dividing cells, induces apoptosis (7). Another bcl-2 binding protein, bag-1 protects cells from apoptosis when bcl-2 is present. BAG-1 or bcl-2 alone are not protective (172).

p53 Induces Apoptosis

p53 induces apoptosis in response to DNA damage from ionizing radiation or drugs (91). The growth suppressive and apoptosis-inducing effects of p53 are likely mediated by separate pathways (16). Deficiencies in p53 may contribute to tumorigenesis by precluding apoptosis as well as by interfering with p53-mediated G1 arrest. The failure to eliminate cells with DNA damage could select for cells that have become transformed (91).

p53 regulation of apoptosis is closely intertwined with bcl-2; increased expression of bcl-2, which interferes with p53-mediated apoptosis without interfering with p53-mediated cell cycle arrest, can induce transcription of bax; this may accelerate apoptosis by increasing the relative amounts of bax-bax homodimers and by decreasing the amounts of bcl-2-bax heterodimers (110). New gene transcription or protein synthesis, however, may not be necessary for p53-mediated apoptosis (10). In fact, p53 itself may not directly induce apoptosis. Instead, it may lower the threshold for inducing apoptosis (110). Both p53-dependent and p53-independent pathways of apoptosis are inhibited by bcl-2 (16).

The Fas Cell Death Pathway

In the immune system, the Fas pathway induces apoptosis in response to an extracellular signal. This pathway involves stimulation of Fas receptors or tumor necrosis factor receptors (TNFRs) by Fas ligand (FasL) or TNF, respectively. It is important to the elimination of autoreactive T cells (T cells which react with self-antigen complexed with self major histocompatibility complex) both in the thymus and, peripherally, to T cell-mediated cytotoxicity and to peripheral suppression of foreign antigen-activated lymphocytes (120). Binding of FasL expressed on activated T cells or released by activated T cells to Fas, expressed on target

B or T cells, rapidly induces apoptosis without new transcription or protein synthesis. Both TNFRs and Fas receptors are transmembrane proteins with an intracellular "death" domain, an amino acid sequence sufficient to cause cell death. FasL itself is a transmembrane protein expressed almost exclusively on the surface of activated T cells (120). The mechanism of Fas-induced cell death is unknown, but the effects of Fas are partially inhibited by bcl-2 (120). Fas activation may lead to formation of a complex lipid, ceramide, which then activates protein kinases that activate other enzymes effecting cell death (120). A variety of proteins bind to the Fas cytoplasmic "death" domain, suggesting that Fas mediates apoptosis through protein-protein interactions (18). Some glioma cell lines may express Fas and are susceptible to Fas-induced apoptosis when treated with anti-Fas antibody. This mechanism of apoptosis may be useful in treating malignant gliomas (188).

Proteases as Effectors of Apoptosis

Proteases, perhaps arranged in an amplifying cascade similar to the coagulation pathway, are the proximate effectors of apoptosis (102). Proteases may activate or disinhibit other proteins that degrade cellular components such as the cytoskeleton or DNA (102). The cell death gene, ced-3, which is required for apoptosis during the development of *C. elegans*, is homologous to a gene called ICE (interleukin-1β-converting enzyme). ICE encodes a cysteine protease that irreversibly initiates apoptosis (167). Pro-IL-1β is cleaved into its active form by ICE. IL-1β cytokine is an important mediator of inflammation (83, 109). The specific role of IL-1β in apoptotic cell death is unknown. However, overexpression of ICE in mammalian cells activates apoptosis; this is partially inhibited by bcl-2. Cell death effectors such as ICE are constitutively expressed, and cell death or survival may be determined by the relative amounts of cell death effectors and protective proteins (167).

Proteins with structural homology to ICE act as both positive and negative regulators of cell death pathways (182). Abnormal regulation of ICE may produce aberrant cell death. High levels of IL-1β occur in pathological states such as Alzheimer's disease, rheumatoid arthritis, septic shock, and head injury (109). In these situations, inhibition of ICE activity may be therapeutic (109). To date, tumorigenesis has not been attributed to inactivation of ICE-like proteases (102).

Apoptosis and Link to the Cell Cycle

During mitosis, chromatin condenses and the lamin intermediate filament component of the nuclear envelope dissolves to facilitate separation of the nuclear material into two daughter cells. Because the nuclear changes of mitosis resemble those of apoptosis, and because CDC2 kinase activation mediates these mitotic changes, activation of CDKs may contribute to apoptosis (161, 162). An apoptotic signal may activate cyclin B1/CDC2 kinase at an inappropriate time in the cell cycle (161) and induce "abortive" mitosis that morphologically resembles apoptosis. Aberrant activation of CDKs may explain the nuclear dissolution occurring at the end of apoptotic cell death. In some situations, the timing of apoptosis in response to an apoptotic stimulus may be cell cycle phase-dependent. In apoptosis induced in T cells by apoptotic agents (concanavalin A or anti-CD3 antibodies, agents which stimulate T-cell surface receptors), cell death occurs only during G2-M transition, even if the apoptotic stimulus is applied at a different phase of the cell cycle (41). The induction of strand breaks characteristic of apoptosis parallel elevation of cyclin B/CDC2 kinase activity and coincide with the associated decline in CDC2 phosphotyrosine. Antisense oligonucleotides to cyclin B inhibit the induction of apoptotic cell death by concanavalin A or anti-CD3 but not that induced by other stimuli. This suggests that cyclin B/CDC2 only mediates certain types of apoptosis in these cells. Cyclin A kinase activity increases in association with CDC2 and CDK2 when HeLa cells are treated with apoptosis-inducing agents (106). Interestingly, in cells transfected with bcl-2, nuclear CDC2 and CDK2 and their associated kinase activity decline. This suggests that bcl-2 may inhibit apoptosis by another mechanism.

The positive cell cycle regulator c-myc may also regulate apoptosis. Apoptosis occurs if the cell receives conflicting growth signals (such as coexpression of p53 and E2F, as described above). As an example, induction of high levels of c-myc proto-oncogene (a transcription factor) expression in cultured cells deprived of growth factors triggers apoptotic cell death in a cell cycle-independent manner (130). The mechanism by which c-myc causes apoptosis is unclear. There is evidence for and against a role for p53 in mediating c-myc-induced apoptosis, and the degree of overlap between the apoptotic and cell cycle progression pathways of c-myc is unknown (130). Mechanisms may vary with cell type. Bcl-2 also suppresses c-myc-associated apoptosis (130), and c-myc-induced apoptosis may be mediated by reactive oxygen species (130).

CONCLUSION

The processes of cell proliferation and cell death are exquisitely complex. A number of important proteins involved in regulating cell proliferation may also be involved in cell death. As an example, the p53 protein can induce G1 cell cycle arrest or apoptosis in response to DNA damage. In addition, positive regulators of the cell cycle, such as CDKs may also be involved in both processes. Despite the rapid pace of discovery, many unanswered questions remain. Currently unexplained is why loss of apparently essential growth inhibitory genes, such as pRb or p53, in humans, through inheritance or in animals through gene knockout, results in tumors in some tissues but not in others. The complexity of regulation of proliferation offers tremendous opportunity for such tissue-specific differences. Although the organism has redundancy of critical genes, such as those that restrain cell growth, to prevent potentially injurious processes, not all members of each family of such critical regulatory genes are found in all tissues. This may explain the tissue specificity in the phenotypic effects of activation or inactivation of these genes.

Despite the deficiencies of present knowledge, a better understanding of the molecular mechanisms of cell proliferation has led to the development of new strategies for cancer treatment. The knowledge that the Ras protein must reside at the cell membrane to activate a signal transduction pathway has prompted the design of drugs that inhibit translocation of Ras to the membrane. Restoration of cell cycle arrest by replacing the gene encoding a cell cycle inhibitor may be antineoplastic, and preventing cell death by inhibiting effectors of apoptosis may retard degenerative diseases. Future advances in molecular diagnosis and in targeting cells with gene therapy should yield new and more effective therapies for both cancer and degenerative diseases.

REFERENCES

1. Afshari, C. A., Vojta, P. J., Annab, L. A., *et al.* Investigation of the role of G1/S cell cycle mediators in cellular senescence. Exp. Cell Res. *209:*231–237, 1993.
2. Allsop, T. E., Wyatt, S., Paterson, H. F., *et al.* The proto-oncogene bcl-2 can selectively rescue neurotrophic factor-dependent neurons from apoptosis. Cell *73:*295–307, 1993.
3. Aprelikova, O., Xiong, Y., and Liu, E. T. Both p16^{INK4A} and p21 families of cyclin-dependent kinase inhibitors block the phosphorylation of cyclin dependent kinases by the CDK-activating kinase. J. Biol. Chem. *270:*18195–18197, 1995.
4. Atjada, P., Wong, H., Veillete, C., *et al.* Overexpression of cyclin D1 blocks proliferation of normal diploid fibroblasts. Exp. Cell Res. *217:*205–216, 1995.
5. Bates, S., Paarry, D., Bonetta, L., *et al.* Absence of cyclin D/CDK complexes in cells lacking functional retinoblastoma protein. Oncogene *9:*1633–1640, 1994.
6. Boguski, M. S., and McCormick, F. Proteins regulating ras and its relatives. Nature *366:*643–654, 1993.
7. Boise, L. H., Gonazalez-Garcia, M., Postema, C. E., *et al.* bcl-x, a bcl-2-related gene that functions as a dominant regulator of apoptotic cell death. Cell *74:*597–608, 1993.
8. Bremner, R., Cohen, B. L., Sopta, M., *et al.* Direct transcriptional repression by pRb and its reversal by specific cyclins. Mol. Cell Biol. *15:*3256–3265, 1995.
9. Buchovich, K., Duffy, L. A., and Harlow, E. The retinoblastoma protein is phosphorylated during specific phases of cell cycle. Cell *58:*1097–1105, 1989.
10. Caelles, C., Heimberg, A., and Karin, M. p53-dependent apoptosis in the absence of transcriptional activation of p53 target genes. Nature *370:*220–223, 1994.
11. Caldas, C., Hahn, S. A., da Costa, L. T., *et al.* Frequent somatic mutations and homozygous deletions of the (MTS1) gene in pancreatic adenocarcinoma. Nature Genet. *8:*27–32, 1994.
12. Cantley, L. C., Auger, K. R., Carpenter, C., *et al.* Oncogenes and signal transduction. Cell *64:*281–302, 1991.
13. Cardoso, M. C., Leonhardt, H., and Nadal-Ginard, B. Reversal of terminal differentiation and control of DNA replication: cyclin A and CDK2 specifically localize at subnuclear sites of DNA replication. Cell *74:*979–992, 1995.
14. Casey, P. J. Protein lipidation and cell signalling. Science *268:*221–225, 1995.
15. Chan, F. K., Zhang, J., Cheng, L., *et al.* Identification of mouse p19, a novel CDK4 and CDK6 inhibitor with homology to p16^{INK4}. Mol. Cell Biol. *15:*2682–2688, 1995.
16. Chiou, S. K., Rao, L., and White, E. Bcl-2 blocks

p53-dependent pathways. Mol. Cell Biol. *14:*2556–2563, 1994.

17. Clark, E. A., and Brugge, J. S. Integrins and signal transduction pathways: the road taken. Science *268:*233–239, 1995.

18. Cleveland, J. L., and Ihle, J. N. Contenders in FasL/TNF signalling. Cell *81:*479–482, 1995.

19. Cohen, G. B., Ren, R., and Baltimore, D. Molecular binding domains of signal transduction proteins. Cell *80:*237–248, 1995.

20. Cohen, J. J. Apoptosis: physiologic cell death. J. Lab. Clin. Med. *124:*761–765, 1994.

21. Counter, C. M., Avilion, A. A., LeFeuvre, C. E., *et al.* Telomere shortening associated with chromosomal instability is arrested in immortal cells which express telomerase activity. EMBO J. *11:*1921–1929, 1992.

22. Crew, C. M., and Erikson, R. L. Extracellular signals and reversible protein phosphorylation: what to Mek of it al. Cell *74:*215–217, 1993.

23. Cross, M., and Dexter, T. M. Growth factors in development, transformation, and tumorigenesis. Cell *64:*271–280, 1991.

24. Darnell, J. E., Kerr, I. M., and Stark, G. R. Jak-STAT pathways and transcriptional activation in response to IFNs and other extracellular signalling proteins. Science *264:*1415–1421, 1994.

25. Davis, R. J. The mitogen-activate protein kinase signal transduction pathway. J. Biol. Chem. *268:*14553–14556, 1993.

25A. DeCaprio, J. A., Furukama, Y., Ajchenbaum, F., et al. The Retinoblastoma-Susceptibility Gene Product Becomes Phosphorylated in Multiple Stages During Cell Cycle Entry and Progression. Proc. Nat. Acad. *89:*1795–1798, 1992.

26. Donehower, L. A., and Bradley, A. The tumor suppressor p53. Biochem. Biophys. Acta *1155:*181–205, 1993.

27. Donehower, L. A., Harvey, M., Slage, B. L., *et al.* Mice deficient for p53 are developmentally normal but susceptible to spontaneous tumors. Nature *356:*215–221, 1992.

28. Dulic, V., Drullinger, L. F., Lees, E., *et al.* Altered regulation of G1 cyclins in senescent human diploid fibroblasts: accumulation of inactive cyclin E-cdk2 and cyclin D2-cdk3 complexes. Proc. Natl. Acad. Sci. U.S.A. *90:*11034–11038, 1993.

29. Dulic, V., Kaufmann, W. K., Wilson, S. J., *et al.* p53 dependent inhibition of cyclin dependent kinase activities in human fibroblasts during radiation induced G1 arrest. Cell *76:*1013–1023, 1994.

30. Dulic, V., Lees, E., and Reed, S. I. Association of human cyclin E with a periodic G1-S phase protein kinase. Science *257:*1958–1961, 1992.

31. Ekstrand, A. J., James, C. D., Cavanee, W. K., *et al.* Genes for epidermal growth factor receptor, transforming growth factor-α, and epidermal growth factor and their expression in human gliomas in vivo. Cancer Res. *51:*2164–2172, 1991.

32. Ekstrand, A. J., Sugawa, N., James, C. D., *et al.* Amplified and rearranged epidermal growth factor receptor genes in human glioblastomas reveal deletions of sequences encoding portions of the N-

and/or C-terminal tails. Proc. Natl. Acad. Sci. *89:*4309–4313, 1992.

33. El-Deiry, Ws., Harper, J. W., O'Connor, P. M., *et al.* WAF1/CIP1 is induced in p53 mediated G1 arrest and apoptosis. Cancer Res. *54:*1169, 1994.

34. El-Deiry, Ws., Tokino, T., Velculescu, V. E., *et al.* WAF 1: a potential mediator of p53 tumor suppression. Cell *75:*817, 1994.

35. Elledge, S. J., and Harper, J. W. Cdk inhibitors: on the threshold of checkpoints and development. Curr. Opin. Cell Biol. *6:*847–852, 1994.

36. Evans, T., Rosenthal, E. T., Youngblom, J., *et al.* Cyclin: a protein specific by maternal mRNA in sea urchin eggs that is destroyed at each cleavage division. Cell *33:*389–396, 1983.

37. Ewen, M. E. The cell cycle and the retinoblastoma protein family. Cancer Metastasis Rev. *13:*45–66, 1994.

38. Farnham, P. J., Slansky, J. E., and Kollmar, R. The role of E2F in the mammalian cell cycle. Biochem. Biophys. Acta *1155:*125–131, 1993.

39. Filmus, J., Robles, A. I., Shi, W., *et al.* Induction of cyclin D1 overexpression by activated ras. Oncogene *9:*3627–3633, 1994.

40. Fisher, R. P., and Morgan, D. O. A novel cyclin associates with MO15/CDK7 to form the CDK-activating kinase. Cell *78:*713–724, 1994.

41. Fotedar, R., Flatt, J., Gupta, S., *et al.* Activation-induced T-cell death is cell cycle dependent and regulated by cyclin B. Mol. Cell Biol. *15:*932–942, 1995.

42. Futreal, P. A., and Barrett, J. C. Failure of senescent cells to phosphorylate the RB protein. Oncogene *6:*1109–1113, 1991.

43. Gibbs, J. B. Ras C-terminal processing enzymes—new drug targets? Cell *65:*1–4, 1991.

44. Girard, F., Struasfield, Fernandez, A., *et al.* Cyclin A is required for the onset of DNA replication in mammalian fibroblasts. Cell *67:*1169–1179, 1991.

45. Glotzer, M., Murray, A. M., and Kirschner, M. W. Cyclin is degraded by the ubiquitin pathway. Nature *349:*132–138, 1991.

46. Goldstein, S. Replicative senescence: the human fibroblast comes of age. Science *249:*1129–1133, 1990.

47. Gu, Y., Rosenblatt, J., and Morgan, D. O. Cell cycle regulation of CDK2 activity by phosphorylation of Thr 160 and Tyr 15. EMBO J. *11:*3995–4005, 1992.

48. Guadagno, T. M., Ohtsubo, M., Roberts, J. M., *et al.* A link between cyclin A expression and adhesion-dependent cell cycle progression. Science *262:*1572–1575, 1993.

49. Guan, K. L., Jenkins, C. W., Li, Y., *et al.* Growth suppression by p18, a p16[INK4] and p14[INK4B]-related CDK6 inhibitor correlates with wild-type pRb function. Genes Dev. *8:*2939–2952, 1994.

50. Hall, A. A biochemical function for Ras-at last. Science *264:*1413–1414, 1994.

51. Han, E. K., Sgambato, A., Jiang, W., *et al.* Stable overexpression of cyclin D1 in a human mammary epithelial cell line prolongs the S-phase and inhibits growth. Oncogene *10:*953–961, 1995.

52. Hannon, G. J., and Beach, D. p15[INK4B] is a potential

effector of TGF-β-induced cell cycle arrest. Nature *371*:257–261, 1994.

53. Harper, J. W., Adami, G. R., Wei, N., *et al.* The p21 Cdk-interacting protein Cip1 is a potent inhibitor of G1 cyclin dependent kinases. Cell *75*:805–816, 1993.

54. Hayflick, L. The limited in vitro lifetime of human diploid cell strains. Exp. Cell Res. *37*:614–636, 1965.

55. Heald, R., and McKeon, F. Mutations of phosphorylation sites in lamin A that prevent nuclear lamina disassembly in mitosis. Cell *61*:579–589, 1990.

56. Heald, R., McLoughlin, M., and McKeon, F. Human Wee1 maintains mitotic timing by protecting the nucleus from cytoplasmically activated cdc2 kinase. Cell *74*:463–474, 1993.

57. Heichman, K. A., and Roberts, J. M. Rules to replicate by. Cell *79*:557–562, 1994.

58. Heim, M. H., Kerr, I. M., Stark, G. R., *et al.* Contribution of the STAT SH2 groups to the specific interferon signalling by the Jak-STAT pathway. Science *267*:1347–1353, 1995.

59. Herber, B., Truss, M., Beato, M., *et al.* Inducible regulatory elements in the human cyclin D1 promotor, 1994.

60. Hill, C. S., and Treisman, R. Transcriptional regulation by extracellular signals: mechanisms and specificity. Cell *80*:199–211, 1995.

61. Hinds, P. W., Dowdy, S. F., Eaton, E. N., *et al.* Function of a human cyclin gene as an oncogene. Proc. Natl. Acad. Sci. U.S.A. *91*:709–713, 1994.

62. Hirai, H., Roussel, M. F., Kato, J. Y., *et al.* Novel INK4 proteins p19 and p18, are specific inhibitors of the cyclin D-dependent kinases CDK4 and CDK6. Mol. Cell Biol. *15*:2672–2681, 1995.

63. Hollstein, M., Sidransky, D., Vogelstein, B., *et al.* p53 mutations in human cancer. Science *253*:49–53, 1991.

64. Huang, H. J., Yee, J. K., Shew, J. Y., *et al.* Suppression of the neoplastic phenotype by replacement of the Rb gene in human cancer cells. Science *242*:1563–1566, 1988.

65. Hunter, T., and Pines, J. Cyclins and cancer II: cyclin D and CDK inhibitors come of age. Cell *79*:573, 1994.

66. Hussussian, C. J., Stuewing, J. P., Golstein, A. M., *et al.* Germline p16 mutations in familial melanoma. Nature Genet. *8*:15–21, 1994.

67. Jacks, T., Fazeli, A., Schmitt, E. M., *et al.* Effects of an Rb mutation in the mouse. Nature *359*:295–300, 1992.

68. Jeffrey, P. D., Russo, A. A., Polyak, K., *et al.* Mechanism of CDK activation revealed by the crystal structure of a cyclin A-CDK2 complex. Nature *376*:313–320, 1995.

69. Jen, J. J., Harper, J. W., Bigner, S., *et al.* Deletion of p16 and p14 in brain tumors. Cancer Res. *54*:6353–6358, 1995.

70. Jiang, W., Kahn, S. M., Zhou, P., *et al.* Overexpression of cyclin D1 in rat fibroblasts causes abnormalities in growth control, cell cycle progression, and gene expression. Oncogene *8*:3447–3457, 1993.

71. Jiang, W., Zhang, Y. J., Kahn, S. M., *et al.* Altered expression of the cyclin D1 and retinoblastoma genes in human esophageal cancer. Proc. Natl. Acad. Sci. U.S.A. *90*:9026, 1993.

72. Johnson, D. G., Schwarz, J. K., Cress, W. D., *et al.* Expression of transcription factor E2F1 induces quiescent cells to enter S phase. Nature *365*:349–352, 1993.

73. Kamb, A., Gruis, N. A., Weaver-Feldhaus, J., *et al.* A cell cycle regulator potentially involved in the genesis of many tumor types. Science *264*:436–440, 1994.

74. Kamb, A., Shattuck-Eidens, D., Eeles, R., *et al.* Analysis of the p16 gene (CDKN2) as a candidate for the chromosome 9p melanoma susceptibility locus. Nature Genet. *8*:22–26, 1994.

75. Kato, J., Matsushime, H., Hiebert, S. W., *et al.* Direct binding of cyclin D to the retinoblastoma gene product (pRb) and pRb phosphorylation by the cyclin D-dependent kinase CDK4. Genes Dev. *7*:331–342, 1993.

76. Kato, J. Y., Matsuoka, M., Polyak, K., *et al.* Cyclic AMP-induced G1 phase arrest mediated by an inhibitor (p27^{kip1}) of cyclin dependent kinase activation. Cell *79*:487–496, 1994.

77. Kerr, J. F., Winterford, C. M., and Harmon, B. V. Apoptosis and its significance in cancer and cancer therapy. Cancer *73*:2013–2026, 1994.

78. Kerr, J. F., Wylie, A. H., and Currie, A. R. Apoptosis: a basic biological phenomenon with wide ranging implications in tissue kinetics. Br. J. Cancer *26*:239–257, 1972.

79. Khosravi-Far, R., and Channing, C. J. The ras signal transduction pathway. Cancer Metastasis Rev. *13*:67–89, 1994.

80. Knudson, A. G. Mutation and cancer. Proc. Natl. Acad. Sci. U.S.A. *68*:820–823, 1971.

81. Koff, A., Giordano, A., Desai, D., *et al.* Formation and activation of cyclin E-cdk2 complex during the G1 phase of the human cell cycle. Science *257*:1689–1694, 1992.

82. Koshland, D. Mitosis: back to basics. Cell *77*:951–954, 1994.

83. Kuida, K., Lippke, J. A., Ku, G., *et al.* Altered cytokine export and apoptosis in mice deficient in interleukin 1β converting enzyme. Nature *267*:2000–2003, 1995.

84. Laskey, R. A., Fairman, M. P., and Blow, J. J. S phase of the cell cycle. Science *246*:609–614, 1989.

85. Lee, E. Y., Chang, C. Y., Hu, N., *et al.* Mice deficient for Rb are nonviable and show defects in neurogenesis and hematopoiesis. Nature *359*:288–294, 1992.

86. Lee, M. H., Reynisdottir, I., and Massague, J. Cloning of p57^{KIP2}, a cyclin-dependent kinase inhibitor with a unique domain structure and tissue distribution. Genes Dev. *9*:639–649, 1995.

87. Leevers, S. J., Paterson, H. F., and Marshall, C. J. Requirement for Ras in Raf activation is overcome by targeting Raf to the plasma membrane. Nature *369*:411–414, 1994.

88. Li, R., Waga, S., Hannon, G. J., *et al.* Differential effects by the p21 CDK inhibitor on PCNA dependent DNA replication and repair. Nature *371*:534–537, 1994.

89. Li, Y., Nichols, M. A., Shay, J. W., *et al.* Transcriptional repression of the D-type cyclin-dependent

kinase inhibitor p16 by the retinoblastoma susceptibility gene product. Cancer Res. *54:*6078–6082, 1994.

90. Liu, J. J., Chao, J. R., Jiang, M. C., *et al.* Ras transformation results in an elevated level of cyclin D1 and acceleration of G1 progression in NIH 3T3 cells. Mol. Cell Biol. *15:*3654–3663, 1995.

91. Lowe, S. W., Ruley, H. E., Jacks, T., *et al.* p53-dependent apoptosis modulates the cytotoxicity of anticancer agents. Cell *74:*957–967, 1993.

92. Lowenstein, E. J., Daly, R. J., Batzer, A. G., *et al.* The SH2 and SH3 domain-containing protein GRB2 links receptor tyrosine kinases to Ras signalling. Cell *70:*431–442, 1992.

93. Lukas, J., Muller, H., Bartkova, J., *et al.* DNA tumor virus oncoproteins and retinoblastoma gene mutations share the ability to relieve the cell's requirement of cyclin D1 function in G1. J. Cell Biol. *125:*625–638, 1994.

94. Lukas, J., Pagano, M., Statkova, Z., *et al.* Cyclin D1 protein oscillates and is essential for cell cycle progression in human tumor cell lines. Oncogene *9:*707–718, 1994.

95. Luo, Y., Hurwitz, J., and Massague. Cell cycle inhibition by independent CDK and PCNA binding domains in p21. Nature *375:*159–161, 1995.

96. Malkin, D. p53 and the Li Fraumeni syndrome. Biochim. Biophys. Acta *1198:*197–213, 1994.

97. Malkin, D., Li, F. P., Strong, L. C., *et al.* Germ line p53 mutations in a familial syndrome of breast cancer, sarcomas, and other neoplasms. Science *250:*1233–1238, 1990.

98. Mango, G., and Joris, I. Apoptosis, oncosis, and necrosis. Am. J. Pathol. *146:*3–15, 1995.

99. Marais, R., Light, Y., Paterson, H. F., *et al.* Ras recruits Raf-1 to the plasma membrane for activation by tyrosine phosphorylation. EMBO J. *13:*3136–3145, 1995.

100. Marshall, C. J. Tumor suppressor genes. Cell *64:*313–326, 1991.

101. Marshall, C. J. Specificity of tyrosine kinase signalling: transient versus sustained extracellular signal-regulated kinase activation. Cell *80:*179–185, 1995.

102. Martin, S. J., and Green, D. R. Protease activation during apoptosis: death by a thousand cuts. Cell *82:*349–352, 1995.

103. Matsuoka, S., Edwards, M. C., Bai, C., *et al.* p57[KIP2], a structurally distinct member of the p21 Cdk inhibitor family, is a candidate tumor suppressor gene. Genes Dev. *9:*650–662, 1995.

104. Matsushime, H., Quelle, D. E., Shurtleff, S. A., *et al.* D-type cyclin dependent kinase activity in mammalian cells. Mol. Cell Biol. *14:*2066–2076, 1994.

105. McIntosh, J. R., and Koonce, M. P. Mitosis. Science *246:*622–628, 1989.

106. Meikrantz, W., Gisselbrecht, S., Tam, S. W., *et al.* Activation of cyclin A-dependent protein kinases during apoptosis. Proc. Natl. Acad. Sci. U.S.A. *91:*3754–3758, 1994.

107. Meyerson, M., and Harlow, E. Identification of G1 kinase activity for cdk6, a novel cyclin D partner. Mol. Cell Biol. *14:*2077, 1994.

108. Michieli, P., Chedid, M., Lin, D., *et al.* Induction of WAF1/CIP1 by a p53 independent pathway. Cancer Res. *54:*3391–3395, 1994.

109. Miura, M., Zhu, H., Rotello, R., *et al.* Induction of apoptosis in fibroblasts by IL-1β-converting enzyme, a mammalian homologue of the C. elegans cell death gene ced-3. Cell *75:*653–660, 1993.

110. Miyashita, T., and Reed, J. C. Tumor suppressor p53 is a direct transcriptional activator of the human bax gene. Cell *80:*293–299, 1995.

111. Mochly-Rosen, D. Localization of protein kinases by anchoring proteins: a theme in signal transduction. Science *268:*247–251, 1995.

112. Morgan, D. O. Principles of CDK regulation. Nature *374:*131–134, 1995.

113. Morrison, R. S., Gross, J. L., Herblin, W. F., *et al.* Basic fibroblast growth factor-like activity and receptors are expressed in a human glioma cell line. Cancer Res. *50:*2524–2529, 1990.

114. Morrison, R. S., Yamaguchi, F., Bruner, J. M., *et al.* Fibroblast growth factor receptor gene expression and immunoreactivity are elevated in human glioblastoma multiforme. Cancer Res. *54:*2794–2799, 1994.

115. Motokura, T., Bloom, T., Kim, H. G., *et al.* A novel cyclin encoded by a bcl-1 linked candidate oncogene. Nature *350:*512–515, 1991.

116. Moulton, T., Samara, G., Chung, W. Y., *et al.* MTS1/p16/CDKN2 lesions in primary glioblastoma multiforme. Am. J. Pathol. *146:*613–619, 1995.

117. Muller, H., Lukas, J., Schneider, A., *et al.* Cyclin D1 expression is regulated by the retinoblastoma protein. Proc. Natl. Acad. Sci. U.S.A. *91:*2945–2949, 1994.

118. Murray, A., and Hunt, A. *The Cell Cycle.* W. H. Freeman, New York, 1993.

119. Mustonen, T., and Alitalo, K. Endothelial receptor tyrosine kinases involved in angiogenesis. J. Cell Biol. 895–898, 1995.

120. Nagata, S., and Goldstein, P. The Fas death factor. Science *267:*1449–1456, 1995.

121. Nevins, J. R. E2F: a link between the Rb tumor suppressor protein and viral oncoproteins. Science *258:*424–429, 1992.

122. Nishikawa, R., Furnari, F. B., Lin, H., *et al.* Loss of p15 expression is frequent in high grade glioma. Cancer Res. *55:*1941–1945, 1995.

123. Noda, A., Ning, Y., Venable, S. F., *et al.* Cloning of senescent derived inhibitors of DNA synthesis using an expression screen. Exp. Cell Res. *211:*90–98, 1994.

124. Nurse, P. Ordering S phase and M phase in the cell cycle. Cell *79:*547–550, 1994.

125. Ohtsubo, M., and Roberts, J. M. Cyclin dependent regulation of G1 in mammalian fibroblasts. Science *259:*1908–1912, 1993.

126. Ohtsubo, M., Theodoras, A. M., Schumacher, J., *et al.* Human cyclin E, a nuclear protein essential for the G1-to-S phase transition. Mol. Cell Biol. *15:*2612–2624, 1995.

127. Okamoto, A., Demetrick, E. A., Spillare, E. A., *et al.* Mutations and altered expression of p16INK4 in human cancer. Proc. Natl. Acad. Sci. U.S.A. *91:*11045–11049, 1994.

128. Oltvai, Z. N., Milliman, C. L., and Korsmeyer, S. J. Bcl-2 heterodimerizes in vivo with a conserved homologue, bax, that accelerates programmed cell death. Cell *74:*609–619, 1993.

129. Otterson, G. A., Kratzke, R. A., Coxon, A., *et al.* Absence of p16 protein is restricted to the subset of lung cancer lines that retains wildtype RB. Oncogene *9:*3375–3378, 1994.

130. Packham, G., and Cleveland, J. L. C-myc and apoptosis. Biochim. Biophys. Acta *1242:*11–28, 1995.

131. Pagano, M., Pepperkok, R., Verde, F., *et al.* Cyclin A is required at two points in the human cell cycle. EMBO J. *11:*961–971, 1992.

132. Pardee, A. B. G1 events and regulation of cell proliferation. Science *246:*603–608, 1989.

133. Parry, D., Bates, S., Mann, D. J., *et al.* Lack of cyclin D-cdk complexes in Rb-negative cells correlates with high levels of p16^{INK4A} tumor suppressor gene product. EMBO J. *14:*503–511, 1995.

134. Paulsson, Y., Bywater, M., Pfeifer-Ohlsson, S., *et al.* Growth factors induce pre-replicative changes in senescent human fibroblasts. EMBO J. *5:*2175–2162, 1986.

135. Pawson, A. Protein molecules and signalling networks. Nature *373:*573–580, 1995.

136. Pawson, T., and Gish, G. SH2 and SH3 domains: from structure to function. Cell *71:*359–362, 1992.

137. Peter, M., Nakagawa, J., Doree, M., *et al.* In vitro disassembly of the nuclear lamina and M phase-specific phosphorylation of lamina by cdc2 kinase. Cell *61:*591–602, 1990.

138. Pines, J. The localization of human cyclins and cdks in the cell cycle. In: *The Cell Cycle: Regulators, Targets, and Clinical Applications,* edited by V. W. Wu, pp. 189–195. Plenum Press, New York, 1994.

139. Polyak, K., Kato, J., Solomon, M. J., *et al.* p27^{kip1}, a cyclin-cdk inhibitor, links transforming growth factor-β and contact inhibition to cell cycle arrest. Genes Dev. *8:*9–22, 1994.

140. Polyak, K., Lee, M. H., Erdjument-Bromage, H., *et al.* Cloning of p27^{kip1}, a cyclin-dependent kinase inhibitor and potential mediator of extracellular signals. Cell *78:*59–66, 1994.

141. Prives, C., and Manfredi, J. J. The tumor suppressor protein: meeting review. Genes Dev. *7:*529–534, 1993.

142. Qio, R. G., Chen, J., Jirn, D., *et al.* An essential role for Rac in Ras transformation. Nature *374:*457–459, 1995.

143. Quelle, D. E., Ashmun, R. A., Hannon, G. J., *et al.* Cloning and characterization of murine p16^{INK4A} and p^{15INK4B} genes. Oncogene *11:*635–645, 1995.

144. Rapp, U. R., Goldsborough, M. D., Mark, G. E., *et al.* Structure and biologic activity of v-raf, a unique oncogene transduced by retrovirus. Proc. Natl. Acad. Sci. U.S.A. *80:*4218–4222, 1983.

145. Reed, J. C. Bcl-2 and the regulation of programmed cell death. J. Cell Biol. *124:*1–6, 1994.

146. Reynisdottir, I., Polyak, K., Iavarone, A., *et al.* KIP/CIP and INK4 CDK inhibitors cooperate to induce cell cycle arrest in response to TGF-β. Genes Dev. *9:*1831–1845, 1995.

147. Ridley, A. J., and Hall, A. The small GTP-binding protein rho regulates assembly of focal adhesions and actin stress fibers in response to growth factors. Cell *70:*389–399, 1992.

148. Ridley, A. J., Paterson, H. F., Johnson, C. L., *et al.* The small GTP-binding protein rac regulates growth factor-induced membrane ruffling. Cell *70:* 401–410, 1992.

149. Rogan, E. M., Bryan, T. M., Hukku, B., *et al.* Alterations in p53 and p16^{INK4} expression and telomere length during spontaneous immortalization of Li-Fraumeni syndrome fibroblasts. Mol. Cell Biol. *15:* 4745–4753, 1995.

150. Ross, R., Raines, E. W., and Bowen-Pope, D. F. The biology of platelet-derived growth factor. Cell *46:* 155–169, 1986.

151. Sasahara, M., Fries, J. W., Raines, E. W., *et al.* PDGF B-chain in neurons of the central nervous system, posterior pituitary, and in a transgenic model. Cell *64:*217–227, 1991.

152. Schneider, E. L., and Fowlikes, B. J. Measurement of DNA content and cell volume in senescent human fibroblasts utilizing flow multiparameter single cell analysis. Exp. Cell Res. *98:*298–302, 1976.

153. Seifert, R. A., Hart, C. E., Phillips, P. E., *et al.* Two different subunits associate to create isoform specific platelet-derived growth factor receptors. J. Biol. Chem. *264:*8771–8778, 1989.

154. Serrano, M., Hannon, G. J., and Beach, D. A new regulatory motif in cell cycle control causing specific inhibition of cyclin D/CDK4. Nature *366:*704–707, 1994.

155. Shamah, S. M., Stiles, C. D., and Guha, A. Dominant-negative mutants of platelet-derived growth factor revert the transformed phenotype of human astrocytoma cells. Mol. Cell Biol. *13:*7203–7212, 1993.

156. Shan, B., and Lee, W. H. Deregulated expression of E2F-1 induces S-phase entry and leads to apoptosis. Mol. Cell Biol. *14:*8166–8173, 1994.

157. Sherr, C. J. Mammalian G1 cyclins. Cell *73:*1059–1065, 1993.

158. Sherr, C. J. G1 phase progression: cycling on cue. Cell *79:*551–555, 1994.

159. Sherr, C. J., and Roberts, J. M. Inhibitors of mammalian G1 cyclin-dependent kinases. Genes Dev. *9:*1149–1163, 1995.

160. Sherwood, S. W., Rush, D., Ellsworth, J. L., *et al.* Defining cellular senescence in IMR-90 cells: a flow cytometric analysis. Proc. Natl. Acad. Sci. U.S.A. *85:*9086–9090, 1988.

161. Shi, L., Nishioka, W. K., Th'ng, J., *et al.* Premature p34cdc2 activation required for apoptosis. Science *263:*1143–1145, 1994.

162. Shimizu, T., O'Connor, P. M., Kohn, K., *et al.* Unscheduled activation of cyclin B1/cdc2 kinase in human promyelocytic leukemia cell line HL 60 cells undergoing apoptosis induced by DNA damage. Cancer Res. *55:*228–231, 1995.

163. Singer, M., and Gottschling, D. E. TLC1: template RNA component of Saccharomyces cervisiae telomerase. Science *266:*404–409, 1994.

164. Singh, P., Wong, S. H., and Hong, W. Overexpression of E2F1 in rat embryo fibroblasts leads to neoplastic transformation. EMBO J. *13:*339–3338, 1994.

165. Stefanik, D. F., Rizkalla, L. R., Soi, A., *et al.* Acidic and basic fibroblast growth factors are present in glioblastoma multiforme. Cancer Res. *51:*5760–5765, 1991.

166. Stein, G. H., Drullinger, L. F., Robetorye, R. S., *et al.* Senescent cells fail to express cdc2, cycA, and cycB

in response to mitogen stimulation. Proc. Natl. Acad. Sci. U.S.A. *88:*11012–11016, 1991.

167. Steller, H. Mechanisms and genes of cellular suicide. Science *267:*1445–1449, 1995.

168. Stoke, D., Macdonald, S. G., Cadwallader, K., *et al.* Activation of raf as a result of recruitment to the plasma membrane. Science *264:*1463–1467, 1994.

169. Strauss, M., Hering, S., Lieber, A., *et al.* Stimulation of cell division and fibroblast focus formation by antisense repression of retinoblastoma protein synthesis. Oncogene *7:*769–773, 1992.

170. Sugawara, O., Oshimura, M., Koi, M., *et al.* Induction of cellular senescence in immortalized cells by human chromosome 1. Science *247:*707–710, 1990.

171. Tahara, H., Sato, E., Noda, A., *et al.* Increase in expression level of p21 sdi1/cip1/waf1 with increasing division age in both normal and SV40 transformed human fibroblasts. Oncogene *10:*835–840, 1995.

172. Takayama, S., Sato, T., Krajewski, S., *et al.* Cloning and functional analysis of bag-1: a novel bcl-2 binding protein with anti-cell death activity. Cell *80:*279–284, 1995.

173. Thompson, C. B. Apoptosis in the pathogenesis and treatment of disease. Science *267:*1456–1462, 1995.

174. Toyoshima, H., and Hunter, T. p27, a novel inhibitor of G1 cyclin-CDK protein kinase activity, is related to p21. Cell *78:*67–74, 1995.

175. Ullrich, A., and Schlessinger, J. Signal transduction by receptors with tyrosine kinase activity. Cell *61:* 203–212, 1990.

176. Ventner, D. J., Bevan, K. L., Ludwig, R. L., *et al.* Retinoblastoma deletions in human glioblastomas. Oncogene *6:*445–448, 1991.

177. Vogelstein, B., and Kinzler, K. W. p53 function and dysfunction. Cell *70:*523–526, 1992.

178. Vojta, P. J., and Barrett, J. C. Genetic analysis of cellular senescence. Biochim. Biophys. Acta *1242:* 29–41, 1995.

179. Votjtek, A. B., Hollengerg, S. M., and Cooper, J. A. Mammalian ras interacts directly with the serine threonine kinase raf. Cell *74:*205–214, 1995.

180. Waga, S., Hannon, G. J., Beach, D., *et al.* The p21 inhibitor of cyclin-dependent kinases inhibits DNA replication by interaction with PCNA. Nature *369:* 574–578, 1994.

181. Wagner, A. J., Kokontis, J. M., and Hay, N. Myc-mediated apoptosis requires wild type p53 in a manner independent of cell cycle arrest and the ability of p53 to induce p21. Genes Dev. *8:*2817–2830, 1994.

182. Wang, L., Miura, M., Bergeron, L., *et al.* Ich-1, and Ice/Ced-3-related gene, encodes both positive and negative regulators of programmed cell death. Cell *78:*739–750, 1994.

183. Ward, G. E., and Kirschner, M. W. Identification of cell cycle regulated phosphorylation sites on nuclear lamin C. Cell *61:*561–577, 1990.

184. Weinberg, R. A. Tumor suppressor genes. Science *254:*1138–1146, 1991.

185. Weinberg, R. A. The retinoblastoma protein and cell cycle control. Cell *81:*323–330, 1995.

186. Weiner, H. L. The role of growth factor receptors in central nervous system development and neoplasia. Neurosurgery *37:*179–194, 1995.

187. Weintraub, S. J., Chow, K. N., Luo, R. X., *et al.* Mechanisms of active transcriptional repression by the retinoblastoma protein. Nature *375:*812–815, 1995.

188. Weller, M., Malipiero, U., Rensing-Ehl, A., *et al.* Fas/APO-1 gene transfer for human malignant glioma. Cancer Res. *55:*2936–2944, 1995.

189. Williams, G. T., and Smith, C. A. Molecular regulation of apoptosis: genetic controls of cell death. Cell *74:*777–779, 1993.

190. Won, K. A., Xiong, Y., Brach, D., *et al.* Growth regulated expression of D-type cyclin genes in human diploid fibroblasts. Proc. Natl. Acad. Sci. U.S.A. *89:*9910–9914, 1992.

191. Wylie, A. H., Morris, R. G., Smith, A. L., *et al.* Chromatin cleavage in apoptosis: association with condensed chromatin morphology and dependence on macromolecular synthesis. J. Pathol. *142:*66–67, 1984.

192. Xiong, Y., Hannon, G. J., Zhang, H., *et al.* p21 is a universal inhibitor of cyclin kinases. Nature *366:* 701–704, 1993.

193. Xiong, X., Zhang, H., and Beach, D. D type cyclins associate with multiple protein kinases and the DNA replication and repair factor PCNA. Cell *71:* 505–514, 1992.

194. Xiong, Y., Zhang, H., and Beach, D. Subunit arrangement of cyclin dependent kinases is associated with cellular transformation. Genes Dev. *7:*1572–1583, 1993.

195. Xu, G., Livingston, D. M., and Krek, W. Multiple members of the E2F transcription family are the products of oncogenes. Proc. Natl. Acad. Sci. U.S.A. *92:*1357–1361, 1995.

196. Yang, E., Zha, J., Jockel, J., *et al.* Bad, a heterodimeric partner for bcl-xL and bcl-2 displaces bax and promotes cell death. Cell *80:*285–291, 1995.

197. Yeh, H. J., Rult, K. G., Wang, Y. X., *et al.* PDGF-A chain is expressed by mammalian neurons during development and in maturity. Cell *64:*209–216, 1991.

198. Yin, X. M., Oltvai, Z. N., and Korsmeyer, S. J. BH1 and BH2 domains of Bcl-2 are required for inhibition of apoptosis and heterodimerization with bax. Nature *369:*321–323, 1994.

199. Zagzag, D. Angiogenic growth factors in neural embryogenesis and neoplasia. Am. J. Pathol. *146:*293–309, 1995.

200. Zambetti, G. P., and Levine, A. J. A comparison of the biologic activities of wild-type and mutant p53. FASEB J. *7:*856–865, 1993.

201. Zhang, H., Hannon, G. J., and Beach, D. p21 containing cyclin kinases exist in both active and inactive states. Genes Dev. *8:*1750–1758, 1994.

202. Zhang, S. Y., Caamano, J., Cooper, F., *et al.* Immunohistochemistry of cyclin D1 in human breast cancer. Am. J. Clin. Pathol. *102:*695–698, 1994.

203. Zhou, P., Jiang, W., Zhang, Y. J., *et al.* Antisense to cyclin D1 inhibits growth and reverses the transformed phenotype of human esophageal cancer cells. Oncogene *11:*571–580, 1995.

CHAPTER 5

Steps Toward a Cellular Biological Analysis of Human Gliomas

MARK NOBLE, Ph.D.

INTRODUCTION

The purpose of this review is to discuss the progress made over the last decade in our particular approach to the study of gliomas. Our research in this arena began with a belief that classification systems rooted solely in morphological analyses of lineage have little chance of being complete and a great likelihood of being largely incorrect. In studies of normal tissues, the rare successes in using morphological analysis to correctly identify cellular lineages have been far outweighed by the failures. It seems reasonable to hypothesize that a similar fate awaits the morphologically based classification systems that are used the world over to analyze gliomas.

There are compelling reasons for having an interest in unraveling the lineages of human glial tumors. For example, the biological analysis of tumor lineage has been of major importance in tumours of the haematopoietic system because of the close association between lineage and response to treatment. In other types of cancers, the identification and differentiation of tumors based on lineage analysis may also identify groups of patients who would benefit from particular treatment strategies. Observations for gliomas consistent with such a possibility are that patients with oligodendrogliomas appear to derive more benefit from chemotherapy than do patients with tumors thought to be of the astrocyte lineage(s) (7, 26). The limitations of conventional neuropathology is demonstrated by the inability to identify the much rarer astrocytoma and glioblastoma patients that derive significant benefit from chemotherapy. Perhaps these rare tumors share a lineage origin with oligodendrogliomas. Such a determination might enable these patients to be diagnosed in a manner with prognostic value.

Another compelling reason to be concerned about identifying the correct cellular origin of human cancers comes from observations that the genetic abnormalities thought to be causal in the generation of gliomas are grouped in constellations that may identify particular families of tumours (25, 59, 60). Is this because particular abnormalities have functional consequences only when they are associated with a specific subset of other abnormalities? Or, alternatively, is this because the ability of a genetic abnormality to alter the normal control of differentiation is dependent upon the cellular lineage in which the abnormality arises? There is substantial support for this second hypothesis. Cell lineage may be very important in determining whether or not a particular genetic lesion will have functional consequences. Hence, the analysis of the means by which oncogenes and suppressor genes exert their effects might be most usefully analyzed in the context of the particular cell of origin for the tumor characterized by a particular abnormality.

Two paths to improving upon morphologically based analytical systems are the ones emerging from molecular biology and from cell biology. Many laboratories have been pursuing the former route, whereas comparatively few have been pursuing the latter. That these two paths must eventually converge is clear, and the studies discussed in this review suggest at least some of the reasons why such convergent analysis will be necessary.

BIOLOGICAL STUDIES ON NORMAL GLIAL PRECURSOR CELLS IN THE OLIGODENDROCYTE-TYPE-2 ASTROCYTE LINEAGE

Our studies began with the cellular analysis of the glial progenitor cells of the rat central nervous system. The biological phenomena of central interest in this research are the same phenomena of interest in cancer. Specifically, we are interested in the lineages that give rise to particular cell types, in the environmental cues that promote the division and differentiation of precursor cells, in understanding the means by which the self-renewal probabilities of precursor cells are regulated, in investigating how precursor cells escape from limited mitotic lifespans, in how they (and their differentiated descendants) escape from programmed cell death, and how it is that glial precursor cells are able to migrate through the tissues of the brain and spinal cord. All of these processes are as relevant to the understanding of glioma cell biology as they are to understanding normal cells, as it is the exaggeration of these processes (allowing greater self-renewal, longer mitotic lifespans, escape from programmed cell death, and migration in the adult nervous system) that makes glioma cells dangerously different from their normal counterparts.

THE ORIGINS OF THE GLIAL CELLS OF THE CENTRAL NERVOUS SYSTEM (CNS)

Several different lineages are able to give rise to the glial cells of the rat CNS, the species in which CNS glial development has been most extensively characterized. At one extreme, it appears that the cells of the rat optic stalk—the embryonic anlage of the optic nerve—give rise only to a single glial population (54), a glial cell-type that has been given the name of the type-1 astrocyte (41). As this name implies, it is thought that the CNS also contains other types of astrocytes, but the true complexity of this family of cells is far from established. Some experiments conducted on spinal cord cultures, for example, have suggested the existence of as

many as five distinct classes of astrocytes just in this single tissue (31). Certainly, it is clear that although the type-1 astrocytes of the optic nerve appear to be similar to astrocytes present in cultures generated from many other regions of the CNS (33, 41, 42), they are not the only source of this category of glia. For example, far at the other extreme from the putatively unipotent cells of the optic nerve are totipotent cells able to give rise to both neuronal and glial lineages, producing a variety of neurons as well as oligodendrocytes and astrocytes (11, 46, 58, 64). Several such precursor populations have been described in the CNS of embryonic, perinatal and adult rats, and the relationship between the cells studied in different laboratories is not yet clear. Still other lineages exist in an intermediate territory, giving rise to a restricted number of different cell types. Of the lineages with restricted developmental potential, the most extensively characterized is called the oligodendrocyte-type-2 astrocyte (O-2A) lineage. The precursor cells of this lineage were first identified in cultures derived from perinatal rat optic nerves (43), where they were found to give rise to two mature glial cell populations: oligodendrocytes and type-2 astrocytes. Oligodendrocytic differentiation of these O-2A progenitor cells occurred when progenitors were grown in chemically defined medium, and progression along this differentiation pathway did not require the presence of inducing factors. In contrast, astrocytic differentiation required the presence of appropriate inducing factors, such as the still unidentified factor(s) present in fetal sera of a number of different species (41, 43, 44).

Although oligodendrocytes, the cells that produce myelin in the central nervous system, are a well-characterized cell-type in vivo, the type-2 astrocyte remains a problem for the developmental neurobiologist. It is not yet clear when and where—and some would say even whether—such cells occur in vivo (Fulton *et al.,* 1991). Some believe that the O-2A progenitor cell should simply be called an oligodendrocyte precursor cell (e.g., 51) while others utilize the O-2A lineage terminology. Because we believe that differentiation pathways that occur *in vitro* are also utilized *in vivo,* we use the latter terminology. That this decision may be warranted is supported by the results of a variety of experiments in which O-2A progenitor cell lines have been implanted in demyelinating lesions of the rat spinal cord and have been found to produce both oligodendrocytes and astrocytes *in vivo* (reviewed in 14).

BIOLOGICAL STUDIES ON THE O-2A PROGENITOR CELL

Having identified a precursor cell for oligodendrocytes, it was next necessary to identify the cellular and molecular signals that controlled division of such cells. Initial studies on generation of oligodendrocytes from O-2A progenitor cells isolated from optic nerves of perinatal rats presented the paradox that the cells were isolated at a time of maximal division of this lineage *in vivo* (52, 53), yet cells did not divide in tissue culture. Resolution of this paradox began with the discovery that cortical astrocytes promoted O-2A progenitor division *in vitro* (33). The astrocytes used in these studies expressed a phenotype like that of type-1 astrocytes of the optic nerve, which are the first identifiable glial cells to appear in the nerve. The similarity of these two populations led us to suggest that the type-1 astrocytes of the optic nerve were responsible for supplying the mitogen(s) required to keep O-2A progenitors in division. Moreover, populations of O-2A progenitors grown in the presence of purified cortical astrocytes were capable of undergoing extended division while also continuing to generate more oligodendrocytes (33), a pattern of behavior similar to that occurring *in vivo*. Thus, the failure of O-2A progenitors to divide in our initial *in vitro* studies was attributable to the lack of necessary mitogens, which appeared to be supplied by another glial cell type.

Purified cortical astrocytes could also promote the correctly timed differentiation *in vitro* of O-2A progenitors isolated from optic nerves of embryonic rats (40). In these experiments, O-2A progenitor cultures were prepared from optic nerves of embryos of various ages and grown on astrocyte monolayers. The number of days that elapsed before the first appearance of oligodendrocytes in these cultures was correlated precisely with the embryonic age from which the cells were isolated, such that cells from younger animals went through a longer period of cell division before generating their first oligodendrocytes. Moreover, regardless of the age from which the cells were isolated, the first oligodendrocytes appeared *in vitro* at a time corresponding to the time when they would have appeared *in vivo* (*i.e.,* the day of birth of the rat). In addition, O-2A progenitor cells stimulated to divide by platelet-derived growth factor, the major O-2A progenitor mitogen produced by astrocytes, (34, 42, 47) generate oligodendrocytes *in vitro* with a timing similar to that observed *in vivo*. (Noble and Murray, 1984; Raff *et al.,* 1985; Temple and Raff, 1986; Raff *et al.,* 1988).

The mechanism by which the timing of oligodendrocyte generation is controlled remains a mystery. More than a decade ago, the observation that clonal families of O-2A progenitor cells dividing under the influence of type-1 astrocytes or PDGF frequently undergo synchronous and symmetrical differentiation throughout a cell family led to the suggestion that the timed generation of oligodendrocytes is regulated by a cell-intrinsic clock that resides within the O-2A progenitor cell (55). For the past decade the intrinsic clock model originally proposed by Temple and Raff (1986) has remained the dominant experimental model for the analysis of timed differentiation in this lineage (30, 42, 55, 69). It is important to note, however, that similarly symmetric and synchronous differentiation has not been observed in studies on O-2A progenitor cells from other CNS regions. Moreover, no previously published data appear to have directly addressed the question of whether the first appearance of oligodendrocytes from dividing embryonic progenitor cells occurs through symmetric clonal differentiation.

Our most recent experiments (21) on the control of the timed generation of oligodendrocytes suggest that the timing of oligodendrocyte differentiation, and the modulation of self-renewal probabilities for dividing O-2A progenitor cells, are both controlled by complex interplays between cell-intrinsic properties and environmental signals. In striking contrast with previous studies, we found that initial generation of oligodendrocytes within a clone of dividing O-2A progenitor cells occurs in association with asymmetric division and differentiation. Once this event occurs, the extent to which oligodendrocytes are produced within a clone is modulated by the proteins and hormones encountered by the dividing cell. Thus, while the initiation of oligodendrocyte generation may be controlled by internal mechanisms, it appears to be the environment that determines the extend to which progenitor cells will undergo self-renewal or generate more oligodendrocytes.

In O-2A progenitor cell populations isolated from the postnatal rat optic nerve, the basal dividing state appears to be that induced by exposure to PDGF and insulin-like growth factor-I. The additional presence of thyroid hormone and/or ciliary neurotrophic factor increases the likelihood that a progenitor cell will cease division and become an oligodendrocyte. The presence of neurotrophin-3 and/or basic fibroblast growth factor (bFGF), in contrast, increases the likelihood of progenitor cell self-renewal. Indeed, exposure of dividing O-2A progenitor cells to the combination of PDGF + bFGF can effectively prevent oligodendrocyte generation while promoting cell division for greatly extended periods, (6).

The regulation of self-renewal probabilities by cell-extrinsic factors may have important implications for understanding this process in cancer cells. The expression of particular growth factor receptors—such as the expression by many glioblastomas of the receptor for bFGF—might not just affect cell division but also play a role in allowing glioma cells to continue replicating beyond their normal mitotic lifespan.

If the mitotic lifespan of a precursor cell can be extended by growing these cells in appropriate cocktails of growth factors, the relationship between this extended mitotic lifespan and the functioning of the internal biological clock that appears to limit the number of divisions that primary cells undergo, at least *in vitro,* can be studied. The intracellular mechanism(s) that controls the timing of oligodendrocyte generation from dividing O-2A progenitor cells can be separated into at least two components, one of which measures time in some form (be this the number of cell divisions or some other phenomenon) and the other of which allows this measurement to have its effect. In these experiments, (4, 5, reviewed in 18) we prevented generation of oligodendrocytes by growing O-2A progenitors in a combination of PDGF + bFGF. After 1, 2, 4 or 6 weeks in this growth condition, we switched cells to growth in the presence of PDGF but not bFGF, a condition that promotes the appropriately timed

generation of oligodendrocytes (42). We found that as cells were forced to divide in the absence of differentiation for longer and longer times, their properties changed in a temporally graded fashion (4, 5). Cells switched from exposure to PDGF + bFGF together to PDGF alone after a short time continued to divide more than cells switched after a longer time. Moreover, in cultures that were maintained for longer periods in PDGF + bFGF, there was an increase in the proportion of the O-2A lineage population that became oligodendrocytes within the first 3 days of growth in the presence of PDGF alone, and the extent of this increase was related to the length of time that cells were first grown in the presence of PDGF + bFGF. These data suggest that measurement of elapsed time continued to occur in the cells prevented from differentiating, but that this measurement was, by itself, unable to induce differentiation; thus, we suggested that the intracellular biological clock could be separated into a measuring component and an effector component. Support for the existence of such a distinction has also been derived from recent studies on conditionally immortalized fibroblasts derived from the H-2K^{b}tsA58 transgenic mouse (22, 23), in which the biological clock that limits the mitotic lifespan of a fibroblast has been found to continue to function normally when cells are immortalized with a conditionally active (thermolabile) mutant of the SV40 large T antigen. Thus, it appears that cells in which terminal differentiation is suppressed, whether by growth factor co-operation or by expression of immortalizing genes, may nonetheless go on to count out their normal mitotic lifespan. Both the effects of astrocytes on promoting O-2A progenitor cell division and differentiation, and the biological clock of the O-2A progenitor cell, are going to be points of particular concern with respect to the biology of human gliomas.

DIFFERENCES BETWEEN O-2A PROGENITOR POPULATIONS OF THE PERINATAL AND ADULT CNS

In the course of our attempts to gain insights into the cellular mechanisms underlying repair of demyelinated lesions in the adult animal, we also initiated studies on O-2A progenitors of the adult CNS. In our initial studies, which were again focused on the rat optic nerve, we found that these O-2A^{adult} progenitor cells differed from their perinatal counterparts in several ways. (65, 66, 67, 68, 69), O-2A^{adult} and O-2A^{perinatal} progenitors differ in morphology, antigen expression, cell-cycle time, migratory rate, time of first appearance *in vivo,* and propensity to undergo asymmetric division and differentiation when grown in the presence of type-1 astrocytes and thyroid hormone. Moreover, our experimental data indicate that the most likely ancestors of O-2A^{adult} progenitors are a subpopulation of the O-2A^{perinatal} progenitor cells (69). Thus, the O-2A^{perinatal} progenitor cell can apparently give rise to a new precursor cell population with fundamentally different properties. Finally, O-2A^{adult} progenitor cells have the important quality of being maintained in the optic nerve throughout life (66, 68). Thus, we would suggest that it is most appropriate to regard O-2A^{adult} progenitors as stem cells, in the specific sense that these cells are capable of functioning as a self-renewing population throughout life, and to regard O-2A^{perinatal} progenitors as cells programmed to differentiate within a limited time span.

The derivation of O-2A^{adult} progenitors from O-2A^{perinatal} progenitors has interesting implications in respect to the possible developmental origin of stem cell populations. Precursor cells with properties appropriate for early development can give rise not only to terminally differentiated end-stage cells, but also to a second generation of precursors with properties appropriate for later developmental periods (for discussion. In the O-2A lineage, it is this second group of precursors that represents the self-renewing stem cells. Whether the ancestral relationship between stem cells and pre-stem cells in other lineages is similar to that seen in the O-2A lineage is not yet known.

In the context of gliomas, there are differences between childhood and adulthood tumors that may relate to the differences between perinatal and adult precursor cells. A particularly striking example of such a difference is found in the pilocytic astrocytomas that occur predominantly in childhood and adolescence, and which have both a different molecular phenotype and a different prognosis than the astrocytomas found in adult patients (48, 61). Is it possible that the differences between the tumors occurring in children and the tumors occurring in adults reflect different lineage origins of tumors in people in different age groups?

THE MESENCHYMAL PARADOX OF GLIOMA BIOLOGY

Recent results of experiments on cells derived from human gliomas suggest that lineage similarities exist between human and rat glial cells. Before discussing these studies, however, it is first necessary to consider results that have been a severe hindrance to the development of a cellular biological analysis of human gliomas.

Like other laboratories interested in human gliomas, we have been generating cell lines for a long time that we have hoped would prove useful both in the study of these human tumours and in the study of human lineages of the central nervous system. And, like other laboratories pursuing these interests, we have run up against the problem that a very large proportion—up to 90%—of human glioma specimens grown in standard tissue culture conditions give rise within several passages to populations that have no glial characteristics and instead resemble mesenchymal cells (3, 24, 62). These mesenchyme-like cells can be derived from tumors of every category and every grade of malignancy. To make matters worse, it is possible to derive such fibronectin-positive and GFAP-negative populations simply by cloning of GFAP-positive parental glioma lines (63). Such populations can also be derived from rat astrocytes immortalized with Simian Virus 40 Large T antigen (17).

The present state of knowledge about the mesenchymal-like derivatives of gliomas is limited. Although some of the mesenchymal-like cells that arise from growth of gliomas in standard tissue culture conditions may be derived from stromal cells rather than from the glioma cells themselves, in some cases these are clearly bona fide tumor cells that display the molecular abnormalities characteristic of gliomas (3, 9, 10). These mesenchymal-like cells can contribute to the tumor mass in the patient (24).

Among the many unanswered questions about the mesenchymal-like cells that can be derived from gliomas, the following strike us as being of particular importance:

(1) *What is the molecular basis for this transition?* How is it that the glial phenotype is supplanted by a mesenchymal phenotype?

Is this transition a one-way pathway, and are there conditions in which the mesenchymal-like cells derived from GFAP$^+$ gliomas can be reconverted to a glial-like phenotype?

(2) *Is this transition associated with an alteration in the biological properties of the resultant cells?* Our own preliminary examination of the mesenchymal-like cells suggest that they may express different surface molecules than those expressed by their GFAP$^+$ counterparts. To our knowledge, however, no studies have been reported in which the mesenchymal derivatives of a GFAP$^+$ glioma have been compared with their glial ancestors in respect to response to growth factors, expression of different cell adhesion molecules or capacity for invasion of neural tissues.

(3) *Does this transition represent an aberrant pathway that becomes accessible to neural tumours or does it instead reflect the developmental potential of the cell of origin of the tumour?* At present, there is insufficient information about CNS development to speculate usefully about the answer to this question.

(4) *What is the frequency of this transition in vivo?*

(5) *Does this transition have any relevance to response to therapy?* These last two questions are closely interconnected. If this transition does not occur *in vivo,* then it is simply a phenomenon of the tissue culture dish and of biological but not therapeutic interest. If one believes that experiments in tissue culture provide a valid insight into what may occur *in vivo,* then there will be more concern about the relevance of this transition to the patient's prognosis and treatment. If this transition does occur frequently *in vivo,* then the differences between the two resulting populations with respect to their growth and survival requirements, migratory behavior, and sensitivity to radiation and chemotherapy become an issue. As increasing numbers of attempts are made to develop therapeutic strategies that involve stimulation of the immune system to kill glioma cells, it becomes important whether the presence of common antigens allows both populations to be the target of a reaction by the immune system or it is necessary to provoke immune reactions against two separate biological entities. Finally, to the extent that *ex vivo* genetic modification is used to make cells immunogenic prior to reimplantation in the patient, it is critical to be able to grow cells in such a manner that the population put back into the patient closely resembles the population taken out in the first place.

A HUMAN GLIOMA OF THE O-2A LINEAGE

Regardless of whether the mesenchymal derivatives of gliomas are of profound or trivial importance, the frequency with which these populations arise has greatly impeded the development of a lineage-based analysis of gliomas that relies on cellular biology rather than histopathology. In order to generate more useful glioma-derived populations for our purposes we have recently changed our approach to the growth of these cells *in vitro* and have abandoned traditional tissue culture techniques.

In an attempt to break through the impasse created by the results described above, glioma-derived cells were grown utilizing the same methods that had enabled us, more than a decade ago, to generate populations of O-2A progenitor cells that would grow in a tissue culture dish. Recreating the micro-environment in which precursor cells find themselves *in vivo* might enable us to conduct meaningful biological experimentation with such cells *in vitro,* an approach that has turned out to be useful not just for the O-2A lineage but for many biological systems.

We believe that we have now isolated a *bona fide* tumor of the O-2A lineage, and thus we have named this cell population Hu-O-2A/Gb-1 (for <u>Hu</u>man <u>O-2A</u> lineage <u>G</u>lioblastoma number <u>1</u>). To grow these cells, tumor specimens were grown in a chemically defined medium that was first conditioned by purified rat cortical astrocytes, precisely as we described a decade ago for the growth of rat O-2A progenitor cells (Noble and Murray, 1984).

Hu-O-2A/Gb-1 cells express antigens characteristic of the O-2A lineage of the rat (and are HNK-1$^+$, A2B5$^+$, and GD3$^+$) and can generate both more progenitor-like cells and O4$^+$GalC$^+$ oligodendrocytes when grown in chemically defined medium conditioned by purified rat cortical astrocytes. When these cells are plated in medium containing fetal calf serum, the oligodendrocyte pathway is suppressed, and differentiation along the astrocyte pathway is enhanced, as also occurs for rodent O-2A progenitor cells. Moreover, the Hu-O-2A/Gb-1 cells are stimulated to divide by both PDGF and bFGF, and simultaneous exposure to both of these mitogens suppresses differentiation along the oligodendrocyte pathway, another characteristic shared with their rodent counterparts. All of these properties have been maintained through at least 20 passages of these cells *in vitro.*

Even more striking are our observations that Hu-O-2A/Gb1 cells express a ^{1}H-NMR spectrum, which is essentially identical to that otherwise uniquely expressed by O-2A^{perinatal} progenitors derived from rat tissues (56, 57) for ^{1}H-NMR characterization of normal glial cells). In these experiments, a perchloric acid extraction is made from cells of interest, and this extract is studied in such a manner as to yield information about the kinds and quantities of free amino acids and other small metabolites contained within the population. We initially found that all of the major cell types of the CNS can be unambiguously distinguished from each other by their ^{1}H-NMR profiles (57). In our current studies we have found that of 10 glioblastoma populations analyzed by ^{1}H-NMR spectroscopy, only the Hu-O-2A/Gb-1 cells possess a metabolite composition like that of rodent O-2A^{perinatal} progenitor cells. The spectra obtained from the other glioblastoma populations, which do not appear on biological grounds to be of the O-2A lineage, are very different from that of either the human or rat O-2A lineage cells.

As indicated by the name given to this cell population, our human O-2A lineage cells were derived from a patient with glioblastoma multiforme. The cells of this tumor are highly invasive, contain many primitive looking cells, and can generate cells of a variety of morphological phenotypes. These terms would also describe accurately the O-2A progenitor cell itself, and possibly any other early precursor cell of the CNS. Thus, it may be that some of the most characteristic features of the malignant tumors of the CNS, such as their capacity to invade the brain and spinal cord, are reflections of the

properties of the precursor cells from which these tumors might be derived.

These current findings are of interest with respect to development and neoplasia of the human CNS for several reasons:

1. The analysis of cells of the rat CNS appears to have considerable potential utility for our attempts to study cells of the human CNS.
2. If cells of the human O-2A lineage behave in the manner of *perinatal* progenitor cells of the O-2A lineage, then the biological clocks that control differentiation of the rat cells derived from optic nerves of perinatal animals may be present in tumors derived from these cells. If such were the case, temporarily interrupting the immortalizing mutation(s) in the tumor cells may cause the cells to rapidly undergo terminal differentiation. Thus, instead of hoping to apply exogenous factors that promote tumor cell differentiation, the mechanisms that can prevent terminal differentiation from taking place could be targeted, and disruption of these mechanisms may lead to cessation of tumor growth.
3. We now have firm ground from which to create a biologically based lineage analysis of human gliomas. We hope that the identification of a single glioma for which the lineage of origin is unambiguously known may be analogous to the importance of the discovery of GFAP as a specific marker of astrocytes (21): once this marker existed, and one cell population existed about whose identity one could be certain, subsequent antigenic markers could be defined much more easily. In the years ahead, it will be necessary to define markers of O-2A lineage tumors that allow all such gliomas to be identified. The defining of this family of gliomas will then make it very much easier to identify the next biological family of tumors.
4. Following on from point three, we would suggest that our ^{1}H-NMR spectroscopic analysis is consistent with the existence of a minimum of two separate lineage contributions to human glioblastoma multiforme. A surprising consistency between the small metabolite profiles expressed by primary cells of the rat CNS and tumors of the human CNS has been seen. For example, our analyses of rodent meningeal cells and human

meningioma cells (13) have provided findings qualitatively similar to our comparisons between rodent O-2A progenitor cells and Hu-O-2A/Gb-1 cells.

5. One of the tools for detecting tumors of the O-2A lineage that may prove most rapidly useful is ^{1}H-NMR spectroscopy of living patients. One of the most important identifying peaks for these cells is N-acetyl-aspartate (NAA), an amino acid detected readily in whole brain scanning procedures. Thus far, our data suggest that any adult patient with a tumor mass containing abundant NAA would be most likely to have a tumor of the O-2A lineage. Although it is clear from *in vivo* studies that gliomas show a reduced NAA content compared with normal brain, there do not yet appear to be any studies examining differences in populations having different levels of NAA.

6. Our results must make one cautious about assigning oligodendrogliomas to the O-2A lineage. Recent studies have suggested that the molecular abnormalities that characterize oligodendrogliomas are distinct from those that characterize glioblastomas. Our own studies have indicated that the molecular abnormalities present in Hu-O-2A/Gb1 cells, in contrast, are like those found in glioblastomas. Perhaps oligodendrogliomas are derived from a separate lineage and not from the oligodendrocyte lineage at all.

7. The simple alterations we have introduced to our tissue culture techniques in the isolation of other gliomas with informative phenotypes may be generally useful. This modification in our strategies for isolating useful cell lines was critical in allowing the isolation of the Hu-O-2A/Gb-1 cells, for had the original tumor biopsy specimen been grown in medium containing fetal sera, there would have been no oligodendrocytes to discover in the cultures. In addition, when cells are grown in the presence of fetal serum, the NAA peak also disappears. Thus, the two most important indicators of a tumor of the O-2A lineage would have been lost had these cells been grown using the tissue culture techniques utilized in most laboratories.

There are still other areas of overlapping interest in the study of normal and neoplastic glial cells. One particularly intriguing area of research concerns determination of the role of gluthathione in modulating programmed cell death in each of these populations. Studies on oligodendrocytes and other cell types have indicated that increasing cellular glutathione levels can profoundly enhance cell survival in the face of cytotoxic agents and also in the presence of what would otherwise be suboptimal amounts of trophic proteins.

Glutathione elevation has also been of great interest in the study of cancer cells, specifically as a means by which cancer cells become resistant to the effects of chemotherapeutic agents. Studies of many different types of cancer cell lines have led to the conclusion that elevations in levels of glutamine-cysteinyl-synthase (the rate-limiting step in glutathione biosynthesis) and/or various members of the gluthathione-S-transferase gene family (a central enzyme in detoxification of xenobiotics) play a central role in the development of chemoresistance (32, 35, 36, 38, 70, 72). The relationship of increased levels of these enzymes and protection from programmed cell death or enhancement of growth factor action has not been established. Study of this relationship may be an area in which to bring together studies on the biology of normal and neoplastic glial cells.

Acknowledgments

Support for the work discussed in this review has come from many sources over the past decade, including the Multiple Sclerosis Society of Great Britain, the Medical Research Council, the Wellcome Trust (NG), the Cancer Research Campaign, Action Research, the Ludwig Institute for Cancer Research, and the Carrie Rudolph Trust. Particular recognition, however, is due to the Preuss Foundation, and in particular to its director, Peter Preuss, and its scientific advisor, Dr. Lorraine Marin, who supported and encouraged this program of research from its very earliest stages.

REFERENCES

1. Barres, B. A., Lazar, M. A., and Raff, M. C. A novel role for thyroid hormone, glucocorticoids and retinoic acid in timing oligodendrocyte development. Development *120:*1097–1108, 1994.
2. Bignami, A., Eng., L. F., Dahl, D., and Uyeda, C. T. Localization of glial fibrillary acidic protein in astrocytes by immunofluorescence. Brain Res. *43:*429–443, 1972.

3. Bigner, D. D., Bigner, S. H., Pegram, C. N. B., et al. Heterogeneity of genotypic and phenotypic characteristics of fifteen permanent cell lines derived from human gliomas. J. Neuropath. Exp. Neurol. *40:*210–229, 1981.

4. Bögler, O., and Noble, M. Studies relating differentiation to a mechanism that measures time in O-2A progenitor cells. Ann. N.Y. Acad. Sci. *633:*505–507, 1991.

5. Bögler, O., and Noble, M. Measurement of time in oligodendrocyte-type-2 astrocyte (O-2A) progenitors is a cellular process distinct from differentiation or division. Dev. Biol. *162,* 525–538, 1994.

6. Bögler, O., Wren, D., Barnett, S. C., *et al.* Cooperation between two growth factors promotes extended self-renewal, and inhibits differentiation, of O-2A progenitor cells. Proc. Natl. Acad. Sci. U.S.A. *87:*6368–6372, 1990.

7. Cairncross, J. G., and Macdonald, D. R. Successful chemotherapy for recurrent malignant oligodendroglioma. Ann. Neurol. *23:*360–364, 1988.

8. Cross, M., and Dexter, T. M. Growth factors in development, transformation and tumorigenesis. Cell *64:* 271–280, 1991.

9. Davenport, R. D., and McCeever, P. E. DNA content and marker expression in human glioma explants. Acta Neuropathologica *74:*362–365, 1987a.

10. Davenport, R. D., and McKeever, P. E. Ploidy of endothelium in high-grade astrocytomas. Analytical and Quantitative Cytology and Histology *9:*25–29, 1987b.

11. Davis, A., and Temple, S. A self-renewing multipotential stem cell in embryonic rat cerebral cortex. Nature *372:*263–266, 1994.

12. Eccleston, A., and Silberberg, D. R. Fibroblast growth factor is a mitogen for oligodendrocytes in vitro. Dev. Brain Res. *21:*315–318, 1985.

13. Florian, C. L., Preece, N. E., Bhakoo, K. K., *et al.* Cell type-specific fingerprinting of meningioma and meningeal cells by proton nuclear magnetic resonance spectroscopy. Cancer Res. *55:*420–427, 1995.

14. Franklin, R. J. M., and Blakemore, W. F. Glial-cell transplantation and plasticity in the O-2A lineage—implications for CNS repair. Trends Neurosci. *18:* 151–156, 1995.

15. Fulton, B. P., Burne, J. F., and Raff, M. C. Glial cells in the rat optic nerve: The search for the type-2 astrocytes. Ann. N.Y. Acad. Sci. *633:*27–34, 1991.

16. Gard, A. L., and Pfeiffer, S. E. Two proliferative stages of the oligodendrocyte lineage (A2B5+O4− and O4+GalC−) under different mitogenic control. Neuron *5:*615–625, 1990.

17. Geller, H. M., and Dubois-Dalcq, M. Antigenic and functional characterization of a rat central nervous system-derived cell line immortalized by a retroviral vector. J. Cell Biol. *107:*1977–1986, 1988.

18. Groves, A., Bögler, O., Jat, P., and Noble, M. The cellular measurement of time. Curr. Opin. Cell Biol. *3:*224–229, 1991.

19. Groves, A. K., Barnett, S. C., Franklin, R. J. M., *et al.* Repair of demyelinated lesions by transplantation of purified O-2A progenitor cells. Nature *362:*453–455, 1993.

20. Hunter, S. F., and Bottenstein, J. E. O-2A glial progenitors from mature brain respond to CNS neuronal cell line-derived growth factors. J. Neurosci. Res. *28:* 574–582, 1991.

21. Ibarrola, N., Mayer-Pröschel, M., Rodriguez-Pena, and Noble, M. Evidence for the existence of at least two timing mechanisms that contribute to oligodendrocyte generation *in vitro.* Dev. Biol., 1996, in press.

22. Ikram, Z., Norton, P., and Jat, P. S. The biological clock that measures the mitotic life-span of mouse embryos fibroblasts continues to function in the presence of simian virus 40 large T antigen. Proc. Nat. Acad. Sci., U.S.A. *91:*6448–6452, 1994.

23. Jat, P. S., Noble, M., Ataliotis, P., *et al.* Transgenic mice harbouring an H-2K^b tsA58 transgene yield conditionally immortalized cell lines. Proc. Natl. Acad. Sci. U.S.A. *88:*5096–5100, 1991.

24. Kennedy, P., Watkins, B., Thomas, D., and Noble, M. Antigenic expression by cells derived from human gliomas does not correlate with morphological classification. J. Neuropathol. Exp. Neurol. *13:*327–347, 1987.

25. Kraus, J. A., Koopmann, J., Kaskel, P., *et al.* Shared allelic losses on chromosomes 1p and 19q suggest a common origin of oligodendroglioma and oligoastrocytoma. J. Neuropath. Exp. Neurol. *54:*91–95, 1995.

26. Macdonald, D. R., Gaspar, L. E., and Cairncross, J. G. Successful chemotherapy for newly diagnosed aggressive oligodendroglioma. Ann. Neurol. *27:*573–574, 1990.

27. Matsui, Y., Zsebo, K., and Hogan, B. L. Cell *70:*841–847, 1992.

28. Mayer, M., and Noble, M. The inhibition of oligodendrocytic differentiation of O-2A progenitors caused by basic fibroblast growth factor is overridden by astrocytes. Glia *8:*12–19, 1992.

29. Mayer, M., Bhakoo, K., and Noble, M. Ciliary neurotrophic factor and leukemia inhibitory factor promote the generation, survival and maturation of oligodendrocytes *in vitro.* Development *120:*143–153, 1994.

30. McKinnon, R. D., Matsui, T., Dubois-Dalcq, M., and Aaronson, S. A. FGF modulates the PDGF-driven pathway of oligodendrocyte development. Neuron *5:*603–614, 1990.

31. Miller, R. H., and Szigeti, V. Clonal analysis of astrocyte diversity in neonatal rat spinal cord cultures. Development *113:*353–362, 1991.

32. Moscow, J. A., and Dixon, K. H. Glutathione-related enzymes, glutathione and multidrug resistance. Cytotechnology *12:*155–170, 1993.

33. Noble, M., and Murray, K. Purified astrocytes promote the division of a bipotential glial progenitor cell. EMBO J *3:*2243–2247, 1984.

34. Noble, M., Murray, K., Stroobant, P., *et al.* Platelet-derived growth factor promotes division and motility, and inhibits premature differentiation, of the oligodendrocyte-type-2 astrocyte progenitor cell. Nature *333:*560–562, 1988.

35. O'Dwyer, P. J., Hamilton, T. C., Yao, K. S., *et al.* Modulation of glutathione and related enzymes in reversal of resistance to anticancer drugs. Hematol. Oncol. Clin. North Am. *9:*383–396, 1995.

36. Pendyala, L., Creaven, P. J., Perez, R., *et al.* Intracellular glutathione and cytotoxicity of platinum com-

plexes. Cancer Chemother. Pharmacol. *36:*271–278, 1995.

37. Port, J. L., Hochwald, S. N., Wang, H. Y., and Burt, M. E. Buthionine sulfoximine pretreatment potentiates the effect of isolated lung perfusion with doxorubicin. Ann. Thorac. Surg. *60:*239–243, 1995.

38. Pratesi, G., Dal-Bo, L., Paolicchi, A., *et al.* The role of the glutathione-dependent system in tumor sensitivity to cisplatin: a study of human tumor xenografts. Ann. Oncol. 6, 283–289, 1995.

39. Raff, M. C. Glial cell diversification in the rat optic nerve. Science *243:*1450–1455, 1989.

40. Raff, M. C., Abney, E. R., and Fok-Seang, J. Reconstitution of a developmental clock in vitro: A critical role for astrocytes in the timing of oligodendrocyte differentiation. Cell *42:*61–69, 1985.

41. Raff, M. C., Abney, E. R., Cohen, J. Two types of astrocytes in cultures of developing rat white matter: differences in morphology, surface properties and growth characteristics. J. Neurosci. *3:*1289–1300, 1983a.

42. Raff, M. C., Lillien, L. E., Richardson, W. D., *et al.* Platelet-derived growth factor from astrocytes drives the clock that times oligodendrocyte development in culture. Nature *333:*562–565, 1988.

43. Raff, M. C., Miller, R. H., and Noble, M. A glial progenitor cell that develops *in vitro* into an astrocyte or an oligodendrocyte depending on the culture medium. Nature *303:*390–396, 1983b.

44. Raff, M. C., Miller, R. H., and Noble, M. Glial cell lineages in the rat optic nerve. Cold Spring Harbor Symp. Quant. Biol. *48:*569–572, 1983c.

45. Raff, M. C., Williams, B. P., and Miller, R. H. The in vitro differentiation of a bipotential glial progenitor cell. EMBO J. *3:*1857–1864, 1984.

46. Reynolds, B. A., and Weiss, S. Generation of neurons and astrocytes from isolated cells of the adult mammalian central nervous system. Science *255:*1707–1710, 1992.

47. Richardson, W. D., Pringle, N., Mosley, M. J., *et al.* A role for platelet-derived growth factor in normal gliogenesis in the central nervous system. Cell *53:*309–319, 1988.

48. Russell, D. S., and Rubinstein, L. J. *Pathology of Tumours of the Nervous System,* 5th Ed. Williams & Wilkins, Baltimore, 1989.

49. Saneto, R. P. and DeVellis, J. Characterization of cultured rat oligodendrocytes proliferating in a serum-free chemically defined medium. Proc. Natl. Acad. Sci. U.S.A. *82:*3509–3513, 1985.

50. Sasahara, M., Fries, J. W. U., Raines, E. W. PDGF B-chain in neurons of the central nervous system, posterior pituitary and in a transgenic model. Cell *64:*217–227, 1991.

51. Skoff, R. P., and Knapp, P. E. Division of astroblasts and oligodendroblasts in postnatal rodent brain: Evidence for separate astrocyte and oligodendrocyte lineages. Glia *4:*165–174, 1991.

52. Skoff, R. P., Price, D. L., and Stocks, A. Electron microscopic autoradiographic studies of gliogenesis in rat optic nerve. 1. Cell proliferation. J. Comp. Anat. *169:*291–311, 1976a.

53. Skoff, R. P., Price, D. L., and Stocks, A. Electron microscopic autoradiographic studies of gliogenesis in rat optic nerve. 2. Time of origin. J. Comp. Anat. *169:*313–323, 1976b.

54. Small, R., Riddle, P., and Noble, M. Evidence for migration of oligodendrocyte-type-2 astrocyte progenitor cells into the developing rat optic nerve. Nature *328:*155–157, 1987.

55. Temple, S., and Raff, M. C. Clonal analysis of oligodendrocyte development in culture: Evidence for a developmental clock that counts cell divisions. Cell *44:*773–779, 1986.

56. Urenjak, J., Williams, S., Gadian, D., and Noble, M. Specific expression of N-acetyl-aspartate in neurones, O-2A progenitors and immature oligodendrocytes in vitro. J. Neurochem. *59:*55–61, 1992.

57. Urenjak, J., Williams, S., Gadian, D., and Noble, M. Proton nuclear magnetic resonance spectroscopy unambiguously identifies different neural cell types. J. Neurosci. *13:*981–989, 1993.

58. Vescovi, A. L., Reynolds, B. A., Fraser, D. D., and Weiss, S. bFGF regulates the proliferative fate of unipotent (neuronal) and bipotent (neuronal/astroglial) EGF-generated CNS progenitor cells. Neuron *11:*951–966, 1993a.

59. von Deimling, A., Louis, D. N., Menon, A. G., *et al.* Deletions on the long arm of chromosome 17 in pilocytic astrocytoma. Acta Neuropathol. *86:*81–85, 1993a.

60. von Deimling, A., Louis, D. N., Schramm, J., and Wiestler, O. D. Astrocytic gliomas: Characterization on a molecular genetic basis. In: *Molecular Neuro-Oncology and Its Impact on the Clinical Management of Brain Tumours,* edited by O. D. Wiestler, U. Schlegel, and J. Schramm, pp. 33–42. Springer-Verlag, London, 1994.

61. von Deimling, A., von Ammon, K., Schoenfeld, D., *et al.* Seizinger, B. R. and Lousi, D. N. Subsets of glioblastoma multiforme defined by molecular genetic analysis. Brain Pathol. *3:*19–26, 1993b.

62. Westphal, M., Nausch, H., and Herrmann, H.-D. Antigenic staining patterns of human glioma cultures: Primary cultures, long term cultures and cell lines. J. Neurocytol. *19:*466–477, 1989.

63. Westphal, M., Hänsel, M., Müller, D., *et al.* Biological and karyotypic characterization of a new cell line derived from a human gliosarcoma. Cancer Res. *48:*731–740, 1988.

64. Williams, B. P., Read, J., and Price, J. The generation of neurons and oligodendrocytes from a common precursor cell. Neuron *7:*685–693, 1991.

65. Wolswijk, G., and Noble, M. Cooperation between PDGF and FGF converts slowly dividing O-2A^{adult} progenitor cells to rapidly dividing cells with characteristics of their perinatal counterparts. J. Cell Biol. *118:*899–900, 1992.

66. Wolswijk, G., Riddle, P., and Noble, M. Co-existence of perinatal and adult forms of a glial progenitor cell during development of the rat optic nerve. Development *109:*691–698, 1990.

67. Wolswijk, G., Riddle, P., and Noble, M. Platelet-derived growth factor is mitogenic for O-2A^{adult} progenitor cells. Glia *4:*495–503, 1991.

68. Woslwijk, G., and Noble, M. Identification of an adult-specific glial progenitor cell. Development *105:*387–400, 1989.

69. Wren, D., Wolswijk, G., and Noble, M. *In vitro* analysis of origin and maintenance of O-2A*adult* progenitor cells. J. Cell Biol. *116*:167–176, 1992.

70. Yao, K. S., Godwin, A. K., Johnson, S. W., *et al.* Evidence for altered regulation of gamma-glutamylcysteine synthetase gene expression among cisplatin-sensitive and cisplatin-resistant human ovarian cancer cell lines. Cancer Res. *55*:4367–4374, 1995.

71. Yeh, J.-J., Ruit, K. G., Wang, Y.-X., *et al.* PDGF A-chain is expressed by mammalian neurons during development and in maturity. Cell *64*:209–219, 1991.

72. Zaman, G. J., Lankelma, J., van Tellingen, O., *et al.* Role of glutathione in the export of compounds from cells by the multidrug resistance-associated protein. Proc. Natl. Acad. Sci. U.S.A. *92*:7690–7694, 1995.

PART III

Molecular Neuro-Oncology

CHAPTER 6

Molecular Biology of Pediatric Brain Tumors

COREY RAFFEL, M.D., Ph.D.

INTRODUCTION

Current theories of oncogenesis suggest that tumors arise as the result of sequential genetic alterations (see Chapter 7). These alterations may activate dominantly acting oncogenes or inactivate genes involved in the regulation of the cell cycle (termed tumor suppressor genes.) Oncogenes are altered or activated forms of normal cellular genes, called proto-oncogenes. Proto-oncogenes encode growth factors, growth factor receptors, transcriptional regulators, or proteins that transmit signals leading to cell division (1, 2, 3, 4). Mutations in these genes lead to increased cell division by a variety of mechanisms.

Tumor suppression genes encode proteins that control entry of a cell into the cell cycle (5). Inactivating mutations in these genes can lead to unregulated entry into the cycle and, thus, to increased cell proliferation. Oncogenes are often referred to as "dominant", as mutation in one allele of the gene serves to activate the transforming properties of the gene. Tumor suppressor genes are called "recessive" because both copies of the gene need to be inactivated to allow unregulated entry into the cell cycle.

MOLECULAR BIOLOGY OF PEDIATRIC BRAIN TUMORS:

While extensive research has been performed to identify the molecular events that lead to adult brain tumors, in particular astrocytomas, less work has been performed on pediatric tumors. In the remainder of this chapter, pediatric brain tumors will be discussed by type and the known molecular biologic features will be presented.

Pilocytic Astrocytomas

Pilocytic astrocytomas are a common pediatric brain tumor; this has permitted a number of studies on tissue removed at the time of operation. These tumors differ from other astrocytic tumors by lacking 17p deletions (6). One study analyzed 20 pilocytic astrocytoma and detected 17p loss in only one. Interestingly, 4 of the twenty (20%) had loss of the long arm of chromosome 17. One of these tumors had an interstitial deletion of 17q that included the gene for type I neurofibromatosis (NF-1). Neither losses on chromosome 10 or 19q nor EGFR amplification were detected in any tumor.

The finding of 17q loss in pilocytic astrocytoma is intriguing, as these tumors can be associated with NF-1 and the gene for NF-1 is located at 17q11.2 (7). *NF1* is a large gene spanning 300kb of genomic DNA with a complex structure of 49 exons (8). Especially interesting is the presence of three other genes embedded in one intron of *NF1* (9, 10, 11). These genes are oriented in the opposite direction to *NF1*. The protein product of the NF1 gene, neurofibromin, is a large protein of 2,818 amino acids.

Neurofibromin is hypothesized to function as a tumor suppressor gene. It may do so by converting *ras,* a protein involved in growth factor mediated cell proliferation, from its active form, containing GTP, to its inactive form, which contains GDP. One portion of neurofibromin, about 360 amino acids, is homologous to mammalian GTPase-activating proteins (GAP) (12, 13, 14). GAP functions to accelerate the conversion of *ras* bound GTP to GDP. If one of the functions of neurofibromin in the cell is to convert *ras* to its inactive form, then mutations in

NF-1 could lead to increased amounts of active *ras*. Increasing *ras* activity could lead to increased cell proliferation, as increased active ras would mimic growth factor stimulation.

Neurofibromin has been shown to be a tumor suppressor in v-ha-ras transformed cells (15). In these experiments, cells were transformed with a viral ras gene that transforms the cells. Addition of the entire NF-1 gene or the GAP portion of the gene reversed the transformed phenotype. Confusing the picture somewhat are studies that demonstrate that the tumor suppressor activity of neurofibromin is independent of its GAP activity (16). The mechanism by which neurofibromin inhibits transformation may involve other currently undefined activities of the protein.

The above evidence favors a role for the NF-1 gene in the genesis of sporadic, as well as NF-1 associated, pilocytic astrocytomas. Confirmation of this hypothesis awaits direct sequencing of the NF-1 gene or cDNA from sporadic tumors, a formidable task, given the large size of the gene.

Pediatric Astrocytomas

Cytogenetic studies of pediatric astrocytomas have been reported, but have been relatively unrevealing. Among a total of 27 pediatric astrocytomas examined, 18 had normal karyotypes (17, 18). Numerical abnormalities noted included increases and decreases in random chromosomes. No specific pattern or marker chromosomes were identified.

Because adult astrocytomas have deletions in the short arm of chromosome 17, LOH analyses of pediatric astrocytomas in this region have been performed. Litofsky, et al, reported LOH on 17p for 5 of 21 astrocytomas, including 2 pilocytic, 1 diffuse, and 2 anaplastic astrocytomas (19). Lanbg et al examined 21 tumors in patients 18 years of age and less and identified LOH on 17p in one glioblastoma (20). Thus, 14% of pediatric astrocytomas of all grades and 16% of non-pilocytic astrocytomas occurring in the pediatric age group have LOH on 17p. These percentages are considerably lower than those seen in adult tumors (21, 22, 23), suggesting that different mechanisms may lead to the generation of pediatric versus adult astrocytomas.

Studies of the p53 gene and protein have also been carried out in pediatric astrocytomas. In one study, an SSCP analysis of p53 exons 5-8 was performed in 35 pediatric astrocytomas

(19). No abnormality was detected in any exon in any tumor. Because more than 90% of p53 mutations in human tumors occur in these exons, these researchers concluded that p53 mutations were rare in pediatric tumors. Indeed, a comparison with the results in adult astrocytomas revealed a statistically significant lower incidence of such mutations in the pediatric tumors, regardless of grade. Interestingly, these workers also performed sequencing of exons 5-8 in 5 tumors with LOH on 17p. No mutation in p53 was detected, suggesting the possibility that another tumor suppressor gene present on 17p other than p53 may be important in the oncogenesis of pediatric astrocytomas. Such a gene has been postulated to be involved in medulloblastoma/PNET (24, 25, 26).

Just as in adult tumors, immunohistochemical studies of p53 in pediatric astrocytomas give somewhat confusing results. As in adult tumors, nuclear p53 accumulation is present in a majority of pediatric astrocytomas, including pilocytic, diffuse, and anaplastic tumors (27). However, between 60 and 80% of the tumors in the three grades had p53 accumulation without any evidence of p53 mutation by SSCP analysis. In addition, these researchers demonstrated an absence of MDM2 amplification in any of the tumors studied. Thus, as with the adult tumors, the meaning of nuclear staining for p53 in some cells of some pediatric astrocytomas is of unclear significance at this time (28).

LOH analysis for chromosome 10 in pediatric astrocytomas revealed positive findings in only 2 of 23 tumors, including 1 of 4 anaplastic astrocytomas and 1 of 7 glioblastomas (20). These investigators examined the same set of tumors for EGFR amplifications; no amplification of EGFR was noted in any pediatric tumor. These results also suggest the possibility of different pathways leading to astrocytic tumors in children versus adults.

Brainstem Gliomas

One of the most malignant pediatric brain tumors is the typical brainstem glioma, seen as a diffuse enlargement of the pons on CT and MR scans (77). These tumors invariably lead to the death of the child, with a median survival of less than one year after presentation. Seven of these tumors have been studied for LOH on chromosome 17p and 10, and for p53 mutations (30). All seven patients were 18 years of age or less and all tumors were classified as glioblastomas on histologic examination. Four of the 7 tumors had LOH on chromosome 17p and four of the seven tumors had LOH on chromosome 10. Three of the tumors had both LOH on 17p and 10. All 4 tumors with 17p loss had p53 mutations in the retained allele; one tumor without a p53 gene deletion had mutation of one allele. These results indicate that pediatric brainstem gliomas differ in their genetic alterations from pediatric malignant astrocytomas found in other parts of the brain. The brainstem gliomas more closely resemble adult glioblastomas in their molecular biology, which may explain the rapidly progressive clinical course in these patients.

Ependymomas

In contrast to pediatric astrocytomas, few studies have been performed in ependymomas. To date, fewer than 25 pediatric tumors have been studied cytogenetically (31, 32, 33, 34, 35, 36). Loss of chromosome 22 is the most frequently detected cytogenetic abnormality and this loss has been confirmed by LOH analysis (36, 37, 38). In addition, these studies indicate that ependymomas lack the typical genetic abnormalities seen in astrocytomas. One patient with a malignant ependymoma was shown to have a germ line p53 mutation (39), but this case appears to be unusual, as no p53 mutations were detected in 15 ependymomas by SSCP analysis (40).

In animals, ependymomas have been induced by injection of SV40 virus into the brain, suggesting a possible role for this virus in the development of these tumors in humans (41). To investigate this possibility, PCR experiments were performed to identify SV40 large T antigen gene sequences in DNA isolated ependymomas (42). Ten of 11 ependymomas had amplification products that specifically hybridized to SV40 probes. Sequencing of the amplification products from 2 of the tumors revealed complete identity with the SV40 large T gene. Three additional tumors yielded amplification products that were identical to a portion of the gene. In 7 of the 11 tumors, immunohistochemical staining for SV40 large antigen was detected in tumor nuclei. The SV40 large T antigen is an oncogene that functions by binding to and inactivating two tumor suppressor genes, p53 and the retinoblastoma susceptibility gene product (p110^{rb})

(43, 44). With these proteins inactivated, cells can enter the cell cycle in an unrestricted fashion. These experiments suggest the possibility that SV40 or related viruses may play a role in the development of ependymomas in humans and that inactivation of p53, p110^{rb}, or both is important in the oncogenesis of ependymomas.

Medulloblastoma/Primitive Neuroectodermal Tumor

Medulloblastoma, the most common malignant brain tumor in children, is the pediatric brain tumor most extensively studied at the molecular level. Initial cytogenetic studies revealed loss of genetic material on the short arm of chromosome 17 in about one third of tumors (17, 18, 45). The loss of heterozygosity on 17p has been confirmed by RFLP analysis. In the initial study, 3 of 13 tumors showed loss of all informative markers on 17p (46). This work was extended to show 17p loss in between 25 and 50% of cases (24, 25, 47). Because the p53 gene is located on 17p, a number of investigators examined the status of this gene in medulloblastoma (24, 26, 48, 49, 50). Taken together, these studies clearly demonstrate that, despite the deletion of one p53 allele in many of the tumors, the p53 gene is rarely mutated in medulloblastoma. Interestingly, a small subset of tumors have only a small area of 17p loss that does not include the p53 gene (24, 25, 26). This finding suggests the possibility that another tumor suppressor gene is present on 17p. This putative suppressor might be important in the oncogenesis of medulloblastoma. Fine mapping of the region has suggested this putative suppressor is located near the abr gene on 17p13.3 (51).

While p53 appears not to be mutated in medulloblastoma, other means of inactivating the protein exist. For example, the mdm2 gene product binds to p53 and inactivates it. Amplification of the mdm-2 gene has been described as a mechanism of p53 inactivation in sarcomas (52,53). However, no evidence for mdm-2 amplification has been detected in medulloblastoma (50).

Besides loss of genetic material on 17p, medulloblastomas have been shown to lose potions of 6q and 16q, but no candidate suppressor genes that may have a role in the development of PNET have been identified in these regions (47).

Medulloblastomas may occur in association with 2 different inherited cancer syndromes, Gorlin syndrome and Turcot syndrome. Gorlin syndrome, also called nevoid basal cell carcinoma syndrome, is an autosomal dominant disorder (54). Affected individuals develop multiple basal cell carcinomas, multiple odontogenic keratocysts of the jaws, palmar and plantar dyskeratoses, and skeletal anomalies, especially rib malformations. In addition, at least 40 cases of medulloblastoma have been reported in patients with this syndrome, indicating that about 3% of Gorlin patients develop medulloblastoma (55, 56). The gene for Gorlin syndrome has been mapped to chromosome 9q31 (57, 58). However, only 5 of 36 cases of medulloblastoma examined had 9q31 loss, and only one of these had loss of the 9q marker most closely linked to the Gorlin gene (59, 60). Work has suggested that 9q deletions occur only in the desmoplastic subtype of medulloblastoma, raising the possibility of a Gorlin syndrome gene mutation being involved in the development of this subclass of tumor (60).

The gene for Gorlin's syndrome has recently been identified as the ptc gene, the human homolog of the Drosophila patched gene (61, 62). This Drosophila gene encodes a protein with 12 putative transmembrane domains; it may function as a receptor or transporter (63, 64). The protein has an essential role in embryonic patterning in Drosophila; a similar role in humans may explain the congenital anomalies associated with Gorlin's syndrome.

The patched protein has an important regulatory role in the "hedgehog" signalling pathway, a complex series of inhibitory elements present in vertebrates as well as in Drosophila (65). The regulatory element, hedgehog, in an undefined fashion upregulates the expression of the wingless and cubitus interruptus. Hedgehog also upregulates patched, which in turn down regulates hedgehog, cubitus interruptus, wingless, and, interestingly, patched itself. Cubitus interruptus plays an essential role between patched and hedgehog (66). Hedgehog up regulates cubitus interruptus, which in turn up regulates other genes in the pathway. Conversely, patched down regulates cubitus interruptus. Over expression of cubitus interruptus is analogous to absence of patched function. All of these proteins have human homologs. The hedgehog gene has three, sonic hedgehog, indian hedgehog, and desert hedgehog. Sonic hedgehog in particular has a tissue distribution similar to patched (67). The human homolog of cubitus interruptus is gli, a transcription factor that may serve as an oncogene in rare glioblasto-

mas (68). The human homolog of wingless is Wnt, a gene whose overexpression causes mammary tumors in mice.

One possible reason for the few 9q deletions seen in medulloblastoma may be that other alterations in the patched/hedgehog pathway are the common alteration in this tumor. This hypothesis suggests that overexpression of any of the proteins normally down regulated by patched could lead to medulloblastoma. In patients with Gorlin's syndrome, down regulation would fail because the patched gene itself is mutated. In spontaneous tumors, alterations leading to overexpression of sonic hedgehog, gli, or Wnt could be responsible. The role of the patched/hedgehog pathway in these tumors awaits further definition of the proteins involved and determination of their function in tumor cells.

Another tumor suppressor gene has been identified on chromosome 9, the MTS-1 gene. This gene encodes an inhibitor of cyclin D-cyclin dependent kinase 4 complex and is mutated or deleted in a large proportion of adult astrocytomas (see chapter 10). In 2 studies of medulloblastomas, however, no mutations of this gene were found in any of 25 medulloblastomas investigated, suggesting that this gene is not involved in medulloblastoma oncogenesis (69, 70).

Turcot's syndrome is a hereditary disorder in which affected individuals have multiple colonic polyps and a brain tumor (71). In one study, mutations in the APC gene were identified in a group of patients with Turcot's syndrome in which the brain tumor was a medulloblastoma (72). The relative risk for developing a medulloblastoma in the patients with Turcot's and an APC gene mutation was 92 times that in the general population. Surprisingly, in light of this association, APC gene mutations have not been identified in spontaneously occurring medulloblastomas. In one study, DNA from 47 medulloblastomas was examined for mutations in the portion of the APC gene that contains at least 2/3 of the mutations seen (73). No tumor had an APC mutation. Interestingly, in the two medulloblastomas that were removed from patients with Turcot's syndrome, the germ line mutation was identified, but no mutation was seen in the other APC allele. In a second study, DNA from 23 medulloblastomas was examined for deletions in the region of the APC gene (74). No LOH was found in this region in any tumor. These results suggest that the APC gene is not important in the development of sporadic medulloblastoma and even suggest that the gene may not be important in the development of medulloblastoma in Turcot's patients.

Close to 20% of medulloblastomas contain double minute chromosomes, suggesting the possibility of gene amplification (45). Gene amplification of 11 oncogenes has been investigated (75). Of 20 primary medulloblastomas studied, only one tumor was found to have amplification of the c-erbB1 proto-oncogene: no other tumor had amplification of any of the oncogenes examined. Interestingly, 4 established medulloblastoma cell lines were also tested and three had proto-oncogene amplification: one had amplified c-myc, one N-myc, and one c-erbB1. These investigators suggest that in vitro culture may select for a small subpopulation of cells within the tumor that have pre-existing amplification (76), or that culture is more successful with tumors that have an amplified proto-oncogene.

Analysis of amplification of the myc family of proto-oncogenes in medulloblastoma has revealed c-myc amplification in 5 of 43 tumors in studies other than the one mentioned above (46, 77, 78). N-myc amplification, N-ras mutations, EGFR c-erbB-2 expression, and bcl-2 expression have all been investigated in medulloblastoma (75, 78, 79, 80, 81). No consistent pattern of expression, mutation, or amplification has been identified. Because EGFR is frequently amplified and/or rearranged in glial tumors (see chapter 10), 7 medulloblastomas were analyzed for EGFR copy number and gene rearrangements (75). No tumor had either finding. Homeobox genes have also been examined in medulloblastoma. Interestingly, the PAX5 gene, which is not expressed during cerebellar development, is expressed in medulloblastoma (82). The significance of this finding is unclear at this time.

Members of the neurotrophin family (nerve growth factor, brain derived neurotroophic factor, NT-3, and NT-4/5) and their family of high affinity receptors (trkA, trkB, and trkC) are important in the proliferation, differentiation, and survival of neuroepithelial cells. In addition to the trk receptors, a low affinity receptor for neurotrophins ($p75^{LNGFR}$) has also been described. Because medulloblastoma is thought to arise from primitive neuroepithelial stem cells, neurotrophins and their receptors may be important in the development and growth of these tumors.

Three studies have examined the status of the low affinity nerve growth factor receptor in medulloblastoma (83, 84, 85). About one third of tumors studied had mRNA for this receptor. Expression of $p75^{LNGFR}$ may be restricted to the subset of PNET demonstrating neuronal differentiation. Addition of NGF had no effect on the growth characteristics or morphology of a PNET cell line expressing the receptor.

Expression of trk receptors and two neurotrophins has been investigated in medulloblastoma specimens immunohistochemically (86). Variable expression of trk receptors was found in the 29 tumors examined. Most tumors expressed at least one functional receptor; some tumors expressed more than one receptor; often one of these was truncated. Brain derived neurotrophic factor and neurotrophin-3 were seen in 22% and 9% of tumors, respectively. Interestingly, one study of a very small number of tumors correlated good clinical outcome with high expression of full length trkC mRNA (87).

Just as the neurotrophins and their receptors have a role in the growth and differentiation of neuroepithelial cells, the insulin-like growth factors, IGF-1 and IGF-2 and the type 1 insulin-like growth factor receptor, IGFR-1, have a role in the growth of many tissues, including those of the central nervous system. In one study of medulloblastoma cell lines, all were found to express IGFR-1 (77). Blocking of ligand binding with a monoclonal antibody to the extracellular portion of the receptor inhibited growth of the cells in vitro. Further work is needed to extend these findings to the tumors themselves.

CONCLUSIONS

A large body of information has been generated concerning the genetic alterations that occur in adult brain tumors. While less information is known about pediatric tumors, considerable progress has been made. Despite this work, the many and complex pathways that lead from a normal cell to tumor initiation and progression are far from completely understood. As new techniques are developed and new genes with potential roles in tumorigenesis are isolated, these pathways will become better delineated.

With current and future information, the diagnostic, prognostic, and therapeutic implications of the genetic alterations in tumor cells will be explored. Certain genetic alterations may be discovered to be restricted to one tumor type. Indeed, molecular tumor typing may eventually supplant histology as a way of identifying tumors. Studies are needed that correlate the presence or absence of specific genetic alterations with patient prognosis. Genetic alterations in tumors may also become important in treatment. Specific genetic deficiencies in tumors could be replaced by gene transfer techniques, and over expression of a gene may be counteracted by drugs that specifically inhibit that gene's protein product.

REFERENCES

1. Solomon, E, Borrw, J, Goddard, AD. Chromosome aberrations and cancer. Science. *254:*1153–1160, 1991.
2. Aaronson, S.A. Growth factors and cancer. Science. *254:* 1146–1153, 1991.
3. Bishop, J.M. The molecular genetics of cancer. Science. *235:*305–311, 1987.
4. Hunter, T. Cooperation between oncogenes. Cell. *64:*249–270, 1991.
5. Sager, R. Tumor suppressor genes: the puzzle and the promise. Science. *246:*1406–1412, 1989.
6. von Deimling A., Louis, D.N., Menon, A.G., von Ammon, K, Petersen, I., Ellison, D., Wiestler, O.D., Seizinger, B.R. Deletions on the long arm of chromosome 17 in pilocytic astrocytoma. Acta Neuropathol. *86:*81–85, 1993.
7. Fountain, J.W., Wallace, R.M., Bruce, M.A., Seizinger, B.R., Menon, A.G., Gusella, J.F., Michels, V.V., Schmidt, M.A., Dewald, G.W., Collins, F.S. Physical mapping of a translocation breakpoint in neurofibromatosis. Science. *244:*1085–1087, 1989.
8. Marchuk, D.A., Saulino, A.M., Tavakkol, R., Swaroop, M., Wallace, M.R., Andersen, L.B., Mitchell, A.L., Gutmann, D.H., Boguski, M., Collins, F.S. cDNA cloning of the Type 1 neurofibromatosis gene: complete sequence of the NF1 gene product. Genomics. *11:*931–940, 1991.
9. Viskochil, D., Cawthon, R., O'Connell, P., Xu, G.F., Stevens, J., Culver, M., Carey, J., White, R. The gene encoding the oligodendrocyte myelin glycoprotein is embedded within the neurofibromatosis Type 1 gene. Mol Cell Biol. *11:*906–912, 1991.
10. O'Connell, P., Viskochil, D., Buchberg, A., Foundation, J., Cawthon, R.M., Culver, M., Stevens, J., Rich, D.C., Ledbetter, D.H., Wallace, M., et al. The human homology of murine EV12 lies between two von Recklinghausen neurofibromatosis translocations. Genomics. *7:*547–554, 1990.
11. Cawthon, R.M., Andersen, L.B., Buchberg, A.M., Xu, G.F., O'Connell, P., Viskochil, D., Weiss, R.B., Wallace, M.R., Marchuk, D.A., Culver, M., Stevens, J., Jenkins, N.A., Copeland, N.G., Collins, F.S., White, R: cDNA sequence and genomic structure of EVI2B, a gene lying within an intron of the neurofibromatosis Type 1 gene. Genomics. *9:*446–460, 1991.
12. Ballester, R., Marchuk, D., Bogushi, M. The NF1 locus encodes a protein functionally related to mammalian GAP and yeast IRA proteins. Cell. *63:*851–859, 1990.
13. Xu, G., Lin, B., Tanaka, K., Dunn, D., Wood, D., Gesteland, R., White, R., Weiss, R., Tamanoi, F. The catalytic domain of the neurofibromatosis Type 1 gene product stimulates ras GTPase and complements IRA mutants of S. Cerevisiae. Cell. *63:*835–841, 1990.
14. Martin, G.A., Viskochil, D., Bollag, G. The GAP-related domain of the neurofibromatosis Type 1 Gene product interacts with ras p21. Cell. *63:*643–849, 1990.
15. Nur-E-Kamal, M.S., Varga, M., Maruta, H. The GTPase-activating NF1 fragment of 91 amino acids reverses v-Ha-Ras induced malignant phenotype. J Biol Chem. *268:*22331–22337, 1993.
16. Johnson, M.R., DeClue, J.E., Felzmann, S., Vass, W.C., Xy, G., White, R., Lowy. D.R. Neurofibromin can inhibit Ras-dependent growth by a mechanism independent of its GTPase-accelerating function. Mol Cell Biol. *14:*641–645, 1994.
17. Griffin, C.A., Hawkins, A.L., Packer, R.J., Rorke, L.B., Emanuel, B.S. Chromosome abnormalities in pediatric brain tumors. Cancer Res. *48:*175–180, 1988.
18. Karnes, P.S., Tran, T.N., Cui, M.Y., Raffel, C., Gilles, F.H., Barranger J.A., Ying, K.L. Cytogenetic analysis of 39 pediatric central nervous system tumors. Cancer Genet Cytogenet. *59:*12–19, 1992.
19. Litofsky, N.S., Hinton, D., Raffel, C. The lack of a role for p53 in astrocytomas in pediatric patients. Neurosurgery. *34:*967–973, 1994.7. Arnoldus EPJ, Noordermeer IA, Boudewijn PAC, Voormolen JHC, Bots GTAM, Raap AK, Pleog VDM. Interphase cytogenetics of brain tumors. Genes Chromosomes Cancer. *3:*101–107, 1991.
20. Lang, F.F., Miller, D.C., Koslow, M., Newcomb, E.W. Pathways leading to glioblastoma multiform: a molecular analysis of genetic alterations in 65 astrocytic tumors. J Neurosurg. *81:*427–436, 1994.
21. El-Azouzi, M., Chung, R.Y., Farmer, G.E., Martuza, R.L., Black, P.M., Rouleau, G.A., Hettlich, C., Hedley-Whyte, E.T., Zervas, N.T., Panagopoulos, K., Nakamura, Y., Gusella, J.F., Seizinger, B.R. Loss of distinct regions on the short arm of chromosome 17 associated with tumorigenesis of human astrocytomas. Proc Natl Acad Sci USA. *86:*7186–7190, 1989.
22. Fults, D., Tippets, R.H., Thomas, G.A., Nakamura, Y., White, R. Loss of heterozygosity for loci on chromosome 17p in human malignant astrocytomas. Cancer Res. *49:*6572–6577, 1989.
23. James, C.D., Carlbom, E., Nordenskjold, M., Collins, V.P., Cavenee, W.K. Mitotic recombination of chromosome 17 in astrocytomas. Proc Natl Acad Sci USA. *86:*2858–2862, 1989.8. Botstein D, White RL, Skolnick M, Davis R. Construction of a genetic linkage map in man using restriction fragment length polymorphisms. Am J Hum Genet. *32:*314–331, 1980.
24. Biegel, J.A., Burk, C.D., Barr, F.G., Emanuel, B.S. Evidence for a 17p tumor related locus distinct from p53 in pediatric primitive neuroectodermal tumors. Cancer Res. *52:*3391–3395, 1992.
25. Cogen, P.H., Daneshvar, L., Metzger, A.K., Cuyk, G., Edwards, M.S.B., Sheffield, V.C. Involvement of multiple chromosome 17p loci in medulloblastoma tumorigenesis. Am J Hum Genet. *50:*584–589, 1992.
26. Raffel, C., Thomas, G.A., Tishler, D.M., Lassoff, S,, Allen, J.C. Absence of p53 mutations in childhood central nervous system primitive neuroectodermal tumors. Neurosurgery. *33:*301–306, 1993.
27. Lang, F.F., Miller, D.C,, Pisharody, S., Koslow, M., New-

comb, E.W. High frequency of p53 protein accumulation without p53 gene mutation in human juvenile pilocytic, low grade and anaplastic astrocytomas. Oncogene. *9:*949–954, 1994.

28. Louis, D.N. The p53 gene and protein in human brain tumors. J Neuropathol Exp Neurol. *53:*11–21, 1994.

29. Stroink, A.R., Hoffman, H.J., Hendrick, E.B., Humphreys, R.P. Diagnosis and management of pediatric brain stem gliomas. J Neurosurg. *65:*744–750, 1986.

30. Louis, D.N., Rubio, M.P., Correa, K.M., Gusella, J.F., von Deimling, A. Molecular genetics of pediatric brain stem gliomas. Application of PCR techniques to small and archival brain tumor specimens. J Neuropathol Exp Neurol. *52:*507–515, 1993.

31. Griffin, C.A., Long, P.P., Carson, B.S., Brem, H. Chromosome abnormalities in low-grade central nervous system tumors. Cancer Genet Cytogenet. *60:*67–73, 1992.

32. Jenkins, R.B., Kimmel, D.W., Moertel, C.A., Schultz, C.G., Scheithauer, B.W., Kelly, P.J., Dewald, G.W. A cytogenetic study of 63 human gliomas. Cancer Genet Cytogenet. *39:*253–279, 1989.

33. Rey, J.A., Bello, M.J., de Campos, J.M., Kusak, M.E., Moreno, S. Chromsomal composition of a series of 22 human low-grade gliomas. Cancer Genet Cytogenet. *29:*223–237, 1987.

34. Sainati, L., Montaldi, A., Putti, M.C., Giangaspero, F., Rigobello, L., Stella, M., Zanesco, L., Basso, G. Cytogenetic t(11;17) (q13;q21) in pediatric epmedymoma: is 11q13 a recurring breakpoint in ependymomas? Cancer Genet Cytogenet. *59:*213–216, 1992.

35. Stratton, M.R., Darling, J., Lantos, P.L., Cooper, C.S., Reeves, B.R. Cytogenetic abnormalities in human ependymomas. Int J Cancer. *44:*579–581, 1989.

36. Weremowicz, S., Kupsky, W.J., Morton, C., Fletcher, J.A. Cytogenetic evidence for a chromosome 22 tumor suppressor gene in ependymoma. Cancer Genet Cytogenet. *61:*193–196, 1992.

37. Bigner, S.H. Cytogenetics of human brain tumors. Cancer Genet Cytogenet. *47:*141–154, 1990.

38. Ransom, D.T., Ritland, S.R., Kimmel, D.W., Moertel, C.A., Dahl, R.J., Scheithauer, B.W., Kelly, P.J., Jenkins, R.B. Cytogenetic and loss of heterozygosity studies in ependymomas, pilocytic astrocytomas, and oligodendrogliomas. Genes Chromosomes Cancer. *5:*348–356, 1992.

39. Metzger, A.K., Sheffield, V.C., Duyk, G., Daneshvar, L., Edwards, M.S.B, Cogen, P.H. Identification of a germline mutation in the p53 gene in a patient with an intracranial ependymoma. Proc Natl Acad Sci USA. *88:*7825–7829, 1991.

40. Ohgaki, H., Eibl, R.H., Wiestler, O.D., Yasargil, M.G., Newcomb, E.W., Kleihues, P. p53 mutations in nonastrocytic human brain tumors. Cancer Res. *51:*6202–6205, 1991.

41. Kirschstein, R.L., Gerber, P. Ependymomas produced after intracerebral inoculation of SV40 into newborn hamsters. Nature. *195:*299–300, 1962.

42. Bergsagel, D.J., Finegold, M.J., Butel, J.S., Kupsky, W.J., Garcea, R.L. DNA sequences similar to those of simian virus 40 in ependymomas and choroid plexus tumors of childhood. N Engl J Med. *326:*988–993, 1992.

43. Linzer, D.I., Levine, A.J. Characterization of a 54K dalton cellular SV40 tumor antigen present in SV40-transformed cells and uninfected embroynal carcinoma cells. Cell. *17:*43–52, 1979.

44. Lane, D.P., Crawford, L.V. T antigen is bound to host protein in SV40 transformed cells. Nature. *278:*261–263, 1979.

45. Bigner, S.H., Mark, J., Friedman, H.S., Biegel, J.A., Bigner, D.D. Structural chromosomal abnormalities in human medulloblastoma. Cancer Genet Cytogenet. *30:*91–101, 1988.

46. Raffel, C., Gilles, F.E., Weinberg, K.I. Reduction to homozygosity and gene amplification in central nervous system primitive neuroectodermal tumors of childhood. Cancer Res. *50:*587–91, 1990.

47. Thomas, G.A., Raffel, C. Loss of heterozygosity on 6q, 16q, and 17p in human central nervous system primitive neuroectodermal tumors. Cancer Res. *51:*639–43, 1991.

48. Saylors, S.L. 3d, Sidransky, D., Friedman, H.S., Bigner, S.H., Bigner, D.D., Vogelstein, B., Brodeur, G.M. Infrequent p53 gene mutations in medulloblastomas. Cancer Res. *51:*4721–3, 1991.

49. Badiali, M., Iolascon, A., Loda, M., Scheithauer, B.W., Baso, G., Trentini, G.P., Giangaspero, F. p53 gene mutations in medulloblastoma. Immunohistochemistry, gel shift analysis, and sequencing. Diagnos Mol Path. *2:*23–8, 1993.

50. Adesina, A.M., Nalbantoglu, J., Cavenee, W.K. p53 gene mutation and mdm2 gene amplification are uncommon in medulloblastoma. Cancer Res. *54:*5649–51, 1994.

51. McDonald, J.D., Daneshvar, L., Willert, J.R., Matsumura, K., Waldman, F., Cogen, P.H. Physical mapping of chromosome 17p13.3 in the region of a putative tumor suppressor gene important in medulloblastoma. Genomics. *23:*229–32, 1994.

52. Oliner, J.D., Kinzler, K.W., Meltzer, P.S., George, D.L., Vogelstein, B. Amplification of a gene encoding a p53-associated protein in human sarcomas. Nature. *358:*80–3, 1992.

53. Ladanyi, M., Cha, C., Lewis, R., Jhanwar, S.C, Huvos, Ag, Healey, J.H. MDM2 gene amplification in metastatic osteosarcoma. Cancer Res. *53:*16–8, 1993.

54. Gorlin, R.J. Nevoid basal-cell carcinoma syndrome. Medicine. *66:*98–113, 1987.

55. Lacombe, D., Chateil, J.F., Fontan, D., Battin, J. Medullobastoma in the nevoid basal-cell carcinoma syndrome: case reports and review of the literature. Genet Counsel. *1:*273–7, 1990.

56. Evans, D.G., Farndon, P.A., Burnell, L.D., Gattamaneni, H.R., Birch, J.M. The incidence of Gorlin syndrome in 173 consecutive cases of medulloblastoma. Brit J Cancer. *64:*959–61, 1991.

57. Farndon, P.A., Del Mastro, R.G., Evans, D.G., Kilpatrick, M.W. Location of gene for Gorlin syndrome. Lancet. *339:*581–2, 1992.

58. Gailani, M.R., Bale, S.J., Leffell, D.J., DiGiovanna, J.J., Peck, G.L., Poliak, S., Drum, M.A., Pastakia, B., McBride, O.W., Kase, R., et al. Developmental defects in Gorlin syndrome related to a putative tumor suppressor gene on chromosome 9. Cell. *69:*111–7, 1992.

59. Albrecht, S., von Deimling, A., Pietsch, T., Giangaspero, F., Brandner, S., Kleihues, P., Wiestler, O.D: Microsatellite analysis of loss of heterozygosity on chromosomes 9q, 11p, and 17p in medullobLastomas. Neuropath Applied Neurobiol. *20:*74–81, 1994.

60. Schofield, D., West, D.C., Anthony, D.C., Marshal, R.,

Sklar, J. Correlation of loss of heterozygosity at chromosome 9q with histological subtype in medulloblastomas. Amer J Path. *146:*472–8, 1995.

61. Johnson RL, Rothman AL, Xie J, Goodrich LV, Bare JW, Bonifas JM, Quinn AG, Myers RM, Cox DR, Epstein EH Jr, Scott MP: Human Homolog of *Patched*, a Candidate Gene for the Basal Cell Nevus Syndrome. Science *272:*1668–1671, 1996.

62. Hahn H, Wicking C, Zaphiropoulos PG, Gailani MR, Shanley S, Chidambaram A, Vorachovsky I, Holmberg E, Unden AB, Giles S, Negus K, Smyth I, Pressman C, Lefell DJ, Gerrard B, Goldstein AM, Dean M, Toftgard R, Chenevix-Trench G, Wainwright B, Bale AE: Mutations of the Human Homolog of Drosophila *Patched* in the Nevoid Basal Cell Carcinoma Syndrome. Cell *85:*841–851, 1996.

63. Hooper JE, Scott MP: The Drosophila Patched Gene Encodes a Putative Membrane Protein Required for Segmental Patterning. Cell *59*(4)*:*751–765, Nov. 17, 1989.

64. Nakano Y, Guerrero I, Hidalgo A, Taylor A, Whittle JR, Ingham PW: A Protein with Several Possible Membrane-Spanning Domains Encoded by the Drosophila Segment Polarity Gene Patched. Nature *341*(6242)*:* 508–513, Oct. 12, 1989.

65. Perrimon N: Hedgehog and Beyond (Review). Cell *80*(4)*:* 517–520, Feb. 24, 1995.

66. Domínguez M, Brunner M, Hafen E, Basler K: Sending and Receiving the Hedgehog Signal: Control by the *Drosophila* Gli Protein Cubitus Interruptus. Science *272:*1621–1624, 1996.

67. Hahn H, Christiansen J, Wicking C, Zaphiropoulos PG, Chidambaram A, Gerrard B, Vorechovsky I, Bale AE, Toftgard R, Dean M, Wainwright B: A Mammalian *Patched* Homolog is Expressed in Target Tissues of *Sonic Hedgehog* and Maps to a Region Associated with Developmental Abnormalities.

68. Kinzler KW, Vogelstein B: The GLI Gene Encodes a Nuclear Protein which Binds Specific Sequences in the Human Genoma. Molecular & Cellular Biology *10*(2)*:* 634–642, Feb. 1990.

69. Jen, J., Harper, J.W., Bigner, S.H., Bigner, D.D., Papadapoulos, N., Markowitz, S., Willson, J.K., Kinzler, K.W., Vogelstein, B. Deletion of p16 and p15 genes in brain tumors. Cancer Res. *54:*6353–8, 1994.

70. Raffel, C., Ueki, K., Harsh, G.R. 4th, Louis, D.N. The multiple tumor suppressor 1/cyclin-dependent kinase inhibitor 2 gene in human central nervous system primitive neuroectodermal tumor. Neurosurg. *36:*971–4, 1995.

71. Turcot, J., Despres, J.-P., St Pierre, F. Malignant tumors of the central nervous system associated with familial polyposis of the colon: report of two cases. Dis Colon Rectum. *2:*465–468, 1959.

72. Hamilton. S.R., Liu, B., Parsons, R.E., Papadopoulos, N., Jen, J., Powell, S.M., Krush, A.J., Berk, T., Cohen, Z., Tetu, B., et al. The molecular basis of Turcot's syndrome. New Engl J Med. *332:*839–47, 1995.

73. Mori, T., Nagase, H., Horii, A., Miyoshi, Y., Shimano, T., Nakatsuru, S., Aoki, T., Arakawa, H., Yanagisawa, A., Ushio, Y., et al. Germ-line and somatic mutations of the APC gene in patients with Turcot syndrome and analysis of APC mutations in brain tumors. Genes Chromosomes Cancer. *9:*168–72, 1994.

74. Yong, W.H., Raffel, C., von Deimling, A., Louis, D.N. The APC gene in Turcot's syndrome. New Engl J Med. *333:*524, 1995.

75. Wasson, J.C., Saylors, R.L. 3d, Zeltzer, P., Friedman, H.S., Bigner, S.H., Burger, P.C., Bigner, D.D., Look, A.T., Douglass, E.C., Brodeur, G.M. Oncogene amplification in pediatric brain tumors. Cancer Res. *50:*2987–90, 1990.

76. Bigner, S.H., Friedman, H.S., Vogelstein, B., Oakes, W.J., Bigner, D.D. Amplification of the c-myc gene in human medulloblastoma cell lines and xenografts. Cancer Res. *50:*2347–50, 1990.

77. MacGregor, D.N., Ziff, E.B. Elevated c-myc expression in childhood medulloblastomas. Ped Res. *28:*63–8, 1990.

78. Badiali, M., Pession, A., Basso, G., Andreini, L., Rigobello, L., Galassi, E., Giangaspero, F. N-myc and c-myc oncogenes amplification in medulloblastomas. Evidence of particularly aggressive behavior of a tumor with c-myc amplification. Tumori. *77:*118–21, 1991.

79. Iolascon, A., Lania, A., Badiali, M., Pession, A., Saglio, G., Giangaspero, F., Miraglia del Giudice, E., Perrotta, S., Cutillo, S. Analysis of N-ras gene mutations in medulloblastomas by polymerase chain reaction and oligonucleotide probes in formalin-fixed, paraffin-embedded tissues. Med Ped Onc. *19:*240–5, 1991.

80. Gilbertson, R.J., Pearson, A.D., Perry, R.H., Jaros, E., Kelly, P.J. Prognostic significance of the c-erbB-2 oncogene product in childhood medulloblastoma. Brit J Cancer. *71:*473–7, 1995.

81. Nakasu, S., Nakasu, Y., Nioka, H., Nakajima, M., Handa, J. bcl-2 protein expression in tumors of the central nervous system. Acta Neuropathologica. *88:*520–6, 1994.

82. Kozmik, Z., Sure, U., Reudi, D., Busslinger, M., Aguzzi, A. Deregulated expression of PAX5 in medulloblastoma. Proc Natl Acad Sci USA. *92:*5709–13, 1995.

83. Pleasure, S.J., Reddy, U.R., Venkatakrishnan, G., Roy, A.K., Chen, J., Ross, A.H., Trojanowski, J.Q., Pleasure, D.E., Lee, V.M. Introduction of nerve growth factor (NGF) receptors into a medulloblastoma cell line results in expression of high- and low-affinity NGF receptors but not NGF-mediated differentiation. Proc Natl Acad Sci USA. *87:*8496–500, 1990.

84. Keles, G.E., Berger, M.S., Schofield, D., Bothwell, M. Nerve growth factor receptor expression in medulloblastomas and the potential role of nerve growth factor as a differentiating agent in medulloblastoma cell lines. Neurosurg. *32:*274–80, 1993.

85. Kokunai, T., Sawa, H., Tatsumi, S., Tamaki, N. Expression of nerve growth factor receptor by human primitive neuroectodermal tumors. Neurologia Medico-Chirurgica. *34:*523–9, 1994.

86. Washiyama, K., Muragaki, Y., Rorke, L.B., Lee, V. M.-Y., Flinstein, S.C., Radeke, M.J., Blumberg, D., Kaplan, D.R., Trojanowski, J.Q. Neurotrophin and neurotrophin receptor proteins in medulloblastomas and other primitive neuroectodermal tumors of the pediatric central nervous system. Amer J Path.

87. Segal, R.A., Goumnerova, L.C., Kwon, Y.K., Stiles, C.D., Pomeroy, S.L. Expression of the neurotrophin receptor TrkC is linked to a favorable outcome in medulloblastoma. Proc Natl Acad Sci USA. *91:*12867–71, 1994.

88. Chin, L.S., Jung, W.K.A., Raffel, C. Two primitive neuroectodermal cell line require an activated insulin-like growth factor receptor for growth in vitro. Neurosurg. In press.

CHAPTER 7

Molecular Genetic Basis of Hereditary Tumor Syndromes of the Nervous System

DAVID N. LOUIS, M.D., HARTMUT P. H. NEUMANN, M.D.,
ANIL G. MENON, M.D. M. PRISCILLA SHORT, M.D.,
BERTON ZBAR, M.D., ANDREAS VON DEIMLING, M.D.

INTRODUCTION

Hereditary tumor syndromes of the nervous system have long captured the imagination of the neurological community. From the initial clinicopathological descriptions more than 100 years ago to the gene cloning successes of the past 5 years, these remarkable conditions have been subject to intense scrutiny by neuropathologists, neurologists, neurosurgeons, and geneticists. This chapter reviews the molecular genetic bases of these tumor syndromes, particularly neurofibromatosis 1, neurofibromatosis 2, tuberous sclerosis, and von Hippel-Lindau disease. The syndromes, their characteristic nervous system lesions, and their known genetic alterations are catalogued in Table 1.

Most of the genes responsible for hereditary tumor syndromes are tumor suppressor genes. Tumor suppressor genes are normal genes that inhibit cell proliferation and growth (100, 114). The loss or inactivation of these genes may, therefore, result in tumor formation or progression. In general, both allelic copies of a tumor suppressor gene must be inactivated to provide an oncogenic stimulus. In the hereditary tumor syndromes, the first allele is inactivated in the germline and the second on a somatic basis. The high likelihood of the second event in at least one susceptible cell explains the apparent dominant inheritance pattern of these tumor syndromes, even though tumor suppressor genes are "recessive" at the genetic level.

In general, the same genes that predispose patients to particular neoplasms when mutated in the germline are involved in the corresponding sporadic tumors as well. Thus, neurofibromatosis 2 patients with inherited NF2 gene mutations are predisposed to meningiomas, schwannomas, and some gliomas; the NF2 gene is, accordingly, inactivated in sporadic meningiomas, schwannomas, and some gliomas (77, 141, 180). In this regard, studies of germline genetic alterations in hereditary tumor syndromes and somatic genetic alterations in sporadic tumors often complement one another. There are some notable exceptions, however, such as the common involvement of the p53 gene in colorectal carcinomas but the lack of colorectal carcinomas in patients with germline p53 gene mutations (90).

There are also a number of variations on the classical tumor suppressor gene paradigm. For some tumor suppressor genes, a single mutant allele may have an oncogenic, "dominant negative" effect without loss of the other allele (70). For instance, patients with Denys-Drash syndrome (intersexual disorders, nephropathy, Wilms' tumor), harboring one mutant copy of the WT1 gene in their germline have a much higher incidence of Wilms' tumor than patients with WAGR syndrome (Wilms' tumor, aniridia,

TABLE 1
Hereditary Tumor Syndromes of the Nervous System

Syndrome	Nervous System Lesions	Chromosomal Locus	Gene	Protein/Function
Neurofibromatosis 1	neurofibroma neurofibrosarcoma optic nerve glioma other astrocytomas pheochromocytoma	17q11	NF1	GTPase-activating (GAP) protein
Neurofibromatosis 2	schwannoma meningioma glioma (ependymoma) glial heterotopia	22q12	NF2	cytoskeletal-cell membrane link
Tuberous sclerosis	subependymal giant cell astrocytoma cortical tuber	16p13 9q34	TSC2 ?	? GAP
von Hippel-Lindau	hemangioblastoma pheochromocytoma	3p25	VHL	?
Retinoblastoma	retinoblastoma pineoblastoma malignant glioma	13q14	RB1	transcription G1 arrest
Li-Fraumeni	malignant glioma	17p13	TP53	transcription G1 arrest apoptosis DNA repair
Familial glioma	malignant glioma	? ?17p13	? ?TP53	
Turcot	medulloblastoma malignant glioma	5q21 2p, 3p, etc.	APC mismatch-	? repair genes
Gorlin	medulloblastoma	9q31	?	
Cowden	Lhermitte-Duclos	?	?	
MEN1	pituitary adenoma	11q13	?	
MEN2A/MEN2B	pheochromocytoma	10q11	RET	transmembrane tyrosine kinase

genitourinary malformations, mental retardation), who lack one WT1 allele in their germline (29). Genomic imprinting, the differential expression of one allele relative to the parental origin of the allele, may also play a role in some hereditary tumor syndromes, e.g., the Beckwith-Wiedemann syndrome (organomegaly, hemihypertrophy, Wilms' tumor, rhabdomyosarcoma, hepatoblastoma) (179) and possibly the retinoblastoma susceptibility syndrome (122). As mentioned briefly above, three hereditary tumor syndromes arise from alterations in a proto-oncogene rather than a tumor suppressor gene: the RET gene in multiple endocrine neoplasia 2A and 2B and hereditary medullary thyroid carcinoma (132). Finally, some hereditary tumor syndromes, such as the hereditary nonpolyposis colorectal carcinoma syndromes (Lynch cancer family syndromes 1 and 2) and some cases of Turcot's syndrome, may be attributable to defects in mismatch repair genes rather than true tumor suppressors (46, 64). As knowledge of the molecular basis of these syndromes advances, countless variations on the general tumor suppressor gene theme will come to the fore and will contribute to a more complete understanding of the genetic basis of tumor predisposition.

NEUROFIBROMATOSIS 1 (NF1)

Clinicopathological Features of NF1

Neurofibromatosis 1 is a hereditary disease transmitted in an autosomal dominant fashion with an incidence of about 1 in 3000 (136). Fifty percent of patients with NF1 do not have a family history of NF1, reflecting the high sporadic mutation rate in the NF1 gene (estimated at 1 in 10000 alleles per generation) (136). The majority of such new mutations are of paternal origin (78). NF1 shows almost 100% penetrance but exhibits considerable variation in clinical severity (variable expressivity), even within the same family (21, 22, 73, 136). Patients suffering from NF1 can present with a wide variety of lesions, and a detailed review of the clinicopathological features has recently been published (175). To meet diagnostic criteria, patients with NF1 must have two or more of the following features (121, 175):

- Six or more cafe-au-lait spots (over 5 mm in greatest diameter in prepubertal individuals and over 15 mm greatest diameter in postpubertal individuals);
- Two or more neurofibromas of any type or one plexiform neurofibroma;
- Freckling in the axillary regions;
- Optic glioma;
- Two or more Lisch nodules;
- A distinctive osseous lesion such as sphenoid dysplasia or thinning of the long bone cortex with or without pseudoarthrosis;
- A first degree relative with NF1 by the above criteria.

Other lesions associated with NF1 include a variety of neoplasms, in particular the malignant peripheral nerve sheath tumor or neurofibrosarcoma.

Molecular Genetics of NF1

Linkage analysis suggested in 1987 that the NF1 gene was located on chromosome 17 (8, 154). Despite the phenotypic variation in NF1, a single locus appeared to be responsible, although such clinical variability suggests that other genetic loci may influence the phenotype (37). Refined genetic mapping placed the NF1 gene on the long arm of the chromosome, close to the centromere (44, 52). The critical breakthroughs that pinpointed the gene were the identification of chromosomal translocations involving the NF1 region on chromosome 17 in two unrelated individuals with the disorder, suggesting that these breakpoints disrupted the function of the NF1 gene (97, 147). Physical mapping techniques were used to identify a 600-kb DNA fragment that spanned both translocation breakpoints and probably contained the NF1 gene (47, 48, 130, 131). Screening of cDNA libraries revealed a gene that showed mutations in DNA from NF1 patients (24, 60, 174, 178).

The NF1 gene spans more than 350 kb of genomic DNA and contains 59 exons, encoding a protein product of 2818 amino acids (10, 11, 102, 113). Three smaller genes—EVI1 (ecotropic virus integration site), EVI2, and OMGP (oligodendrocyte myelin glycoprotein)—are

embedded in one of the larger introns of the NF1 gene, although whether these genes or their products play any role in the regulation of NF1 is not yet known. The NF1 gene appears to be ubiquitously expressed (31–34, 53, 60), and it is abundantly expressed in tissues such as Schwann cells, that are affected in NF1 in both normal and afflicted individuals with the disorder (59, 89). Some of the exons that comprise the 11 to 13 kb NF1 transcript are spliced alternatively, yielding different NF1 transcripts (10, 119, 169). The primary isoform, sometimes called the type I isoform, was the first one described in the cloning of the NF1 gene (24, 178). An alternative isoform (type II), originally isolated from tumor RNA, contains a 63-bp exon spliced 5' to the exon coding for the GAP-related domain (128, 169); however, this isoform is not restricted to tumors and has comparable GAP activity (4). A third isoform (type III) contains an additional 54 bases that encode an 18 amino acid insert near the C terminus of the protein (23). In staged mouse embryos, the NF1 gene was expressed as early as 8 days post-coitum (E8) (32, 74). A significant increase in neurofibromin in all tissues was observed in 11-day (E11) embryos. Interestingly, the type I and type II isoforms were expressed at different times and in different tissues, depending on the differentiation of the tissue. The type I isoform was mainly expressed in the early stages (E8 through E11), whereas type II was predominant after day 11 (74).

The protein product of the NF1 gene has been termed neurofibromin. Sequence analysis of the NF1 gene and its predicted protein product revealed a domain shared by GTP-ase activating proteins (GAPs) of both vertebrates and invertebrates (7, 20, 34, 184, 185). The proposed involvement of neurofibromin in a *ras*-associated signal transduction pathway suggests that neurofibromin may localize with *ras*. Immunohistochemical studies in rat tissues and cultured human cell lines have demonstrated neurofibromin possibly sublocalizing with microtubules (32, 53, 58). However, other immunohistochemical studies and differential centrifugation (where NF1-GAP activity had a 60:40 cytoplasmic:particulate/nuclear fractions ratio) have questioned this assumption (15).

Genetic and biochemical approaches using the GAP-related domain of the NF1 gene (NF1-GRD) have supported the hypothesis that neurofibromin is involved in the *ras* pathway, possibly by stimulating ras-GTPase activity (7, 184, 185). A complex regulatory pathway of *ras* activation involves NF1-GRD and p120-GAP (the other major activator of ras GTPase); at high concentrations of N-*ras* GTP, p120-GAP is the major stimulator of GTPase activity, whereas at low concentrations of N-*ras* GTP, p120 and NF1-GRD stimulation is comparable, suggesting that NF1-GRD has a higher affinity for N-*ras* (115). Recent studies have also proposed that molecules such as arachidonate and phosphotidylinositol 4,5-biphosphate, which are mitogenic in vitro, differentially inhibit p120GAP and NF1-GRD (54, 65). This observation would corroborate the earlier hypothesis that neurofibromin acts in signal transduction in the *ras*-dependent mitogenic pathway (15, 35). It has also been suggested that neurofibromin might have two different roles: as a negative regulator of p21Ras mediated signalling pathway for proliferation; and as a downstream effector of p21Ras possibly in a pathway of differentiation (149).

NF1 gene mutations have now been documented in a number of NF1 patients and in some sporadic tumors. The NF1 gene can apparently be inactivated by a number of mechanisms. However, the large size of the NF1 gene has made the detection of mutations a Herculean effort. An international NF1 Genetic Analysis Consortium has been established with the specific purpose of collecting and organizing information regarding these mutations. Some of the germline mutations have recently been tabulated (175). These include point mutations and deletions (24, 178) as well as insertions (177). At the present, distinct genotype-phenotype correlations have not yet emerged from this analysis, and will have to await more extensive collections of both clinical and mutation data.

NF1 patients develop benign neurofibromas and malignant peripheral nerve sheath tumors (MPNSTs)/neurofibrosarcomas. Given the two-hit hypothesis of tumor suppressor gene inactivation, it was predicted that these tumors would have loss of the remaining copy of chromosome 17q. In fact, deletions of chromosome 17q were interpreted early on to indicate that the NF1 was a classic tumor suppressor (159). Mutations in the NF1 gene and/or loss of the remaining copy of chromosome 17q have now been demonstrated in many tumors associated with NF1 (98, 101, 176)—in both NF1 patients and, importantly, in sporadic cases. Curiously, however, unequivocal proof of inactivation of both alleles of the NF1 gene in neurofibromas, the hallmark tumor of NF1, is still missing, and it remains possible that some neurofibromas are inherently polyclonal lesions (116, 160). In addition, NF1 mutations have been noted in tumors not traditionally associated with NF1, such as neuroblastoma and melanoma (81, 149). Some tumors (neurofibrosarcomas and MPNSTs) obtained from NF1 patients also have abnormalities in the ratio of bound/unbound GTP Ras (9, 35), underlining the importance of the NF1-related pathway in the genesis of these tumors.

Knockout mice have provided an important avenue for the investigation of the physiological role of the NF1 gene. Mice that are homozygously mutant for the NF1 gene lack neurofibromin in all tissues, show widespread developmental abnormalities, and do not survive beyond the 14-day (postconception) embryo stage (18). Mice that are heterozygous, i.e., have only one copy of the mutant NF1 gene, often develop tumors that are seen in some NF1 patients, notably pheochromocytomas and myeloid leukemias. Other tumors that were disproportionately seen in this population of heterozygous mutant mice included lymphoma, lymphoid leukemia, lung adenocarcinoma, hepatoma, and fibrosarcoma, corroborating the role of the NF1 gene as a tumor suppressor (76).

NEUROFIBROMATOSIS 2 (NF2)

Clinicopathological Features of NF2

Neurofibromatosis 2, previously known as central neurofibromatosis or bilateral acoustic neurofibromatosis, is an uncommon disorder, affecting approximately 1 in 40,000 individuals (43). The condition is inherited in an autosomal dominant manner with high penetrance, although about one-half of cases have no family history and most likely represent new mutations. Patients with NF2 are genetically predisposed to a number of characteristic tumors, as well as some non-neoplastic conditions such as posterior subcapsular lens opacities. The neuropathological abnormalities are generally low-grade neoplasms or malformative conditions of Schwann cells (schwannomas and schwannosis), meningothelial cells (meningiomas and meningioangiomatosis) and glia (gliomas and glial hamartomas). A detailed review of the clinical and pathological features of NF2 has been recently published (104). The current diagnostic criteria (43, 72, 157) for NF2 are either:

1) bilateral vestibular schwannomas; or
2) a first degree relative with NF2, and either
   a unilateral vestibular schwannoma or
   two of the following: meningioma, schwannoma, glioma, neurofibroma, posterior subcapsular lens opacity, or cerebral calcification; or
3) two of the following
   unilateral vestibular schwannoma
   multiple meningiomas
   either schwannoma, glioma, neurofibroma, posterior subcapsular lens opacity, or cerebral calcification.

As molecular genetic analyses of the NF2 gene become more commonplace, however, diagnostic criteria may shift, perhaps bringing a variety of NF2-variants into the fold.

Molecular Genetics of NF2 and Related Tumors

In 1986 and 1987, molecular genetic studies of sporadic and NF2-associated schwannomas and meningiomas showed frequent allelic loss of chromosome 22, suggesting that the NF2 gene resided on chromosome 22 (151, 152). This hypothesis was confirmed when molecular genetic analyses of large NF2 pedigrees demonstrated linkage of NF2 to chromosome 22q12 (140, 181). Subsequent analyses have shown that all studied NF2 pedigrees link to chromosome 22q, implying that defects in one gene account for all families with NF2 (120). Additional linkage studies were used to narrow the location of the NF2 gene, and in 1993, the gene was cloned by two independent groups (139, 166).

The NF2 gene spans 110 kb, comprising 16 constitutive exons and one alternatively spliced exon. NF2 mRNA transcripts occur in three different size ranges, approximately 7 kb, 4.4 kb, and 2.6 kb, and encode at least two major alternative protein forms (12, 77, 139, 166). The alternatively spliced exon 16 alters the C-terminus of the protein, replacing 16 amino acids with 11 novel residues (12, 77). Additional alternative splices predicting other minor species have also been described (5, 133). The mouse homologue, which maps to mouse chromosome 11, is similarly alternatively spliced and predicts a protein that is 98% identical to the human gene product (27, 61, 67).

The NF2 gene is expressed in most studied normal human tissues, including heart, lung, skeletal muscle, kidney, breast, ovary and placenta, brain, pancreas, and liver (139, 166). High expression has been noted in mouse fetal brain (139). The predicted protein product of the NF2 gene shows a strong similarity to the highly conserved protein 4.1 family of cytoskeleton-associated proteins, which includes protein 4.1, talin, moesin, ezrin, radixin, and two protein tyrosine phosphatases, PTP-MEG and PTP-H1. Because the NF2-encoded protein is most similar to moesin, ezrin, and radixin, it was named merlin, for moesin-ezrin-radixin-like protein (166). The alternative name schwannomin was subsequently suggested by a second group (139). Merlin can be detected immunohistochemically in the cytoplasm of many cells, including Schwann cells, fibroblasts, neurons, and histiocytes (unpublished data) (146).

While members of the protein 4.1 family probably have a number of functions, their primary role may be in mediating communication between the extracellular milieu and the cytoskeleton, by acting as a link between integral membrane proteins and the scaffolding proteins of the filamentous submembrane lattice (106). For instance, moesin, ezrin, and radixin interact with CD44 as a membrane target (167). The 4.1 family proteins are defined by a homologous domain of approximately 270 amino acids near the amino-terminus (106). In merlin and its most closely related proteins, moesin, ezrin, and radixin, this domain is followed by a long α-helical segment and a charged carboxyl-terminal domain. The similarity between merlin and these other three proteins suggests that merlin may also associate with both membrane and cytoskeletal structures. However, the distinct localization and behavior of moesin, ezrin and radixin make it likely that merlin also has a unique cellular role. At least five proteins, varying in size from 70 to 165 kD, appear to bind merlin at its amino-terminal, moesin-ezrin-radixin homology domain (162). Since most of the described NF2 mutations (see below) would probably alter such merlin-protein binding, these proteins may be important for merlin to effect tumor suppression.

Unlike the search for NF1 gene mutations, analysis of the NF2 gene has revealed a plethora of germline and somatic mutations that are predicted to affect protein expression, supporting the hypothesis that NF2 functions as a tumor suppressor gene (5, 12, 16, 17, 75, 77, 108, 109, 117, 139, 141, 143–146, 166, 180). These have largely been inactivating genetic alterations, such as frameshift and nonsense mutations, although rare missense mutations have also been detected.

The initial identification of merlin as the NF2 suppressor was based on four non-overlapping interstitial deletions in four unrelated NF2 patients (166). Subsequently, a large number of additional mutations have been defined in NF2 patients (16, 17, 108, 109, 117, 139, 145, 166). Most germline mutations are predicted to truncate the protein product. As noted above, the majority of these mutations are point mutations that alter splice junctions or create new stop codons, but small and large deletions have also been documented. These alterations have been documented throughout the gene, with the exception of the alternatively spliced exons 16 and 17, but one large series has suggested that germline mutations occur preferentially in exons 1 through 8 (117). A possible hot spot for mutations may be position 169, in exon 2, in which a C to T transition at a CpG dinucleotide results in a stop at codon 57 (16, 117). Other CpG dinucleotides are also commonly targets for C to T transitions (146), presumably from deamination of 5-methylcytosine to thymine, as has been documented in other tumor suppressor genes such as p53 (103). In the NF2 gene, these transitions typically convert an arginine to a stop codon (145).

Some authors have suggested that there are two phenotypes for NF2: the milder "Gardner" phenotype, in which patients develop bilateral vestibular schwannomas later in life without many other nervous system tumors, and the severe "Wishart" phenotype, in which multiple meningiomas and ependymomas accompany early bilateral vestibular schwannomas (43). Since all families with NF2 link to chromosome 22 (120), implying a single responsible gene, the phenotypic subtypes raise the possibility of allelic variants of NF2. However, although most families display relative homogeneity, "Wishart" and "Gardner" phenotypes can occur in the same families, making the possibility of allelic variants less likely. Recently, two unrelated NF2 patients, one with the severe "Wishart" and the other with the mild "Gardner" phenotype, have been reported to have the same constitutional NF2 mutation (17). This observation suggests that factors other than the specific NF2 mutation must regulate phenotypic expression of a mutant NF2 gene. One such factor may be somatic mosaicism for the NF2 mutation. Somatic mosaicism occurs when a mutation occurs early in embryogenesis rather than in the germline; as a result, only some cells bear the mutation. In the above-mentioned report of two phenotypically dissimilar patients with the same NF2 mutation, the patient with the mild "Gardner" phenotype was mosaic for the NF2 mutation (17). On the other hand, one recent study has suggested that patients with milder phenotypes are associated with mutations that preserve the carboxyl-terminus of the protein, whereas grossly truncating mutations result in the more severe phenotype (117). Further correlative analyses of NF2 phenotype and genotype will be necessary to clarify the complicated and perhaps multifactorial issue of phenotypic variation.

Interestingly, the types of mutations that occur in the germline of NF2 patients are somewhat different from those that occur somatically in sporadic schwannomas and meningiomas. Somatic alterations in sporadic tumors are usually small deletions, or occasionally insertions, that either produce a frameshift and a premature stop codon or disrupt proper splicing. NF2 gene mutations have now been detected in numerous schwannomas, confirming the prediction that this tumor suppressor is integral to schwannoma formation (13, 75, 77, 99, 145, 146, 168). Most studies have identified mutations in at least 50% of schwannomas, in vestibular tumors as well as schwannomas from other sites. For instance, our initial study of the entire coding region of the NF2 gene found mutations in 19 of 30 sporadic schwannomas (77). Our continued analysis of a second cohort of 60 vestibular schwannomas using combined screening methods, however, has revealed an additional 63 mutations. These recent findings suggest that NF2 mutations may be present in the vast majority of schwannomas (L. B. Jacoby, personal communication). Most somatic changes are small deletions or insertions that create either frameshifts and premature stop codons or altered splicing. Inactivating mutations have been detected in all exons except exons 16 and 17, which encode the alternative carboxyl-termini, and are relatively evenly distributed across the first 15 exons with no outstanding hot spots. In schwannomas, germline NF2 mutations in NF2 patients and somatic NF2 mutations in sporadic schwannomas are often accompanied by allelic loss of the other chromosome 22q, in accordance with the "two-hit" model of tumor suppressor gene inactivation. Thus, inactivation of NF2 is a common feature underlying both inherited and sporadic forms of schwannoma. One study has confirmed such inactivation at the protein level, showing loss of merlin expression by immunohistochemistry in schwannomas (146).

The distribution of mutations may also differ between schwannomas and meningiomas, since meningioma mutations cluster primarily in the first half of the coding sequence (99, 144, 180). As in schwannomas, NF2 gene alterations result predominantly in immediate truncation, splicing abnormalities or altered reading frames. The NF2 gene may also functions as a tumor suppressor in some other tumors, such as ependymoma, melanoma, breast cancer, and colorectal cancer (5, 12, 141, 143). Finally, in the long-standing debate over whether intracranial hemangiopericytomas are subtypes of meningiomas, NF2 gene analysis supports the prevalent clinical, immunohistochemical, and ultrastructural impression that hemangiopericytomas are not biologically related to meningiomas (82).

TUBEROUS SCLEROSIS (TS)

Clinicopathological Features of TS

Tuberous sclerosis is an autosomal dominant hereditary tumor syndrome and is the second most common such syndrome after neurofibromatosis 1. In contrast with neurofibromatosis, TS involves tissues derived from all primary germ layers, and the majority of the lesions are classified as either hamartomas or hamartias rather than as frank neoplasms (55). Diagnostic criteria have been divided into primary, secondary, and tertiary features. The most common lesion of TS, although not specific, is the hypopigmented "ashleaf spot." Diagnostic cutaneous lesions are multiple facial angiofibromas and subungual fibromas. The finding of a fibrous forehead plaque and a shagreen patch are secondary features, and the hypomelanotic macules (ashleaf spots) and confetti skin lesions are considered tertiary lesions consistent with a diagnosis of TS in the presence of a single primary feature (138). Other secondary features that support a diagnosis of TS include cardiac rhabdomyomas, pulmonary lymphangiomatosis, renal angiomyolipomas, and renal cysts. Tertiary features include hamartomatous rectal polyps, bone cysts, gingival fibromas, and hamartomas involving other organs.

Almost all patients meeting these primary to tertiary diagnostic criteria have central nervous system involvement. The major nervous system lesions are cortical tubers and subependymal giant cell astrocytomas. Neurologic symptoms occur in between 30% and 90%, of persons with TS. (55, 156). The neurological manifestations of TS vary widely between families and within families. Severe involvement may cause intractable seizures, severe mental retardation, or progressive hydrocephalus secondary to growth of a subependymal giant cell astrocytoma, whereas mild involvement may be a readily controlled seizure disorder. In the absence of seizures, the incidence of mental retardation is low; conversely, patients with mental retardation invariably have seizures (55). The famous Vogt triad of mental retardation, seizures, and facial angiofibromas is now recognized to apply to only a minority of patients (55). Detailed accounts of the neurological, psychiatric, ophthalmological (158), and neuropathological (137) features of TS have recently been published.

Molecular Genetics of TS

In 1987, linkage analysis of large TS families showed that a gene for tuberous sclerosis resided on the long arm of chromosome 9, near the locus for the ABO blood groups (28, 50, 129). Linkage to chromosome 9q was confirmed by other groups, but in 1991, there was strong evidence that despite the potential for significant lod scores, a number of families did not show linkage to chromosome 9 markers, suggesting that TS, unlike NF1, NF2 or VHL, demonstrated genetic heterogeneity (62, 63, 79, 80, 85, 156). Smith et al. reported a family that demonstrated significant linkage to a marker on chromosome 11 (161), but this could not be confirmed in other families. In 1992, a consortium of US researchers reported linkage to the autosomal dominant polycystic kidney (ADPKD) gene on the short arm of chromosome 16 (16p13.3) using pedigrees not linked to the chromosome 9 markers (84). Using markers from this region, and a family with both ADPKD and TS segregating with a 16:22 translocation, a European consortium successful identified the chromosome 16 TS gene, designated TSC2, in 1993 (40). The TSC2 gene encodes a 5.5 kb transcript with a wide range of expression. The protein product, tuberin, has a region of homology to the Rap 1 activator Rap 1-GAP. However, whether or not this homology accounts for TSC2 function as a tumor suppressor gene awaits further investigation.

No conclusive evidence has been found for a third TS locus in addition to the loci on chromosomes 9q and 16p. Initially 30 to 40% of cases linked to the chromosome 9 locus. Using the additional chromosome 16 data, however, a better current estimate is that the chromosome 9q and 16p loci each account for about 50% of TS. Interestingly, the percentage varies in data from different research groups (62). Chromosome 16p13 deletions have been demonstrated in a number of TS-associated hamartomas, a cortical tuber, several angiomyolipomas, a cardiac rhabdomyomas, and a single subependymal giant cell astrocytoma (57), supporting the notion that TSC2 functions as a tumor suppressor gene. Somatic TSC2 mutations have been reported in TS-associated tumors (E. P. Henske, personal communication). Allele loss in the region of TSC1 (the chromosome 9 gene) has also been demonstrated in a single subependymal giant cell astrocytoma and angiomyolipoma (56). Currently, ongoing studies are attempting to localize the chromosome 9 gene, with the exclusion of a number of candidate genes isolated by exon trapping from the suspect region on 9q (68). Whether or not the two TS genes interact also awaits further investigation after the cloning of the chromosome 9q gene. The lack of clinical distinction between those families linked to chromosome 9q and those families linked to chromosome 16p suggests that the two gene products converge in a cascade that controls both migration and growth at a very early stage of development. In such a scenario, inactivation of either TSC1 or TSC2 would have the same predicted effect.

VON HIPPEL-LINDAU SYNDROME (VHL)

Clinicopathological Features of VHL

Von Hippel-Lindau syndrome is a dominantly inherited tumor syndrome with a high penetrance (90%) that primarily involves six different organ systems: the eyes, the central nervous system, the kidneys, the pancreas, the adrenal glands and paraganglia, and the epididymis (123, 127). Studies in South Baden (Germany), and East Anglia (Great Britain) have suggested a VHL prevalence of 1 in 31,000 to 53,000 (111, 124, 126). VHL may occur in individuals without a family history of the illness, but this is much less common than in NF1 and TS (only six of 114 cases at the National Cancer Institute (127)). Morphologically, VHL has two typical features: first, affected tissues often have multiple lesions; second, three different types of lesions occur: benign cysts, vascular tumors, and carcinomas. The eyes are affected by retinal angiomata. In the central nervous system, hemangioblastomas may occur in any location, but they primarily affect the cerebellum and spinal cord (45, 125). Visceral lesions consist of renal cysts and cancers, pancreatic cysts and perhaps pancreatic cancers, pheochromocytoma, and epididymal cystadenoma. Clinical heterogeneity, however, is a well known feature of VHL; for instance, some VHL families contain members affected with pheochromocytomas, while other VHL families do not. A detailed account of the clinical, pathological, radiological, and therapeutic aspects of VHL has recently been published (127).

Molecular Genetics of VHL

Although clinical heterogeneity is common between VHL families, a single genetic locus near the tip of the short arm of chromosome 3 (3p25-26) appears responsible for the disorder. Linkage analysis demonstrated in the late 1980s that the VHL gene was linked to RAF1, a proto-oncogene located near the tip of the short arm of chromosome 3 (3p25-26) (153). Refined linkage studies over the next few years confirmed and narrowed the most likely location for the VHL gene (71, 110, 155, 172), and a pulsed field gel electrophoresis (PFGE) map of the VHL region was generated (186). PFGE studies of more than 100 VHL families identified three families with germline deletions in the VHL gene (186). These germline deletions were overlapping and provided a precise physical localization for the VHL disease gene. Additional positional cloning strategies identified a cosmid with conserved sequences that was located entirely within the three nested deletions and that was used to isolate two cDNAs. The gp7 cDNA detected intragenic mutations in the germline of affected individuals and was shown to be the VHL gene (93, 96).

The VHL gp7 cDNA detects a 5-kb message expressed in all adult tissues that have been tested (brain, heart, kidney). The VHL gene encodes a novel protein, with homology only to a cell surface component of Trypanosoma brucei. Notably, the sequence lacks domains to suggest a DNA binding protein, enzymatic activity, nuclear localization, or membrane localization. The VHL gene contains 3 exons with a long 3' untranslated region. The open reading frame encodes a putative protein of 852 amino acids (but see below). The region 5' to the cloned DNA has been examined for additional exons, but none have been identified to date. The transcription start sites and promoter of the VHL gene are located within exon 1, with transcription initiated around a putative SP1 binding site about 60 bp upstream from the first AUG codon. Several putative transcription factor binding sites, notably for nuclear respiratory factor 1 and PAX were found upstream of the transcription start sites. A minimal region of 106 bp was delineated. The promoter sequence does not contain TATA and CCAAT boxes (92).

Recent work has focused on determining the location of the translation start sites of the VHL gene. Exon 1 contains two possible translation start sites. These two AUG codons were evaluated for ability to support translation in an in vitro coupled transcription/translation assay and an in vivo transient transfection assay. Three proteins, 18, 30, and 36 kd, were expressed from the VHL cDNA, both in vitro and in vivo (Stackhouse et al., submitted). Based on the pattern of antisera reactivity, the 30- and 18-kd proteins were considered to be the products of translation from the first and the second AUG codons, respectively, with the 36-kd protein most likely a posttranslationally modified derivative of the 30 kd protein. The predicted size of the protein initiated at the first AUG codon is 213 amino acids and from the second AUG, 160

amino acids. These proteins would be predicted to be 23 kb and 18 kd. The VHL gene also shows alternative splicing; a VHL message is expressed with or without exon 2. Thus, at least four different proteins can be expressed, consisting of 119, 160, 172, and 213 amino acids. The functional differences and tissue distributions of the various proteins are being investigated inasmuch as differences in distribution of VHL isoforms might contribute to the tissue specific pattern of neoplasia in VHL.

The VHL gene is a tumor suppressor gene for specific cell types in the retina, central nervous system, adrenal gland, kidney, pancreas, and epididymis. Loss of heterozygosity for chromosome 3p has been demonstrated in clear cell carcinomas of the kidney, pheochromocytomas, and central nervous system hemangioblastomas. In VHL families where it was possible to trace the parental origin of the chromosome 3p sequences, the chromosome 3p bearing the wild-type allele was lost in tumors (165). Somatic mutations of the VHL gene have also been demonstrated in sporadic cerebellar hemangiomas (86). Furthermore, by analogy with sporadic renal cell carcinoma, in which hypermethylation of exon 1 is a mechanism of VHL gene inactivation, some sporadic hemangioblastomas may be inactivated by similar types of alterations.

In patients with VHL, there is a remarkable correlation between disease classification and the type of VHL mutation. VHL mutations are scattered throughout the gene, and about 40% of germline mutations are predicted to produce a truncated VHL protein. At the National Cancer Institute, germline mutations were detected in 75% of 114 VHL families (25, 127). Large deletions account for about 21% of mutations; missense, 58%; microdeletions/insertions, 14%; and nonsense, 7%. Strikingly, 96% of VHL type 2 families (those having pheochromocytomas) have missense mutations in the VHL gene. VHL type 1 families (those without pheochromocytomas), on the other hand, have large deletions, missense mutations, nonsense mutations, and microdeletions/insertions. Specific phenotypes are also associated with mutations at nucleotides 505, 686, and 712 (25, 127). For instance, members of a large family with a 505 T to C mutation have pheochromocytomas, angiomas, and hemangioblastomas without renal cell carcinomas or pancreatic cysts. This mutation has been found to be quite frequent in families with VHL in the Black Forest and was also present in two families in Pennsylvania (19). The 686 T to C mutation, on the other hand, does not predispose to pheochromocytomas but does result in renal cell carcinomas. Members of a large family with a 712 C to T mutation (a mutational hot spot) define another VHL phenotype, with pheochromocytomas, angiomas, hemangioblastomas, renal cell carcinomas, and pancreatic cysts—VHL type 2B (25, 30).

RARER SYNDROMES

Retinoblastoma Syndrome

The hereditary retinoblastoma syndrome, while rare, is the prototypical hereditary tumor syndrome. From the original, seminal suggestion that retinoblastomas arise after two oncogenic events (91), to the cloning and analysis of the Rb gene (49), this rare syndrome has been integral to understanding tumor suppressor genes and human cancer susceptibility. In addition to developing retinoblastomas and osteosarcomas, patients with germline Rb mutations have an increased incidence of nervous system tumors, particularly the pineoblastomas that characterize so-called "trilateral" retinoblastoma (6). Supporting a role for the Rb gene in pineoblastoma tumorigenesis has been the observation that some human pineoblastomas harbor Rb gene mutations (D. W. Yandell, personal communication). In addition, pineoblastomas have been noted in 40% of mice with germline inactivation of both the Rb and p53 genes (183), providing experimental evidence that Rb is involved in pineal oncogenesis. Some studies have also suggested that patients who survive retinoblastoma have a higher incidence of malignant gliomas (39). In this regard, it is interesting to note that the Rb gene is mutated in malignant astrocytomas and may play a role in astrocytoma progression (69). Clearly, the integral function of the Rb protein in cell cycle control extends to a variety of nervous system cells in addition to those of the retina.

Li-Fraumeni and Familial Glioma Syndromes

In the Li-Fraumeni syndrome, patients inherit a predisposition to breast carcinoma, soft tissue sarcoma, glioma, osteosarcoma, leukemia, lymphoma, and adrenocortical carcinoma, as well as other malignancies. Mutational analyses have implicated the p53 gene on 17p13.1 (112), which encodes a nuclear phosphoprotein involved in many cellular functions, including cell cycle arrest, DNA damage and repair, apoptosis, and angiogenesis. Analyses of the p53 gene in human brain tumors have been numerous and have shown that p53 mutations occur primarily in diffuse astrocytomas, and less commonly in other nervous system tumors (103).

For those families with a predisposition to malignant gliomas but without the full Li-Fraumeni syndrome, the situation is far less clear. Some studies have not found germline p53 mutations in patients from families with multiple malignant gliomas (171). We have not detected p53 germline mutations in eight glioma families (unpublished data), including one family with four of ten siblings affected (36), although we have noted a germline p53 mutation in a patient with neurofibromatosis type 1 and a glioblastoma multiforme (26). One recent report, on the other hand, has noted a germline p53 mutation, a deletion of codon 236, in a Swiss family with four astrocytomas in two generations (105). This family, however, had a history of leukemia and adrenocortical carcinoma and may represent a forme fruste of Li-Fraumeni syndrome. One group has reported that germline p53 mutations may be common in patients with "multifocal" glioma, glioma with another primary malignancy, and glioma associated with a family history of cancer (94). In this study, however, some of the affected pedigrees featured tumors such as breast cancer and sarcomas, again raising the possibility that such families are formes fruste of Li-Fraumeni syndrome. Consequently, while germline p53 mutations occur in some families whose cancer predisposition includes malignant gliomas, the true biological distinction between these families and the Li-Fraumeni syndrome remains unclear. Most glioma families, however, do not harbor germline p53 mutations, and their tumors presumably result from inherited defects in another tumor suppressor gene. We have assayed the MTS1/CDKN2 gene, which encodes the p16 cycle dependent kinase-inhibitor protein, in five families with malignant glioma, but we have not detected germline alterations ((36) and unpublished data); furthermore, the MTS1/CDKN2 gene is only rarely involved in astrocytoma and medulloblastoma formation (134, 170), making it an unlikely candidate for a glioma syndrome gene.

As mentioned above, while complete concordance between the types of hereditary tumors resulting from a germline mutation in a tumor suppressor gene and the types of sporadic tumors resulting from a sporadic mutation in the same gene is lacking, there is nonetheless a fairly good correlation (90). For these reasons, it is unlikely that germline p53 or MTS1/CDKN2 mutations would predispose patients only to gliomas; indeed, as mentioned above, patients with germline p53 mutations usually have the full Li-Fraumeni syndrome. In this regard, the chromosome 19q glioma tumor suppressor gene may be a particularly attractive candidate for the hereditary glioma syndrome gene, since chromosome 19q alterations are associated with different types of malignant glioma, but not with other human tumors (142, 150).

Turcot Syndrome

In Turcot syndrome, patients develop polyposis coli along with nervous system tumors, both malignant gliomas and medulloblastomas. Although the clinically related familial adenomatous polyposis and Gardner's syndromes are associated with germline mutations in the APC gene on chromosome 5q, initial studies failed to show linkage of the Turcot phenotype to the APC locus (164). Recent investigations, however, have demonstrated linkage of at least some families to markers close to APC (95), and germline APC mutations have been documented in patients with Turcot syndrome (118). Hamilton et al. have recently shown that most families with Turcot syndrome have mutations in the APC tumor suppressor gene, but other families with Turcot syndrome have defects in the mismatch-repair genes hMLH1 or hPMS2. Interestingly, medulloblastoma segregates those families with APC gene mutations, while glioblastoma multiforme occurs in those families with mismatch-repair gene defects (64). Interestingly, no APC mutations have been detected in sporadic malignant gliomas and medulloblastomas (118), which agrees with our finding of only rare 5q allelic loss in medulloblastomas and malignant gliomas (187). These data raise the possibility that a second gene, distinct from APC, may be responsible for the brain tumors seen in Turcot syndrome and perhaps for other

cases of Turcot syndrome. On the other hand, as already noted, a strict correlation between germline and sporadic mutations in individual tumor types does not always exist (90). If there is a second responsible gene, it does not appear to be p53, since Turcot syndrome patients do not harbor germline p53 gene mutations (88).

Gorlin Syndrome

Gorlin or basal cell nevus syndrome is a hereditary tumor syndrome in which patients have a variety of dysmorphic features as well as a predisposition to basal cell carcinomas, keratocysts of the jaw, ovarian fibromas, and medulloblastomas. Rarely, other nervous system tumors have been noted in patients with Gorlin syndrome, including astrocytoma (41) and meningioma (1). Of the various hereditary tumor syndromes of the nervous system, Gorlin syndrome is the most clearly associated with medulloblastomas, and one study has estimated that as many as 2% of medulloblastomas may arise in the setting of Gorlin syndrome (42). The Gorlin syndrome locus has been mapped to chromosome 9q31 (51), although the gene remains to be identified. Studies of 9q loss in sporadic medulloblastomas have shown allelic chromosome 9q loss in a small percentage of medulloblastomas, particularly in tumors from adults (3) and in desmoplastic variants (148). The cloning of the Gorlin syndrome gene will clarify the probable role of this gene in medulloblastoma tumorigenesis.

Cowden Syndrome

Cowden syndrome predisposes patients to tricholemmomas, hamartomas, and benign tumors of the skin and other organs, as well as breast, uterine, and thyroid carcinoma. The chromosomal locus and gene for Cowden syndrome have not yet been identified. Recently, an association has been noted between Cowden syndrome and Lhermitte-Duclos disease (dysplastic gangliocytoma of the cerebellum) (2), with one review of the literature suggesting that one-third of reported cases of Lhermitte-Duclos occurred in the setting of Cowden syndrome (173). In addition, a few families have been reported with Cowden syndrome and macrocephaly (66). The association of Cowden syndrome with cerebellar and cerebral dysplastic "overgrowth" lesions is reminiscent of the hypertrophy of other organs that may accompany

Beckwith-Weidemann syndrome; if analogous, Cowden syndrome may also arise from alterations in a proto-oncogene, rather than a tumor suppressor gene. Some families with Cowden syndrome have also shown increasing severity of disease over subsequent generations. Such genetic "anticipation" is characteristic of the "triplet repeat" diseases (182) and has not yet been described in any of the classical hereditary tumor syndromes. Furthermore, differential phenotypes have been noted depending on maternal or paternal transmission, possibly suggesting a role for genomic imprinting in this disorder (66). An association between Cowden syndrome and meningiomas has been noted although this observation was based on few patients (107).

Multiple Endocrine Neoplasia Syndromes

The multiple endocrine neoplasia (MEN) syndromes are a varied group of hereditary tumor syndromes which include some tumors of the nervous system and its surrounds (132). MEN 1 predisposes patients to pancreatic, parathyroid, and pituitary neoplasia, particularly pituitary adenomas. While the MEN 1 locus has been mapped to chromosome 11q13, the gene has not yet been identified. Interestingly, from a neuropathological point of view, allelic loss of chromosome 11q in the MEN 1 region has been noted in sporadic pituitary adenomas of different types, implying that the MEN 1 gene is probably a tumor suppressor involved in pituitary adenoma formation (14, 163).

Patients with MEN 2A have a high incidence of pheochromocytomas, as well as medullary thyroid carcinoma and parathyroid neoplasia, whereas the less common MEN 2B patients inherit the predisposition to pheochromocytomas, medullary thyroid carcinoma, and mucosal neuromas. Another uncommon variant of MEN 2 is familial medullary thyroid carcinoma syndrome (FMTC), in which patients are predisposed only to medullary thyroid carcinoma. The MEN2 locus was mapped to the pericentromeric region of the long arm of chromosome 10, and appeared to be the same locus for both MEN 2A, MEN 2B and FMTC. Curiously, however, studies of sporadic and hereditary pheochromocytomas and medullary thyroid carcinomas failed to demonstrate allelic loss of chromosome 10q, leading some investigators to

suspect that the MEN2 gene was not a classical tumor suppressor. This hypothesis was borne out when the RET proto-oncogene, a transmembrane tyrosine kinase, was identified as the culprit behind MEN 2A, MEN 2B and FMTC (132). In addition, the RET gene turned out to be responsible for Hirschsprung's disease (38), illustrating the sometimes close relationship between hereditary tumor syndromes and developmental defects of the neural crest. Subsequent studies have demonstrated a strong correlation between the type of RET alteration and the disease phenotype (119, 132). For instance, MEN 2A patients with a cysteine to arginine substitution at codon 634 have a much higher incidence of parathyroid disease. Such studies mark the beginning of a new genetic approach to clinicopathological correlations, which will no doubt be extended to all of the above hereditary tumor syndromes in the near future. The identification of the MEN2 gene also has practical sequelae since it facilitates identification of patients with germline mutations, which in turn allows more directed genetic counseling and therapies such as prophylactic thyroidectomy.

Other Syndromes

Less studied, rarer hereditary tumor syndromes abound in the recesses of the medical literature, and some of these conditions feature nervous system tumors. For example, syndromes that predispose to melanocytic tumors of the nervous system, such as neurocutaneous melanosis (Touraine syndrome), an autosomal dominant condition in which patients have large cutaneous nevi, leptomeningeal pigmentation, and a marked predisposition to leptomeningeal melanomas have been described (83). Other families have a predisposition to both cutaneous melanomas and astrocytomas (87), perhaps suggesting the MTS1/CDKN2 gene or a second astrocytoma gene on chromosome 9p as the responsible gene in such a family. Other rare syndromes have characteristic "cutaneous neuropathologies," such as the psammomatous melanotic schwannomas of Carney's complex (135). Most of these rarities, however, have not been studied extensively and are beyond the scope of this overview.

CONCLUSIONS

The progress that has been made in identifying the molecular genetic basis of the hereditary tumor syndromes of the nervous system has a number of important ramifications. While prospects of gene therapy and molecular pharmacological interventions may hold promise for treating these disorders in the future, the availability of genetic testing is already having an impact on the clinical management of these patients. For instance, distinguishing disease gene carriers from their normal relatives spares normal individuals the expense and inconvenience of repeated medical testing and firmly identifies those patients who will require close follow-up. The correlation between genotype and phenotype, particularly in VHL, will guide the physician in choice of screening tests and in prognosis; some patients will require close monitoring for pheochromocytomas, others for renal cell carcinoma. Prognostic information can also be provided: VHL patients with the 505 mutation appearing to have a better prognosis than patients with the 712–713 mutation. Furthermore, treatments are available that may reduce the morbidity and mortality of some of these diseases, and the ability to identify asymptomatic gene carriers provides an opportunity to test chemoprevention agents in a high risk population. Clearly, the identification of these genes has opened up exciting prospects for the clinical evaluation and management of these remarkable conditions.

REFERENCES

1. Albrecht, S., Goodman, J. C., Rajagopolan, S., et al. Malignant meningioma in Gorlin's syndrome: Cytogenetic and p53 gene analysis. Case report. J. Neurosurg. 81:466–471, 1994.
2. Albrecht, S., Haber, R. M., Goodman, J. C., and Duvic, M. Cowden syndrome and Lhermitte-Duclos disease. Cancer 70:869–876, 1992.
3. Albrecht, S., von Deimling, A., Pietsch, T., et al. Microsatellite analysis of loss of heterozygosity on chromosomes 9q, 11p and 17p in medulloblastomas. Neuropathol. Appl. Neurobiol. 20:74–81, 1994.
4. Andersen, L. B., Ballester, R., Marchuk, D. A., et al. A conserved alternative splice in the von Recklinghausen neurofibromatosis (NF1) gene produces two neurofibromin isoforms, both of which have GTPase-activating protein activity. Mol. Cell. Biol. 13:487–495, 1993.
5. Arakawa, H., Hayashi, N., Nagase, H., et al. Alternative splicing of the NF2 gene and its mutation analysis of breast and colorectal cancers. Hum. Molec. Genet. 3:565–568, 1994.
6. Bader, J. L., Meadows, A. T., Zimmerman, L. E., et al. Bilateral retinoblastoma with ectopic intracranial retinoblastoma: trilateral retinoblastoma. Cancer Genet. Cytogenet. 5:203–213, 1982.
7. Ballester, R., Marchuk, D., Boguski, M., et al. The NF1 locus encodes a protein functionally related to mammalian GAP and yeast IRA proteins. Cell 63: 851–859, 1990.
8. Barker, D., Wright, E., Nguyen, K., et al. Gene for von Recklinghausen neurofibromatosis is in the pericentromeric region of chromosome 17. Science 236: 1100–1102, 1987.
9. Basu, T. N., Gutmann, D. H., Fletcher, J. A., et al. Aberrant regulation of ras proteins in malignant tumour cells from type 1 neurofibromatosis patients. Nature 356:713–715, 1992.
10. Bernards, A., Haase, V. H., Murthy, A. E., et al. Complete human NF1 cDNA sequence: Two alternatively spliced mRNAs and absence of expression in a neuroblastoma line. Dna Cell Biol. 11:727–734, 1992.
11. Bernards, A., Snijders, A. J., Hannigan, G. E., et al. Mouse neurofibromatosis type 1 cDNA sequence reveals high degree of conservation of both coding and non-coding mRNA segments. Hum. Mol. Genet. 2:645–650, 1993.
12. Bianchi, A. B., Hara, T., Ramesh, V., et al. Mutations in transcript isoforms of the neurofibromatosis 2 gene in multiple human tumour types. Nature Genet. 6:185–192, 1994.
13. Bijlsma, E. K., Merel, P., Bosch, D. A., et al. Analysis of mutations of the SCH gene in schwannomas. Genes Chromosomes Cancer 11:7–14, 1994.
14. Boggild, M. D., Jenkinson, S., Pistorello, M., et al. Molecular genetic studies of sporadic pituitary tumors. J. Clin. Endocrinol. Metab. 78:387–392, 1994.
15. Bollag, G., and McCormick, F. Differential regulation of rasGAP and neurofibromatosis gene product activities. Nature 351:576–579, 1991.
16. Bourn, D., Carter, S., Mason, S., et al. Germline mutations in the neurofibromatosis type 2 tumour suppressor gene. Hum. Mol. Genet. 3:813–816, 1994.
17. Bourn, D., Carter, S. A., Evans, D. R. G., et al. A mutation in the neurofibromatosis type 2 tumorsuppressor gene, giving rise to widely different clinical phenotypes in two unrelated individuals. Am. J. Hum. Genet. 55:69–73, 1994.
18. Brannan, C. I., Perkins, A. S., Vogel, K. S., et al. Targeted disruption of the neurofibromatosis type-1 gene leads to developmental abnormalities in heart and various neural crest-derived tissues. Genes Dev. 8:1019–1029, 1994.
19. Brauch, H., Kishida, T., Glavac, D., et al. Von Hippel-Lindau (VHL) disease with pheochromocytoma in the Black Forest region of Germany: Evidence for a founder effect. Hum. Genet. 95:551–556, 1995.
20. Buchberg, A. M., Cleveland, L. S., Jenkins, N. A., and Copeland, N. G. Sequence homology shared by neurofibromatosis type 1 gene and IRA-1 and IRA-2 negative regulators of the ras cyclic AMP pathway. Nature 347:291–294, 1990.
21. Carey, J. C., Baty, B. J., Johnson, J. P., et al. The genetic aspects of neurofibromatosis. Ann. NY Acad. Sci. 486:45–56, 1986.

22. Carey, J. C., Laub, J. M., and Hall, B. D. Penetrance and variability in neurofibromatosis: a genetic study of 60 families. Birth Defects: Original Article Series 15:271–281, 1979.
23. Cawthon, R. M., O'Connell, P., Buchberg, A. M., et al. Identification and characterization of transcripts from the neurofibromatosis 1 region: The sequence and genomic structure of EVI2 and mapping of other transcripts. Genomics 7:555–565, 1990.
24. Cawthon, R. M., Weiss, R., Xu, G., et al. A mayor segment of the neurofibromatosis type 1 gene: cDNA sequence, genomic structure, and point mutations. Cell 62:193–201, 1990.
25. Chen, F., Kishida, T., Yao, M., et al. Germline mutations in the von Hippel-Lindau disease tumor suppressor gene: correlations with phenotype. Hum. Mutat. 5:66–75, 1995.
26. Chung, R. Y., Whaley, J., Kley, N., et al. TP53 mutation and 17p deletion in human astrocytomas. Genes Chromosomes Cancer 3:323–331, 1991.
27. Claudio, J. O., Marineau, C., and Rouleau, G. A. The mouse homologue of the neurofibromatosis 2 gene is highly conserved. Hum. Mol. Genet. 3:185–190, 1994.
28. Connor, J. M., Pirrit, L. A., Yates, J. R., et al. Linkage of the tuberous sclerosis locus to a DNA polymorphism detected by v-abl. J. Med. Genet. 24:544–546, 1987.
29. Coppes, M. J., Haber, D. A., and Grundy, P. E. Genetic events in the development of Wilms' tumor. N. Engl. J. Med. 331:586–590, 1994.
30. Crossey, P. A., Richards, F. M., Foster, K., et al. Identification of intragenic mutations in the von Hippel-Lindau disease tumour suppressor gene and correlation with disease phenotype. Hum. Mol. Genet. 3:1303–1308, 1994.
31. Daston, M. M., and Ratner, N. Expression of P30, a protein with adhesive properties, in Schwann cells and neurons of the developing and regenerating peripheral nerve. J. Cell Biol. 112:1229–1239, 1991.
32. Daston, M. M., and Ratner, N. Neurofibromin, a predominantly neuronal GTPase activating protein in the adult, is ubiquitously expressed during development. Dev. Dynamics 195:216–226, 1992.
33. Daston, M. M., Scrable, H., Nordlund, M., et al. The protein product of the neurofibromatosis type 1 gene is expressed in highest abundance in neurons, schwann cells, and oligodendrocytes. Neuron 8:415–428, 1992.
34. DeClue, J. E., Cohen, B. D., and Lowy, D. R. Identification and characterization of the neurofibromatosis type 1 protein product. Proc. Natl. Acad. Sci. USA 88:9914–9928, 1991.
35. DeClue, J. E., Papageorge, A. G., Fletcher, J. A., et al. Abnormal regulation of mammalian p21ras contributes to malignant tumor growth in von Recklinghausen (type 1) neurofibromatosis. Cell 69:265–273, 1992.
36. Dirven, C. M. F., Tuerlings, J., Molenaar, W. M., et al. Glioblastoma multiforme in four siblings: A cytogenetic and molecular genetic study. J. Neuro-Oncol. (in press), 1995.
37. Easton, D. F., Ponder, M. A., Huson, S. M., and Ponder, B. A. An analysis of variation in expression of neurofibromatosis (NF) type 1 (NF1): Evidence for modifying genes. Am. J. Hum. Genet. 53:305–313, 1993.
38. Edery, P., Lyonnet, S., Mulligan, L. M., et al. Mutations of the RET proto-oncogene in Hirschsprung's disease. Nature 367:378–380, 1994.
39. Eng, C., Li, F. P., Abramson, D. H., et al. Mortality from second tumors amoung long-term survivors of retinoblastoma. J. Natl. Cancer Inst. 85:1121–1128, 1993.
40. European Chromosome 16 Tuberous Sclerosis Consortium. Identification and characterization of the tuberous sclerosis gene on chromosome 16. Cell 75:1305–1315, 1993.
41. Evans, D. G., Birch, J. M., and Orton, C. I. Brain tumours and the occurrence of severe invasive basal cell carcinoma in first degree relatives with Gorlin syndrome. Br. J. Neurosurg. 5:643–646, 1991.
42. Evans, D. G., Farndon, P. A., Burnell, L. D., et al. The incidence of Gorlin syndrome in 173 consecutive cases of medulloblastoma. Br. J. Cancer 64:959–961, 1991.
43. Evans, D. G. R., Huson, S. M., Donnai, D., et al. A clinical study of type 2 neurofibromatosis. Q. J. Med. 304:603–618, 1992.
44. Fain, P. R., Goldgar, D. E., Wallace, M. R., et al. Refined physical and genetic mapping of the NF1 region on chromosome 17. Am. J. Hum. Genet. 45:721–728, 1989.
45. Filling-Katz, M. R., Choyke, P. L., Oldfield, E., et al. Central nervous system involvement in Von Hippel-Lindau disease. Neurology 41:41–6, 1991.
46. Fishel, R., Lescoe, M. K., Rao, M. R., et al. The human mutator gene homolog MSH2 and its association with hereditary nonpolyposis colon cancer. Cell 75:1027–1038, 1993.
47. Fountain, J. W., Wallace, M. R., Brereton, A. M., et al. Physical mapping of the von Recklinghausen Neurofibromatosis on chromosome 17. Am. J. Hum. Genet. 44:58–67, 1989.
48. Fountain, J. W., Wallace, M. R., Bruce, M. A., et al. Physical mapping of a translocation breakpoint in neurofibromatosis. Science 244:1085–1087, 1989.
49. Friend, S. H., Bernards, R., Rogelj, S., et al. A human DNA segment with properties of the gene that predisposes to retinoblastoma and osteosarcoma. Nature 323:643–646, 1986.
50. Fryer, A. E., Chalmers, A., Connor, J. M., et al. Evidence that the gene for tuberous sclerosis is on chromosome 9. Lancet 1:659–661, 1987.
51. Gailani, M. R., Bale, S. J., Leffell, D. J., et al. Developmental defects in Gorlin syndrome related to a putative tumor suppressor gene on chromosome 9. Cell 69:111–117, 1992.
52. Goldgar, D. E., Green, P., Parry, D. M., and Mulvihill, J. J. Multipoint linkage analysis in neurofibromatosis type I: an international collaboration. Am. J. Hum. Genet. 44:6–12, 1989.
53. Golubic, M., Roudebush, M., Dobrowolski, S., et al. Catalytic properties, tissue and intracellular distribution of neurofibromin. Oncogene 7:2151–2159, 1992.
54. Golubic, M., Tanaka, K., Dobrowolski, S., et al. The

GTPase stimulatory activities of the neurofibromatosis type 1 and the yeast IRA2 proteins are inhibited by arachidonic acid. EMBO J. 10:2897–2903, 1991.

55. Gomez, M. R. *Tuberous Sclerosis*, 2nd Ed. Raven Press, New York, 1988.

56. Green, A. J., Johnson, P. H., and Yates, J. R. The tuberous sclerosis gene on chromosome 9q34 acts as a growth suppressor. Hum. Mol. Genet. 3:1833–1834, 1994.

57. Green, A. J., Smith, M., and Yates, J. R. W. Loss of heterozygosity on chromosome 16p13.3 in hamartomas from tuberous sclerosis patients. Nature Genet. 6:193–196, 1994.

58. Gregory, P. E., Gutmann, D. H., Mitchell, A., et al. Neurofibromatosis type 1 gene product (neurofibromin) associates with microtubules. Somatic Cell Mol. Genet. 19:265–274, 1993.

59. Gutmann, D. H., Tennekoon, G. I., Cole, J. L., et al. Modulation of the neurofibromatosis type 1 gene product, neurofibromin, during Schwann cell differentiation. J. Neurosci. Res. 36:216–223, 1993.

60. Gutmann, D. H., Wood, D. L., and Collins, F. S. Identification of the neurofibromatosis type 1 gene product. Proc. Natl. Acad. Sci. USA 88:9658–9662, 1991.

61. Haase, V., Trofatter, J. A., MacCollin, M., et al. The murine NF2 homologue encodes a highly conserved merlin protein with alternative forms. Hum. Mol. Genet. 3:407–411, 1994.

62. Haines, J. L., Amos, J., Attwood, J., et al. Genetic heterogeneity in tuberous sclerosis. Study of a large collaborative dataset. Ann. NY Acad. Sci. 615:256–264, 1991.

63. Haines, J. L., Short, M. P., Kwiatkowski, D. J., et al. Localization of one gene for tuberous sclerosis within 9q32–9q34, and further evidence for heterogeneity. Am. J. Hum. Genet. 49:764–772, 1991.

64. Hamilton, S. R., Liu, B., Parsons, R. E., et al. The molecular basis of Turcot's syndrome. N. Engl. J. Med. 332:839–847, 1995.

65. Han, J.-W., McCormick, F., and Macara, I. G. Regulation of ras-GAP and the neurofibromatosis 1 gene product by eicosanoids. Science 252:576–579, 1991.

66. Hanssen, A. M., Werquin, H., Suys, E., and Fryns, J. P. Cowden syndrome: report of a large family with macrocephaly and increased severity of signs in subsequent generations. Clin. Genet. 44:281–286, 1993.

67. Hara, T., Bianchi, A. B., Seizinger, B. R., and Kley, N. Molecular cloning and characterization of alternatively spliced transcripts of the mouse neurofibromatosis 2 gene. Cancer Res. 54:330–335, 1994.

68. Henske, E. P., Short, M. P., Jozwiak, S., et al. Identification of VAV2 on 9q34 and its exclusion as the tuberous sclerosis gene TSC1. Ann. Hum. Genet. 1995.

69. Henson, J. W., Schnitker, B. L., Correa, K. M., et al. The retinoblastoma susceptibility (Rb) gene is involved in the malignant progression of human astrocytomas. Ann. Neurol. 36:714–721, 1994.

70. Herskowitz, I. Functional inactivation of genes by dominant negative mutations. Nature 329:219–222, 1987.

71. Hosoe, S., Brauch, H., Latif, F., et al. Localization of the von Hippel-Lindau disease gene to a small region of chromosome 3. Genomics 8:634–640, 1990.

72. Huson, S. M. Neurofibromatosis: Historical perspective, classification and diagnostic criteria. In: *The neurofibromatoses: A pathogenetic and clinical overview*. Chapman & Hall Medical, London, 1994.

73. Huson, S. M., Haper, P. S., and Compston, D. A. von Recklinghausen's neurofibromatosis: a clinical and population study in south-east Wales. Brain 111: 1355–1381, 1988.

74. Huynh, D. P., Nechiporuk, T., and Pulst, S. M. Differential expression and tissue distribution of type I and type II neurofibromins during mouse fetal development. Dev. Biol. 161:538–551, 1994.

75. Irving, R. M., Moffat, D. A., Hardy, D. G., et al. Somatic NF2 gene mutations in familial and non-familial vestibular schwannoma. Hum. Mol. Genet. 3:347–350, 1994.

76. Jacks, T., Shih, T. S., Schmitt, E. M., et al. Tumour predisposition in mice heterozygous for a targeted mutation in Nf1. Nature Genet. 7:353–361, 1994.

77. Jacoby, L. B., MacCollin, M., Louis, D. N., et al. Exon scanning for mutation in the NF2 gene in schwannomas. Hum. Molec. Genet. 3:413–419, 1994.

78. Jadayel, D., Fain, P., Upadhyaya, M., et al. Paternal origin of new mutations in von Recklinghausen neurofibromatosis. Nature 343:558–559, 1990.

79. Janssen, L. A., Povey, S., Attwood, J., et al. A comparative study on genetic heterogeneity in tuberous sclerosis: evidence for one gene on 9q34 and a second gene on 11q22-23. Ann. NY Acad. Sci. 615:306–315, 1991.

80. Janssen, L. A., Sandkuyl, L. A., Merkens, E. C., et al. Genetic heterogeneity in tuberous sclerosis. Genomics 8:237–242, 1990.

81. Johnson, M. R., Look, A. T., DeClue, J. E., et al. Inactivation of the NF1 gene in human melanoma and neuroblastoma cell lines without impaired regulation of GTP. Ras. Proc. Natl. Acad. Sci. USA. 90:5539–5543, 1993.

82. Joseph, J. T., Lisle, D. K., Jacoby, L. B., et al. NF2 gene analysis distinguishes hemangiopericytoma from meningioma. Am. J. Pathol. 1995, (in press).

83. Kadonaga, J. N., and Frieden, I. J. Neurocutaneous melanosis: definition and review of the literature. J. Am. Acad. Dermatol. 1991.

84. Kandt, R. S., Haines, J. L., Smith, M., et al. Linkage of an important gene locus for tuberous sclerosis to a chromosome 16 marker for polycystic kidney disease. Nature Genet. 2:37–41, 1992.

85. Kandt, R. S., Pericak, V. M., Hung, W. Y., et al. Absence of linkage of ABO blood group locus to familial tuberous sclerosis [published erratum appears in Exp. Neurol. 105:320, 1989]. Experimental Neurology 104:223–8, 1989.

86. Kanno, H., Kondo, K., Ito, S., et al. Somatic mutations of the von Hippel-Lindau tumor suppressor gene in sporadic central nervous system hemangioblastomas. Cancer Res. 54:4845–4847, 1994.

87. Kaufman, D. K., Kimmel, D. W., Parisi, J. E., and Michels, V. V. A familial syndrome with cutaneous malignant melanoma and cerebral astrocytoma. Neurology 43:1728–1731, 1993.

88. Kikuchi, T., Rempel, S. A., Rutz, H. P., et al. Turcot's syndrome of glioma and polyposis occurs in the absence of germ line mutations of exons 5 to 9 of the p53 gene. Cancer Res. 53:957–961, 1993.

89. Kim, H., Rosenbaum, T., Kombrinck, K., et al. Neurofibromin-deficient and v-ras expressing Schwann cells show decreased proliferation in response to rhGGF2 and axons: increased ras-GTP and morphologic change. Oncogene 1995, (in press).

90. Knudsen, A. G. All in the (cancer) family. Nature Genet. 5:103–104, 1993.

91. Knudson, A. G. Mutation and cancer: Statistical study of retinoblastoma. Proc. Natl. Acad. Sci. USA 68: 820–823, 1971.

92. Kuzmin, I., Duh, F.-M., Latif, F., et al. Identification of the promoter of the human von Hippel-Lindau gene. Oncogene 1995, (in press).

93. Kuzmin, I., Stackhouse, T., Latif, F., et al. One-megabase yeast artificial chromosome and 400-kilobase cosmid-phage contigs containing the von Hippel-Lindau tumor suppressor and Ca(2+)-transporting adenosine triphosphatase isoform 2 genes. Cancer Res. 54:2486–2491, 1994.

94. Kyritsis, A. P., Bondy, M. L., Xiao, M., et al. Germline p53 gene mutations in subsets of glioma patients. JNCI 86:344–349, 1994.

95. Lasser, D. M., DeVivo, D. C., Garvin, J., and Wilhelmsen, K. C. Turcot's syndrome: Evidence for linkage to the adenomatous polyposis (APC) locus. Neurology 44:1083–1086, 1994.

96. Latif, F., Tory, K., Gnarra, J., et al. Identification of the von Hippel-Lindau disease tumor suppressor gene. Science 260:1317–1320, 1993.

97. Ledbetter, D. H., Rich, D. C., O'Connell, P., et al. Precise localization of NF1 to 17q11.2 by balanced translocation. Am. J. Hum. Genet. 44:20–24, 1989.

98. Legius, E., Marchuk, D. A., Collins, F. S., and Glover, T. W. Somatic deletion of the neurofibromatosis type 1 gene in a neurofibrosarcoma supports a tumour suppressor gene hypothesis. Nature Genet. 3:122–126, 1993.

99. Lekanne Deprez, R. H., Bianchi, A. B., Groen, N. A., et al. Frequent NF2 gene transcript mutations in sporadic meningiomas and vestibular schwannomas. Am. J. Hum. Genet. 54:1022–1029, 1994.

100. Levine, A. J. The tumor suppressor genes. Ann. Rev. Biochem. 62:623–651, 1993.

101. Li, Y., Bollag, G., Clark, R., et al. Somatic mutations in the neurofibromatosis 1 gene in human tumors. Cell 69:275–281, 1992.

102. Li, Y., O'Connell, P., Breidenbach, H. H., et al. Genomic organization of the neurofibromatosis 1 gene. Genomics 25:9–18, 1995.

103. Louis, D. N. The p53 gene and protein in human brain tumors. J. Neuropathol. Exp. Neurol. 53:11–21, 1994.

104. Louis, D. N., Ramesh, V., and Gusella, J. F. Neuropathology and molecular genetics of neurofibromatosis 2 and related tumors. Brain Pathol. 5:163–172, 1995.

105. Lübbe, J., von Ammon, K., Watanabe, K., et al. Familial brain tumour syndrome associated with a p53 germline deletion of codon 236. Brain Pathol. 5:15–23, 1995.

106. Luna, E. J., and Hitt, A. L. Cytoskeleton-plasma membrane interactions. Science 258:955–964, 1992.

107. Lyons, C. J., Wilson, C. B., and Horton, J. C. Association between meningioma and Cowden's disease. Neurology 43:1436–1437, 1993.

108. MacCollin, M., Mohney, T., Trofatter, J., et al. DNA diagnosis of neurofibromatosis 2. JAMA 270: 2316–2320, 1993.

109. MacCollin, M., Ramesh, V., Jacoby, L. B., et al. Mutational analysis of patients with neurofibromatosis 2. 1994.

110. Maher, E. R., Bentley, E., Yates, J. R., et al. Mapping of the von Hippel-Lindau disease locus to a small region of chromosome 3p by genetic linkage analysis. Genomics 10:957–960, 1991.

111. Maher, E. R., Iselius, L., Yates, J. R. W., et al. Von Hippel-Lindau disease: A genetic study. J. Med. Genet. 28:443–447, 1991.

112. Malkin, D., Li, F. P., Strong, L. C., et al. Germ line p53 mutations in a familial syndrome of breast cancer, sarcomas, and other neoplasms. Science 250:1222–1228, 1990.

113. Marchuk, D. A., Saulino, A. M., Tavakkol, R., et al. cDNA cloning of the type 1 neurofibromatosis gene: complete sequence of the NF1 gene product. Genomics 11:931–940, 1991.

114. Marshall, C. J. Tumor suppressor genes. Cell 64:313–326, 1991.

115. Martin, G. A., Viskochil, D., Bollag, G., et al. The GAP-related domain of the neurofibromatosis type 1 gene product interacts with ras p21. Cell 63:843–849, 1990.

116. Menon, A. G., Anderson, K. M., Riccardi, V. M., et al. Chromosome 17p deletions and p53 gene mutations associated with the formation of malignant neurofibrosarcomas in Recklinghausen neurofibromatosis. Proc. Natl. Acad. Sci. USA 87:5435–5439, 1990.

117. Merel, P., Hoang-Xuan, K., Sanson, M., et al. Screening for germ-line mutations in the NF2 gene. Genes Chromosomes Cancer 12:117–127, 1995.

118. Mori, T., Nagase, H., Horii, A., et al. Germ-line and somatic mutations of the APC gene in patients with Turcot syndrome and analysis of APC mutations in brain tumors. Genes Chromosomes Cancer 9:168–172, 1994.

119. Mulligan, L. M., Eng, C., Healey, C. S., et al. Specific mutations of the RET proto-oncogene are related to disease phenotype in MEN 2A and FMTC. Nature Genet. 6:70–74, 1994.

120. Narod, S. A., Parry, D. M., Parboosingh, J., et al. Neurofibromatosis type 2 appears to be a genetically homogeneous disease. Am. J. Hum. Genet. 51:486–496, 1992.

121. National Institutes of Health. National Institutes of Health Consensus Development Conference: Neurofibromatosis Conference Statement. Arch. Neurol. 45:575–578, 1988.

122. Naumova, A., and Sapienza, C. The genetics of reti-

noblastoma, revisited. Am. J. Hum. Genet. 54:264–273, 1994.

123. Neumann, H. P. Basic criteria for clinical diagnosis and genetic counselling in von Hippel-Lindau syndrome. Vasa 16:220–226, 1987.

124. Neumann, H. P., Berger, D. P., Sigmund, G., et al. Pheochromocytomas, multiple endocrine neoplasia type 2, and von Hippel-Lindau disease. N. Engl. J. Med. 329:1531–1538, 1993.

125. Neumann, H. P., Eggert, H. R., Weigel, K., et al. Hemangioblastomas of the central nervous system. A 10-year study with special reference to von Hippel-Lindau syndrome. J. Neurosurg. 70:24–30, 1989.

126. Neumann, H. P., and Wiestler, O. D. Clustering of features of von Hippel-Lindau syndrome: Evidence for a complex genetic locus. Lancet 337:1052–1054, 1991.

127. Neumann, H. P. H., Lips, C. J. M., Hsia, Y. E., and Zbar, B. Von Hippel Lindau syndrome. Brain Pathol. 5:181–193, 1995.

128. Nishi, T., Lee, P. S., Oka, K., et al. Differential expression of two types of the neurofibromatosis 1 (NF1) gene transcripts related to neuronal differentiation. Oncogene 6:1555–1559, 1991.

129. Northrup, H., Beaudet, A. L., O'Brien, W. E., et al. Linkage of tuberous sclerosis to ABO blood group. Lancet (letter) 2:804 805, 1987.

130. O'Connell, P., Leach, R., Cawthon, R. M., et al. Two NF1 translocations map within a 600-kilobase segment of 17q11.2. Science 244:1087–1088, 1989.

131. O'Connell, P., Leach, R. J., Ledbetter, D. H., et al. Fine structure DNA mapping studies of the chromosomal region harboring the genetic defect in neurofibromatosis type I. Am. J. Hum. Genet. 44:51–57, 1989.

132. Ponder, B. A. The gene causing multiple endocrine neoplasia type 2 (MEN 2). Ann. Med. 26:199–203, 1994.

133. Pykett, M. J., Murphy, M., Harnish, P. R., and George, D. The neurofibromatosis 2 (NF2) tumor gene encodes multiple alternatively spliced transcripts. Hum. Mol. Genet. 3:559–564, 1994.

134. Raffel, C., Ueki, K., Harsh, G. R., and Louis, D. N. The multiple tumor suppressor 1/cyclin dependent kinase inhibitor 2 gene (MTS1/CDKN2) in human central nervous system primitive neuroectodermal tumor. Neurosurgery 36:971–974, 1995.

135. Reznik, M. Cutaneous neuropathology: Neurofibromas, schwannomas and other neural neoplasms with cutaneous and extracutaneous expressions. Clin. Neuropathol. 10:225–231, 1991.

136. Riccardi, V. M. *Neurofibromatosis. Phenotype, Natural History, and Pathogenesis*, 2nd Ed. Johns Hopkins University Press, Baltimore, 1992.

137. Richardson, E. P. J. Pathology of tuberous sclerosis. Ann. NY. Acad. Sci. 615:128–139, 1991.

138. Roach, E., Smith, M., Huttenlocher, P., et al. Diagnostic criteria: Tuberous sclerosis complex. J. Child. Neurol. 7:221–224, 1992.

139. Rouleau, G. A., Merel, P., Lutchman, M., et al. Alteration in a new gene encoding a putative membrane-organizing protein causes neurofibromatosis type 2. Nature 363:515–521, 1993.

140. Rouleau, G. A., Wertelecki, W., Haines, J. L., et al.

141. Rubio, M.-P., Correa, K. M., Ramesh, V., et al. Analysis of the neurofibromatosis 2 (NF2) gene in human ependymomas and astrocytomas. Cancer Res. 54:45–47, 1994.

142. Rubio, M.-P., Correa, K. M., Ueki, K., et al. The putative glioma tumor suppressor gene on chromosome 19q maps between APOC2 and HRC. Cancer Res. 54:4760–4763, 1994.

143. Rustgi, A. K., Xu, L., Pinney, D., et al. The neurofibromatosis 2 gene in human colorectal cancer. Cancer Genet. Cytogenet. 1995, (in press).

144. Ruttledge, M. H., Sarrazin, J., Rangaratnam, S., et al. Evidence for the complete inactivation of the NF2 gene in the majority of sporadic meningiomas. Nature Genet. 6:180–184, 1994.

145. Sainz, J., Figueroa, K., Baser, M. E., et al. High frequency of nonsense mutations in the NF2 gene caused by C to T transitions in five CGA codons. Hum. Mol. Genet. 4:137–139, 1995.

146. Sainz, J., Huynh, D. P., Figueroa, K., et al. Mutations of the neurofibromatosis type 2 gene and lack of the gene product in vestibular schwannomas. Hum. Mol. Genet. 3:885–891, 1994.

147. Schmidt, M. A., Michels, V. V., and Dewald, G. W. Cases of neurofibromatosis with rearrangements of chromosome 17 involving band 17q11.2. Am. J. Med. Genet. 28:771–777, 1987.

148. Schofield, D., West, D. C., Anthony, D. C., et al. Correlation of loss of heterozygosity at chromosome 9q with histologic subtype in medulloblastomas. Am. J. Pathol. 146:472–480, 1995.

149. Seizinger, B. R. NF1: A prevalent cause of tumorigenesis in human cancers? Nature Genet. 3:97–99, 1993.

150. Seizinger, B. R., Klinger, H. P., Junien, C., et al. Report of the committee on chromosome and gene loss in human neoplasia. Cytogenet. Cell Genet. 58:1080–1096, 1991.

151. Seizinger, B. R., Martuza, R. L., and Gusella, J. F. Loss of genes on chromosome 22 in tumorigenesis of human acoustic neuroma. Nature 322:644–647, 1986.

152. Seizinger, B. R., Rouleau, G., Ozelius, L. J., et al. Common pathogenetic mechanism for three tumor types in bilateral acoustic neurofibromatosis. Science 236:317–319, 1987.

153. Seizinger, B. R., Rouleau, G. A., Ozelius, L. J., et al. Von Hippel-Lindau disease maps to the region of chromosome 3 associated with renal cell carcinoma. Nature 332:268–269, 1988.

154. Seizinger, B. R., Rouleau, G. A., Ozelius, L. J., et al. Genetic linkage of von Recklinghausen neurofibromatosis to the nerve growth factor receptor gene. Cell 49:589–594, 1987.

155. Seizinger, B. R., Smith, D. I., Filling, K. M., et al. Genetic flanking markers refine diagnostic criteria and provide insights into the genetics of Von Hippel Lindau disease. Proc. Natl. Acad. Sci. USA. 88:2864–2868, 1991.

156. Short, M. P., Haines, J., Jewell, A., et al. Clinical

findings and linkage studies in familial tuberous sclerosis. Ann. NY Acad. Sci. 615:380–381, 1991.

157. Short, M. P., Martuza, R. L., and Huson, S. M. Neurofibromatosis 2: Clinical features, genetic counselling and management issues. In: *The neurofibromatoses: A pathogenetic and clinical overview.* Chapman & Hall Medical, London, 1994.

158. Short, M. P., Richardson, E. P., Haines, J. L., and Kwiatkowski, D. J. Clinical, neuropathological, and genetic aspects of the tuberous sclerosis complex. Brain Pathol. 5:173–180, 1995.

159. Skuse, G. R., Kosciolek, B. A., and Rowley, P. T. Molecular genetic analysis of tumors in von Recklinghausen neurofibromatosis: loss of heterozygosity for chromosome 17. Genes Chromosomes Cancer 1:36–41, 1989.

160. Skuse, G. R., Kosciolek, B. A., and Rowley, P. T. The neurofibroma in von Recklinghausen neurofibromatosis has a unicellular origin. Am. J. Hum. Genet. 49:600–607, 1991.

161. Smith, M., Smalley, S., Cantor, R., et al. Mapping of a gene determining tuberous sclerosis to human chromosome 11q14–11q23. Genomics 6:105–114, 1990.

162. Takeshima, H., Izawa, I., Lee, P. S. Y., et al. Detection of cellular proteins that interact with the NF2 tumor suppressor gene product. Oncogene 9:2135–2144, 1994.

163. Thakker, R. V., Pook, M. A., Wooding, C., et al. Association of somatotrophinomas with loss of alleles on chromosome 11 and with gsp mutations. J. Clin. Invest. 91:2815–2821, 1993.

164. Tops, C. M., Vasen, H. F., van Berge Henegouwen, G., et al. Genetic evidence that Turcot syndrome is not allelic to familial adenomatous polyposis. Am. J. Med. Genet. 43:888–893, 1992.

165. Tory, K., Brauch, H., Linehan, M., et al. Specific genetic change in tumors associated with von Hippel-Lindau disease. JNCI 81:1097–1101, 1989.

166. Trofatter, J. A., MacCollin, M. M., Rutter, J. L., et al. The neurofibromatosis 2 tumor suppressor gene encodes a novel moesin-ezrin-radixin-like protein. Cell 72:791–800, 1993.

167. Tsukita, S., Oishi, K., Sato, N., et al. ERM family members as molecular linkers between the cell surface glycoprotein CD44 and actin-based cytoskeletons. J. Cell Biol. 126:391–401, 1994.

168. Twist, E. C., Ruttledge, M. H., Rousseau, M., et al. The neurofibromatosis type 2 gene is inactivated in schwannomas. Hum. Mol. Genet. 3:147–151, 1994.

169. Uchida, T., Matozaki, T., Suzuki, T., et al. Expression of two types of neurofibromatosis type 1 gene transcripts in gastric cancers and comparison of GAP activities. Biochem. Biophys. Res. Commun. 187:332–339, 1992.

170. Ueki, K., Rubio, M.-P., Ramesh, V., et al. MTS1/CDKN2 gene mutations are rare in primary human astrocytomas with allelic loss of chromosome 9p. Hum. Mol. Genet. 3:1841–1845, 1994.

171. van Meyel, D. J., Ramsay, D. A., Chambers, A. F., et al. Absence of hereditary mutations in exons 5 through 9 of the p53 gene and exon 24 of the neurofibromin gene in families with glioma. Ann. Neurol. 35:120–122, 1994.

172. Vance, J. M., Small, K. W., Jones, M. A., et al. Confirmation of linkage in von Hippel-Lindau disease. Genomics 6:565–567, 1990.

173. Vinchon, M., Blond, S., Lejeune, J. P., et al. Association of Lhermitte-Duclos and Cowden disease: Report of a new case and review of the literature. J. Neurol. Neurosurg. Psychiatry 57:699–704, 1994.

174. Viskochil, D., Buchberg, A. M., Xu, G., et al. Deletions and a translocation interrupt a cloned gene at the neurofibromatosis type 1 locus. Cell 62:187–192, 1990.

175. von Deimling, A., Krone, W., and Menon, A. G. Neurofibromatosis type 1: Pathology, clinical features, and molecular genetics. Brain Pathol. 5:153–162, 1995.

176. von Deimling, A., Louis, D. N., Menon, A. G., et al. Allelic loss on the long arm of chromosome 17 in pilocytic astrocytoma. Acta. Neuropathol. 86:81–85, 1993.

177. Wallace, M. R., Andersen, L. B., Saulino, A. M., et al. A de novo Alu insertion results in neurofibromatosis type 1. Nature 353:864–866, 1991.

178. Wallace, M. R., Marchuk, D. A., Andersen, L. B., et al. Type 1 neurofibromatosis gene: identification of a large transcript disrupted in three NF1 patients [published erratum appears in Science 21:250(4988):1749, 1990]. Science 249:181–186, 1990.

179. Weksberg, R., Shen, D. R., Fei, Y. L., et al. Disruption of insulin-like growth factor factor 2 imprinting in Beckwith-Wiedemann syndrome. Nature Genet. 5:143–150, 1993.

180. Wellenreuther, R., Kraus, J. A., Lenartz, D., et al. Analysis of the neurofibromatosis 2 gene reveals molecular variants of meningioma. Am. J. Pathol. 146:827–832, 1995.

181. Wertelecki, W., Rouleau, G. A., Superneau, D. W., et al. Neurofibromatosis 2: Clinical and DNA linkage studies of a large kindred. N. Engl. J. Med. 319:278–283, 1988.

182. Willems, P. J. Dynamic mutations hit double figures. Nature Genet. 8:213–215, 1994.

183. Williams, B. O., Remington, L., Albert, D. M., et al. Cooperative tumorigenic effects of germline mutations in Rb and p53. Nature Genet. 7:480–484, 1994.

184. Xu, G., O'Connell, P., Viskochil, D., et al. The neurofibromatosis type 1 gene encodes a protein related to GAP. Cell 62:599–608, 1990.

185. Xu, G. F., Lin, B., Tanaka, K., et al. The catalytic domain of the neurofibromatosis type 1 gene product stimulates ras GTPase and complements ira mutants of S. cerevisiae. Cell 63:835–841, 1990.

186. Yao, M., Latif, F., Orcutt, M. L., et al. von Hippel-Lindau disease: identification of deletion mutations by pulsed-field gel electrophoresis. Hum. Genet. 92:605–614, 1993.

187. Yong, W. H., Raffel, C., von Deimling, A., and Louis, D. N. Lack of allelic loss at APC in sporadic medulloblastomas. N. Engl. J. Med. (letter). 333:524, 1995.

CHAPTER 8

Molecular Biology of Meningiomas and Peripheral Nerve Sheath Tumors

MATTHIAS KIRSCH, M.D., THOMAS SANTARIUS, M.D.,
PETER McL. BLACK, M.D., Ph.D.

INTRODUCTION

Meningiomas and peripheral nerve sheath tumors (pNST) demonstrate common clinical characteristics: they are generally benign, slow growing tumors that are well demarcated from the surrounding tissue and can be cured by surgical intervention. However, their developmental origin, function, and molecular characteristics reveal that they represent very different entities. Over the past 2 decades, major advances have been made toward the understanding of the pathogenesis of meningiomas and pNSTs at the molecular level. This chapter will discuss genetic aberrations, epigenetic effects, hormone and growth factor dependency, and clonal composition of these tumors as well as methodological aspects.

CELLULAR ORIGIN

Meningioma

Meningiomas are mostly benign primary tumors of the meninges and comprise approximately 18% and 25% of intracranial and spinal neoplasms, respectively (1, 156). They are most commonly located on the surface of the brain and inside the spinal canal, although rare cases of extraneuraxial meningiomas have been reported (171). Histologically, meningiomas are classified as typical (WHO grade I) comprising more than 90% of all meningiomas, atypical (WHO grade II), papillary (WHO grade II-III), and anaplastic (WHO grade III) (see Table 1).

The cellular origin of meningiomas has been an area of controversy for many years. This is reflected in the development of the nomenclature, where terms, such as fungus (Louis in 1774, ref. (112)) or sarcoma (Virchow in 1864, ref. (191)) of the dura mater, and dural endothelioma (Golgi in 1869, ref. (62)) were proposed. It is now widely accepted that meningiomas arise from arachnoid cap cells, also known as meningocytes. These cells are scattered throughout the arachnoid, with highest concentrations in the Paccionian granulations. They are thought to be of mesodermal origin. Extraneuraxial meningiomas are also believed to arise from meningocytes, although the mechanisms of their ectopic occurrence, *e.g.*, in dermis of a finger (39), remains obscure. Arachnoid cells function as a part of the protective leptomeningeal cover of the CNS without direct contact with neuroglial structures. However, the developmental origin of meningocytes and the neoplastic transformation to meningioma are not well characterized because of the current unavailability of specific histopathological markers.

Peripheral Nerve Sheath Tumors (Schwannomas and Neurofibromas)

Peripheral nerve sheath tumors arise from Schwann-cells that develop as a distinct lineage from the neural crest and can be subdivided into schwannomas, neurofibromas, and malignant pNSTs (see Table 1). Schwann cells surround peripheral nerve axons and are essential for conduction of nerve impulses. Although schwannomas consist only of neoplastic Schwann cells, neurofibromas are composed of neoplastic Schwann cells, fibroblasts and perineural cells (91). It is not clear whether the multicellular appearance of neurofibromas results from neoplastic transformation of Schwann cells followed by consecutive recruitment of normal cells or whether several cell types are affected by the oncogenic process at the same time.

Intracranial schwannomas are responsible for 8 to 12% of all primary intracranial tumors. The majority arises from the vestibular part of the acoustic nerve. Less common are schwannomas of cranial nerves V, IX, X, or XI. Schwannomas occur preferentially at the border between the central and peripheral myelin sheets. The extraordinary long intradural margin between white matter and pia mater might contribute to the susceptibility of the vestibular nerve for neoplastic transformation although the mechanism remains to be investigated. Peripheral nerve schwannomas are less common than spinal schwannomas, which most commonly arise from dorsal sensory root fibers. pNSTs are well circumscribed, encapsulated and demarcated from surrounding tissue, which accounts for their expanding but generally non-infiltrating growth pattern. Their histological appearance has been classified according to Antoni, where the Antoni A pattern is characterized by compact elongated cells arranged in a palisading fashion, and the Antoni B pattern displays lipidization and less cellularity (91). Another histological classification distinguishes cellular, plexiform, and melanotic schwannomas. There are no highly specific and sensitive markers for pNSTs available, but both schwannomas and neurofibromas are usually positive for Leu-7 and S-100 proteins. Neurofibromas occur as solitary tumors or as plexiform neurofibromas involving several nerve branches. In contrast to meningiomas and intracranial schwannomas which occur predominantly in females, the incidence of spinal and peripheral neurofibromas does not reveal a gender preference. Malignant peripheral nerve sheath tumors are not common and mostly represent malignant transformation of neurofibromas associated with neurofibromatosis I (for review see ref. (155)).

CLONALITY

The analysis of the clonal derivation of tumors lays at the heart of oncological research since it provides insight into etiology and pathogenesis. Moreover, clonal analysis may be of diagnostic value and improve monitoring of disease progression. Tumors of clonal origin arise from a single progenitor cell as a result of transforming cellular events that confer a growth advantage over adjacent normal cells. These aberrations include activation of oncogenes or inactivation of tumor suppressor genes. According to Nowell's clonal evolution theory of tumorigenesis, additional aberrations may accumulate during tumor progression leading to genetic heterogeneity and selection of more aggressive sublines (133). The relative proportion of tumor cell subpopulations depends on the growth advantage conferred by the cumulative genetic changes in the clone. The majority of tumors analyzed to date, including astrocytic CNS tumors, are monoclonal in origin (83, 196). It is important to note that polyclonality observed in some cases may be the result of different processes: first, polyclonal tumors may arise as a result of multiple initiation events in two or more parental cells at early stages of tumorigenesis. The initiating events may be caused by different somatic mutations or, more likely, by exogenous or endogenous factors, such as viral infection, hormonal stimulation, or environmental factors that affect several cells at the same time. Second, polyclonality may be the result of contamination of normal cells in the tumor tissue, caused either by recruitment of normal cells, such as chemotactic endothelial cell proliferation during tumor-neovascularization, infiltration of reactive inflammatory cells as an immunological response, or infiltration of the tumor into surrounding normal parenchyma. Third, results from clonal analysis may be skewed as a result of differences in sensitivity of different assay systems as discussed below.

Methodological Aspects

Clonal derivation can be analyzed by screening a tumor for the presence of genetic heterogeneity using cytogenetic, molecular genetic, or viral integration approaches. Analysis of clonality in females heterozygous for specific genetic markers on the X-chromosome has been employed widely (82, 196). Because of random inactivation of the X-chromosome by selective methylation in early embryogenesis, normal tissue will be polyclonal in this assay, whereas clonally derived tissues exhibit only one X-chromosomal inactivation pattern. The predictive value of early markers employed, such as the X chromosome-linked glucose-6-phosphate dehydrogenase (G6PD) gene (50), was limited due to the low frequency of heterozygosity in females. The use of differential methylation of cytosine residues within X-chromosomes linked genes in combination with DNA restriction fragments length polymorphisms (RFLP) (193), *e.g.*, the hypoxanthine guanine phosphoribosyl-transferase (HPRT) and phosphoglycerate kinase (PGK) genes (194), or with variable number tandem repeat (VNTR) markers; *e.g.*, M27β at the DXS255 locus (2), has increased the percentage of informative cases up to 90% but require large amounts of DNA (5–10 μg) for Southern blot analysis.

Highly polymorphic di-, tri-, or tetranucleotide repeats, so-called microsatellite markers, can be analyzed easily by PCR and require only minute amounts of DNA. Such a trinucleotide

repeat is located in the coding region of the first exon of the human androgen receptor gene on the X chromosome (HUMARA) (7). It exhibits a high frequency of heterozygosity (90%) and reliable methylation patterns (122). As one allele is inactivated by methylation, analysis of the methylation pattern of this gene in tumor specimens reveals information regarding clonal derivation. Another technique is to evaluate the mRNA expression by reverse transcription (RT) and polymerase chain reaction (PCR). The combination of this methylation-based clonality assay with a transcription based assay using RT-PCR at the same locus increases the sensitivity and specificity of clonal analysis (21). However, the technique is limited by the level of transcription of the androgen receptor gene in the tissue of investigation.

Meningioma

Based on the finding that the androgen receptor is expressed in most meningiomas (28), Zhu *et al.* compared methylation- and transcription-based clonality assays at the human androgen receptor gene locus (HUMARA) in sporadic meningiomas (211). Their data from 19 informative patients demonstrated that clonality results obtained with the two techniques were concordant in most cases. Discordant data were attributed to normal tissue contamination or variable methylation and expression patterns within the tumor. Interestingly, only 60% of meningiomas were monoclonal in origin, whereas 40% were polyclonal. A similar frequency (35%) of polyclonality in sporadic meningiomas has been observed by Wu *et al.* (personal communication). Jacoby *et al.* (82) reported monoclonality in nine informative meningioma patients, based on a methylation-based HPRT assay. However, using the grading criteria of clonality of Zhu *et al.* (211), 2/9 to 4/9 cases would be acknowledged to be polyclonal, consistent with the former two studies. The comparison of multiple meningiomas within the same patients using the PGK and androgen receptor methylation-based clonality assays revealed monoclonality for 4/4 cases (102). Similarly, analysis of the NF-2 gene in two patients with sporadic multiple meningioma by single strand conformation polymorphism (SSCP) and direct sequencing demonstrated the same mutations in all nodules from a given patient (195). The latter two studies suggest the origin from a single progenitor cell. In contrast, comparison of eight meningioma nodules from one patient using LOH analysis of chromosome 22 and the HUMARA clonality assay found that at least one nodule was of different origin (Zhu J., Wu J., *et al.*, personal communication). Polyclonality may be explained by the observation that both meningiomas and schwannomas can be influenced by hormonal stimuli. This is further supported by the observation of a higher incidence of meningiomas and schwannomas in females than in males, as well as an increased level of expression and nuclear localization of steroid hormone receptors, including the progesterone and androgen receptors (24, 28). These findings suggest that hormone receptor activation may be important as an adjunctive mechanism (see below).

Schwannoma

Using the methylation-based HPRT assay, monoclonality has been demonstrated in seven informative cases of sporadic schwannomas (82). However, the combination of the transcription based assay at the HUMARA locus and LOH analysis of chromosome 22 revealed that the majority of sporadic schwannomas are polyclonal (Zhu *et al.* personal communication). Since both meningiomas and schwannomas frequently exhibit LOH on chromosome 22q, one may speculate that loss of a tumor suppressor gene, such as the neurofibromin/NF2 gene, may represent a common primary event during neoplastic transformation.

Neurofibroma

Neurofibromas usually appear as solitary, slow growing tumors, either sporadic or hereditary, associated with neurofibromatosis type 1. The fact that neurofibromas are composed of different cell types might argue against monoclonality. As with malignant gliomas, which are histologically very heterogenous but mostly clonal in origin, morphological appearance does not allow any conclusion as to the clonal origin of these tumors. For example, most studies on the clonality of neurofibromas were conducted in multiple neurofibromas from NF1 patients. Although the study by Fialkow *et al.* (51), who introduced clonal analysis using the G6PD isozyme polymorphism, reported polyclonality in multiple neurofibromas, more recent reports

employing methylation-based RFLP analysis at the PGK locus suggested monoclonality (174).

Clonality is an important issue in tumor pathogenesis. The development of more specific markers for clonal analysis would facilitate the study of the origin and progression of neoplastic disease as well as the development of tools for new therapeutic strategies. A polyclonal tumor is more likely to survive cytotoxic therapy because of the presence of diverse populations of cells with various susceptibility for treatment. Studies on initially polyclonal tumors that have been treated may lead to the identification of phenotypic characteristics of cell populations that survive the selection of cytotoxic/cytoreductive treatment.

GENETIC ABERRATIONS

Advances in molecular biology and molecular genetics have led to the formulation of the oncogene/tumor suppressor gene concept, which explains oncogenesis by two principal mechanisms: The pathological activation of normal cellular genes, called proto-oncogenes, leads to abnormal growth by gain of function, whereas loss of tumor suppressor gene activity leads to derepressed cell growth. Activation of oncogenes can be caused either by mutations or by introduction of oncogenes by viral transduction. Several classes of oncogenes can lead to induction or potentiation of proliferation: growth factors, growth factor receptors, and apoptosis inhibiting factors. Oncogenes activated in brain tumors include c-sis or c-erbB, which encode the B subunit of platelet-derived growth factor and the epidermal growth receptor, respectively, and bcl-2 which encodes an apoptosis inhibitor (6, 109, 140). Tumor suppressor genes in a normal cell control suppress proliferation to maintain the physiological equilibrium of growth, differentiation, and cell death in normal tissue. These genes act in a recessive fashion; both alleles have to be functionally disabled in order to lose their anti-proliferative effects and enable neoplastic growth. Therefore, two independent cellular events have to occur to produce complete inactivation, a theory known as the two-hit-hypothesis (92). The initiating genetic aberrations leading to neoplastic transformation appear to be relatively cell specific, as demonstrated in neurofibromatosis type 2 for Schwann cells and in retinoblastoma for retinal cells, although some overlapping is seen as in Li-Fraumeni syndrome which displays multiple cancer types of different organs.

Peripheral Nerve Sheath Tumors

Neurofibromas and schwannomas are among the characteristic features of the hereditary disorders neurofibromatosis types 1 and 2 (NF1 and NF2, see table 2). NF1 and 2 belong to the group of neurocutaneous disorders and are inherited in a autosomal dominant fashion. Whereas NF1 is characterized by multiple peripheral nerve neurofibromas, patients with NF2 develop multiple schwannomas, most commonly bilateral acoustic schwannomas. In addition, patients with neurofibromatosis are at increased risk for other primary intracranial tumors, such as gliomas and meningiomas, as well as for malignant neurofibrosarcomas (MPNST). Identification of genetic aberrations in the hereditary form of schwannomas and neurofibromas have to some extent provided further insight into pathogenetic mechanisms underlying sporadic cases. Certain genetic aberrations are common in both hereditary and sporadic tumors and will be summarized here.

Neurofibromatosis Type 1 (NF1)

The incidence of NF1 is ten times higher than that of NF2. Neurofibromatosis type 1 (NF-1) is characterized by cafe-au-lait spots, hamartomas of the iris (Lisch nodules), and multiple cutaneous and plexiform neurofibromas. Other neoplasms associated with NF-1 include schwannomas, pheochromocytomas, rhabdomyo- sarcomas, optic gliomas, and astrocytomas. The NF1 gene has been mapped by linkage analysis and by chromosomal breakpoint analysis to chromosome 17q11.2 and consists of 33 different exons (178, 206). At least two transcripts have been identified that are differentially expressed in fetal or adult brain or in normal human periph-

TABLE 2
Molecular Genetics of Meningioma, Schwannoma, and Neurofibroma

Name/Syndrome	Common Findings and Symptoms	Other Tumors	Genetics	Gene Product/ Function	Reference
Meningioma	Intracranial, less frequent intraspinal, rarely multiple meningioma, anaplastic meningioma		Monosomy chr 22, LOH 22q, 1p, 10	NF2 ?	(105, 141, 157, 158)
Neurofibromatosis type 1 (NF-1) von Recklinghausen's disease	Neurofibromas, café-au-lait spots, hyperpigmentation, Lisch nodules (iris hamartomas), acoustic neuroma	Malignant schwannoma, neurofibrosarcoma, pheochromocytoma, rhabdomyosarcoma, optic glioma, astrocytoma, glioblastoma	Incidence 1: 3,500 autosomal dominant, chr 17q11.2	Neurofibromin; homology to ras-GTPase-activating protein	(128, 131, 192, 197)
Neurofibromatosis type 2 (NF-2) Bilateral acoustic Neurofibromatosis	Bilateral acoustic neuromas, less frequent skin stigmata than NF-1: skin nodules, dermal neurofibromas, cafe-au-lait spots, posterior subcapsular cataracts, schwannoma, rarely spinal nerve root neurofibroma	Multiple cerebral, spinal and peripheral neurofibroma, meningioma, ependymoma, less frequent glioma and neurofibrosarcoma	Incidence: 1: 40,000 autosomal dominant; deletions or LOH of 22q, monosomie chr 22	Merlin (moesin-ezrin-radixin like protein)/ schwannoma; tumor suppressor, cytoskeleton-associated protein, signal transducer	(46, 119, 169, 170, 187)
Sporadic schwannoma	Solitary schwannoma, not NF related		LOH chr.22	NF-2 gene	(55, 105)

eral nerve (30, 38) (for review see ref. (31)). The NF1 gene product, neurofibromin, comprises 2818 amino acids domain that contain a 360 amino acid with strong homology to the catalytic domains of *ras*-GTPase-activating proteins (206). This domain, termed NF1-GRD, has the ability to interact with the *ras* protein, a GTP-dependent signal transducer with oncogenic properties. Neurofibromin is associated with microtubules at this domain (66) suggesting a role in microtubule-mediated intracellular signal transduction. Therefore, inactivation of the NF1 gene may induce tumorigenic transformation. Convincing evidence for its tumor-suppressive properties has been obtained by gene-transfer of the NF1-GRD and other domains of the neurofibromin-gene into v-Ha-*Ras* transformed 3T3 fibroblasts (56, 135). It has been demonstrated that the NF1 protein can diminish the oncogenic effects of *ras* by stimulating its intrinsic GTPase activity (134). If the NF1 gene acts as a tumor suppressor gene, both alleles have to be functionally inactivated for initiation of malignant transformation. Indeed, germline mutations always affect only one allele, whereas the other allele is inactivated by a somatic mutation. Recently, LOH analysis in 22 neurofibromas from five unrelated NF1 patients revealed somatic deletions in eight tumors (36%) from two patients (34). In contrast to NF-1 associated neurofibromas, benign sporadic neurofibromas do not display loss of heterozygosity (LOH) at the NF1 locus (173). In addition, other tumors, such as colon cancer and myelodysplasia, which often show high levels of activated *ras*, do not occur more frequently in NF1 patients than in the general population (for review see (31)). Absence of LOH at the NF1 locus does not necessarily exclude a pathogenetic role of the NF1 gene for sporadic cases, since other means of gene inactivation such as small point mutations in both alleles, mutation of the promoter region (cis-acting elements) or gene-regulating factors (trans-acting elements), imprinting, or translational dysregulation may be involved. Furthermore, neurofibromin may have additional, yet unknown tumor-suppressive functions that are independent of *ras*. Transgenic knock-out mice homozygous for a mutation in the NF1 gene did not survive beyond 14 days of gestation mainly because of cardiac outflow tract malformations (80). Heterozygous mice, however, display an increased cancer predisposition and develop tumors such as pheochromocytoma and leukemia, which do occur in the human disease, although the full spectrum of human NF1 symptoms was not observed.

Neurofibromatosis Type 2 (NF2)

NF2 is characterized clinically by bilateral acoustic schwannomas. Dermatological symptoms are less prominent than in NF-1. NF2 is also associated with other brain tumors, including meningiomas, schwannomas, and astrocytomas. The NF2 gene has been mapped to chromosome 22q11 (154, 169) and encodes merlin/schwannomin, a cytoskeleton associated protein (153, 187) that is involved in intracellular signal transduction. The N-terminus of the 595 amino acid protein has similarities to the F-actin-binding protein family called TERM, which includes the talin, ezrin, radixin, and moesin family of proteins. These proteins link the cell membrane with the cytoskeleton (153, 187). Thus, NF2 is part of the tumor suppressor family of actin- cytoskeleton-associated proteins, which includes vinculin, alpha-actinin, tropomyosin-1, gelsolin, and tensin (184). Several alternatively spliced forms have been described in normal cells (148), whose importance in neoplasia has to be evaluated. Similar to NF1, merlin/schwannomin may act as a tumor suppressor gene as expression of the NF2-cDNA in 3T3 cells slows proliferation and changes morphology. Furthermore, expression of the NF-2 cDNA in v-Ha-*Ras* transfected 3T3 fibroblasts has been shown to reverse the *Ras*-induced malignant phenotype (184), suggesting that NF2 regulates proliferation along the *Ras* pathway. Immunohistochemical studies demonstrated that tumor Schwann cells do not express merlin/schwannomin, compared with normal vestibular nerve tissue (159), supporting the contention that the NF2 gene acts as a tumor suppressor gene in human tumors. Interestingly, both familial and sporadic tumors frequently display loss of genetic material from chromosome 22. LOH of chromosome 22 or mutations of the NF2 gene were reported in 20 to 56% of sporadic and NF2 related pNSTs (81, 159, 189).

Meningiomas

In 1967 Zang and Singer first linked monosomy of chromosome 22 with the development of meningiomas (208). Cytogenetic studies have repeatedly shown monosomy of chromosome 22 in up to 70% of cases (209). LOH of chromosome 22 is present in almost all tumor samples with multiple chromosomal aberrations (42), suggesting that loss of chromosome 22 is an early event in the development of meningiomas. Loss of genetic material on chromosomes 1, 3, 5, 10, 7, 14, and Y has also been observed less frequently (reviewed in (13, 175)).

Based on the observation that meningiomas may occur as NF-2 related tumors and that sporadic cases exhibit a high frequency of loss of genetic material of chromosome 22, several studies have investigated NF2 gene mutations in sporadic meningiomas. Whereas one study suggests that the NF2 gene is not the target for LOH of chromosome 22 (43), others found LOH of chromosome 22 at the chromosomal location of the NF2 gene in more than 60% of sporadic meningiomas, with monosomy of chromosome 22 accounting for half of the cases (158). Furthermore, analysis of the NF2 gene by SSCP indicated mutations in 15 to 60% of meningiomas (141, 157, 201) were more frequent in fibroblastic and transitional meningiomas than in meningiothelial meningiomas (70–83% vs. 25%, respectively) (201). Most of the mutations were found in tumors that had already lost one chromosome 22 allele (141, 157), which is consistent with the requirement of two hits for the inactivation of the NF2 tumor suppressor gene. In contrast to sporadic cases, analysis of the NF2 gene in a family with multiple meningiomas and ependymomas did not reveal significant genetic linkage (146). These studies suggest that in up to 40% of meningiomas, genes other than NF2 are responsible for tumor development.

The progression from a benign (WHO grade I) to a more malignant (WHO grades II and III) meningioma appears to be associated with loss of heterozygosity of chromosome 1 and 10 (see Table 5). All meningiomas with LOH of chromosome 10 or 1p also had LOH of chromosome 22 (11, 150). These data support the concept that alterations of chromosome 22 represent an early event in meningeal neoplasia, whereas alterations of chromosome 1p and 10 coincide with malignant progression. Therefore, specific genetic aberrations can be correlated with malignancy changes.

GENOMIC IMPRINTING AND DNA METHYLATION

Activation of oncogenes and inactivation of tumor suppressor genes can be caused by events that interfere with their transcriptional or translational regulation. An epigenetic process, referred to as genomic imprinting, has recently been implicated in tumorigenesis. Genomic imprinting (GI) is the specific inactivation of maternal or paternal alleles attributable to gamete-specific modification causing parental-specific gene expression in diploid cells (49). Imprinted genes are functionally inactive and lack transcription. The inactivation of one X-chromosome in females appears to be mediated by genomic imprinting. Evidence for the importance of allele-specific gene expression from a parent of origin was first obtained in mice by demonstrating that androgenic embryos carrying two paternal chromosomal sets or parthenogenic embryos carrying two maternal chromosomal sets failed to develop normally (33, 181).

Genetic imprinting has been implicated in the etiology of Prader-Willie syndrome and Angelman syndrome, both revealing uniparental disomy of the maternal or paternal chromosome 15q11-12, respectively (116, 160). GI can be associated with malignant transformation, including some cases of Beckwith-Wiedemann syndrome, an overgrowth syndrome predisposing to cancer, particularly Wilms tumor (87). This syndrome is associated with paternal uniparental disomy at chromosome 11p15 or mutation of the maternal chromosome 11p15, suggesting that the maternal allele is imprinted, whereas the paternal allele codes for a growth factor, most likely insulin growth factor-2 (IGF-2). This is supported by the observation that in most Wilms' tumors that retain both alleles, loss of imprinting occurs leading to expression of both alleles (136, 149).

One process by which otherwise genetically identical alleles may be rendered functionally different is physical modification of the DNA by methylation, most often of cytosine residues within CpG dinucleotides by the enzyme methyltransferase. While most of the cytosine residues in the human genome are methylated, nonmethylated clusters of CpG dinucleotides, called CpG islands, are frequently located in the 5′-region of housekeeping genes (100). Approximately 60% of genes in mammalian genomes contain GC-rich regions that regulate gene expression by binding to specific transcription factors, and a correlation between hypomethylation and increased gene activity has been observed. Furthermore, *de novo* methylation of CpG islands occurring in cultured cells indicates a role for methylation in the suppression of growth impeding gene activity (9). Interestingly, methylated cytosine residues tend to mutate more commonly than non-methylated residues because of spontaneous deamination (100). Overall DNA methylation decreases with age *in vivo* and during senescense *in vitro*, but not in immortalized cells (9, 100).

Hypo- and hypermethylation of DNA has also been implicated in tumorigenesis (see Table 3). Hypomethylation has been associated frequently most with the activation of proto-oncogenes, such as c-*fos*, c-*myc*, and *bcl*-2 genes, and with tumor progression (100). The overall level of DNA methylation is generally lower in neoplastic than in normal cells despite the presence of higher levels of methyltransferase (44, 48). Hypermethylation may represent an important mechanism of tumor initiation because it can inactivate tumor suppressor genes. Laird *et al.* demonstrated that in mice with multiple intestinal neoplasia (MIN), a model for human adenomatous polyposis coli, hypomethylation suppressed the formation of polyps (99). In this study, hypomethylation was induced either by crossing MIN mice with methyltransferase knockout mice or by treatment with a methyltransferase inhibitor. Recent evidence suggests that hypermethylation of a structural gene or its promoter region plays an important role in the inactivation of a number of tumor suppressor genes such as the Rb gene, the von-Hippel-Lindau gene (VHL), the PDGF-A gene promotor region, and the p16 gene, all of which have been implicated in brain tumor growth (47, 57, 74, 103, 110, 129). The p16 gene rarely shows intragenic mutations in many tumor types, including brain tumors, but it is commonly inactivated by homozygous deletion (190). In tumor cell lines, a normal p16 gene can be transcriptionally repressed if the corresponding CpG island at exon 1 is methylated (129). Furthermore, pharmacological inhibition of methyltransferase was capable of restoring p16 gene expression. *De novo* methylation of the Rb gene or its promoter region has been shown in up to 16% of sporadic retinoblastomas (161, 202), whereas changes in the methylation pattern of the VHL gene have been reported in some cases of sporadic renal cell carcinomas (74). DNA hypermethylation on chromosome 17p has been detected in 84% (17/20) of all grades of astrocytomas, and in 80% (4/5) of medulloblastomas, but not (0/12) in neuroblastomas (115).

Analysis of the parental origin of NF-1 gene mutations revealed that in all families studied the paternally derived allele was mutated (179). This finding suggests a role for genomic imprinting that may either enhance mutation of the paternal allele or protect the maternal allele from mutation. In a small number of sporadic and NF-2-associated acoustic schwannomas, a threefold preference for LOH of the maternally derived chromosome 22q was observed (54). However, the analysis of sporadic meningiomas did not show such a correlation, and LOH of 22q seemed to be independent of paternal or maternal origin (53, 177). Although further investigations are necessary, these data point to the role of methylation or genomic imprinting as an important pathogenetic mechanism in tumorigenesis of sporadic and NF-related neurofibromas and schwannomas.

TABLE 3
Genomic Imprinting in Nervous System Tumors (49)

Tumor Type	Gene	Parental Allele Affected	Chromosome	Aberration	References
Neurofibromatosis type I (NF1)	NF1	Paternal allele	17	Mutation	(179)
Neurofibromatosis type II (NF2)	Multiple loci	Maternal 3:1 paternal	22	LOH	(54)
Sporadic neuroma	Multiple loci	Maternal 3:1 paternal	22	LOH	(54)
Meningioma	Multiple loci	Maternal or paternal	22	LOH	(53, 177)
Bilateral retinoblastoma	Rb	Maternal	13	LOH	(41, 212)
Unilateral retinoblastoma	Rb	Maternal	13	LOH	(41, 103, 212)
Neuroblastoma	Multiple loci	Maternal	1	LOH	(23, 32)
Neuroblastoma	N-myc	Paternal	2	Amplification	(32)

TABLE 4
Summary of Estrogen and Progesterone Detection in Meningiomas

Series (Ref. No.)	Technique	Specimen	Patient No.	Estrogen	Progesteron
Blaauw (12)	Binding assay	Tissue	67	few	80%
Blankenstein (16)	Binding assay	Cytosol, tissue	45	15%	89%
Blankenstein (17)	Binding assay	Cytosol	140	9%	
	Enzyme immunoassay	Cytosol	21	84%	
Blankenstein (15)	Binding assay	Culture	20	none	90%
Bouillot (18)	Immunohistochemistry	Meningioma tissue	52	none	53%
Brentani (19)	Density gradient	Meningioma tissue	6	33%	100%
Cahill (22)	Density gradient	Tissue	23	17%	34%
Carroll (24)	Northern blot,	Meningioma mRNA	33	N/A	64%
	immunohistochemistry		13	N/A	61%
Concolino (35)	Density gradient	Spinal meningioma	6	yes	no
Courriere (36)	Binding assay	Cytosol	12	none	83%
Donnell (40)	Binding assay		6	67%	N/A
Glick (60)	Binding assay	Cytosol	21	62%	N/A
Grunberg (68)	Binding assay	Cytosol	17	6%	69%
Halper (71)	Nuclear binding assay,		52	33%	69%
	binding assay,			2%	76%
	immunohistochemistry			none	89%
Hayward (73)	Radioreceptor	Spinal meningioma	22	none	77%
Hinton (77)	Radioreceptor	Spinal meningioma	11	36%	54%
Ironside (79)	Isoelectric focussing	Cryostat section	45	none	53%
Khalid (90)	Immunohistochemistry	Meningioma tissue	34	none	100%
Kobayashi (93)	Binding assay	Cytosol	8	37%	none
Kornblum (94)	Binding assay	Cytosol	29	none	27%
Kuratsu (96)	Binding assay	Cytosol	19	none	89%
Lee (104)	Binding assay		20	35%	82%
Lesch (106)	Enzyme immunoassay	Cytosol	70	51% minor	76%
	Binding assay	Cytosol		40% minor, 11% distinct	
Lesch (107)	Binding assay	Cytosol	54%		89%
Magdelenat (113)	Binding assay	Meningioma tissue	42	30/38 (79%)	93%
Markwalder (117)	Binding assay	Meningioma tissue	44	miniscule	77%
Martuza (121)	Binding assay	Meningioma tissue	42	25 (60% minor, 19% distinct) cytosolic, 16/28 (57% minor, 21% distinct) nuclear	16/22 (73% minor, 41% distinct) cytosolic
Martuza (120)	Binding assay	Meningioma tissue	10	70%	N/A
Maxwell (124)	Northern blot	Meningioma mRNA	9	none	55%
Meixenberger (127)	Binding assay	Cytosol	28	11%	64%
Moguilewsky (132)	Binding assay		21	35% cytosol 60% nuclear	90% cytosol 76% nuclear

Perrot-Applanat (142)	Immunohistochemistry	Meningioma tissue	36		72%
Poisson (143)	Binding assay	Meningioma tissue	25	?	96%
Punnonen (147)	Binding assay	Cytosol	4	none	75%
Schnegg (163)	Binding assay	Meningioma tissue	10	none	40%
Schrell (166)	Binding assay,	Cytosol,	50	20%	98%
	enzyme immunoassay,	Cytosol,	50	2%	100%
	immunohistochemistry,	Meningioma tissue,	50	none	N/A
	in situ hybridization	meningioma tissue	50	none	N/A
Schwartz (168)	Binding assay	Meningioma tissue	26	31%	30%
Tilzer (185)	Binding assay	Cytosol	6	low 66%	66%
Whittle (204)	Binding assay	Meningioma tissue	20	none	55%
Whittle (203)	Binding assay	Meningioma tissue	29	none	55%
Yu (207)	Binding assay	Meningioma tissue	16	94%	9/11 (82%)
Zava (210)	Binding assay	Culture	10	none	70%

Table compiled and updated with information from Black (13) and Smith & Cahill (175). Binding assay comprises competitive binding, charcoal adsorption, nuclear binding, and saturation binding assays.

HORMONES, GROWTH FACTORS, AND THEIR RECEPTORS

Steroid Hormone Receptors in Meningiomas

In his monograph on meningiomas, Cushing noted a significant female predominance in the occurrence of meningiomas and postulated involvement of hormones in meningioma development and growth (37). More recent epidemiological data confirms a greater incidence of meningiomas in women with a female to male ratio of approximately 2:1. Furthermore, a positive correlation between breast cancer and meningiomas has been reported (8, 20, 45, 98, 164, 176). Occult meningiomas may become symptomatic during pregnancy; symptoms may cease after delivery (130). These observations have been addressed in numerous experimental studies linking meningiomas with steroid hormones since Donnel *et al.* reported estrogen binding sites on four of six meningiomas (40).

Several studies confirmed the presence of steroid binding receptors in meningiomas. Using competitive binding assays, binding sites for progesterone and estrogen have been reported in 40 to 100% and 0 to 94% of meningiomas, respectively (see Table 4). More recent studies, using more specific binding criteria and alternative techniques such as immunohistochemistry and mRNA analysis have corroborated expression of progesterone receptors, whereas there is still controversy about whether estrogen receptors are present (13, 175). Although progesterone receptor positive tumors occur more frequently in females than in males, the presence of receptor, does not correlate with plasma progesterone levels (*i.e.*, the menstrual status), progesterone receptor activity, age, histological subtype, or clinical behavior (13, 24, 27, 175). Although most studies have demonstrated the presence of progesterone receptors in meningiomas, the data regarding their function in meningiomas remains inconclusive. Schwartz *et al.* suggested that progesterone receptors and estrogen receptors in meningiomas may not meet the specific criteria for true steroid receptor proteins (168), such as a high affinity to the ligand, a finite binding capacity, specificity of the binding site for the ligand, and a correlation of the binding with a meaningful biological response.

The biological effects of steroid hormones are mediated by the interaction between the ligand-receptor complex with responsive DNA sequences. This interaction usually results in increased transcription of genes located downstream of these sequences. Using immunohistochemistry or *in situ* hybridization, nuclear localization of the progesterone receptor in meningiomas has been demonstrated (24, 142, 145). However, the effects of progesterone stimulation *in vitro* on meningioma cell proliferation are still unresolved (3, 114, 138).

Evidence for the functional role of progesterone receptors has recently been obtained by transfection of primary meningioma cell cultures with a construct that contained two palindromic progesterone/glucocorticoid (PRE/GRE) responsive elements in front of the thymidine kinase promoter and the chloramphenicol acetyl sequence of the tyrosine aminotransferase reporter gene (CAT) (27). Transfected cells were stimulated separately with a progesterone agonist, R5020, and dexamethasone, a glucocorticoid agonist. Changes in transcription were measured by the changes in CAT activity. An increase in CAT activity after dexamethasone stimulation was noted in all eight cultures tested. An increase in CAT activity in response to the addition of progesterone was observed only in those four of eight meningiomas cultures positive for progesterone receptor mRNA, suggesting that the progesterone receptor in meningiomas is functional.

In vivo evidence for the biological activity or progesterone receptors in meningiomas has been provided by Olson *et al.* (139), who implanted nude mice with freshly resected human meningiomas. One group of these mice received 10 mg/kg of the antiprogesterone mifepristone (RU486) daily; the other group received placebo. After 3 months, tumor volume was 154% of baseline in the control group and 25% of baseline in the group receiving RU486, demonstrating an inhibitory effect of RU486 on meningioma growth.

Initial clinical trials using a variety of hormonal preparations have so far produced inconclusive results. The antiestrogen tamoxifen was applied to treat unresectable meningiomas without convincing results (63, 118). Similarly, progesterone supplementation (megasterol acetate 40–30 g four times a day for up to 2 years) showed no effect in nine patients (67). Administration of mifepristone for treatment of unresectable meningiomas in 28 patients with a me-

TABLE 5
Loss of Heterozygosity Associated with Malignant Progression in Meningiomas

Meningioma Type	LOH of chr. 22 ref (11, 150)	LOH of 1p (19, 22)	LOH of 10 (247)
Typical	9/33 (18%), 5/15 (33%)	1/33 (3%)	0/20
Atypical	12/15 (80%), 2/2 (100%)	10/15 (67%)	1/2 (50%)
Anaplastic	2/2 (100%), 5/10 (50%)	2/2 (100%)	4/13 (31%)

dian observation time of 24 months revealed objective responses in eight and subjective improvements in five patients (68), confirming similar effects of mifepristone by other groups (70, 101).

There is also substantial evidence for the presence of androgen, glucocorticoid, and mineralocorticoid receptors in meningiomas based on DCC, immunocytochemistry, and Northern blot analysis (19, 27, 28, 124, 143). Expression of the androgen receptor has been detected in 69% and 31% of meningiomas in females and males, respectively, which correlates with immunohistochemical data on nuclear receptor staining (28).

Although nuclear localization of androgen receptors suggests their functional relevance (28, 124), studies on the effect of androgens on meningioma proliferation *in vitro* have produced mixed results. Whereas low concentrations of testosterone inhibited cell growth in one of two meningioma cell culture examined (58), dihydrotestosterone had a small stimulatory effect in two separate studies (137, 210).

The presence of D-1 and D-2 dopamine receptors (D1R, D2R) in cultured meningioma cells has been demonstrated by RT-PCR in 80% or 100%, respectively. Ligand binding studies suggest only the D1R (25) is functional. Micromolar concentrations of the dopamine agonist bromocriptine resulted in a significant decrease of proliferation of cultured meningiomas (167), whereas bromocriptine inhibits prolactin secretion and proliferation of prolactin positive cells (111). Prolactin has been shown to stimulate meningioma cell growth in vitro (84), and its mRNA has been detected in 50 to 60% of meningioma tissue specimens (25). Whether the inhibition of meningioma proliferation by bromocriptine *in vitro* is caused by direct inhibitory effect of dopamine on meningioma cells, or is attributable to an interference with the inhibitory effect on the prolactin signaling system, or both, remains to be determined.

Growth Factors in Meningiomas

A variety of growths factors and their receptors, such as platelet derived growth factor (PDGF), fibroblast growth factors (FGF), epidermal growth factor (EGF), insulin like growth factors (IGF), and many more, have been implicated in tumorigenesis. Autonomous proliferation is one of the most important features of neoplastic growth. Unresponsiveness to physiologic growth regulating signals from close or distant sources may be caused by autocrine stimulation, when tumor cells produce a growth factor as well as its corresponding receptor. Three such autocrine circuits have been described in meningiomas for PDGF (4, 123, 182, 183), acidic and basic FGF (182, 183), and IGF (59, 188).

The platelet derived growth factor (PDGF) family contains two subunits, A and B, which are active either as heterodimer (PDGF-AB) or homodimers (PDGF-AA and PDGF-BB). PDGF-B is encoded by *c-sis*, an oncogene thought to be part of an autocrine stimulation loop during malignant transformation in astrocytomas (for review see in ref. (65)) and meningiomas (14, 123, 198). PDGF acts through receptors designated α and β. PDGF-α-R is responsive to all three PDGF isoforms, whereas PDGF-β-R preferentially binds PDGF-BB (65). Both receptors have tyrosine kinase activity and cause *c-fos* activation as part of the induction cascade (95). In gliomas, PDGF-A and PDGF-α-R are predominantly found in tumor cells, whereas PDGF-B and PDGF-β-R are mainly detected within endothelial cells of the tumor vasculature (69, 75, 76, 125). In meningiomas, both PDGF-A and PDGF-B mRNA expression have been demonstrated (14). Although none of these tumors revealed PDGF-α-R expression, PDGF-β-R was expressed in 19/20 meningiomas. Furthermore, in most meningioma cell cultures, PDGF-BB, but not PDGF-AA, induced stimulation of cell growth and increased *c-fos* expression (14, 198). These results provided evidence for an upregulated autocrine mechanism involving PDGF-BB and PDGF-β-R in meningiomas.

The fibroblast growth factor (FGF) family of proteins act as potent mitogens, differentiation factors, and angiogenic agents (52). It includes at least nine members. Two types of FGF receptors encoded by the *flg* and *bek* genes selectively binding either acidic or basic FGF have been described (183). While both basic and acidic FGF mRNA have been detected by *in situ* hybridization in 4/4 meningiomas (5), larger studies (182, 183) using Northern blot analysis found basic and acidic FGF mRNA expression in 20 of 22 and in 3 of 22 meningiomas, respectively. Similarly, immunohistochemical analysis revealed positive staining for basic FGF in almost all meningioma cells. No significant difference in *flg* and *bek* expression level in meningiomas versus normal brains and meninges were found, but expression of basic FGF was elevated in meningiomas compared with normal tissue. In addition to autocrine stimulation, basic FGF has been shown to interact with other angiogenic factors. It interacts synergistically with PDGF upon induction of mitogenesis of vascular smooth muscle cells and upregulation of PDGF-α-R (165). Synergistic properties of VEGF and basic FGF induce proliferation of bovine capillary endothelial cells (64) and suggest a direct involvement in neovascularization.

The insulin-like growth factors (IGF-I and IGF-II) exhibit structural homology with proinsulin. Their actions are mediated through two types of receptors: IGF-IR and IGF-IIR. IGF-IR has high affinity for IGF-I and a lower affinity for IGF-II and insulin, whereas IGF-IIR has high affinity for IGF-II, lower affinity for IGF-I and does not bind to insulin (61). The IGF-IR has tyrosine kinase activity that is stimulated by ligand binding. The IGF-II receptor has no such activity. IGF-I is a potent inducer of oligodendrocyte development (126) and stimulates growth of meningioma and astrocytoma cells in culture (59). Stiles and coworkers conceptualized the synergistic growth stimulatory action of IGFs and PDGF by showing that both factors are needed for optimal growth of cultured 3T3 fibroblasts (180). Using *in situ* hybridization and immunohistochemistry, Antoniades *et al.* (10) demonstrated mRNA and protein expression of both IGF-I and IGF-II in meningioma samples. They also found IGF-I mRNA in normal brain and pachymeninges, but failed to detect presence of either IGF-II mRNA or protein in these tissues. They proposed that the abnormal expression of IGF-II is coupled with the expression of IGF-IIR, which is present in fetal and neonatal tissues (72) but absent in adult pachymeninges and may be the basis of an autocrine stimulatory loop in meningiomas. Binding studies have shown that both IGF and epidermal growth receptors are expressed in meningiomas (97).

The epidermal growth factor (EGF) receptor is a transmembrane receptor tyrosine kinase whose ligands include EGF and TGF-α (transforming growth factor alpha). The amplification and overexpression of EGF-R has been shown in up to 40% of malignant gliomas (205). Up to 100% of meningiomas demonstrate staining for EGF-R by immunohistochemistry, immunoblot, or radionuclide binding (78, 85, 86, 96, 151). Staining is confined to the cytoplasm and cell membrane of the meningioma cells (86). Soluble EGF was able to stimulate meningioma cell growth in culture (3, 151), whereas varying results were obtained by co-incubation of EGF and PDGF with cultured meningioma cells (199, 200). The presence of fetal calf serum in the culture media seemed to be necessary to obtain growth stimulatory effects (199). EGF induced growth was partially blocked by bromocriptine and the anti-androgene northisterone, but not by estrogen or progesterone (3) whereas the combined proliferative effect of EGF and PDGF could be blocked by the partial PDGF antagonist trapidil (186).

Oncogenes (such as *c-cis* encoding PDGF-B, and *int-2*, *FGF-5*, *hst-2/FGF-6* encoding FGF-related proteins) have been implicated in the pathogenesis of meningiomas suggested (for review see ref. (144)). *c-fos*, *erb*B, Ha-*ras*, K-*ras* and *c-myc* oncogenes are overexpressed in meningiomas (reviewed in (175)). The finding that all meningiomas expressing *c-sis* were also positive for *c-fos* suggests that the PDGF autocrine loop may have *c-fos* as its nuclear target (152). Expression of *k-ras* was six- to eightfold greater in meningiomas than in meningeal cells or fibroblasts (29), and *c-myc* is 5- to 20-fold higher expressed in meningiomas than in normal tissue (89). The level of *c-myc* expression was higher in tumors with loss of heterozygosity on chromosome 22, suggesting that loss of a putative tumor suppressor gene may induce or be accompanied by activation of the *c-myc* oncogene. Although cases of *c-myc* and *N-myc* amplification were reported (162), the exact mechanisms for enhanced expression of these oncogenes in meningiomas remains obscure.

Steroid Hormone Receptors in Vestibular Schwannomas

Although the role of steroid hormones in meningiomas has been intensively investigated, no conclusive studies have been performed in schwannomas or neurofibromas. Several studies using immunohistochemistry or competitive ligand binding studies report inconsistent results (88, 172, 204). Expression analysis by Northern blotting and RT-PCR in 21 vestibular schwannomas demonstrated that all specimens were positive for glucocorticoid receptor mRNA, whereas none of the schwannomas revealed expression of estrogen receptor mRNA (26). Progesterone receptor mRNA was detectable in one-third of cases. Androgen receptor expression was detectable in two male specimens but not in any of the female specimens. In contrast to findings in meningiomas, this study does not support a critical role of steroid receptors in the majority of schwannomas.

CONCLUSION

Advances in molecular biology and molecular genetics have provided further insight into the biology of meningiomas, neurofibromas, and schwannomas. Tumorigenesis is a multistep process and displays many different facets of altered cell growth. We are only beginning to understand the complexity of neoplastic growth and further investigations are necessary to dissect the pathogenetic mechanisms responsible for tumorigenesis. Detailed knowledge of the subcellular and molecular events underlying neoplasia is a prerequisite for more accurate classification, diagnostic studies, and monitoring of disease progression, as well as the development of new adjunct, causally targeted therapeutic strategies for the benefit of our patients.

Acknowledgments

The authors thank Dr. Rona S. Carroll and Dr. Jiguang Zhu for their help.

REFERENCES

1. Burger, P. C., and Vogel, F. S., editors. *Surgical Pathology of the Nervous System and Its Coverings.* pp. 67–68. J. Wiley, New York, 1991.
2. Abrahamson, G., Fraser, N. J., Boyd, J., *et al.* A highly informative X-chromosome probe, M27 beta, can be used for the determination of tumour clonality. Br. J. Haematol. *74:*371–372, 1990.
3. Adams, E. F., Schrell, U. M., Fahlbusch, R., and Thi-

erauf, P. Hormonal dependency of cerebral meningiomas. Part 2: In vitro effect of steroids, bromocriptine, and epidermal growth factor on growth of meningiomas. J. Neurosurg. *73:*750–755, 1990.

4. Adams, E. F., Todo, T., Schrell, U. M., *et al.* Autocrine control of human meningioma proliferation: secretion of platelet-derived growth-factor-like molecules. Int. J. Cancer *49:*398–402, 1991.

5. Akutsu, Y., Aida, T., Nakazawa, S., and Asano, G. Localization of acidic and basic fibroblast growth factor mRNA in human brain tumors. Jpn. J. Cancer Res. *82:*1022–1027, 1991.

6. Alderson, L. M., Castleberg, R. L., Harsh, G. R. 4th, *et al.* Human gliomas with wild-type p53 express bcl-2. Cancer Res. *55:*999–1001, 1995.

7. Allen, R. C., Zoghbi, H. Y., Moseley, A. B., *et al.* Methylation of HpaII and HhaI sites near the polymorphic CAG repeat in the human androgen-receptor gene correlates with X chromosome inactivation. Am. J. Hum. Genet. *51:*1229–1239, 1992.

8. Annegers, J. F., Schoenberg, B. S., Okazaki, H., and Kurland, L. T. Epidemiologic study of primary intracranial neoplasms. Arch. Neurol. *38:*217–219, 1981.

9. Antequera, F., Boyes, J., and Bird, A. High levels of de novo methylation and altered chromatin structure at CpG islands in cell lines. Cell *62:*503–514, 1990.

10. Antoniades, H. N., Galanopoulos, T., Neville-Golden, J., and Maxwell, M. Expression of insulin-like growth factors I and II and their receptor mRNAs in primary human astrocytomas and meningiomas; in vivo studies using in situ hybridization and immunocytochemistry. Int. J. Cancer *50:*215–222, 1992.

11. Bello, M. J., De Campos, J. M., Kusak, M. E., *et al.* Allelic loss at 1p is associated with tumor progression of meningiomas. Genes Chromosomes Cancer *9:*296–298, 1994.

12. Blaauw, G., Blankenstein, M. A., and Lamberts, S. W. Sex steroid receptors in human meningiomas. Acta Neurochir. *79:*42–47, 1986.

13. Black, P. M. Meningiomas (Review). Neurosurgery *32:*643–657, 1993.

14. Black, P. M., Carroll, R., Glowacka, D., *et al.* Platelet-derived growth factor expression and stimulation in human meningiomas. J. Neurosurg. *81:*388–393, 1994.

15. Blankenstein, M. A., Blaauw, G., and Lamberts, S. W. Progestin and estrogen receptors in human meningioma. Clin. Neuropharmacol. *7:*363–367, 1984.

16. Blankenstein, M. A., Blaauw, G., Lamberts, S. W., and Mulder, E. Presence of progesterone receptors and absence of oestrogen receptors in human intracranial meningioma cytosols. Eur. J. Cancer Clin. Oncol. *19:*365–370, 1983.

17. Blankenstein, M. A., van der Meulen-Dijk, C., and Thijssen, J. H. Assay of oestrogen and progestin receptors in human meningioma cytosols using immunological methods. Clin. Chim. Acta *165:*189–195, 1987.

18. Bouillot, P., Pellissier, J. F., Devictor, B., *et al.* Quantitative imaging of estrogen and progesterone receptors, estrogen-regulated protein, and growth fraction: immunocytochemical assays in 52 meningiomas. Corre-

lation with clinical and morphological data. J. Neurosurg. *81:*765–773, 1994.

19. Brentani, M. M., Lopes, M. T., Martins, V. R., and Plese, J. P. Steroid receptors in intracranial tumors. Clin. Neuropharmacol. *7:*347–350, 1984.

20. Burns, P. E., Jha, N., and Bain, G. O. Association of breast cancer with meningioma: report of five cases. Cancer *58:*1537–1539, 1986.

21. Busque, L., Zhu, J. G., Dehart, D., *et al.* An expression based clonality assay at the human androgen receptor locus (HUMARA) on chromosome X. Nucleic Acids Res. *22:*697–698, 1994.

22. Cahill, D. W., Bashirelahi, N., Solomon, L. W., *et al.* Estrogen and progesterone receptors in meningiomas. J. Neurosurg. *60:*985–993, 1984.

23. Caron, H., van Sluis, P., van Hoeve, M., *et al.* Allelic loss of chromosome 1p36 in neuroblastoma is of preferential maternal origin and correlates with N-myc amplification (published erratum appears in Nat. Genet. *4:*431, 1993.). Nat. Genet. *4:*187–190, 1993.

24. Carroll, R. S., Glowacka, D., Dashner, K., and Black, P. M. Progesterone receptor expression in meningiomas. Cancer Res. *53:*1312–1316, 1993.

25. Carroll, R. S., Schrell, U. M. H., Zhang, J., *et al.* Dopamine-D1, dopamine-D2 and prolactin receptor mRNA expression by the polymerase chain reaction in human meningiomas. Neurosurgery 1996, In press.

26. Carroll, R. S., Zhang, J., and Black, P. M. Steroid hormone receptors in vestibular schwannomas. 1995, Personal communication.

27. Carroll, R. S., Zhang, J., Dashner, K., and Black, P. M. Progesterone and glucocorticoid receptor activation in meningiomas. Neurosurgery *37:*92–97, 1995.

28. Carroll, R. S., Zhang, J. P., Dashner, K., *et al.* Androgen receptor expression in meningiomas. J. Neurosurg. *82:*453–460, 1994.

29. Carstens, C., Messe, E., Zang, K. D., and Blin, N. Human KRAS oncogene expression in meningioma. Cancer Lett. *43:*37–41, 1988.

30. Cawthon, R. M., Weiss, R., Xu, G. F., *et al.* A major segment of the neurofibromatosis type 1 gene: cDNA sequence, genomic structure, and point mutations (published erratum appears in Cell *62:*following 608, 1990.). Cell *62:*193–201, 1990.

31. Cawthon, R., and White, R. Neurofibromatosis 1. In: *Molecular Genetics of Nervous System Tumors,* edited by A. J. Levine and H. H. Schmidek, pp. 319–327. Wiley-Liss, New York, 1993.

32. Cheng, J. M., Hiemstra, J. L., Schneider, S. S., *et al.* Preferential amplification of the paternal allele of the N-myc gene in human neuroblastomas. Nature Genet. *4:*191–194, 1993.

33. Clarke, H. J., Varmuza, S., Prideaux, V. R., *et al.* The development potential of parthenogenetically derived cells in chimeric mouse embryos: implications of action of imprinted genes. Development *104:*175–182, 1988.

34. Colman, S. D., Williams, C. A., and Wallace, M. R. Benign neurofibromas in type 1 neurofibromatosis (NF1) show somatic deletions of the NF1 gene. Nature Genet. *11:*90–92, 1995.

35. Concolino, G., Giuffre, R., Margiotta, G., *et al.* Steroid receptors in CNS: estradiol (ER) and progesterone (PR) receptors in human spinal cord tumors. J. Steroid Biochem. *20:*491–494, 1984.

36. Courriere, P., Tremoulet, M., Eche, N., and Armand, J. P. Hormonal steroid receptors in intracranial tumours and their relevance in hormone therapy. Eur. J. Cancer Clin. Oncol. *21:*711–714, 1985.

37. Cushing, H., and Eisenhart, L. *Meningiomas: Their Classification, Regional Behaviour, Life History, and Surgical End Results.* Charles C. Thomas, Springfield, Illinois, 1938.

38. Danglot, G., Teinturier, C., Duverger, A., and Bernheim, A. Tissue-specific alternative splicing of neurofibromatosis 1 (NF1) mRNA. Biomed. Pharmacother. *48:*365–372, 1994.

39. Daugaard, S. Ectopic meningioma of a finger. Case report. J. Neurosurg. *58:*778–780, 1983.

40. Donnell, M. S., Meyer, G. A., and Donegan, W. L. Estrogen-receptor protein in intracranial meningiomas. J. Neurosurg. *50:*499–502, 1979.

41. Dryja, T. P., Mukai, S., Petersen, R., *et al.* Parental origin of mutations of the retinoblastoma gene. Nature *339:*556–558, 1989.

42. Dumanski, J. P., Carlbom, E., Collins, V. P., and Nordenskjüld, M. Deletion mapping of a locus on human chromosome 22 involved in the oncogenesis of meningioma. Proc. Natl. Acad. Sci. U. S. A. *84:*9275–9279, 1987.

43. Dumanski, J. P., Rouleau, G. A., Nordenskjüld, M., and Collins, V. P. Molecular Genetic Analysis of Chromosome 22 in 81 Cases of Meningioma. Cancer Res. *50:*5863–5867, 1990.

44. el-Diery, W. S., Nelkin, B. D., Celano, P., *et al.* High expression of the DNA methyltransferase gene characterizes human neoplastic cells and progression stages of colon cancer. Proc. Natl. Acad. Sci. U. S. A. *88:*3470–3474, 1991.

45. Emry, J. K. *The Association Between Breast Cancer and Meningioma.* University of Southern California, Los Angeles, 1984.

46. Evans, D. G., Huson, S. M., Donnai, D., *et al.* A genetic study of type 2 neurofibromatosis in the United Kingdom. I. Prevalence, mutation rate, fitness and confirmation of maternal transmission effect on severity. J. Med. Genet. *29:*841–846, 1992.

47. Evans, H. J., and Prosser, J. Tumor-suppressor genes: cardinal factors in inherited predisposition to human cancers (Review). Environ. Health Perspect. *98:*25–37, 1992.

48. Feinberg, A. P. Alterations in DNA methylation in colorectal polyps and cancer (Review). Prog. Clin. Biol. Res. *279:*309–317, 1988.

49. Feinberg, A. P. Genomic imprinting and gene activation in cancer. Nature Genet. *4:*110–113, 1993.

50. Fialkow, P. J. Use of genetic markers to study cellular origin and development of tumors in human females. Adv. Cancer Res. *15:*191–226, 1972.

51. Fialkow, P., Sagebiel, R., Gartler, S., and Rimoin, D. Multiple cell origin of hereditary neurofibromas. N. Engl. J. Med. *284:*298–300, 1971.

52. Folkman, J., and Klagsburn, M. Angiogenic factors (Review). Science *235:*442–447, 1987.

53. Fontaine, B., Rouleau, G. A., Seizinger, B., *et al.* Equal parental origin of chromosome 22 losses in human sporadic meningioma: no evidence for genomic imprinting. Am. J. Hum. Genet. *47:*823–827, 1990.

54. Fontaine, B., Sanson, M., Delattre, O., *et al.* Parental origin of chromosome 22 loss in sporadic and NF2 neuromas. Genomics *10:*280–283, 1991.

55. Fontaine, B., Hanson, M. P., VonSattel, J. P., *et al.* Loss of Chromosome 22 Alleles in Human Sporadic Spinal Schwannomas. Ann. Neurol. *29:*183–186, 1991.

56. Fridman, M., Tikoo, A., Varga, M., *et al.* The minimal fragments of c-Raf-1 and NF1 that can suppress v-Ha-Ras-induced malignant phenotype. J. Biol. Chem. *269:*30105–30108, 1994.

57. Furnari, F. B., Huang, H. J. S., and Cavenee, W. K. Genetics and malignant progression of human brain tumors. Cancer Surv. 1995, In press.

58. Gibelli, N., Zibera, C., Butti, G., *et al.* Hormonal modulation of brain tumour growth: a cell culture study. Acta Neurochirurgica *101:*129–133, 1989.

59. Glick, R. P., Gettleman, R., Patel, K., *et al.* Insulin and insulin-like growth factor I in brain tumors: binding and in vitro effects. Neurosurgery *24:*791–797, 1989.

60. Glick, R. P., Molteni, A., and Fors, E. M. Hormone binding in brain tumors. Neurosurgery *13:*513–519, 1983.

61. Glick, R. P., Unterman, T. G., Blaydes, L., and Hollis, R. Insulin-like growth factors in central nervous system tumors (Review). Ann. NY Acad. Sci. *692:*223–229, 1993.

62. Golgi, C. *Sulla struttura sullo sviluppo degli psammomi.* Morgagni, Napoli, 1869.

63. Goodwin, J. W., Crowley, J., Eyre, H. J., *et al.* A phase II evaluation of tamoxifen in unresectable or refractory meningiomas: a Southwest Oncology Group study. J. Neurooncol. *15:*75–77, 1993.

64. Goto, F., Goto, K., Weindel, K., and Folkman, J. Synergistic effects of vascular endothelial growth factor and basic fibroblast growth factor on the proliferation and cord formation of bovine capillary endothelial cells within collagen gels. Lab. Invest. *69:*508–517, 1993.

65. Goumnerova, L., and Guha, A. Oncogenes and Growth Factors in Human Astrocytomas. In: *Astrocytomas: Diagnosis, Treatment, and Biology,* edited by P. M. Black, W. L. Schoene, and L. A. Lampson, pp. 211–227. Blackwell Scientific Publications, Boston, 1993.

66. Gregory, P. E., Gutmann, D. H., Mitchell, A., *et al.* Neurofibromatosis type 1 gene product (neurofibromin) associates with microtubules. Somatic Cell Mol. Genet. *19:*265–274, 1993.

67. Grunberg, S. M., and Weiss, M. H. Lack of efficacy of megestrol acetate in the treatment of unresectable meningioma. J. Neurooncol. *8:*61–65, 1990.

68. Grunberg, S. M., Weiss, M. H., Spitz, I. M., *et al.* Treatment of unresectable meningiomas with the antiprogesterone agent mifepristone. J. Neurosurg. *74:*861–866, 1991.

69. Guha, A., Dashner, K., Black, P. M., *et al.* Expression of PDGF and PDGF receptors in human astrocy-

toma operation specimens supports the existence of an autocrine loop. Int. J. Cancer *60:*168–173, 1995.

70. Haak, H. R., de Keizer, R. J., Hagenouw-Taal, J. C., *et al.* Successful mifepristone treatment of recurrent, inoperable meningioma (letter). Lancet *336:*124–125, 1990.

71. Halper, J., Colvard, D. S., Scheithauer, B. W., *et al.* Estrogen and progesterone receptors in meningiomas: comparison of nuclear binding, dextran-coated charcoal, and immunoperoxidase staining assays. Neurosurgery *25:*546–552, 1989.

72. Han, V. K., Lund, P. K., Lee, D. C. and D'Ercole, A. J. Expression of somatomedin/insulin-like growth factor messenger ribonucleic acids in the human fetus: identification, characterization, and tissue distribution. J. Clin. Endocrinol. Metab. *66:* 422–429, 1988.

73. Hayward, E., Whitwell, H., Paul, K. S., and Barnes, D. M. Steroid receptors in human meningioma. Clin. Neuropharmacol. *7:*351–356, 1984.

74. Herman, J. G., Latif, F., Weng, Y., *et al.* Silencing of the VHL tumor-suppressor gene by DNA methylation in renal carcinoma. Proc. Natl. Acad. Sci. U. S. A. *91:*9700–9704, 1994.

75. Hermanson, M., Funa, K., Hartman, M., *et al.* Platelet-derived growth factor and its receptors in human glioma tissue: expression of messenger RNA and protein suggests the presence of autocrine and paracrine loops. Cancer Res. *52:*3213–3219, 1992.

76. Hermansson, M., Nister, M., Betsholtz, C., *et al.* Endothelial cell hyperplasia in human glioblastoma: coexpression of mRNA for platelet-derived growth factor (PDGF) B chain and PDGF receptor suggests autocrine growth stimulation. Proc. Natl. Acad. Sci. U. S. A. *85:*7748–7752, 1988.

77. Hinton, D., Mobbs, E. G., Sima, A. A., and Hanna, W. Steroid receptors in meningiomas: a histochemical and biochemical study. Acta Neuropathol. *62:*134–140, 1983.

78. Horsfall, D. J., Goldsmith, K. G., Ricciardelli, C., *et al.* Steroid hormone and epidermal growth factor receptors in meningiomas. Aust. N. Z. J. Surg. *59:*881–888, 1989.

79. Ironside, J. W., Battersby, R. D., Dangerfield, V. J., *et al.* Cryostat section assay of oestrogen and progesterone receptors in meningiomas: a clinicopathological study. J. Clin. Pathol. *39:*44–50, 1986.

80. Jacks, T., Shih, T. S., Schmitt, E. M., *et al.* Tumour predisposition in mice heterozygous for a targeted mutation in Nf1. Nature Genet. *7:*353–361, 1994.

81. Jacoby, L. B., MacCollin, M., Louis, D. N., *et al.* Exon scanning for mutation of the NF2 gene in schwannomas. Hum. Mol. Genet. *3:*413–419, 1994.

82. Jacoby, L. B., Pulaski, K., Rouleau, G. A., and Martuza, R. L. Clonal analysis of human meningiomas and schwannomas. Cancer Res. *50:*6783–6786, 1990.

83. Jacoby, L. B. Clonal origin of nervous system tumors. In: *Molecular Genetics of Nervous System Tumors*, edited by A. J. Levine and H. Schmidek, pp. 209–215 Wiley-Liss, Inc, New York, 1993.

84. Jimenez-Hakim, E., El-Azouzi, M., and Black, P. M. The effect of prolactin and bombesin on the growth of meningioma-derived cells in monolayer culture. J. Neurooncol. *16:*185–190, 1993.

85. Johnson, M. D., Horiba, M., Winnier, A. R., and Arteaga, C. L. The epidermal growth factor receptor is associated with phospholipase C-gamma1 in meningiomas. Hum. Pathol. *25:*146–153, 1994.

86. Jones, N. R. Epidermal growth factor receptor and its ligands in human brain tumors. Dissertation Abstracts International *52:*151-B(Abstract), 1991.

87. Junien, C., and Henry, I. Genetics of Wilms' tumor: a blend of aberrant development and genomic imprinting (Review). Kidney Int. *46:*1264–1279, 1994.

88. Kansantikul, V., and Brown, K. J. Estrogen receptors in acoustic neurilemmomas. Surg. Neurol. *15:*105–109, 1995.

89. Kazumoto, K., Tamura, M., Hoshino, H., and Yuasa, Y. Enhanced expression of the sis and c-myc oncogenes in human meningiomas. J. Neurosurg. *72:* 786–791, 1990.

90. Khalid, H., Yasunaga, A., Kishikawa, M., Shibata, S. Immunohistochemical expression of the estrogen receptor-related antigen (ER-D5) in human intracranial tumors. Cancer *75:*2571–2578, 1995.

91. Kleihues, P., Burger, P. C., and Scheithauer, B. W. *Histological Typing of Tumors of the Central Nervous System.* 2nd ed. Springer Verlag, Berlin, 1993.

92. Knudson, A. G. Mutation and cancer: statistical study of retinoblastoma. Proc. Natl. Acad. Sci. U. S. A. *68:*820–823, 1971.

93. Kobayashi, S., Mizuno, T., Tobioka, N., *et al.* Sex steroid receptors in diverse human tumors. Gann *73:*439–445, 1982.

94. Kornblum, J. A., Bay, J. W., and Gupta, M. K. Steroid receptors in human brain and spinal cord tumors. Neurosurgery *23:*185–188, 1988.

95. Kruijer, W., Cooper, J. A., Hunter, T., *et al.* Platelet-derived growth factor induces rapid but transient of the sis and c-myc oncogenes in human meningiomas. Nature *312:*711–791, 1985.

96. Kuratsu, J. I., Seto, H., Kochi, M., and Ushio, Y. Expression of PDGF, PDGF-receptor, EGF-receptor and sex hormone receptors on meningioma. Acta Neurochir. *131:*289–293, 1994.

97. Kurihara, M., Tokunaga, Y., Tsutsumi, K., *et al.* Characterization of insulin-like growth factor I and epidermal growth factor receptors in meningioma. J. Neurosurg. *71:*538–544, 1989.

98. Kurland, L. T., Schoenberg, B. S., Annegers, J. F., *et al.* The incidence of primary intracranial neoplasms in Rochester, Minnesota, 1935–1977. Ann. NY Acad. Sci. *381:*6–16, 1982.

99. Laird, P. W., Jackson-Grusby, L., Fazeli, A., *et al.* Suppression of intestinal neoplasia by DNA hypomethylation. Cell *81:*1–20, 1995.

100. Laird, P. W., and Jaenisch, R. DNA methylation and cancer (Review). Hum. Mol. Genet. 1487–1495, 1994.

101. Lamberts, S. W., Tanghe, H. L., Avezaat, C. J., *et al.* Mifepristone (RU 486) treatment of meningiomas. J. Neurol. Neurosurg. Psychiatry *55:*486–490, 1992.

102. Larson, J. J., Tew, J. M., Simon, M., and Menon, A. G. Evidence for clonal spread in the develop-

ment of multiple meningiomas. J. Neurosurg. *83:* 705–709, 1995.

103. Leach, R. J., Magewu, A. N., Buckley, J. D., *et al.* Preferential retention of paternal alleles in human retinoblastoma: evidence for genomic imprinting. Cell Growth Differ. *1:*401–406, 1990.

104. Lee, L. S., Chi, C. W., Chang, T. J., *et al.* Steroid hormone receptors in meningiomas of Chinese patients. Neurosurgery 25:541–545, 1989.

105. Lekanne Deprez, R. H., Bianchi, A. B., Groen, N. A., *et al.* Frequent NF2 gene transcript mutations in sporadic meningiomas and vestibular schwannomas. Am. J. Hum. Genet. *54:*1022–1029, 1994.

106. Lesch, K. P., and Gross, S. Estrogen receptor immunoreactivity in meningiomas. Comparison with the binding activity of estrogen, progesterone, and androgen receptors. J. Neurosurg. *67:*237–243, 1987.

107. Lesch, K. P., Schott, W., Engl, H. G., *et al.* Gonadal steroid receptors in meningiomas. J. Neurol. *234:* 328–333, 1987.

108. Levine, A. J. Tumor suppressor genes. In: *The Molecular Basis of Cancer,* edited by J. Mendelsohn, P. M. Howley, M. A. Israel, and L. A. Liotta, pp. 86–104. W.B. Saunders, Philadelphia, 1995.

109. Liberman, T. A., Nusbaum, H. R., Razon, N., *et al.* Amplification, enhanced expression and possible rearrangement of EGF receptor gene in primary human brain tumors of glial origin. Nature *313:* 144–147, 1985.

110. Lin, X., Guo, L., Gu, L., and Deuel, T. Site-specific methylation inhibits transcriptional activity of platelet-derived growth factor A-chain promoter. J. Biol. Chem. *268:*17334–17340, 1993.

111. Lloyd, H. M., Meares, J. D., and Jacobi, J. Effects of oestrogen and bromocriptine on in vivo secretion and mitosis in prolactin cells. Nature *255:*497–498, 1975.

112. Louis, A. *Memoire surles tumeurs fungueuses de la dure-mere.* Paris: Mem. Acad. Roy.Chir. Paris, pp. 1–59, 1774.

113. Magdelenat, H., Pertuiset, B. F., Poisson, M., *et al.* Progestin and oestrogen receptors in meningiomas. Biochemical characterization, clinical and pathological correlations in 42 cases. Acta Neurochir. *64:*199–213, 1982.

114. Maiuri, F., Montagnani, S., Gallicchio, B., *et al.* Oestrogen and progesterone sensitivity in cultured meningioma cells. Neurol. Res. *11:*9–13, 1989.

115. Makos, M., Nelkin, B. D., Chazin, V. R., *et al.* DNA hypermethylation is associated with 17p allelic loss in neural tumors. Cancer Res. *53:*2715–2718, 1993.

116. Malzac, P., Moncla, A., Voelckel, M. A., *et al.* Prader-Willi syndrome: diagnostic strategy with a cytogenetic and molecular approach. Neuromusc. Disord. *3:*493–496, 1993.

117. Markwalder, T. M., Gerber, H. A., Waelti, E., *et al.* Hormonotherapy of meningiomas with medroxyprogesterone acetate. Immunohistochemical demonstration of the effect of medroxyprogesterone acetate on growth fractions of meningioma cells using the monoclonal antibody Ki-67. Surg. Neurol. *30:* 97–101, 1988.

118. Markwalder, T. M., Seiler, R. W., and Zava, D. T. Antiestrogenic therapy of meningiomas—a pilot study. Surg. Neurol. 24:245–249, 1985.

119. Martuza, R. L., and Eldridge, R. Neurofibromatosis 2 (bilateral acoustic neurofibromatosis). N. Engl. J. Med. *318:*684–688, 1988.

120. Martuza, R. L., MacLaughlin, D. T., and Ojemann, R. G. Specific estradiol binding in schwannomas, meningiomas, and neurofibromas. Neurosurgery *9:*665–671, 1981.

121. Martuza, R. L., Miller, D. C., MacLaughlin, D. T. Estrogen and progestin binding by cytosolic and nuclear fractions of human meningiomas. J. Neurosurg. *62:*750–756, 1985.

122. Mashal, R. D., Lester, S. C., and Sklar, J. Clonal analysis by study of X chromosome inactivation in formalin-fixed paraffin-embedded tissue. Cancer Res. *53:*4676–4679, 1993.

123. Maxwell, M., Galanopoulos, T., Hedley-Whyte, E. T., *et al.* Human meningiomas co-express platelet-derived growth factor (PDGF) and PDGF-receptor genes and their protein products. Int. J. Cancer *46:*16–21, 1990.

124. Maxwell, M., Galanopoulos, T., Neville-Golden, J., and Antoniades, H. N. Expression of androgen and progesterone receptors in primary human meningiomas. J. Neurosurg. *78:*456–462, 1993.

125. Maxwell, M., Naber, S. P., Wolfe, H. J., *et al.* Coexpression of platelet-derived growth factor (PDGF) and PDGF-receptor genes by primary human astrocytomas may contribute to their development and maintenance. J. Clin. Invest. *86:*131–140, 1990.

126. McMorris, F. A., Smith, T. M., DeSalvo, S., and Furlanetto, R. W. Insulin-like growth factor I/somatomedin C: a potent inducer of oligodendrocyte development. Proc. Natl. Acad. Sci. U. S. A. *83:* 822–826, 1986.

127. Meixensberger, J., Caffier, H., Naumann, M., and Hofmann, E. Sex hormone binding and peritumoural oedema in meningiomas: is there a correlation? Acta Neurochir. *115:*98–102, 1992.

128. Menon, A. G., Ponder, B. A., and Seizinger, B. R. The neurofibromatosis genes: from molecular cloning to cellular function. Cancer Cells *3:*147–152, 1991.

129. Merlo, A., Herman, J. G., Mao, L., *et al.* 5′ CpG island methylation is associated with transcriptional silencing of the tumour suppressor p16/CDKN2/ MTS1 in human cancers. Nature Med. *1:*686–692, 1995.

130. Michelsen, J. J., New, P. F. Brain tumour and pregnancy. J. Neurol. Neurosurg. Psychiatry *32:*305–307, 1969.

131. Mochizuki, H., Nishi, T., Bruner, J. M., *et al.* Alternative splicing of neurofibromatosis type 1 gene transcript in malignant brain tumors: PCR analysis of frozen-section mRNA. Mol. Carcinogen *6:*83–73, 1992.

132. Moguilewsky, M., Pertuiset, B. F., Verzat, C., *et al.* Cytosolic and nuclear sex steroid receptors in meningioma. Clin. Neuropharmacol. *7:*375–381, 1984.

133. Nowell, P. C. The clonal evolution of tumor cell population. Science *194:*23–28, 1976.

134. Nur-E-Kamal, M. S., and Maruta, H. The role of Gln61 and Glu63 of Ras GTPases in their activation

by NF1 and Ras GAP. J. Biol. Chem. *3:*1437–1442, 1992.

135. Nur-E-Kamal, M. S., Varga, M., and Maruta, H. The GTPase-activating NF1 fragment of 91 amino acids reverses v-Ha-Ras-induced malignant phenotype. J. Biol. Chem. *30:*22331–22337, 1993.

136. Ogawa, O., Eccles, M. R., Szeto, J., *et al.* Relaxation of insulin-like growth factor II gene imprinting implicated in Wilms' tumour. Nature *362:*749–751, 1993.

137. Olson, J. J., Beck, D. W., MacIndoe, J. W., and Min-Loh, P. Androgen receptors in meningiomas. Cancer *61:*952–955, 1988.

138. Olson, J. J., Beck, D. W., Schlechte, J., and Loh, P. M. Hormonal manipulation of meningiomas in vitro. J. Neurosurg. *65:*99–107, 1986.

139. Olson, J. J., Beck, D. W., Schlechte, J. A., and Loh, P. M. Effect of the antiprogesterone RU-38486 on meningioma implanted into nude mice. J. Neurosurg. *66:*584–587, 1987.

140. Pantazis, P., Pelicci, P. G., Dalla-Favera, R., and Antoniades, H. N. Synthesis and secretion of proteins resembling platelet-derived growth factor by human glioblastoma and fibrosarcoma cells in culture. Proc. Natl. Acad. Sci. U. S. A. *82:*2404–2408, 1985.

141. Papi, L., De Vitis, L. R., Vitelli, F., *et al.* Somatic mutations in the neurofibromatosis type 2 gene in sporadic meningiomas. Hum. Genet. *95:*347–351, 1995.

142. Perrot-Applanat, M., Groyer-Picard, M. T., and Kujas, M. Immunocytochemical study of progesterone receptor in human meningioma. Acta Neurochir. *115:*20–30, 1992.

143. Poisson, M., Pertuiset, B. F., Hauw, J. J., *et al.* Steroid hormone receptors in human meningiomas, gliomas and brain metastases. J. Neurooncol. *1:*179–189, 1983.

144. Poulsgard, L., Ronne, M., and Schmidek, H. H. The cytogenetic and molecular genetic analysis of meningiomas. In: *Molecular Genetics of Nervous System Tumors*, edited by A. J. Levine, H. Schmidek, pp. 249–254. Wiley-Liss Inc, New York, 1993.

145. Press, M. F., Greene, G. L. Localization of progesterone receptor with monoclonal antibodies to the human progestin receptor. Endocrinology *122:*1165–1175, 1988.

146. Pulst, S. M., Rouleau, G. A., Marineau, C., *et al.* Familial meningioma is not allelic to neurofibromatosis 2. Neurology *43:*2096–2098, 1993.

147. Punnonen, R., and Kuurne, T. Estrogen and progestin receptors in intracranial tumors. Horm. Res. *27:*74–77, 1987.

148. Pykett, M. J., Murphy, M., Harnish, P. R., and George, D. L. The neurofibromatosis 2 (NF2) tumor suppressor gene encodes multiple alternatively spliced transcripts. Hum. Mol. Genet. *3:*559–564, 1994.

149. Rainier, S., Johnson, L. A., Dobry, C. J., *et al.* Relaxation of imprinted genes in human cancer. Nature *362:*747–749, 1993.

150. Rempel, S. A., Schwechheimer, K., Davis, R. L., *et al.* Loss of heterozygosity for loci on chromosome 10 is associated with morphologically malignant men-

ingioma progression. Cancer Res. *53:*2386–2392, 1993.

151. Reubi, J. C., Maurer, R., Klijn, J. G., *et al.* High incidence of somatostatin receptors in human meningiomas: biochemical characterization. J. Clin. Endocrinol. Metab. *63:*433–438, 1986.

152. Riva, P., and Larizza, L. Expression of c-sis and c-fos genes in human meningiomas and neurinomas. Int. J. Cancer *51:*873–877, 1992.

153. Rouleau, G. A., Merel, P., Lutchman, M., *et al.* Alteration in a new gene encoding a putative membrane-organizing protein causes neuro-fibromatosis type 2. Nature *363:*515–521, 1993.

154. Rouleau, G. A., Wertelecki, W., Haines, J. L., *et al.* Genetic linkage of bilateral acoustic neurofibromatosis to a DNA marker on chromosome 22. Nature *329:*246–248, 1987.

155. Russell, D. S., and Rubinstein, L. J. Tumours of the cranial, spinal and peripheral nerve sheaths. In: *Pathology of Tumours of the Nervous System*, 5th ed., pp. 533–538. Williams & Wilkins, Baltimore, 1989.

156. Russell, D. S., and Rubinstein, L. J. Tumours of the meninges and related tissues. In: *Pathology of Tumours of the Nervous System*. 5th ed., pp. 449–532. Williams & Wilkins, Baltimore, 1989.

157. Ruttledge, M. H., Sarrazin, J., Rangaratnam, S., *et al.* Evidence for the complete inactivation of the NF2 gene in the majority of sporadic meningiomas. Nature Genet. *6:*180–184, 1994.

158. Ruttledge, M. H., Xie, Y. G., Han, F. Y., *et al.* Deletions on chromosome 22 in sporadic meningioma. Genes Chromosomes Cancer *10:*122–130, 1994.

159. Sainz, J., Huynh, D. P., Figueroa, K., *et al.* Mutations of the neurofibromatosis type 2 gene and lack of the gene product in vestibular schwannomas. Hum. Mol. Genet. *3:*885–891, 1994.

160. Saitoh, S., Harada, N., Jinno, Y., *et al.* Molecular and clinical study of 61 Angelman syndrome patients (Review). Am. J. Med. Genet. *52:*158–163, 1994.

161. Sakai, T., Toguchida, J., Ohtani, N., *et al.* Allele-specific hypermethylation of the retinoblastoma tumor-suppressor gene. Am. J. Hum. Genet. *48:*880–888, 1991.

162. Sauceda, R., Ocadiz, R., Gutierrez, A. L., *et al.* Novel combination of c-myc, N-myc and N-ras oncogene alterations in brain tumors. Mol. Brain Res. *3:*123–132, 1988.

163. Schnegg, J. F., Gomez, F., LeMarchand-Beraud, T., and de Tribolet, N. Presence of sex steroid hormone receptors in meningioma tissue. Surg. Neurol. *15:*415–418, 1981.

164. Schoenberg, B. S., Christine, B. W., and Whisnant, J. P. Nervous system neoplasms and primary malignancies of other sites. The unique association between meningiomas and breast cancer. Neurology *25:*705–712, 1975.

165. Schollmann, C., Grugel, R., Tatje, D., *et al.* Basic fibroblast growth factor modulates the mitogenic potency of the platelet-derived growth factor (PDGF) isoforms by specific upregulation of the PDGF alpha receptor in vascular smooth muscle cells. J. Biol. Chem. *267:*18032–18039, 1992.

166. Schrell, U. M., Adams, E. F., Fahlbusch, R., *et al.*

Hormonal dependency of cerebral meningiomas. Part 1: Female sex steroid receptors and their significance as specific markers for adjuvant medical therapy. J. Neurosurg. *73:*743–749, 1990.

167. Schrell, U. M., Fahlbusch, R., Adams, E. F., *et al.* Growth of cultured human cerebral meningiomas is inhibited by dopaminergic agents. Presence of high affinity dopamine-D1 receptors. J. Clin. Endocrinol. Metab. *71:*1669–1671, 1990.

168. Schwartz, M. R., Randolph, R. L., Cech, D. A., *et al.* Steroid hormone binding macromolecules in meningiomas. Failure to meet criteria of specific receptors. Cancer *53:*922–927, 1984.

169. Seizinger, B. R., Martuza, R. L., Gusella, J. F. Loss of genes on chromosome 22 in tumorigenesis of human acoustic neuroma. Nature *322:*644–647, 1986.

170. Seizinger, B. R., Rouleau, G., Ozelius, L. J., *et al.* Common pathogenetic mechanism for three tumor types in bilateral acoustic neurofibromatosis. Science *236:*317–319, 1987.

171. Shuangshoti, S. Primary meningiomas outside the central nervous system. In: *Meningiomas,* edited by O. Al-Mefty pp. 107–128 Raven Press, New York, 1991.

172. Siglock, T. J., Rosenblatt, S. S., Finck, F., *et al.* Sex hormone receptors in acoustic neuromas. Am. J. Otol. *11:*237–239, 1990.

173. Skuse, G. R., Kosciolek, B. A., and Rowley, P. T. Molecular genetic analysis in von Recklinghausen neurofibromatosis: loss of heterozygosity for chromosome 17. Genes Chromosomes Cancer *1:*36–41, 1989.

174. Skuse, G., Kosciolek, B., and Rowley, P. The neurofibroma in von Recklinghausen neurofibromatosis has a unicellular origin. Am. J. Hum. Genet. *49:*600–607, 1991.

175. Smith, D. A., and Cahill, D. W. The biology of meningiomas. Neurosurg. Clin. North Am. *5:*201–215, 1994.

176. Smith, F. P., Slavik, M., and MacDonald, J. S. Association of breast cancer with meningioma. A report of two cases and review of the literature. Cancer *42:*1992–1994, 1978.

177. Snason, M., Delattre, O., Couturier, J., *et al.* Parental origin of chromosome 22 alleles lost in meningioma. Am. J. Hum. Genet. *47:*877–880, 1990.

178. Stephens, K., Green, P., Riccardi, V. M., *et al.* Genetic analysis of eight loci tightly linked to neurofibromatosis 1. Am. J. Hum. Genet. *44:*13–19, 1989.

179. Stephens, K., Kayes, L., Riccardi, V. M., *et al.* Preferential mutation of the neurofibromatosis type 1 gene in paternally derived chromosomes. Hum. Genet. *88:*279–282, 1992.

180. Stiles, D. D. The Molecular Biology of Platelet-Derived Growth Factor. Cell *33:*653–655, 1983.

181. Surani, M. A. Genomic imprinting: developmental significance and molecular mechanism (Review). Curr. Opin. Genet. Dev. *1:*241–246, 1991.

182. Takahashi, J. A., Mori, H., Fukumoto, M., *et al.* Gene expression of fibroblast growth factors in human gliomas and meningiomas: demonstration of cellular source of basic fibroblast growth factor mRNA and peptide in tumor tissues. Proc. Natl. Acad. Sci. U. S. A. *87:*5710–5714, 1990.

183. Takahashi, J. A., Suzui, H., Yasuda, Y., *et al.* Gene expression of fibroblast growth factor receptors in the tissues of human gliomas and meningiomas. Biochem. Biophys. Res. Commun. *177:*1–7, 1991.

184. Tikoo, A., Varga, M., Ramesh, V., *et al.* An anti-Ras function of neurofibromatosis type 2 gene product (NF2/Merlin). J. Biol. Chem. *269:*23387–23390, 1994.

185. Tilzer, L. L., Plapp, F. V., Evans, J. P., *et al.* Steroid receptor proteins in human meningiomas. Cancer *49:*633–636, 1982.

186. Todo, T., and Fahlbusch, R. Accumulation of inositol phosphates in low-passage human meningioma cells following treatment with epidermal growth factor. J. Neurosurg. *80:*890–896, 1994.

187. Trofatter, J. A., MacCollin, M. M., Rutter, J. L., *et al.* A novel moesin-, ezrin-, radixin-like gene is a candidate for the neurofibromatosis 2 tumor suppressor. Cell *72:*791–800, 1993.

188. Tsutsumi, K., Niwa, M., Kitagawa, N., *et al.* Enhanced expression of an endothelin ETA receptor in capillaries from human glioblastoma: a quantitative receptor autoradiographic analysis using a radioluminographic imaging plate system. J. Neurochem. *63:*2240–2247, 1994.

189. Twist, E. C., Ruttledge, M. H., Rousseau, M., *et al.* The neurofibromatosis type 2 gene is inactivated in schwannomas. Hum. Mol. Genet. *3:*147–151, 1994.

190. Ueki, K., Rubio, M. P., Ramesh, V., *et al.* MTS1/CDKN2 gene mutations are rare in primary human astrocytomas with allelic loss of chromosome 9p. Hum. Mol. Genet. *3:*1841–1845, 1994.

191. Virchow, R. *Die krankhaften Geschwülste.* Hirschwald, Berlin, 1863.

192. Viskochil, D., Buchberg, A. M., Xu, G., *et al.* Deletions and a translocation interrupt a cloned gene at the neurofibromatosis type 1 locus. Cell *62:*187–192, 1990.

193. Vogelstein, B., Fearon, E. R., Hamilton, S. R., and Feinberg, A. P. Use of a restriction fragment length polymorphism to determine the clonal origin of human tumors. Science *227:*642–645, 1985.

194. Vogelstein, B., Fearon, E. R., Hamilton, S. R., *et al.* Clonal analysis using recombinant DNA probes from the X-chromosome. Cancer Res. *47:*4806–4813, 1987.

195. von Deimling, A., Kraus, J. A., Stangl, A. P., *et al.* Evidence for subarachnoid spread in the development of multiple meningiomas. Brani Pathol. *5:*11–14, 1995.

196. Wainscoat, J. S., and Fey, M. F. Assessment of clonality in human tumors: a review. Cancer Res. *50:*1355–1560, 1990.

197. Wallace, M. R., Marchuk, D. A., Andersen, L. B., *et al.* Type I neurofibromatosis gene identification of a large transcript disrupted in three NF1 patients. Science *245:*181–186, 1990.

198. Wang, J. L., Nister, M., Hermansson, M., *et al.* Expression of PDGF beta-receptors in human meningioma cells. Int. J. Cancer *46:*772–778, 1990.

199. Weisman, A. S., Villemure, J. G., and Kelly, P. A. Regulation of DNA synthesis and growth of cells derived from primary human meningiomas. Cancer Res. *46:*2545–2550, 1986.

200. Weisman, A. S., Raguet, S. S., and Kelly, P. A. Characterization of epidermal growth factor receptor in human meningioma. Cancer Res. *47:*2172–2176, 1987.

201. Wellenreuther, R., Kraus, J. A., Lenartz, D., *et al.* Analysis of the neurofibromatosis 2 gene reveals molecular variants of meningioma. Am. J. Pathol. *146:*827–832, 1995.

202. White, E. p53, guardian of Rb. Nature *371:*21–22, 1994.

203. Whittle, I. R., Foo, M. S., Besser, M., and Vanderfield, G. K. Progesterone and oestrogen receptors in meningiomas: biochemical and clinicopathological considerations. Aust. N. Z. J. Surg. *54:*325–330, 1984.

204. Whittle, I. R., Hawkins, R. A., and Miller, J. D. Sex hormone receptors in intracranial tumours and normal brain. Eur. J. Surg. Oncol. *13:*303–307, 1987.

205. Wong, A. J., Bigner, S. H., Bigner, D. D., *et al.* Increased expression of the epidermal growth factor receptor gene in malignant gliomas is invariably associated with gene amplification. Proc. Natl. Acad. Sci. U. S. A. *84:*6899–6903, 1987.

206. Xu, G. F., O'Connell, P., Viskochil, D., *et al.* The neurofibromatosis type 1 gene encodes a protein related to GAP. Cell *62:*599–608, 1990.

207. Yu, Z. Y., Wrange, O., Haglund, B., *et al.* Estrogen and progestin receptors in intracranial meningiomas. J. Steroid Biochem. *16:*451–456, 1982.

208. Zang, K. D., and Singer, H. Chromosomal constitution of meningiomas. Nature *216:*84–85, 1967.

209. Zankl, H., and Zang, K. D. Cytological and cytogenetical studies on brain tumors. 4. Identification of the missing G chromosome in human meningiomas as no. 22 by fluorescence technique. Humangenetik *14:*167–169, 1972.

210. Zava, D. T., Markwalder, T. M., and Markwalder, R. V. Biological expression of steroid hormone receptors in primary meningioma cells in monolayer culture. Clin. Neuropharm. *7:*382–388, 1984.

211. Zhu, J., Frosch, M. P., Busque, L., *et al.* Analysis of meningiomas by methylation- and transcription-based clonality assays. Cancer Res. *55:*3865–3872, 1995.

212. Zhu, X. P., Dunn, J. M., Phillips, R. A., *et al.* Preferential germline mutation of the paternal allele in retinoblastoma. Nature *340:*312–313, 1989.

CHAPTER 9

Molecular Pathogenesis of Human Pituitary Tumors

JOSEPH M. ALEXANDER, Ph.D., BROOKE SWEARINGEN, M.D.

INTRODUCTION

Pituitary adenomas are the most common adult intracranial neoplasms. They comprise approximately 10% of diagnosed brain tumors. However, the molecular events leading to their formation are largely unknown. Pituitary tumors are categorized by the pituitary hormone they secrete, the syndrome of clinical hormone excess, and the pituitary cell type of origin. The most common pituitary tumor type, prolactinoma, is lactotroph derived. Patients with these tumors typically present with galactorrhea, amenorrhea, and hirsutism associated with clinical hyperprolactinemia. Growth hormone secreting pituitary adenomas are somatotroph-derived; they cause the clinical features of acromegaly, with acral enlargement, altered facial characteristics, visual fields defects, and hypogonadism. Corticotroph tumors synthesize and secrete excess adrenocorticotropin (ACTH), leading to clinical symptoms of Cushing's disease due to hypercortisolemia. Thyrotroph-derived adenomas are rare. Their clinical manifestations of secondary hyperthyroidism arise from overproduction of thyroid-stimulating hormone (TSH). Endocrine-inactive pituitary adenomas often secrete intact gonadotropins and/or their free subunits (16, 53) and are therefore considered to be of gonadotroph cell origin, although they do not cause a recognized syndrome of excess hormone overproduction. Such tumors are slow-growing macroadenomas with extrasellar extension and present with symptoms of mass effect, including headache, visual field deficits, cranial nerve palsies, and associated hypopituitarism.

Molecular genetic assessments of X-chromosome inactivation and tumor mutations have established the clonal basis of human pituitary adenomas. Historically, theories of pituitary tumorigenesis have posited two alternative hypotheses: hormone regulatory dysfunction versus somatic mutation (Fig. 1). Until recently, evidence favoring one theory over the other was largely inferential and relied on tumor histology and serum hormone data. Hypothalamic dysregulation has long been invoked as a primary pathogenetic mechanism of pituitary adenoma formation, and several studies have demonstrated that hypothalamic and circulating regulatory peptides may act as pituitary cell growth factors to stimulate both tumor proliferation and hormone secretion (18, 83, 107, 118). However, molecular biological techniques have repeatedly demonstrated that the vast majority of both benign and malignant human tumors are monoclonal in origin. These data demonstrate that many human tumors result from genomic mutations that confer a selective growth advantage to a single cell. If pituitary adenomas have pathogenetic mechanisms similar to those of other human tumors, they likely arise *de novo* as a result of genomic mutation, a genetic event that may be potentiated by hypothalamic or hormonal dysregulation.

PROLIFERATION THEORY OF PITUITARY NEOPLASIA

The proliferation hypothesis of pituitary tumorigenesis argues that pituitary adenomas are caused by hypothalamic or hormonal dysregulation. An imbalance in a specific endocrine axis stimulates the growth of many normal pituitary cell subtypes. The resultant chronic pituitary hypertrophy establishes a heterogeneous

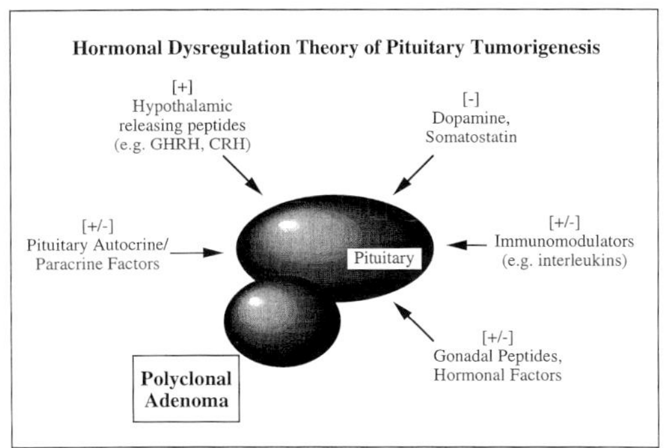

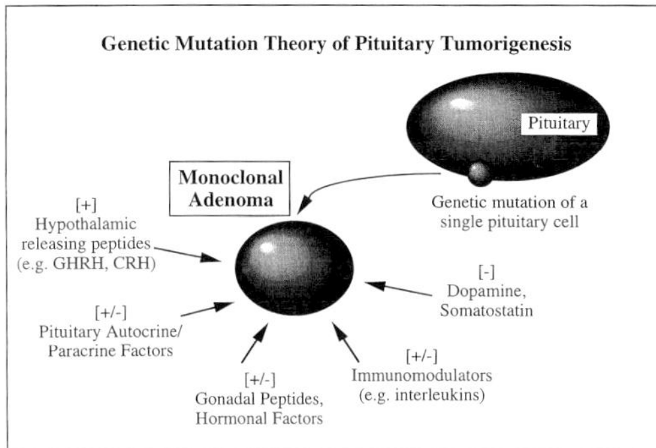

Figure 1. Pathogenetic theories of pituitary neoplasia. The hormonal dysregulation theory states that pituitary tumors arise because of hypothalamic or hormonal imbalances that act directly on large fields of pituicytes. This produces a heterogeneous, and genetically polyclonal, pituitary adenoma. The genetic mutation theory states that sporadic oncogenic mutations arise spontaneously and offer a selective growth advantage to a single pituitary cell. Once a monoclonal adenoma has been established, hypothalamic and hormonal factors may modulate its growth and/or phenotype.

population of mitogenic cells that generate a tumor. A prolonged phase of pituitary hypertrophy-hyperplasia would, therefore, be required for tumor development. Several lines of evidence support this theory. First, the varied histological appearance of tumors and their production of multiple pituitary hormones (demonstrated by immunocytochemical staining within single-tumor sections) are consistent with a multicellular origin (63, 81, 95, 96). Second, patients with ectopic biosynthesis of hypothalamic releasing factors (specifically, corticotropin-releasing hormone (CRH) and growth hormone-releasing hormone (GHRH)) often have multifocal pituitary hyper plasia as well as syndromes of clinical hormone

excess (12, 23, 26, 112). Third, transgenic studies and *in vitro* data strongly suggest that hypothalamic-releasing peptides function as pituitary cell growth factors and identify excessive hypothalamic stimulation as a contributor to pituitary adenoma formation (18, 83, 107, 116, 118). These data would argue that adenomas arise not from spontaneous mutations in individual pituitary cells but, rather, from hypothalamic dysregulation or other as yet unidentified imbalances in endocrine regulatory mechanisms that affect multiple cells simultaneously.

MUTATIONAL THEORY OF PITUITARY NEOPLASIA

The spontaneous genetic mutation hypothesis states that a sporadic oncogenic mutation within a single pituitary cell confers a selective growth advantage. This proliferating cell then establishes a monoclonal neoplasm with a homogeneous genetic endowment. Several observations support this theory. First, chronic primary endocrine end organ failure (*i.e.*, premature ovarian failure or hypothyroidism from thyroid disease resulting in chronic pituitary overstimulation from loss of feedback inhibition) is rarely associated with adenoma development. Second, histological examination of pituitary neoplasms seldom reveals the regions of hyperplasia that would be expected if hyperplasia from overstimulation preceded neoplastic transformation (63). Third, pituitary tumors rarely recur after surgical resection (13). Fourth, pituitary tumors occur in patients with multiple endocrine neoplasia type I (21). Multiple endocrine neoplasia (MEN-1) exhibits an autosomal dominant pattern of genetic inheritance of an altered tumor suppressor allele at 11q13; presumably this genomic alteration underlies development of MEN-1-associated pituitary tumors. Fifth, specific mutations in the signaling pathway of GHRH have been identified in up to 40% of GH-secreting adenomas. These mutations constitutively activate the Gs-α subunit associated with the GHRH receptor in somatotrophs, providing an uninterrupted stimulus to GH secretion and somatotroph proliferation (68). Although a number of base substitutions in either of two codons able to constitutively activate the G protein have been identified, only one specific substitution occurs in each tumor, even when multiple sites within the tumor are assayed. This argues strongly for monoclonality of this subset of growth hormone-secreting tumors. These observations in aggregate suggest that pituitary tumor formation begins with a genetic lesion in a single pituitary cell.

Clonality Studies in Pituitary Tumors

Although almost all types of human tumors are monoclonal in origin, there are a few notable exceptions; some neurofibromas (38) and trichoepitheliomas (73) are polyclonal. Molecular genetic techniques permit analysis of patterns of X-inactivation in genomic DNA from human pituitary tumors. This analysis demonstrates that most pituitary tumors are monoclonal in origin and arise *de novo* from oncogenic transformation of a single pituitary cell.

Assay of patterns of X-chromosome inactivation in clinically nonfunctioning tumors first demonstrated the monoclonal nature of pituitary adenomas (3, 48, 52). However, many clinically nonfunctioning adenomas exhibit immunocytochemical heterogeneity of gonadotropin subunit synthesis. Radioimmunoassay, immunocytochemistry, and analysis of mRNA have shown that most nonfunctioning adenomas synthesize and secrete intact follicle-stimulating hormone (FSH), as well as free a- and b-gonadotropin subunits. Fewer secrete intact luteinizing hormone (LH) (53, 101). They occasionally exhibit TSH*b* biosynthesis and/or TSH secretion but rarely secrete ACTH, prolactin (PRL), or GH (42). This heterogeneity of subunit secretion may arise from later tumorigenic events, such as differential expression of hormonal cell-surface receptors or synthesis of autocrine-paracrine regulatory factors, which may foster the observed heterogeneous tumor phenotype (4, 41).

Studies of human somatotroph and lactotroph adenomas have shown that sporadic tumors are monoclonal in origin (28). In animal models, however, hypothalamic and hormonal factors may initiate and continue to promote extensive proliferative responses in both tumor types. Transgenic mouse models of GHRH overproduction and constitutively activated GHRH cytoplasmic signaling pathways (36, 51, 71), and a case report of an acromegalic patient with ectopic GHRH-producing tumors (58), have demonstrated GHRH to be a potent inducer of somatotroph hyperplasia. In a transgenic mouse model of GHRH overproduction, chronic GHRH exposure for 10–12 months promotes

adenoma formation (116). Chronic estrogen administration induces proliferation that leads to lactotroph hyperplasia and hyperprolactinemia in animal models (19, 31, 34). Long-term estrogen treatment may produce lactotroph adenomas. These proliferative effects of hypothalamic and hormonal factors would argue that these pituitary tumor subtypes arise from polyclonal proliferation of pituitary cells, but the clonality of pituitary hyperplasia and associated adenomas in animal models is unknown. Given the apparent monoclonal origin of human somatotroph and lactotroph adenomas (28), however, if hypothalamic or hormonal stimulation of proliferation contributes to human pituitary tumorigenesis, it must occur very early and perhaps even before oncogenic transformation.

In patients with either Cushing's disease or Nelson's syndrome, data aggregated from four separate studies show that 87% (27/31) of pituitary adenomas are monoclonal in origin (28, 35, 45, 126). One of the four polyclonal tumor specimens had interspersed normal tissue within tumor (28). The remaining three (two macro- and one microadenomas) were examined for contaminating normal cells but none were detected (45). Other circumstantial evidence, as well, favors a primary pituitary oncogenic mutation rather than hypothalamic overstimulation as the underlying cause of corticotroph adenomas. The vast majority of patients with Cushing's disease are cured surgically by adenomectomy (13). The typical persistence of hypoadrenalism several months after surgery suggests that there is no chronic source of excess CRH (79), and, subsequently, patients may re-establish normal hypothalamic-pituitary-adrenal axis function. Clinical hypercortisolism was not reversed by pituitary stalk section in a patient with Cushing's disease; this is also consistent with intrinsic pituitary, rather than hypothalamic, pathogenesis (115). Some data suggest, however that hypothalamic overstimulation may play a role in corticotroph hyperplasia and tumorigenesis (117). Tumor recurrence after surgical cure (1), the diffuse corticotroph hyperplasia found in surgical specimens (95, 96) and cases of ectopic CRH-producing tumors leading to corticotroph hyperplasia and Cushing's disease (7, 35, 113) all argue that hypothalamic overstimulation may play a role in tumorigenesis, although the relation between corticotroph hyperplasia and adenoma formation remains unclear. Animal models that test the effects of chronic CRH excess on corticotroph proliferation and secretion have yielded conflicting results. Corticotroph hyperplasia occurs in rats injected daily with CRH (18). However, transgenic mouse models of CRH overproduction exhibit symptoms of Cushing's disease without concomitant corticotroph proliferation (69). In a patient with an ectopic CRH-producing bronchial carcinoid and Cushing's disease, polymerase chain reaction (PCR)-based determination of X-chromosome inactivation patterns showed a polyclonal pattern, consistent with a multicellular proliferative response to excess levels of circulating CRH (35). In summary, most corticotroph adenomas appear to result from spontaneous mutations in a single cell, but a small minority may develop from a multicellular field of proliferating cells.

Role of Cell Surface Receptors in the Pathogenesis of Human Pituitary Adenomas

Specific defects in genes controlling the cell cycle have been identified for other tumor types; the transformation to neoplasia is thought to be a multi-step process. In pituitary neoplasms, the transformation may include mutations in genes controlling responsiveness to hypothalamic stimulatory hormones, as well as in those controlling the cell-cycle. The best characterized cell surface receptors potentially involved in pituitary tumorigenesis include 1) GHRH receptors, 2) GnRH receptors, 3) activin transforming growth factor B (TGFB) receptors and 4) somatostatin receptors.

GHRH Receptors

The foremost example of linkage of pituitary tumorigenesis to a specific molecular defect is the discovery of activating mutations in the G protein associated with the receptor for GH-releasing hormone in GH-secreting adenomas. In normal pituitary somatotrophs GHRH promotes growth hormone secretion and proliferation through Gs-α-mediated stimulation of adenylyl cyclase and intracellular cyclic AMP accumulation. To date, activating mutations have been localized to two sites within Gs, codon 201 and codon 227. Both mutations diminish GTP hydrolysis, stabilize Gs-α- in the GTP-bound state, and thus produce a constitutively activated stimulatory G-protein trimeric complex. This leads to increased adenylyl cyclase activity, and elevated intracellular cAMP levels. In the pituitary, such constitutive activation of G-protein-signaling pathways can lead to hypersecretion of hormones (such as that documented in somatotroph adenomas) and/or increased cellular proliferation (that might be neoplastic). These mutations were discovered following the observation that some human somatotroph tumors have constitutive activation of pathways stimulated by GHRH in primary tumor cell culture. Although a number of base substitutions in either of two codons able to constitutively activate the G-protein, adenylyl cyclase activity, cAMP production, and GH release have been identified, only one specific substitution occurs in each tumor. This strongly suggests the monoclonality of each tumor.

Gonadotropin-releasing Hormone Receptor (GnRH) Receptors

In contrast to the intact LH and intact FSH produced by normal gonadotrophs, uncombined FSHβ- or α-subunits are frequently secreted by neoplastic gonadotrophs (32, 60, 93, 103–104). Elevation of free FSHβ subunit is most commonly observed clinically and in the laboratory; it occurs in up to one third of patients with gonadotroph tumors (60). Gonadotroph tumors may also secrete excessive intact, bioactive gonadotropins, commonly FSH and, rarely, LH (61). Men with FSH-producing tumors have elevated levels of serum FSHβ relative to α-subunit, compared with normal or hypogonadal men (103). Gonadotropin subunit mRNA expression is found in 77% of human gonadotroph tumors. In 33% of tumors, FSHβ steady-state mRNA levels are higher than levels of α-subunit mRNA (60). These data demonstrate that, in contrast to normal pituitary or placental tissue, pituitary adenomas have imbalanced gonadotropin subunit steady-state mRNA levels. FSHβ hypersecretion may reflect on the biosynthesis of gonadotropin subunit abnormalities in neoplastic gonadotrophs.

In tissue culture, cells from human gonadotroph tumors have the same abnormalities of gonadotropin biosynthesis and secretion found in the intact tumor; the secretory phenotype is maintained in the absence of hypothalamic and hormone stimuli. A substantial subset of gonadotroph adenomas continues to secrete FSHβ-subunit in excess of α-subunit in primary tissue culture (5, 67, 124). Although rare, *in vitro* production of LHβ in excess of α-subunit at both mRNA and protein levels also occurs (61). These data suggest that underlying gonadotropin biosynthetic defects result in aberrant gonadotropin gene expression and subunit secretion in neoplastic human pituitary cells. The factors responsible for these abnormalities of control of gonadotropin biosynthesis and secretion may also underlie a tumor's abnormal growth.

The amplitude and frequency of the hypothalamic GnRH pulse regulate production of LH and FSH by normal pituitary gonadotrophs and, thus, serum LH and FSH levels. Changes in the GnRH pulse produce different patterns of gonadotropin subunit gene expression and secretion in normal gonadotrophs. Alterations of GnRH pulse amplitude and frequency in the rat pituitary creates imbalances in the expression of α- and β-subunit genes. Pituitary perfusion systems in experimental animals have facilitated study of the regulation of hormone and subunit production by GnRH (100, 119–121). GnRH administration to normal perfused rat pituitary cells for 30–120 minutes decreases gonadotropin secretion (121). Recovery of secretion is delayed, and complete recovery can require 30 minutes. Administration of GnRH antagonist to normal human (74) and normal rat pituitary cells *in vitro* (30) consistently decreases intact gonadotropin and α-subunit secretion without a stimulatory agonist phase. Some gonadotroph tumors are GnRH-responsive *in vitro*: GnRH induces mobilization of intracellular Ca^{2+} and subunit secretion from cultured pituitary tumor cells (65, 67, 105). Although these experiments confirm *in vivo* clinical studies documenting GnRH-responsiveness of a subset of human gonadotroph adenomas, they do not address the physiological regulation of neoplastic gonadotrophs by pulsatile GnRH. In addition, the mechanism underlying GnRH responsiveness in neoplastic gonadotrophs is unknown.

The clinical and *in vitro* data demonstrating that some gonadotroph tumors are unresponsive to GnRH despite their gonadotroph secretory phenotype raises the possibility that abnormal tumor GnRH responsiveness reflects dysregulation of GnRH-receptor (GnRH-Rc) biosynthesis and/or cell-signaling pathways. The cloning of human hypothalamus-releasing peptide receptors opens new opportunities for investigating receptor expression and function in neoplastic pituitary cells (28, 39, 78). GnRH-Rc biosynthesis is regulated by gonadal steroids and GnRH itself (10, 56). Investigation of GnRH-Rc gene expression may help decipher GnRH regulation and reveal cell-signaling defects in human gonadotroph tumors. Sequence analysis of the human GnRH-Rc shows that it is a G-protein coupled receptor (28). The conserved structure of the cloned GnRH-Rc confirms biochemical data showing that its stimulation of phospholipase-C and phosphatidylinositol hydrolysis is mediated by its interactions with Gqα GTP-binding proteins (49, 57). Constitutive activation of this cell-signaling pathway has mitogenic and transforming effects in NIH3T3 mouse fibroblasts (59). Therefore, GnRH-Rc may modulate tumor growth as well as gonadotropin biosynthesis and secretion.

Study of gonadotropin responsiveness to GnRH in perfused gonadotroph adenomas with reverse transcriptase-PCR evidence of FSHβ and α-subunit biosynthesis found that 9 of 13 tumors were unresponsive to pulsatile GnRH (4). There were no significant differences in the mean baseline secretion of intact gonadotropins or α-subunit between responders and nonresponders. However, FSHβ was undetectable in all GnRH-unresponsive tumors. Mean secretory rates of LH, FSH, and α-subunit ranged from <0.8–4.2 IU/liter (min^{-1}), 1.1–5.1 IU/L (min^{-1}), and 0.2–0.6 μg/L (min^{-1}), respectively. Secretory profiles and GnRH receptor gene expression in representative responsive and unresponsive tumors are shown in Figure 2. A membrane-depolarizing pulse of 60 mM KCl was administered to four of the nine GnRH-unresponsive tumors to confirm that lack of response was not caused by absence of intracellular gonadotropins. In each case, a significant transient secretory burst of gonadotropins and/or free subunits occurred. GnRH-Rc mRNA was detected in all GnRH-responsive tumors and was comparable to that seen in normal human pituitary tissue. In contrast, gonadotroph tumors unresponsive to pulsatile GnRH had no detectable GnRH-Rc mRNA. Responsiveness of perfused tumors to exogenous GnRH could be predicted by the presence of GnRH-Rc mRNA expression. GnRH responsiveness is thus critically dependent on GnRH-Rc mRNA expression.

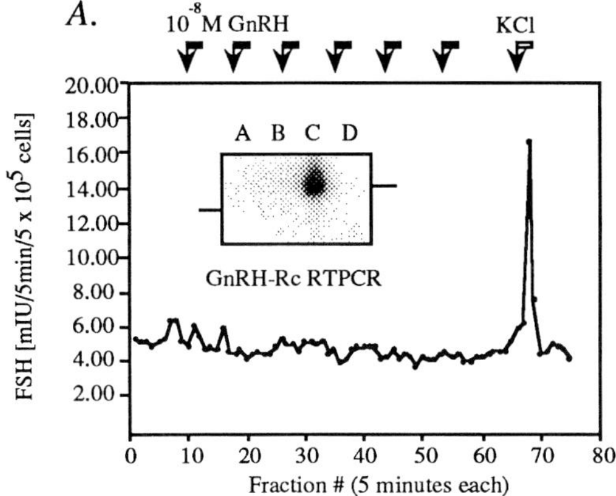

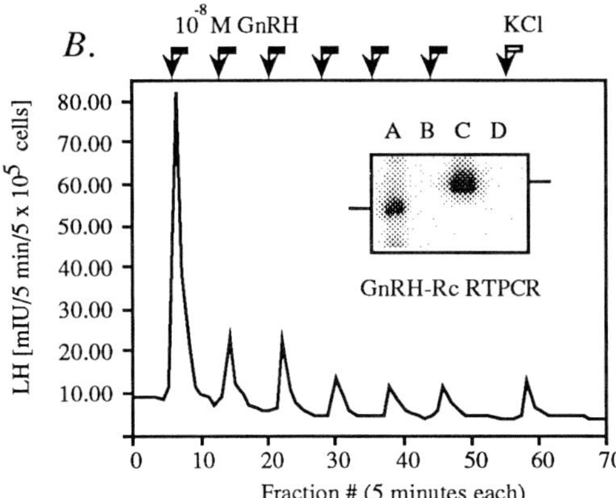

Figure 2. GnRH receptor biosynthetic defects in human gonadotroph tumors. Secretion of FSH and LH in perfusion by GnRH-unresponsive (*A*) and responsive (*B*) pituitary tumors, respectively. RTPCR results are shown for GnRH-Rc mRNA. Lane A: GnRH-RC (+ reverse transcriptase); Lane B: GnRH-RC (− reverse transcriptase); Lane C: GapDH (+ reverse transcriptase); Lane D: GapDH (− reverse transcriptase). Note the lack of GnRH-Rc mRNA in Lane A of the unresponsive tumor. Ten-minute GnRH pulses were given every 45 minutes, followed by a single 10-minute pulse of 60 mM KCl at the conclusion of the experiment. *Arrows* indicate the timing and duration of each GnRH pulse.

These data indicate that GnRH-Rc biosynthesis is deficient in most human gonadotroph adenomas. Alterations in GnRH-Rc biosynthesis in neoplastic gonadotrophs may reflect defects in cell signaling. In one model of constitutive activation of GnRH pathways, continuous *in vitro* administration of GnRH to normal rat pituitary cells decreased pituitary GnRH-Rc mRNA levels (56). This suggests that long-term desensitization of GnRH responses after application of GnRH agonists results from downregulation of constitutive GnRH-Rc gene expression and steady-state mRNA levels. Therefore, mutations that activate gonadotroph-specific GnRH second-messenger pathways can chronically downregulate GnRH-Rc biosynthesis and desensitize neoplastic gonadotrophs to GnRH stimulation. It is unknown whether mutations that activate second-messenger systems stimulate cell proliferation as well as desensitize the GnRH-signaling pathways that modulate gonadotropin biosynthesis and secretion. Studies of tumor responses to hypothalamic peptides such as GnRH may help identify mutations underlying biosynthetic and secretory defects.

Activin Transforming Growth Factor β (TGFβ) Receptors

Activins are sulfhydryl-linked dimers comprised of two distinct protein subunits (βA and βB) which are encoded by separate genes and are structurally related to a diverse family of growth factors in the TGFβ gene family (72, 76). Locally secreted activin potently and selectively induces growth and differentiation in pituitary cells and regulates FSHβ biosynthesis and secretion (24, 25). Activin binds to a heterotetromeric transmembrane receptor complex with serine/threonine (*ser/thr*) kinase activity (77). The activin-signaling pathway modulates the expression and activity of several nuclear factors important in gene regulation and cell cycling, such as the immediate early gene junB (44) and the tumor suppressor protein retinoblastoma (Rb) (99). Growth-inhibition by activin occurs in a number of cell types, including human K562 erythroleukemic cells (99), human fetal adrenal cells (106), and epidermal growth factor (EGF)-stimulated hepatocytes (125). However, activins can stimulate cell proliferation in a number of endocrine cells, including human granulosa cells (40, 89), a testicular tumor cell line (94), and fetal rat osteoblast cells (27). In the pituitary, activin inhibits basal and GHRH-stimulated GH secretion and decreases intracellular cAMP levels in somatotrophs (15). Exogenous activin-A has an antimitogenic effect on somatotroph cells in primary rat pituitary cultures (15). Activin-A also inhibits POMC mRNA biosynthesis, ACTH secretion, and cell proliferation in AtT20 cells, a mouse corticotroph cell line (14). Therefore, autocrine biosynthesis of activin may regulate proliferation of both normal and neoplastic cells. Human pituitary tumors synthesize activin mRNAs and secrete bioactive activin (6). The effects of activin are downregulated by follistatin (24), a monomeric glycoprotein that binds activin and is expressed in normal rat pituitary (33, 55). Endogenous follistatin mRNAs have been identified in gonadotroph adenomas (86), but tumor-specific follistatin biosynthesis has not been found in any other secretory pituitary tumor subtype.

In contrast to the arrest of growth and regulation of hormone production by activin in normal animals, unresponsiveness to exogenous activin occurs in some human gonadotroph tumors (5). This difference suggests that there are defects in activin receptors and/or intracellular

signaling in human gonadotroph tumors. Cloning of activin receptors has revealed a novel class of transmembrane receptors with *ser/thr* kinase activity and varying affinities for activin and/or TGF-β (77). The loss of activin-responsiveness by many gonadotroph tumors may reflect loss of functional activin cell-surface receptors similar to that in human lymphoid (54) and colorectal tumors (75), Hep2B, and Mv1Lu cell lines (85). The activin receptor family has two classes, designated type I and type II. Non-covalent interactions between type I and type II receptors generate active signaling receptor complexes (Fig. 3). Type I receptors (Alk1–5) function primarily as intracellular signal transducers, while binding specificity for TGFβ or activin resides in the type II receptors (122). Therefore, receptor complexes comprised of

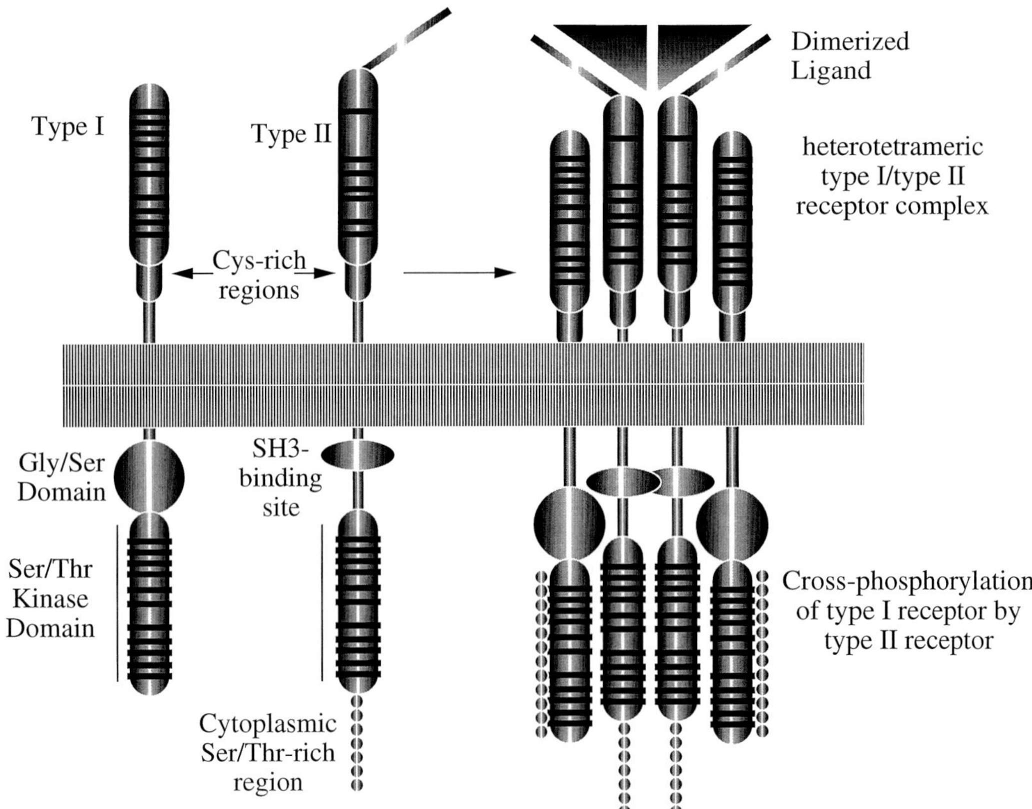

Figure 3. Schematic of the activin receptor-signaling complex. Dimeric ligand (*triangles*) associates with type II receptor, initiating the formation of a heterotetrameric receptor complex. Type II receptor cross-phosphorylates type I receptor at intracellular serine and threonine residues (*stars*). Type I receptors then activate, via their endogenous kinase domains, specific downstream signaling cascades that modulate cell proliferation. *SKR, ser/thr* kinase region. *Horizontal bars* on the intracellular region of type I and II receptor represent the 11 kinase subdomains responsible for signaling.

both receptor classes are required for functional activin or TGFβ signaling. For TGFβ signaling, the type I receptor is activated by TGFβ-bound type II receptor cross-phosphorylation at intracellular *ser/thr* residues. This activated complex then stimulates specific intracellular signaling cascades via type I receptor-specific *ser/thr* kinase activity (122). The identification of these receptors for TGFβ-related growth factors such as activin in human neoplastic pituitary tissue is a first step in investigating their role as signal transducers in tumor pathogenesis, hormone secretion, and control of cellular proliferation. Findings regarding activin may be applicable to a number of human endocrine neoplasms.

Alk2 and Alk4 are the human type I activin receptors critical to modulation of activin signaling. Functional complementation studies in mink lung epithelial (Mv1Lu) cell lines that lack type I or type II receptors show that only specific heteromeric complexes mediate intracellular signaling in response to activin and TGFβ. Type I activin receptors Alk2 and Alk4 increase expression of an activin-responsive reporter gene construct (p3TP-lux) when coexpressed with activin type II receptor (ActRII) in Mv1Lu cells treated with activin (8, 22). The coexpression of TβRII and either Alk2 or Alk4 does not confer responsiveness when cells are treated with TGFβ, confirming that these type I receptors are activin specific. Analogously, the Alk5 receptor is specific for TGFβ. In Mv1Lu(R) mutant cell lines lacking type I receptors (9, 22), expression of Alk5 increased expression of both the TGFβ responsive endogenous plasminogen activator inhibitor I gene and cotransfected p3TP-lux reporter constructs. In addition, activated Alk5/TβRII complexes suppress Mv1Lu(R) cell proliferation and upregulate TGFβ-gene expression. Using this complementation strategy, Alk3 has been demonstrated to be a bone morphogenetic protein (BMP-2/4)-specific type I receptor (62, 111). Alk1 has not been linked to any known TGFβ-related ligand and remains classified as a type I orphan receptor.

Messenger RNAs for type I and type II activin/TGFβ receptor mRNAs are present in human pituitary adenomas (2). ALK2 and ALK5, specific mediators of activin and TGFβ signals, respectively, are expressed in tumors but not in normal human pituitary cells. ALK2 receptor mRNA expression was further restricted to mam-mosomatotroph tumors. In contrast, mRNA-encoding ALK1, a type I orphan receptor, is present in all normal human pituitaries studied and highly prevalent in all tumor types except corticotroph adenomas. ALK3 mRNA is prevalent in both neoplastic and normal pituitary. ALK3, a bone morphogenetic protein (BMP)-2/4 type I receptor, complexes with TβRII but cannot transmit TGFβ signals (62, 109–111). Type II receptor mRNAs encoding ActRII and TβRII are found in both normal and neoplastic pituitary tissue. In contrast, ActRIIB mRNA is highly prevalent in all tumors but scarce in normal human pituitary tissues.

Alternate splicing of the cytoplasmic domain of ALK4 mRNA generates truncated forms of the receptor that lack specific carboxyl kinase subdomains (Fig. 4) (123). By forming inactive type I-type II signaling complexes, truncated forms of the ALK4 cytoplasmic domain attenuate activin signal transduction and have a dominant negative phenotype for growth arrest by activin. The full-length ALK4 receptor mRNA, as well as three truncated ALK4 mRNA variants generated by alternate splicing of the cytoplasmic *ser/thr* kinase, occur in most pituitary tumors of all types. Two of these mRNA variants (ALK4-2 and ALK-3) do not occur in normal pituitary tissue. Another ALK4 splice variant (ALK4-5) generated by alternate splicing that eliminates exon 9 is also found only in tumors.

TGFβ mediates growth arrest late in G1 phase of the cell cycle of Mv1Lu cells by inhibiting biosynthesis of cyclin-dependent kinase 4 (cdk4) and downregulating cdk2/cyclinE complexes critical for progression through the G1/S transition (37, 88). TGFβ also increases transcription of p15, a cell-cycle inhibitor that produces G1 growth arrest by binding and inactivating cdk4 and cdk6 (43). Activin may have similar effects as it induces differentiation in a number of cell lines and tissues, but its nuclear effects are poorly understood. The identification of receptors for TGFβ-related growth factors such as activin in human neoplastic pituitary tissue is a first step in investigating their role as signal transducers in tumor pathogenesis, hormone secretion, and cell proliferation.

Somatostatin Receptors

Somatostatin (SRIF) is a widely distributed peptide with diverse biological effects, includ-

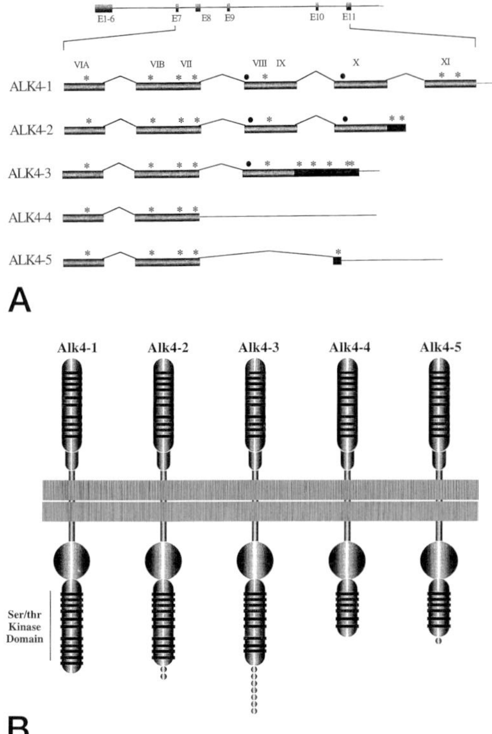

Figure 4. Alternate splice variants of ALK4 in pituitary tumors. Panel *A*: Schematic representation of the genomic organization of ALK4 exons 7 through 11. Kinase subdomains (*ser/thr*) are listed in roman numerals above each exon. Serine or threonine (*) residues and tyrosine residues (O) are also shown above each exon. *Black boxes* indicate coding sequence while *stippled areas* represent novel coding sequences generated by alternate splicing of ALK4. The alternate splice for the novel ALK4-5 mRNA is shown at the *bottom* of the panel. Panel *B*: Predicted protein structure of truncated ALK4 receptor isoforms. *Horizontal bars* on the intracellular region of ALK4 receptor represent the 11 kinase subdomains responsible for signaling. *Stars* represent *ser/thr* residues.

ing inhibition of hormone release from the anterior pituitary and gastrointestinal tract and neuromodulation of brain function (79). The SRIF analog, octreotide, has antiproliferative effects both *in vitro* and *in vivo* (17, 66, 108) and is an effective treatment for several endocrine neoplasms (29, 50, 80, 107). Octreotide is used for GH-secreting pituitary tumors and some clinically nonfunctioning pituitary adenomas (47, 80, 118). However, it fails to suppress GH in some somatotroph adenomas, (47) and other somatotroph tumors fail to shrink, even though GH levels decline. The contribution of

transcriptional regulation of expression of somatostatin receptor (SSTR) genes and alteration of signal transduction to these phenomena are unknown. In addition, it is unknown if the subtype of SSTR expressed reflects underlying mechanisms of tumorigenesis or if it determines the type of hormone secreted by a tumor.

SRIF activates a family of G protein-coupled membrane receptors that possess differing intrinsic affinities for specific SRIF analogs and activates several second-messenger pathways (31, 64, 84, 90, 97, 114). The cloning of five SSTRs (36, 70, 90, 98) facilitates specific analyses of SSTR gene expression. SSTR subtypes 1 through 4 are expressed in a number of nonpituitary endocrine neoplasms (98). Differential expression of SSTR subtypes in pituitary adenomas and other tumors may predict clinical response to octreotide and other potentially therapeutic SRIF analogs. SSTR subtypes 1, 2, and 5 exist in most tumors, regardless of secretory phenotype, and in all normal pituitary controls. In contrast, SSTR3 mRNA is present in only one somatotroph adenoma and SSTR4 mRNA has not been detected in any tissues studied. SSTR2 and SSTR5 mRNAs have been detected in somatotroph tumors in which SRIF inhibits secretion of both GH and free α-subunit (Fig. 5). In addition, such inhibition occurs in the absence of SSTR1 mRNA, indicating that although this receptor subtype mRNA is frequently expressed in somatotroph tumors, it is not required for SRIF to affect production of either GH or α-subunit.

Although SSTR genes are also expressed in nonpituitary endocrine tumors, the SSTR subtype expressed may differ. SSTR1 and SSTR2 mRNAs are common to both pituitary and nonpituitary human endocrine neoplasms. RT-PCR techniques have identified SSTR1 mRNA in all endocrine tumors studied, including glucagonomas, insulinomas, pheochromocytomas, and a carcinoid (98). SSTR2 mRNA is expressed by these same tumor types with the exception of the one carcinoid tumor studied. SSTR3 and SSTR4 mRNA expression is commonly found in glucagonomas and insulinomas (98). In contrast, SSTR3 mRNA is rarely present in pituitary tumors and is never found in normal pituitary tissue. SSTR4 mRNA expression is found in neither neoplastic nor normal pituitary tissue. These data suggest that the expression of SSTR3 and SSTR4 mRNA is relatively specific

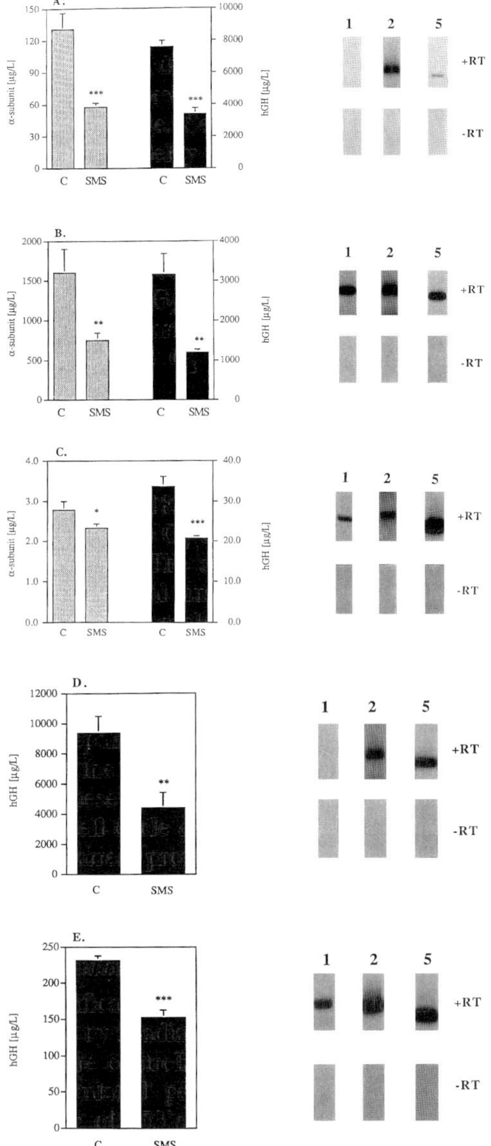

Figure 5. Growth hormone-free α-subunit responses to SRIF and SSTR subtype gene expression *in vitro*. Triplicate wells of enzymatically dispersed GH-secreting adenomas, three of which also hypersecreted free α-subunit (*A*, *B*, and *C*), were incubated with 10^{-7} M SRIF or control media. Culture media were collected at 24 hours and assayed for GH and α-subunit secretion. RTPCR results for specific SSTR subtype gene expression for the five tumors are summarized to the *right* of the secretion *graphs*. All tumors were negative for SSTR3 and SSTR4 RTPCR amplification. All RNA samples were negative for SSTR transcript amplification when reverse transcriptase was excluded from the reactions ($-$ RT lanes). *, $P < .05$; **, $p < .01$; ***, $p < .001$.

to nonpituitary endocrine tumors. Furthermore, nonpituitary endocrine tumors do not express SSTR5 mRNA (98), whereas most pituitary tumors and normal pituitary tissue do.

SRIF and/or SRIF analogs have antiproliferative effects on a number of human tumors, and octreotide is widely used as an adjuvant medical therapy after resection of GH-secreting tumors. In addition, although most patients with clinically nonfunctioning tumors are unresponsive to octreotide, few patients with α-subunit secreting pituitary adenomas exhibit improved visual fields or decreases in glycoprotein hormone subunit secretion during octreotide administration (80). In addition, functional SSTR cell-surface receptor binding is detected in patients with clinically nonfunctioning pituitary tumors using labeled SRIF analogs (70). Glycoprotein hormone subunit secretion is suppressed by SRIF in some clinically nonfunctioning tumors studied *in vitro* (87). However, a subset of acromegalic patients remains unresponsive to therapy with SRIF analog, and there is currently no means of determining which somatotroph or clinically nonfunctioning tumors will respond to octreotide. Mechanisms of tumor unresponsiveness are complex; possibilities include a change of the SSTR subtype expressed, alteration of the SSTR profile, or modification of postreceptor events. The identification of receptor subtypes will be critical in elucidating these mechanisms and may be useful in predicting tumor responsiveness to octreotide *in vivo*. In future studies, the correlation between SSTR subtype mRNA expression, the function of specific functional SSTR receptor proteins, and clinical responses such as suppression of GH levels and reduction in tumor size will integrate molecular diagnosis and somatostatin analog treatment.

SSTR density correlates with clinical response to octreotide in acromegaly (92). Expression of SSTR2 and SSTR5 mRNA correlates with SRIF inhibition of secretion of both GH and free α-subunit *in vitro* (82). In addition, SSTR1 mRNA expression is not required for this inhibition of GH and free α-subunit *in vitro*, suggesting that a functional SSTR1 is also unnecessary. Therefore, SSTR2 and/or SSTR5 may mediate SRIF's inhibition of GH and free α-subunit secretion. This is consistent with the clinical actions of octreotide, which has a high affinity for SSTR2 (11, 91). It will be important to determine how SSTR mRNA expression correlates with the hormone-suppressive effects of octreotide in human tumors *in vitro*. Alternatively, other SSTR subtypes that have not yet been cloned may be important mediators of SRIF's actions. In fact, SRIF-28 binding sites in the mouse pituitary AtT20 cell line distinct from SRIF-28-selective SSTR5 have been identified (86).

Alterations in the expression of receptors for hypothalamic peptides may underlie the abnormalities of hormone production found in human pituitary adenomas. However, many patients with pituitary tumors show no clinical response to octreotide, and the presence of SSTR mRNA does not predict the clinical effects of octreotide on any type of pituitary adenoma. Therefore, specific SSTR mRNA expression may not correlate with the presence of functional receptor proteins. Alternatively, other receptor subtypes not yet identified may be important mediators of the clinical effects of octreotide. The expression of specific SSTR mRNAs in different types of pituitary tumor has been established. An important future line of investigation will be the detection and functional characterization of SSTR subtype protein expression. These studies should provide both a further understanding of the pathogenetic mechanisms of pituitary tumorigenesis and the rationale for the clinical use of specific SRIF analogs.

CONCLUSIONS

Recent studies have yielded new insights into the role of altered expression of genes for hypothalamic peptides and pituitary receptors in the development of pituitary tumors and the response of these tumors to treatment with hormone analogs. The discovery of activating mutations of the stimulatory α-subunit of heterotrimeric G-proteins (Gs-alpha) of the GHRH receptor in up to 40% of growth hormone-secreting human pituitary adenomas is the foremost example of linkage of pituitary tumorigenesis to a specific molecular defect (68). Analogous abnormalities of the GnRH receptor in gonadotroph tumors suggest that alterations in Gq/11α or other components of the phospholipase-C (PLC) intracellular signaling pathway could contribute to the development of human gonadotroph tumors. Approximately one third of human gonadotroph tumors are unresponsive

to activin, and many tumors express truncated forms of the type I activin receptor, which could function as dominant-negative suppressors of TGFβ antiproliferative pathways. Finally, the analysis of patterns of SSTR gene expression patterns in somatotroph and clinically nonfunctioning pituitary adenomas may prove to be clinically useful in designing therapeutic SRIF analogs.

In the majority of human tumor models, the transformation from normal cells to neoplastic ones is a multistep process (20). The current model of human neoplasia invokes a number of genomic alterations, including allelic loss of tumor suppressor genes, changes in DNA methylation patterns, faulty DNA editing and repair enzymes, and oncogene activation at many points along intracellular signaling and mitogenic pathways. Thus, although somatic mutation is clearly a pathogenetic mechanism in the majority of pituitary tumors, there are still many important unanswered questions regarding the molecular pathogenetic mechanisms of human pituitary neoplasia. Does a period of hyperplasia predispose pituitary cells to acquire genetic lesions, or do they truly arise spontaneously from mitotically quiescent pituitary cells? It is unknown whether factors, such as the loss of TGFβ-related antiproliferative pathways, that increase rates of pituitary cell growth, concomitantly affect the frequency of oncogenic mutations. Are alterations in the expression of genes for cell surface receptors of hormones and neurotransmitters such as GnRH and somatostatin, causal or coincidental events in the pathogenesis of these tumors? A subset of pituitary tumors shows allelic loss at 11q13, a chromosomal region that includes the MEN-1 gene (29, 46). What role do tumor suppressor genes, such as MEN-1, play in the pathogenesis of these tumors? Pathogenetic studies using modern molecular genetic tools can now concentrate on documenting the genomic changes that are associated with pituitary tumor formation. Characterization of tumoral responses to hypothalamic and hormonal factors have already provided potential insights into the pathogenesis of these tumors. Future studies will need to investigate the genomic mechanisms that give rise to pituitary tumors and will lead to a greater understanding of the multistep process of pituitary neoplasia.

REFERENCES

1. Adashi, E. Y., Resnick, C. E., Vera, A., *et al.* In vivo regulation of granulosa cell type I insulin-like growth factor receptors: evidence for an inhibitory role for the putative endogenous ligand(s) of the ovarian gonadotropin-releasing hormone receptor. Endocrinology *128:*3130–3137, 1991.
2. Alexander, J. M., Bikkal, H. A., Zervas, N. T., *et al.* Tumor-specific expression and alternate splicing of mRNAs encoding activin/transforming growth factor-beta receptors in human pituitary adenomas. J. Clin. Endocrinol. Metab. *81:*783–790, 1996.
3. Alexander, J. M., Biller, B. M., Bikkal, H., *et al.* Clinically nonfunctioning pituitary tumors are monoclonal in origin. J. Clin. Invest. *86:*336–340, 1990.
4. Alexander, J. M., and Klibanski, A. Gonadotropin-releasing hormone receptor mRNA expression by human pituitary tumors in vitro. J. Clin. Invest. *93:*2332–2339, 1994.
5. Alexander, J. M., Jameson, J. L., Bikkal, H. A., *et al.* The effects of activin on follicle-stimulating hormone secretion and biosynthesis in human glyco-protein hormone-producing pituitary adenomas. J. Clin. Endocrinol. Metab. *72:*1261–1267, 1991.
6. Alexander, J. M., Swearingen, B., Tindall, G. T., *et al.* Human pituitary adenomas express endogenous inhibin subunit and follistatin messenger ribonucleic acids. J. Clin. Endocrinol. Metab. *80:*147–152, 1995.
7. Anderson, L., Milligan, G., and Eidne, K. A. Characterization of the gonadotrophin-releasing hormone receptor in alpha T3-1 pituitary gonadotroph cells. J. Endocrinol. *136:*51–58, 1993.
8. Attisano, L., Carcamo, J., Ventura, F., *et al.* Identification of human activin and TGF beta type I receptors that form heteromeric kinase complexes with type II receptors. Cell *75:*671–680, 1993.
9. Bassing, C. H., Yingling, J. M., Howe, D. J., *et al.* A transforming growth factor beta type I receptor that signals to activate gene expression. Science *263:* 87–89, 1994.
10. Bauer-Dantoin, A. C., Weiss, J., and Jameson, J. L. Roles of estrogen, progesterone, and gonadotropin-releasing hormone (GnRH) in the control of pituitary GnRH receptor gene expression at the time of the preovulatory gonadotropin surges. Endocrinology *136:*1014–1019, 1995.
11. Bell, G. I., and Reisine, T. Molecular biology of somatostatin receptors. Trends Neurosci. *16:*34–38, 1993.
12. Belsky, J. L., Cuello, B., Swanson, L. W., *et al.* Cushing's syndrome due to ectopic production of corticotropin-releasing factor. J. Clin. Endocrinol. Metab. *60:*496–500, 1985.
13. Bercu, B. B., Yang, S. W., Masuda, R., *et al.* Role of selected endogenous peptides in growth hormone-releasing hexapeptide activity: analysis of growth hormone-releasing hormone, thyroid hormone-releasing hormone, and gonadotropin-releasing hormone. Endocrinology *130:*2579–2586, 1992.
14. Bilezikjian, L. M., Blount, A. L., Campen, C. A., *et al.* Activin-A inhibits proopiomelanocortin messenger RNA accumulation and adrenocorticotropin secretion of AtT20 cells. Mol. Endocrinol. *5:*1389–1395, 1991.
15. Billestrup, N., Gonzalez-Manchon, C., Potter, E., *et al.* Inhibition of somatotroph growth and growth hormone biosynthesis by activin in vitro. Mol. Endocrinol. *4:*356–362, 1990.
16. Black, P. M., Hsu, D. W., Klibanski, A., *et al.* Hormone production in clinically nonfunctioning pituitary adenomas. J. Neurosurg. *66:*244–250, 1987.
17. Bogden, A. E., Taylor, J. E., Moreau, J. P., *et al.* Treatment of R-3327 prostate tumors with a somatostatin analogue (somatuline) as adjuvant therapy following surgical castration. Cancer Res. *50:*2646–2650, 1990.
18. Bookstaff, R. C., Kamel, F., Moore, R. W., *et al.* Altered regulation of pituitary gonadotropin-releasing hormone (GnRH) receptor number and pituitary responsiveness to GnRH in 2,3,7,8-tetrachlorodibenzo-p-dioxin-treated male rats. Toxicol. Appl. Pharmacol. *105:*78–92, 1990.
19. Braden, T. D., and Conn, P. M. Altered rate of synthesis of gonadotropin-releasing hormone receptors: effects of homologous hormone appear independent of extracellular calcium. Endocrinology *126:*2577–2582, 1990.
20. Braden, T. D., Farnworth, P. G., Burger, H. G., *et al.* Regulation of the synthetic rate of gonadotropin-releasing hormone receptors in rat pituitary cell cultures by inhibin. Endocrinology *127:*2387–2392, 1990.
21. Brandi, M. L., Marx, S. J., Aurbach, G. D., *et al.* Familial multiple endocrine neoplasia type. I. A new look at pathophysiology. Endocr. Rev. *8:*391–405, 1987.
22. Carcamo, J., Weis, F. M., Ventura, F., *et al.* Type I receptors specify growth-inhibitory and transcriptional responses to transforming growth factor beta and activin. Mol. Cell Biol. *14:*3810–3821, 1994.
23. Carey, R. M., Varma, S. K., Drake, C. R., Jr., *et al.* Ectopic secretion of corticotropin-releasing factor as a cause of Cushing's syndrome: a clinical, morphologic, and biochemical study. N. Engl. J. Med. *311:*13–20, 1984.
24. Carroll, R. S., Corrigan, A. Z., Gharib, S. D., *et al.* Inhibin, activin, and follistatin: regulation of follicle-stimulating hormone messenger ribonucleic acid levels. Mol. Endocrinol. *3:*1969–1976, 1989.
25. Carroll, R. S., Corrigan, A. Z., Vale, W., *et al.* Activin stabilizes follicle-stimulating hormone-beta messenger ribonucleic acid levels. Endocrinology *129:* 1721–1726, 1991.
26. Caselitz, J., and Saeger, W. The ultrastructure of the pituitary gland under chronic stimulation of the ACTH-cells in human pathology and animal experiments. *Endokrinologie 74:*163–176, 1979.
27. Centrella, M., McCarthy, T. L., and Canalis, E. Activin-A binding and biochemical effects in osteoblast-enriched cultures from fetal-rat parietal bone. Mol. Cell. Biol. *11:*250–258, 1991.
28. Chi, L., Zhou, W., Prikhozhan, A., *et al.* Cloning and characterization of the human GnRH receptor. Mol. Cell Endocrinol. *91:*R1–6, 1993.
29. Dan-Cohen, H., Ben-Menahem, D., and Naor, Z. The gonadotropin-releasing hormone receptor: signals

involved in gonadotropin secretion and biosynthesis. Horm. Res. *33:*76–86, 1990.

30. Danforth, D. R., Williams, R. F., Gordon, K., *et al.* Inhibition of pituitary gonadotropin secretion by the gonadotropin-releasing hormone antagonist antide. I. In vitro studies on mechanism of action. Endocrinology *128:*2036–2040, 1991.

31. De-Leeuw, R., Habibi, H. R., Nahorniak, C. S., *et al.* Dopaminergic regulation of pituitary gonadotrophin-releasing hormone receptor activity in the goldfish (Carassius auratus). J. Endocrinol. *121:*239–247, 1989.

32. Demura, R., Jibiki, K., Kubo, O., *et al.* The significance of alpha-subunit as a tumor marker for gonadotropin-producing pituitary adenomas. J. Clin. Endocrinol. Metab. *63:*564–569, 1986.

33. DePaolo, L. V., Mercado, M., Guo, Y., *et al.* Increased follistatin (activin-binding protein) gene expression in rat anterior pituitary tissue after ovariectomy may be mediated by pituitary activin. Endocrinology *132:*2221–2228, 1993.

34. Eidne, K. A., McNiven, A. I., Taylor, P. L., *et al.* Functional expression of rat pituitary gonadotrophin-releasing hormone receptors in Xenopus oocytes. J. Mol. Endocrinol. *1:*R9–12, 1988.

35. Eidne, K. A., Sellar, R. E., Couper, G., *et al.* Molecular cloning and characterisation of the rat pituitary gonadotropin-releasing hormone (GnRH) receptor. Mol. Cell Endocrinol. *90:*R5–9, 1992.

36. Evans, J. J., Robinson, G., and Catt, K. J. Gonadotrophin-releasing activity of neurohypophysial hormones. I. Potential for modulation of pituitary hormone secretion in rats. J. Endocrinol. *122:*99–106, 1989.

37. Ewen, M., Sluss, H., Whitehouse, L., *et al.* Cdk4 modulation by TGF-B leads to cell cycle arrest. Cell *74:*1009–1020, 1993.

38. Fialkow, P. J., Sagebiel, R. W., Gartler, S. M., *et al.* Multiple cell origin of hereditary neurofibromas. N. Engl. J. Med. *284:*298–300, 1971.

39. Gaylinn, B. D., Harrison, J. K., Zysk, J. R., *et al.* Molecular cloning and expression of a human anterior pituitary receptor for growth hormone-releasing hormone. Mol. Endocrinol. *7:*77–84, 1993.

40. Gonzalez-Manchon, C., and Vale, W. Activin-A, inhibin and transforming growth factor-beta modulate growth of two gonadal cell lines. Endocrinology *125:*1666–1672, 1989.

41. Greenman, Y., and Melmed, S. Heterogeneous expression of two somatostatin receptor subtypes in pituitary tumors. J. Clin. Endocrinol. Metab. *78:*398–403, 1994.

42. Habibi, H. R., Marchant, T. A., Nahorniak, C. S., *et al.* Functional relationship between receptor binding and biological activity for analogs of mammalian and salmon gonadotropin-releasing hormones in the pituitary of goldfish (Carassius auratus). Biol. Reprod. *40:*1152–1161, 1989.

43. Hannon, G. J., and Beach, D. p15INK4B is a potential effector of TGF-beta-induced cell cycle arrest (see comments). Nature *371:*257–261, 1994.

44. Hashimoto, M., Gaddy-Kurten, D., and Vale, W. Protooncogene junB as a target for activin actions. Endocrinology *133:*1934–1940, 1993.

45. Hawes, B. E., Barnes, S., and Conn, P. M. Cholera toxin and pertussis toxin provoke differential effects on luteinizing hormone release, inositol phosphate production, and gonadotropin-releasing hormone (GnRH) receptor binding in the gonadotrope: evidence for multiple guanyl nucleotide binding proteins in GnRH action. Endocrinology *132:*2124–2130, 1993.

46. Hazum, E. Purification of gonadotropin releasing hormone receptors using the avidin-biotin technique. J. Chromatogr. *510:*233–238, 1990.

47. Hazum, E., and Conn, P. M. Molecular mechanism of gonadotropin releasing hormone (GnRH) action. I. The GnRH receptor. (Published erratum appears in Endocr. Rev. 10(2):229, 1989.) Endocr. Rev. *9:*379–386, 1988.

48. Herman, V., Fagin, J., Gonsky, R., *et al.* Clonal origin of pituitary adenomas. J. Clin. Endocrinol. Metab. *71:*1427–1433, 1990.

49. Hsieh, K-P., and Martin, T. F. J. Thyrotropin-releasing hormone and gonadotropin-releasing hormone receptors activate phospholipase C by coupling to the guanosine triphosphate-binding proteins Gq and G11. Mol. Endocrinol. *6:*1673–1681, 1992.

50. Hurbain-Kosmath, I., Berault, A., Noel, N., *et al.* Gonadotropes in a novel rat pituitary tumor cell line, RC-4B/C: establishment and partial characterization of the cell line. In Vitro Cell. Dev. Biol. *26:*431–440, 1990.

51. Iwashita, M., Hirota, K., Izumi, S. I., *et al.* Solubilization and characterization of the rat pituitary gonadotrophin-releasing hormone receptor. J. Mol. Endocrinol. *1:*187–196, 1988.

52. Jacoby, L. B., Hedley-Whyte, E. T., Pulaski, K., *et al.* Clonal origins of pituitary adenomas. J. Neurosurg. *73:*731–735, 1990.

53. Jameson, J. L., Klibanski, A., Black, P. M., *et al.* Glycoprotein hormone genes are expressed in clinically nonfunctioning pituitary adenomas. J. Clin. Invest. *80:*1472–1478, 1987.

54. Kadin, M. E., Cavaille-Coll, M. W., Gertz, R., *et al.* Loss of receptors for transforming growth factor beta in human T-cell malignancies. Proc. Natl. Acad. Sci. U. S. A. *91:*6002–6006, 1994.

55. Kaiser, U. B., and Chin, W. W. Regulation of follistatin messenger ribonucleic acid levels in the rat pituitary. J. Clin. Invest. *91:*2523–2531, 1993.

56. Kaiser, U. B., Jakubowiak, A., Steinberger, A., *et al.* Regulation of rat pituitary gonadotropin-releasing hormone receptor mRNA levels in vivo and in vitro. Endocrinology *133:*931–934, 1993.

57. Kaiser, U. B., Katzenellenbogen, R. A., Conn, P. M., *et al.* Evidence that signalling pathways by which thyrotropin-releasing hormone and gonadotropin-releasing hormone act are both common and distinct. Mol. Endocrinol. *8:*1038–1048, 1994.

58. Kakar, S. S., Musgrove, L. C., Devor, D. C., *et al.* Cloning, sequencing, and expression of human gonadotropin releasing hormone (GnRH) receptor. Biochem. Biophys. Res. Commun. *189:*289–295, 1992.

59. Kalinec, G., Nazarali, A. J., Hermouet, S., *et al.* Mutated alpha subunit of the Gq protein induces ma-

lignant transformation in NIH 3T3 cells. Mol. Cell Biol. *12:*4687–4693, 1992.

60. Katznelson, L., Alexander, J. M., Bikkal, H. A., *et al.* Imbalanced follicle-stimulating hormone beta-subunit hormone biosynthesis in human pituitary adenomas. J. Clin. Endocrinol. Metab. *74:*1343–1351, 1992.

61. Klibanski, A., Deutsch, P. J., Jameson, J. L., *et al.* Luteinizing hormone-secreting pituitary tumor: biosynthetic characterization and clinical studies. J. Clin. Endocrinol. Metab. *64:*536–542, 1987.

62. Koenig, B. B., Cook, J. S., Wolsing, D. H., *et al.* Characterization and cloning of a receptor for BMP-2 and BMP-4 from NIH 3T3 cells. Mol. Cell Biol. *14:*5961–5974, 1994.

63. Kovacs, K., and Horvath, E. Pathology of pituitary tumors. Endocrinol. Metab. Clin. North Am. *16:* 529–551, 1987.

64. Koves, K., Gottschall, P. E., and Arimura, A. Gonadotropin-releasing hormone binding sites in ovaries of normal cycling and persistent-estrus rats. Biol. Reprod. *41:*505–511, 1989.

65. Kwekkeboom, D. J., De Jong, F. H., and Lamberts, S. W. J. Gonadotropin release by clinically nonfunctioning and gonadotroph pituitary adenomas in vivo and in vitro: relation to sex and effects of thyrotropin-releasing hormone, gonadotropin-releasing hormone, and bromocriptine. J. Clin. Endocrinol. Metab. *68:*1128–1135, 1989.

66. Lamberts, S. W., Krenning, E. P., and Reubi, J. C. The role of somatostatin and its analogs in the diagnosis and treatment of tumors. Endocr. Rev. *12:*450–482, 1991.

67. Lamberts, S. W., Verleun, T., Oosterom, R., *et al.* The effects of bromocriptine, thyrotropin-releasing hormone, and gonadotropin-releasing hormone on hormone secretion by gonadotropin-secreting pituitary adenomas in vivo and in vitro. J. Clin. Endocrinol. Metab. *64:*524–530, 1987.

68. Landis, C. A., Masters, S. B., Spada, A., *et al.* GTPase inhibiting mutations activate the alpha chain of Gs and stimulate adenylyl cyclase in human pituitary tumours. Nature *340:*692–696, 1989.

69. Laws, S. C., Webster, J. C., and Miller, W. L. Estradiol alters the effectiveness of gonadotropin-releasing hormone (GnRH) in ovine pituitary cultures: GnRH receptors versus responsiveness to GnRH. Endocrinology *127:*381–386, 1990.

70. Lee, L. R., Haisenleder, D. J., Marshall, J. C., *et al.* Expression of alpha-subunit and luteinizing hormone (LH) beta messenger ribonucleic acid in the rat during lactation and after pup removal: relationship to pituitary gonadotropin-releasing hormone receptors and pulsatile LH secretion. Endocrinology *124:*776–782, 1989.

71. Lee, L. R., Paul, S. J., and Smith, M. S. Dose response effects of pulsatile GnRH administration on restoration of pituitary GnRH receptors and pulsatile LH secretion during lactation. Neuroendocrinology *49:* 664–668, 1989.

72. Ling, N., Ying, S.-Y., Ueno, N., *et al.* Pituitary FSH is released by a heterodimer of the β-subunits from the two forms of inhibin. Nature *321:*779–782, 1986.

73. Liscovitch, M., and Amsterdam, A. Gonadotropin-releasing hormone activates phospholipase D in ovarian granulosa cells: possible role in signal transduction. J. Biol. Chem. *264:*11762–11767, 1989.

74. Mansfield, J. M., Beardsworth, D. E., and Loughlin, J. S. Long-term treatment of central precocious puberty with a long-acting analogue of luteinizing hormone-releasing hormone: effects on somatic growth and skeletal maturation. N. Engl. J. Med. *309:*1286–1291, 1983.

75. Markowitz, S., Wang, J., Myeroff, L., *et al.* Inactivation of the type II TGF-beta receptor in colon cancer cells with microsatellite instability. Science *268:* 1336–1338, 1995.

76. Mason, A. J., Hayflick, J. S., Ling, N., *et al.* Complementary DNA sequences of ovarian follicular fluid inhibin show precursor structure and homology with transforming growth factor-β. Nature *318:*659–663, 1985.

77. Mathews, L. S. Activin receptors and cellular signaling by the receptor serine kinase family (review). Endocr. Rev. *15:*310–325, 1994.

78. Mayo, K. E. Molecular cloning and expression of a pituitary-specific receptor for growth hormone-releasing hormone. Mol. Endocrinol. *6:*1734–1744, 1992.

79. McArdle, C. A., Cragoe, E. J., Jr., and Poch, A. Na+ dependence of gonadotropin-releasing hormone action: characterization of the Na+/H+ antiport in pituitary gonadotropes. Endocrinology *128:*771–778, 1991.

80. McArdle, C. A., Gorospe, W. C., Huckle, W. R., *et al.* Homologous down-regulation of gonadotropin-releasing hormone receptors and desensitization of gonadotropes: lack of dependence on protein kinase C. Mol. Endocrinol. *1:*420–429, 1987.

81. McNicol, A. M. Patterns of corticotropic cells in the adult human pituitary in Cushing's disease. Diagn. Histopathol. *4:*335–341, 1981.

82. Miller, G. M., Alexander, J. M., Bikkal, H. A., *et al.* Somatostatin receptor subtype gene expression In pituitary adenomas. J. Clin. Endocrinol. Metab. *80:* 1386–1392, 1995.

83. Naor, Z. Signal transduction mechanisms of Ca2+ mobilizing hormones: the case of gonadotropin-releasing hormone. Endocr. Rev. *11:*326–353, 1990.

84. Omeljaniuk, R. J., Habibi, H. R., and Peter, R. E. Alterations in pituitary GnRH and dopamine receptors associated with the seasonal variation and regulation of gonadotropin release in the goldfish (Carassius auratus). Gen. Comp. Endocrinol. *74:*392–399, 1989.

85. Park, K., Kim, S. J., Bang, Y. J., *et al.* Genetic changes in the transforming growth factor beta (TGF-beta) type II receptor gene in human gastric cancer cells: correlation with sensitivity to growth inhibition by TGF-beta. Proc. Natl. Acad. Sci. U. S. A. *91:*8772–8776, 1994.

86. Patel, Y. C., Panetta, R., Escher, E., *et al.* Expression of multiple somatostatin receptor genes in AtT-20 cells: evidence for a novel somatostatin-28 selective

receptor subtype. J. Biol. Chem. *269:*1506–1509, 1994.

87. Perrin, M. H., Haas, Y., Porter, J., *et al.* The gonadotropin-releasing hormone pituitary receptor interacts with a guanosine triphosphate-binding protein: differential effects of guanyl nucleotides on agonist and antagonist binding. Endocrinology *124:*798–804, 1989.

88. Polyak, K., Kato, J. Y., Solomon, M. J., *et al.* p27Kip1, a cyclin-Cdk inhibitor, links transforming growth factor-beta and contact inhibition to cell cycle arrest. Genes Dev. *8:*9–22, 1994.

89. Rabinovici, J., Spencer, S. J., and Jaffe, R. B. Recombinant human activin-A promotes proliferation of human luteinized preovulatory granulosa cells in vitro. J. Clin. Endocrinol. Metab. *71:*1396–1398, 1990.

90. Reinhart, J., Mertz, L. M., and Catt, K. J. Molecular cloning and expression of cDNA encoding the murine gonadotropin-releasing hormone receptor. J. Biol. Chem. *267:*21281–21284, 1992.

91. Rens-Domiano, S., Law, S. F., Yamada, Y., *et al.* Pharmacological properties of two cloned somatostatin receptors. Mol. Pharmacol. *42:*28–34, 1992.

92. Reubi, J. C., and Landolt, A. M. The growth hormone responses to octreotide in acromegaly correlate with adenoma somatostatin receptor status. J. Clin. Endocrinol. Metab. *68:*844–850, 1989.

93. Ridgway, E. C., Klibanski, A., Ladenson, P. W., *et al.* Pure alpha-secreting pituitary adenomas. N. Engl. J. Med. *304:*1254–1259, 1981.

94. Roberts, V., Meunier, H., Sawchenko, P. E., *et al.* Differential production and regulation of inhibin subunits in rat testicular cell types. Endocrinology *125:*2350–2359, 1989.

95. Saeger, W., and Ludecke, D. K. Pituitary hyperplasia: definition, light and electron microscopical structures and significance in surgical specimens. Virchows Arch. A. Pathol. Anat. Histopathol. *399:*277–287, 1983.

96. Schnall, A. M., Kovacs, K., Brodkey, J. S., *et al.* Pituitary Cushing's disease without adenoma. Acta Endocrinol. *94:*297–303, 1980.

97. Sealfon, S. C., Gillo, B., Mundamattom, S., *et al.* Gonadotropin-releasing hormone receptor expression in Xenopus oocytes. Mol. Endocrinol. *4:*119–124, 1990.

98. Sealfon, S. C., Laws, S. C., Wu, J. C., *et al.* Hormonal regulation of gonadotropin-releasing hormone receptors and messenger RNA activity in ovine pituitary culture. Mol. Endocrinol. *4:*1980–1987, 1990.

99. Sehy, D. W., Shao, L. E., Yu, A. L., *et al.* Activin A-induced differentiation in K562 cells is associated with a transient hypophosphorylation of RB protein and the concomitant block of cell cycle at G1 phase. J. Cell Biochem. *50:*255–265, 1992.

100. Shupnik, M. A. Effects of gonadotropin-releasing hormone on rat gonadotropin gene transcription in vitro: requirement for pulsatile administration for luteinizing hormone-beta gene stimulation. Mol. Endocrinol. *4:*1444–1450, 1990.

101. Snyder, P. Gonadotroph cell adenomas of the pituitary. Endocr. Rev. *6:*552, 1985.

102. Snyder, P. J., Bashey, H. M., Kim, S. U., *et al.* Secretion of uncombined subunits of luteinizing hormone by gonadotroph cell adenomas. J. Clin. Endocrinol. Metab. *59:*1169–1175, 1984.

103. Snyder, P. J., Johnson, J., and Muzyka, R. Abnormal secretion of glycoprotein alpha subunit and follicle-stimulating (FSH) hormone beta subunit in men with pituitary adenomas and FSH hypersecretion. J. Clin. Endocrinol. Metab. *51:*579–584, 1980.

104. Snyder, P. J., Muzyka, R., Johnson, J., *et al.* Thyrotropin-releasing hormone provokes abnormal follicle-stimulating hormone (FSH) and luteinizing hormone responses in men who have pituitary adenomas and FSH hypersecretion. J. Clin. Endocrinol. Metab. *51:*744–748, 1980.

105. Spada, A., Reza-Elahi, F., Lania, A., *et al.* Hypothalamic peptides modulate cytosolic free Ca2+ levels and adenylyl cyclase activity in human nonfunctioning pituitary adenomas. J. Clin. Endocrinol. Metab. *73:*913–918, 1991.

106. Spencer, S. J., Rabinovici, J., and Jaffe, R. B. Human recombinant activin-A inhibits proliferation of human fetal adrenal cells in vitro. J. Clin. Endocrinol. Metab. *71:*1678–1680, 1990.

107. Stojilkovic, S. S., Merelli, F., Iida, T., *et al.* Endothelin stimulation of cytosolic calcium and gonadotropin secretion in anterior pituitary cells. Science *248:*1663–1666, 1990.

108. Taylor, J. E., Bogden, A. E., Moreau, J. P., *et al.* In vitro and in vivo inhibition of human small cell lung carcinoma (NCI-H69) growth by a somatostatin analogue. Biochem. Biophys. Res. Commun. *153:*81–86, 1988.

109. ten Dijke, P., Ichijo, H., Franzen, P., *et al.* Activin receptor-like kinases: a novel subclass of cell-surface receptors with predicted serine/threonine kinase activity. Oncogene *8:*2879–2887, 1993.

110. ten Dijke, P., Yamashita, H., Ichijo, H., *et al.* Characterization of type I receptors for transforming growth factor-beta and activin. Science *264:*101–104, 1994.

111. ten Dijke, P., Yamashita, H., Sampath, T. K., *et al.* Identification of type I receptors for osteogenic protein-1 and bone morphogenetic protein-4. J. Biol. Chem. *269:*16985–16988, 1994.

112. Thorner, M. O., Perryman, R. L., Cronin, M. J., *et al.* Somatotroph hyperplasia. Successful treatment of acromegaly by removal of a pancreatic islet tumor secreting a growth hormone-releasing factor. J. Clin. Invest. *70:*965–977, 1982.

113. Trudeau, V. L., Murthy, C. K., Habibi, H. R., *et al.* Effects of sex steroid treatments on gonadotropin-releasing hormone-stimulated gonadotropin secretion from the goldfish pituitary. Biol. Reprod. *48:*300–307, 1993.

114. Virmani, M. A., Stojilkovic, S. S., and Catt, K. J. Stimulation of luteinizing hormone release by gamma-aminobutyric acid (GABA) agonists: mediation by GABAA-type receptors and activation of chloride and voltage-sensitive calcium channels. Endocrinology *126:*2499–2505, 1990.

115. Wang, Q. F., Farnworth, P. G., Burger, H. G., *et al.* Acute inhibitory effect of follicle-stimulating hormone-suppressing protein (FSP) on gonadotropin-

releasing hormone-stimulated gonadotropin secretion in cultured rat anterior pituitary cells. Mol. Cell Endocrinol. *72:*33–42, 1990.

116. Wang, Q. F., Farnworth, P. G., Burger, H. G., *et al.* Effect of inhibin on activators of protein kinase-C and calcium-mobilizing agents which stimulate secretion of gonadotropins in vitro: implication of a postgonadotropin-releasing hormone receptor effect of inhibin on gonadotropin release. Endocrinology *126:*3210–3217, 1990.

117. Waters, S. B., and Conn, P. M. Regulation of the pituitary gonadotrope by gonadotropin-releasing hormone: multiple intracellular effectors. (Published erratum appears in Chin. J. Physiol. 34(2): 241, 1991.) Chin. J. Physiol. *34:*1–26, 1991.

118. Waters, S. B., Hawes, B. E., and Conn, P. M. Stimulation of luteinizing hormone release by sodium fluoride is independent of protein kinase-C activity and unaffected by desensitization to gonadotropin-releasing hormone. Endocrinology *126:*2583–2591, 1990.

119. Weiss, J., Duca, K. A., and Crowley, W. F., Jr. Gonadotropin-releasing hormone-induced stimulation and desensitization of free alpha-subunit secretion mirrors luteinizing hormone and follicle-stimulating hormone in perifused rat pituitary cells. Endocrinology *127:*2364–2371, 1990.

120. Weiss, J., Harris, P. E., Halverson, L. M., *et al.* Dynamic regulation of follicle-stimulating hormone-beta messenger ribonucleic acid levels by activin and gonadotropin-releasing hormone in perifused

rat pituitary cells. Endocrinology *131:*1403–1408, 1992.

121. Weiss, J., Jameson, J. L., Burrin, J. M., *et al.* Divergent responses of gonadotropin subunit messenger RNAs to continuous versus pulsatile gonadotropin-releasing hormone in vitro. Mol. Endocrinol. *4:*557–564, 1990.

122. Wrana, J. L., Attisano, L., Wieser, R., *et al.* Mechanism of activation of the TGF-beta receptor. Nature *370:*341–347, 1994.

123. Xu, J., Matsuzaki, K., McKeehan, K., *et al.* Genomic structure and cloned cDNAs predict that four variants in the kinase domain of serine/threonine kinase receptors arise by alternative splicing and poly(A) addition. Proc. Natl. Acad. Sci. U. S. A. *91:*7957–7961, 1994.

124. Yamada, S., Asa, S. L., Kovacs, K., *et al.* Analysis of hormone secretion by clinically nonfunctioning human pituitary adenomas using the reverse hemolytic plaque assay. J. Clin. Endocrinol. Metab. *68:*73–80, 1989.

125. Yasuda, H., Mine, T., Shibata, H., *et al.* Activin A: an autocrine inhibitor of initiation of DNA synthesis in rat hepatocytes. J. Clin. Invest. *92:*1491–1496, 1993.

126. Young Lai, E. V., and Todoroff, E. C. The pituitary gonadotropin-releasing hormone (GnRH) receptor of the female rabbit: characterization and developmental aspects. Can. J. Physiol. Pharmacol. *70:* 1639–1646, 1992.

CHAPTER 10

Molecular Themes in Glial Tumors

DAN FULTS, M.D.

INTRODUCTION

The fundamental cause of cancer is loss of cell growth control. Normally, cells are governed by two countervailing molecular programs, one promoting and the other inhibiting cell proliferation. The central nervous system (CNS) is the stage on which cell growth control is played out with the greatest drama. In early embryogenesis, the primitive neuroepithelial cells within the germinal matrix multiply rapidly. During differentiation, however, growth inhibitory influences become so dominant that these highly prolific stem cells shut down their mitotic machinery almost completely to become slowly dividing glia and post-mitotic neurons. Failure of neuroepithelial stem cells to differentiate properly might explain the development of primitive neuroectodermal tumors (PNETs) in children. Reactivation of repressed cell proliferation programs later in life might lead to gliomas in adults.

The evidence that cancer is a genetic disease is now incontrovertible. Not only the initiating events in carcinogenesis, but also the individual steps in tumor progression, are the direct result of mutations that either turn on growth-stimulatory genes (proto-oncogenes) or turn off growth-inhibitory ones (tumor suppressor genes). Although the fundamental cause of CNS cancer is also genetic, few brain tumor cases are heritable. That is, the overwhelming majority of brain tumors in adults are sporadic in that they result from acquired, somatic mutations in growth control genes and not from inherited, germ-line mutations. This is consistent with observations that the incidence of cerebral gliomas increases with advancing age and that few if any family pedigrees exist where brain tumors alone

are prevalent (80). My goal in writing this chapter is to sketch some of the aberrant cell growth control mechanisms that have been discovered in human glial tumors (astrocytoma, oligodendroglioma, and ependymoma) and to introduce some of the key molecular players involved. This discourse is certainly not exhaustive or even adequate to explain fully the formation of human gliomas or their recalcitrant behavior, which has frustrated neurosurgeons since the beginning of our specialty.

TUMOR SUPPRESSOR GENES

Chromosome Deletions Point to Multiple Tumor Suppressor Genes in Human Glioma Progression

An intrinsic feature of cerebral gliomas, which is shared by many other solid tumors, is the tendency to progress through stages of increasing malignancy with the passage of time, often in spite of treatment. Tumor progression is widely regarded as a multi-step process that begins with a single altered cell whose clonal descendants are forced to undertake a program of increasingly deregulated growth. Inactivation of genes that function normally to suppress cell proliferation (tumor suppressor genes) are now known to define critical steps in tumor progression. Mutations that inactivate tumor suppressor genes behave in a genetically recessive fashion. That is, both copies of the gene must be knocked out by some mechanism before the mutant phenotype (loss of cell growth control) becomes evident. Since one mechanism for inactivating genes is chromosome loss or deletion, the loss of a specific chromosomal region, when found frequently in a particular type of tumor, is a signpost for a tumor suppressor gene on the missing part of the chromosome.

The first clues to the chromosomal location of tumor suppressor genes in brain tumors came from cytogenetic studies showing that loss of certain chromosomes was non-random (reviewed in (4)). In glioblastoma multiforme (GBM), for example, two of the most consistent chromosome changes were loss of whole copies of chromosome 10 and deletions or translocations affecting the short arm of chromosome 9 (9p). Cancer cells are expected to have a certain background of chromosome loss—a secondary effect of their high mitotic index. However, the observed non-random chromosome deletions strongly suggested that loss of specific genes from the missing chromosome regions might be directly responsible for malignant transformation.

Later, when the loss of heterozygosity (LOH) test was developed, a more sensitive assay for finding chromosome deletions was in hand. LOH studies not only confirmed the suspicions of cytogeneticists regarding the possible location of tumor suppressor genes, they also revealed additional chromosome regions that were missing in tumor cells. In malignant astrocytomas, LOH studies showed hot spots for chromosome deletions on 9p, 10p, 10q, 11p, 17p, 19q, and 22q (reviewed in (52)). In low grade astrocytomas, a low level of LOH has been reported on 6p (48). LOH on 19q is not a genetic event unique to purely astrocytic tumors but is observed in oligodendrogliomas (WHO grade II and III) as well as in mixed oligoastrocytomas (WHO grade III) (98). In the other major type of glioma, ependymoma, both cytogenetic and LOH studies have shown deletions on 22q. The gene implicated in type 2 neurofibromatosis (*NF2*) has been cloned and considered a candidate gene in ependymoma (91). This was a reasonable prediction given the location of *NF2* on chromosome 22 (band q12) where deletions occur in ependymomas and the prevalence of other glial tumors in *NF2* patients. However, *NF2* gene mutations are rare in ependymomas, suggesting that another tumor suppressor gene, not yet discovered, is present there (75).

Genetic Models of Astrocytoma Progression Based on Loss of Heterozygosity

Working from the assumption that LOH is an accurate measure of gene inactivation, tumor biologists have used LOH data to construct genetic models of glioma progression (reviewed in (59), (52), (7)). The genetic changes that occur during glioma progression are best studied in diffuse fibrillary astrocytomas because of their prevalence in the population and the greater number of histopathologically definable stages (grades). When DNA from patients with various astrocytoma grades is tested for LOH with markers on chromosome 10, LOH is seen almost exclusively in GBM (>60% of cases), but seldom in anaplastic astrocytomas (AA) (<25%), and never in low grade astrocytomas (LGA), suggesting that loss of a tumor suppressor gene located on chromosome 10 is a terminal genetic event associated with end-stage disease. With markers on chromosome 17, LOH is seen in both AA and GBM with equal frequency (approximately one-third of cases), suggesting that inactivation of a gene on chromosome 17 signals the transition from benign to malignant tumor growth. Similarly, LOH on 9p, 11p, 13q, and 19q, seen in the earliest malignant astrocytoma stages, predicts that loss of genes from these chromosome regions conspire to bring about malignant transformation in astrocytomas.

Before the actual genes are isolated from these chromosome regions, LOH data must be viewed only as a first approximation of gene inactivation and used cautiously in predicting tumor behavior or patient prognosis. In point of fact, the *P53* gene, which is the target for 17p deletions in human astrocytomas (discussed below), may be inactivated in tumors that do not show LOH (by point mutation or formation of dysfunctional complexes with other cellular proteins, for example). Furthermore, the LOH test, an assay usually performed on total genomic DNA extracted from tumor specimens, may not be sufficiently sensitive to detect allelic loss in low grade gliomas, which are usually mixtures of normal and neoplastic cells. Immunocytochemistry, which assays protein levels in individual cells, has shown abnormal accumulation of p53 protein even in minor subpopulations of cells within low grade astrocytomas (53). Taken together, the LOH data support a model for astrocytoma progression wherein sequential inactivation of multiple tumor suppressor genes located on different chromosomes forces the astrocytoma cell into a pathway of increasingly disinhibited growth. This is similar to and based on the more detailed multi-step model of colorectal carcinogenesis (15). In that system, the pathway connecting the benign adenomatous polyp with end-stage adenocarcinoma is marked by many more intermediate stages than in gliomas. We do not know whether this difference simply reflects the greater accessibility of colorectal tumor intermediates via the fiberoptic endoscope or whether gliomas progress so rapidly that few histopathologically discrete intermediates even exist.

While many low grade and anaplastic astrocytomas progress along the above-described pathway in a step-wise manner, many GBMs appear to arise *de novo* without apparent progression from a less malignant precursor stage, especially in elderly patients. An important, unanswered question is whether these *de novo* GBMs have simply progressed rapidly through clinically occult intermediate stages or whether they have arisen by an alternative pathway governed by a different set of altered gene products (99).

Cloning Tumor Suppressor Genes from Chromosome Regions Deleted in Tumors

If a tumor-specific chromosome deletion can be mapped accurately to small enough region of the chromosome, then molecular cloning strategies can be used to isolate the disease-causing gene. In this approach, called positional cloning, chromosome markers are used to pinpoint deletions in patient tumor DNA samples to a small chromosome region, ideally containing only a few megabases of DNA sequence. Genomic clones spanning this region are isolated, and the region is then scanned for genes that are expressed in normal tissues. The deleted chromosome region will contain numerous genes, so the goal is to distinguish the disease-causing gene from the innocent bystanders. To that end, the candidate genes are cloned and tested for the presence of mutations in DNA from patient tumors. In cases where one copy of the gene has been lost from the tumor cell by chromosome deletion (as manifest by LOH) the finding of a point mutation in the remaining copy of the gene strongly implicates that candidate as the tumor-causing gene. That is, by identifying a two-hit mechanism for inactivating both copies (alleles) of the gene in the tumor cell, one has powerful evidence that the gene in

question is actually a tumor suppressor. Once the gene is cloned, its sequence is determined and compared with the sequence of known genes by searching computer databases. Regions of sequence homology shared with genes that have been studied previously provide important clues to the new gene's function. In some instances, the deleted chromosome region will contain genes that have already been cloned, sequenced, and proven to be players in oncogenesis. This candidate gene approach greatly simplifies to task of gene identification by obviating the need for positional cloning, which is an extremely labor-intensive endeavor.

P53 is a Tumor Suppressor Gene in Human Astrocytomas

The *P53* gene was first identified as a tumor suppressor gene in human gliomas by the candidate gene approach. From the outset, *P53* was a likely suspect because of its well-known involvement in cellular transformation. The p53 protein was first discovered as a mysterious 53-kilodalton phosphoprotein that formed tight complexes with the SV40 large T antigen in cells transformed by infection with the SV40 tumor virus (45), (50). In these infected cells, p53 was a product of the host cell, not the viral genome. When the *P53* gene was cloned, mutant copies of the gene were shown to immortalize normal cells when introduced by transfection and to induce full neoplastic transformation when cotransfected with an activated *RAS* oncogene ((33) and references therein). Moreover, normal (wild-type) copies of the *P53* gene could inhibit the transforming activity of mutant *P53* clones in these cotransfection assays (16).

The evidence incriminating *P53* as a tumor suppressor gene in human gliomas centered on the localization of the human *P53* gene to the short arm of chromosome 17 (in chromosome band p13.1), precisely where deletions had been observed so frequently in malignant astrocytomas. Direct support for a two-hit mechanism of *P53* gene inactivation in human brain tumors was provided by several laboratories that reported point mutations within the *P53* coding sequence in a majority (>60%) of malignant astrocytomas with LOH on 17p (22), (19), (96). The ultimate proof that p53 functioned as a tumor suppressor in human gliomas came from experiments where expression of exogenous, wild-type p53 in GBM cell lines lacking endogenous p53 protein (or expressing only mutant forms) caused these transformed cells to assume a more normal phenotype (58), (94).

A prodigious body of experimental evidence now places p53 at center stage in human oncology. In fact, 60% of human tumors carry *P53* gene mutations. Many outstanding reviews on p53 have been published (95), (47), (35); therefore, only current models of p53 function in cell growth control will be summarized here, and the consequences of p53 dysfunction in gliomas will be emphasized.

The *P53* Gene Encodes a Cell Cycle Checkpoint Regulator

When cells sustain DNA damage by exposure to radiation or treatment with various chemotherapeutic agents, the intracellular concentration of p53 protein rises sharply (Figure 1). As a result, the damaged cell is prevented from progressing through its cell cycle. Specifically, p53 arrests the cell in the G1 phase, thereby blocking entry into S phase when DNA synthesis occurs. This cell cycle checkpoint serves a protective function, enabling the cell to repair its genome before the damaged DNA is replicated and mutations are perpetuated into the next cell generation. This role for p53 as "guardian of the genome" (44) draws strong support from experiments showing that when cells with no p53 protein are irradiated they acquire gene amplifications one million times more readily than cells with normal levels of p53 (51), (104). Inactivation of p53 then sets the stage for tumor progression, destabilizing the tumor cell genome and increasing the chance of amplifying growth-stimulatory oncogenes or deleting chromosome regions that contain tumor suppressor genes. In human gliomas, tumor progression and genomic instability go hand in hand. Chromosome deletions are more frequent and more widespread throughout the genome in GBM compared with less malignant tumor stages (25). In one study of *P53* mutations in sequential tumor specimens from individual patients with progressive disease, histologic progression from LGA to GBM occurred concomitant with clonal expansion of *P53*-mutant cells that comprised only a small subpopulation in the initial low grade tumor (86).

When a cell has incurred irreparable DNA damage, it may be eliminated by apoptosis, a genetically encoded cell death program (re-

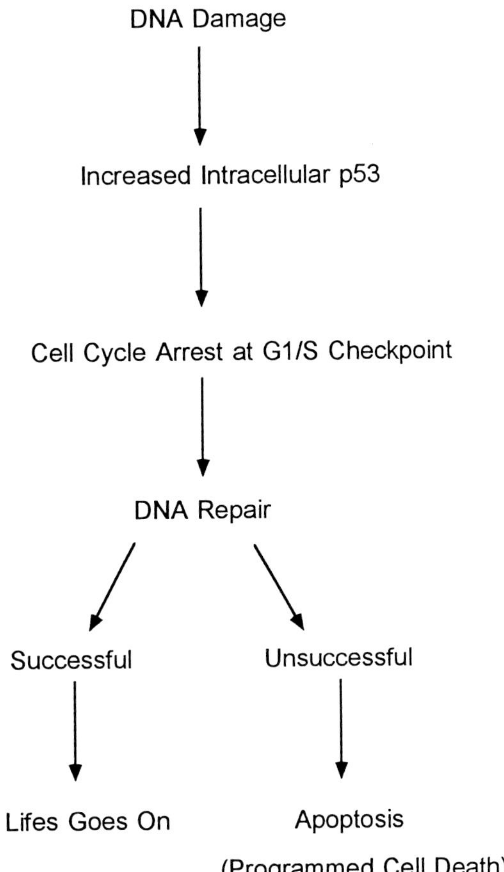

Figure 1. Model of p53 as guardian of the genome. After DNA damage, high p53 levels cause G1 arrest. If DNA repair is unsuccessful, crippled cells are diverted into a pathway of apoptosis. Adopted from Lane, D. P. *Nature 358:*15–16, 1992.

viewed in (18)). Apoptosis has evolved as a way for organisms to eliminate nonessential and potentially harmful cell types, like cancer cells, that arise by mutation. It is the rise in intracellular p53 consequent to DNA damage that triggers the apoptosis response. Moreover, aberrant apoptosis is now viewed as an important cause of cancer treatment resistance. Ionizing radiation, when delivered in therapeutic doses, may not kill cancer cells by direct cytotoxic mechanisms but rather by damaging DNA sufficiently to elicit apoptosis. This hypothesis predicts accurately that tumors with *P53* mutations respond less favorably to treatment (54). Given the prevalence of *P53* mutations in human gliomas and the fact that conventional radiation and chemotherapy work by marshaling the forces of apoptosis, improved brain tumor treatments in the future may need to target the undiscovered apoptosis effectors downstream of p53.

Tumor Suppressor Genes on Chromosome 9p Encode Cell Cycle Inhibitors Important in Human Gliomas

Positional cloning was used successfully to isolate a pair of genes, *MTS1* and *MTS2*, located in tandem on the short arm of chromosome 9 (in band p21) that appear to be targets for the 9p deletions found frequently in malignant astrocytomas and other human cancers. The fact that homozygous deletion (loss of both alleles) in *MTS1* and *MTS2* was observed in a wide variety of human tumor cell lines (gliomas, breast carcinomas, melanomas) indicated that these were likely tumor suppressor genes involved in multiple cancer types—hence the genetic designation, MTS, for multiple tumor suppressor (41). *MTS1* and *MTS2* encode proteins designated p16^{INK4} and p15^{INK4B} (p16 and p15 for short) that play key roles in regulating the passage of cells through the cell cycle (83), (29). Like p53, p16 halts cell cycle progression at the G1/S boundary, but its effect is mediated through a different set of growth control proteins. Figure 2 shows a model of how p16 interacts with these other cell cycle regulatory proteins to suppress cell proliferation.

Progression through the cell cycle is governed by a set of nuclear protein kinases, the cyclin-dependent kinases (CDKs), which become active when joined in complexes with cyclins, another family of nuclear proteins (re-

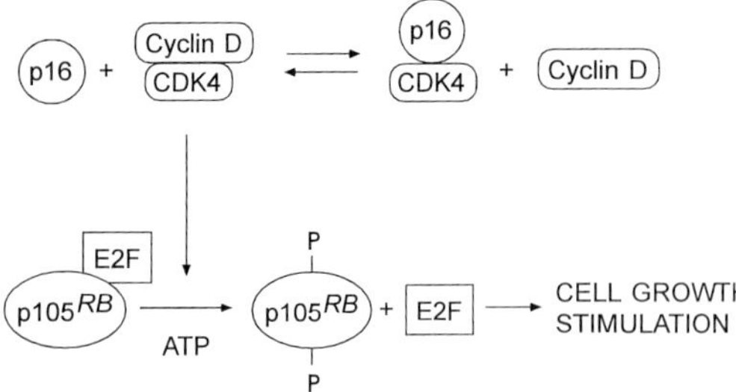

Figure 2. A molecular mechanism for cell growth suppression by p16. By binding to CDK4, p16 blocks the formation of active Cyclin D-CDK4 complexes. Inactive p16-CDK4 complexes cannot phosphorylate p105^{RB} to release transcription factor, E2F.

viewed in (36) and (85)). The expression of the various CDKs is held constant while their catalytic activity is regulated by changes in the level of the cyclins, which rise and fall as the cell traverses the stages of its growth cycle. In mammalian cells, the cyclin-CDK complexes most heavily involved with regulating the G1/S checkpoint are three D-type cyclins (D1, D2, D3) and their partner CDKs, primarily CDK4. Cyclin D-CDK4 complexes transduce cell growth stimulatory signals, allowing cells to move past the G1/S checkpoint and onward through the cell cycle.

The physiological substrate for the Cyclin D-CDK4 kinase is p105^{RB}, the product of the retinoblastoma gene, *RB*. *RB*, was the first tumor suppressor gene identified (20). Individuals who inherit a mutant allele of the *RB* gene are predisposed to retinoblastomas as well as non-ocular, second tumors, especially osteosarcomas. In keeping with its role as a tumor suppressor, the RB protein functions normally to inhibit cell proliferation. However, the precise activity of p105^{RB} in regulating cell growth depends upon its state of phosphorylation (reviewed in (34)). In the G1 phase of the cell cycle, p105^{RB} exists in a hypophosphorylated state. Just before S phase, it becomes phosphorylated and remains so until late in mitosis. Thus, phosphorylation of p105^{RB} is a molecular trigger that starts the cell cycle rolling. How, then, is cell growth control lost in tumors completely devoid of RB protein, like retinoblastomas with deletions in both copies of the *RB* gene? One possible explanation is that p105^{RB} might convey its growth inhibitory signal via a downstream effector molecule. A good candidate for this effector is transcription factor E2F. E2F forms complexes with p105^{RB} and, when acting alone, can induce mitotically quiescent cells to enter the S phase of the cell cycle, probably by turning on genes required for DNA synthesis like thymidine kinase and dihydrofolate reductase. In this model, p105^{RB} suppresses cell growth by binding E2F. When sequestered in a complex with p105^{RB}, E2F is unable to transactivate genes encoding key cell cycle proteins. Phosphorylation of p105^{RB} by Cyclin D-activated CDK4 releases E2F thereby restoring normal cell cycling. In cells lacking p105^{RB} altogether, like tumors with inactivating *RB* gene mutations, the growth stimulatory effect of E2F goes unchecked.

Another layer of control has been applied to this system by the CDK inhibitor proteins (CDIs), which inhibit CDK activity by binding in competition with cyclins. The *MTS1* and *MTS2* gene products, p16 and p15, are CDIs that bind with CDK4 and diminish its catalytic activity by preventing association with D-type cyclins. The overall effect of p16 and p15 is to convey a growth inhibitory signal to the cell—the defining feature of a tumor suppressor gene.

A growing body of experimental evidence indicates that defects in this cell cycle regulatory pathway promote human glioma formation. Initial reports showed that homozygous deletions in the *MTS1* gene were present in 80% of human glioma cell lines (41). After some early suspicion that this was an *in vitro* effect unique to cultured cell lines, more recent studies have demonstrated convincingly that both *MTS1* and *MTS2* genes are defective in primary tumors as well (39), (79), (26), (101). Specifically, homozygous deletions in *MTS1* have been reported in 41 to 59% of primary GBMs, 68% of GBM xenografts, and 19 to 52% of primary AAs. *MTS2* deletions have been observed in 71% of GBM xenografts. Definitive proof that *MTS1* is a tumor suppressor gene came from transfection experiments wherein expression of p16 in glioma cell lines lacking p16 protein caused cell growth suppression (2). In tumors, *MTS1* and *MTS2* appear to be knocked out by large deletions that remove one or both genes rather than by intragenic point mutation. A careful sequence analysis of 30 primary malignant astrocytomas revealed only a single case of a point mutation in the protein coding portion of the *MTS1* gene (93). This phenomenon stands in sharp contrast to the way in which the *P53* tumor suppressor gene is inactivated. In the latter case, point mutations in many different parts of the gene either terminate protein synthesis prematurely or produce a defective cellular p53 protein. One possible explanation for the prevalence of whole gene deletion as a mechanism of inactivating *MTS1* and *MTS2* is that loss of both gene products, p16 and p15, might be required for full neoplastic transformation to take place. Certainly their tandem arrangement on the chromosome makes these two genes highly vulnerable to elimination by chromosome deletion.

The mechanism for cell growth suppression by p16 schematized in Figure 2 accurately predicts that defective versions of any one of these interacting proteins might subvert normal control of glial cell growth. Amplification and/or overexpression of *CDK4* (30), (79) and inactivating mutations in *RB* (32) have been reported in human malignant astrocytomas. LOH on 13q, reported in 47% of malignant astrocytomas, most likely promotes tumor growth by deleting the *RB* gene (located on 13q14). The overall effect of these changes is to interfere with the growth suppressing agenda of the retinoblastoma gene.

Unidentified Tumor Suppressor Genes in Human Gliomas

The high frequency of LOH on chromosomes 10, 11, and 19 suggests strongly that additional tumor suppressor genes participate in human glioma formation. Although these genes have not yet been identified, deletion mapping studies have, in some cases, narrowed the search to smaller chromosome regions containing some likely candidates. For example, on chromosome 19 a region has been defined in band q13 that contains several genes involved in DNA repair (*ERCC1*, *ERCC2*, *XRCC*) (98). As discussed below, mutations in genes that encode DNA repair enzymes could promote tumor progression by destabilizing the genome.

On chromosome 11, deletions have been mapped to band p15.5 not only in malignant astrocytomas in adults, but also in PNETs in children (24). The Wilms' tumor susceptibility gene (*WT1*) is not a likely candidate gene since it is located much more proximal on chromosome 11, in band p13. The *HRAS* gene, which does map inside the deleted region, has been considered a candidate suppressor gene in brain tumors because its encoded protein, p21^{RAS}, can induce differentiation or growth arrest in cells of neural crest origin (reviewed in (55)). The fact that *RAS* gene mutations have not been found in either astrocytomas or PNETs argues against this alternative role for p21^{RAS} as a growth suppressor protein.

Several lines of experimental evidence indicate that one or more tumor suppressor genes located on chromosome 10 are important determinants for high grade glioma formation. First, both cytogenctic studies (5), (40) and LOH studies (38), (21) have shown that loss of sequences from chromosome 10 is a common genetic event in GBM, detectable in over 60%

of cases. Second, introduction of a normal copy of chromosome 10 into a GBM cell line by microcell transfer suppresses tumor cell growth (70). Regrettably, progress toward identifying candidate genes has been impeded by the large deletions typically found in patient tumor DNA samples. In fact, glioblastoma cells have a striking tendency to lose one entire copy of chromosome 10. For example, in 69 GBM patients that we tested for LOH with RFLP markers for 31 distinct loci on chromosome 10, LOH was found in 42 (61%). In 33 of these 42 patients (79%), LOH was seen with every informative marker, indicating whole chromosome loss (reduction to hemizygosity). Although a small number of GBM cases have been reported with subchromosomal deletions, the smallest deleted regions remain too vast for identifying candidate genes using positional cloning methods. The complexity of this problem is heightened by claims that deletions cluster in three different regions of chromosome 10: one near the q telomere, a second at the p telomere, and the third near the q centromere (42). The presence of multiple suppressor genes on chromosome 10 could explain the prevalence of whole chromosome loss in GBM tumors and the paucity of submicroscopic deletions. That is, loss of multiple, syntenic growth control genes might be required for astrocytomas to progress to end-stage GBM. To date, the 10q deletions have been mapped in greatest detail (73), (72), (23). Even so, the genetic distance spanned by the smallest 10q deletions exceeds 17% of the entire chromosome. Moreover, the complex chromosomal rearrangements (translocations, multiple interstitial deletions) that are seen in GBMs diminish the reliability of deletion mapping as a tool for narrowing the search for candidate genes.

Given the enormous genetic territory covered by chromosome 10 deletions in GBMs, any gene on that chromosome must be viewed as a tumor suppressor suspect. Mutations in *MXI1*, a gene that maps to the q24-q25 region of chromosome 10 and that encodes a protein with negative regulatory effects on the MYC oncoprotein, have been reported in prostatic carcinomas, tumors that also show frequent LOH on 10q (13). Exploring the possibility that *MXI1* is a target for the 10q deletions in GBMs, we used single strand conformation polymorphism (SSCP) analysis (described in an earlier chapter) to look for *MXI1* mutations in DNA from 63 GBMs and 5 AAs (37 GBMs and all 5 AAs had LOH on chromosome 10). We examined the two exons coding for helix-loop-helix and leucine zipper domains thinking that mutations there would be most likely to alter MYC regulatory function. We found no evidence for *MXI1* mutation in any of these cases (unpublished data). Since the reported *MXI1* mutations in prostatic carcinomas were found only in a small fraction of cells within the tumor specimens, the possibility remains that our SSCP analysis simply failed to detect mutations in the brain tumors. Nevertheless, it seems unlikely that *MXI1* is the major target for chromosome 10 deletions present in the majority of GBMs.

Another candidate suppressor gene on chromosome 10 is *MGMT* which encodes a DNA repair enzyme, O^6-methylguanine-DNA methyltransferase. Although gene mutation studies have not been reported, enzyme activity is subnormal in primary GBM tumors (87), and both protein and mRNA levels are reduced in GBM cell lines (65). Another hypothetical candidate is *CDC2*, a 10q21 gene that, like *CDK4*, regulates cell cycling. The CDC2 protein complexes with Cyclin B to form an active kinase that stimulates cells to move past the G2/M checkpoint to begin mitosis. As new genes are cloned and mapped to chromosome 10, mutation studies in primary brain tumors will be needed to identify this long-sought glioma suppressor gene, keeping in mind that multiple genes may be inactivated by the large deletions typically found in these tumors.

Aberrant DNA Mismatch Repair in Brain Tumors—Lessons from Colorectal Cancer

The long-held notion that cancer is a disease of genetic instability has now been proven by the discovery that mutations in genes encoding DNA repair enzymes cause hereditary non-polyposis colorectal cancer (HNPCC, Lynch syndrome). The molecular mechanisms of DNA repair have been the subject of intense scientific inquiry over the past several decades. One major repair program, methyl-directed mismatch repair, corrects errors in Watson-Crick (purine-pyrimidine) base pairing during DNA synthesis. In *E. Coli*, the products of four genes (MutH, MutL, MutS, MutU) are essential for mismatch repair (reviewed in (61)). Bacterial mutants with defective versions of these genes show a marked increase in spontaneous mutation rate. In addition to correcting simple DNA biosynthetic errors during replication of individual DNA molecules, these repair enzymes also block crossovers between genetically divergent regions on different DNA molecules. Overall, mismatch repair genes work to maintain the fidelity of DNA replication and genetic recombination and, therefore, function as tumor suppressors.

The first clue that DNA mismatch repair was defective in human cancer came from the observation that tumors from HNPCC patients showed a phenomenon called microsatellite instability (1), (90). Microsatellite instability is observed when PCR is used to amplify regions of the genome containing microsatellite sequences, short DNA segments (2–4 basepairs in length) repeated in tandem many times. These microsatellites are dispersed widely throughout the human genome. During replication of a DNA strand containing a microsatellite sequence the replication enzymes may become confused by the long stretch of redundant sequence and synthesize more or fewer of these repeat units than was present on the template strand. Under normal conditions, the cell's mismatch repair system will correct this replication error. By contrast, a faulty repair system will permit replication of the erroneous DNA molecules. When PCR is used to amplify a microsatellite region in a cell which is mismatch repair defective, DNA fragments longer or shorter than normal become apparent. These DNA replication errors (microsatellite instability) were observed frequently in colonic tumors from patients with HNPCC, a genetic syndrome known to be linked to chromosome 2 (69). When cloned, the disease-causing gene (*hMSH2*) was found to be the human homologue of the bacterial MutS gene (17), (46). To date, mutations in four DNA mismatch repair genes (*hMSH2, hMLH1, hPMS1*, hPMS2) have been discovered in HNPCC tumors (reviewed in (61)). Biochemical analysis of cell lines derived from tumors with microsatellite instability has consistently shown an associated deficiency in mismatch repair (66).

Microsatellite instability is also seen in sporadic (non-hereditary) colorectal tumors (13%) although much less frequently than in HNPCC (79%), indicating that mismatch repair defects may be a more general cause of genetic instability in cancer cells (1). In one survey of 196 sporadic cancers of various types, microsatellite instability was found in 8% of cases overall, with the lowest frequency in brain tumors (2%) (103). In another study of 16 astrocytomas, microsatellite instability was seen more frequently (37%) (11).

Inherited, germ-line mutations in mismatch repair genes may be the cause of certain familial brain tumors that arise in Turcot's syndrome, a rare autosomal dominant condition in which brain tumors (medulloblastomas and GBMs) occur in association with familial adenomatous polyposis coli (APC). APC differs from HNPCC in several ways: (1) it is less common, (2) APC patients have multiple adenomatous polyps lining the entire colon, and (3) the responsible gene, located on chromosome 5, does not encode a DNA repair enzyme. In a study of 14 Turcot's syndrome families, germ-line mutations in two different genes were identified: the *APC* gene in 10 families and a mismatch repair gene (*hPMS2* or *hMLH1*) in two others (28). *APC* and mismatch repair gene mutations did not occur together in the same family. The brain tumors in the mismatch repair deficient families were all GBMs with microsatellite instability, whereas those in the *APC*-mutant families were predominantly medulloblastomas without microsatellite instability. An unexpected finding was the unusually long survival in three GBM patients with DNA-replication errors. Coupled with the rather low incidence of microsatellite instability in sporadic gliomas, these data indicate that defective DNA mismatch repair programs, while possibly involved in certain familial brain tumors, do not account for all the genetic derangements that accumulate during malignant glioma progression.

Mutation studies do not support a major role for the *APC* gene in sporadic gliomas. In one study, no somatic mutations in *APC* were found among 91 brain tumors of various histologic types (medulloblastomas, GBMs, oligodendrogliomas), including two medulloblastomas in patients with Turcot's syndrome (62). In 32 sporadic malignant astrocytomas that we tested, *APC* mutations were found in only two tumors: a chain-terminating point mutation in codon 332 in one AA and a hemizygous deletion of the entire *APC* gene in a GBM (unpublished data).

CELL GROWTH PROMOTING GENES

Growth Factor Receptors Transduce Mitogenic Signals via the RAS-MAP Kinase Pathway

So far I have discussed molecular systems that restrain cell proliferation within the CNS and some consequences of losing this normal braking mechanism. Equally important are forces that promote cell growth. Polypeptide growth factors interacting with specific cell surface receptors convey a message that the surrounding environment is favorable for cell division. A molecular paradigm for cell growth stimulation by polypeptide growth factors that is highly relevant to the human glioma problem is the epidermal growth factor (EGF) and its receptor (EGFR). Like other growth factor receptors, EGFR is a transmembrane protein with three main components: an extracellular region that binds ligand, a transmembrane region that anchors the receptor protein to the cell membrane, and a cytoplasmic region that transmits to intracellular molecules the message that a growth factor has engaged its receptor. The cytoplasmic portion of EGFR is itself an enzyme (a tyrosine-specific protein kinase) that transfers a phosphate group to a tyrosine residue on another protein. When ligand binds receptor at the cell surface, two receptor molecules dimerize (reviewed in (31)). Consequently, the partner kinases autophosphorylate each other, an event that increases the tyrosine kinase activity of each receptor monomer. The activated receptor is then poised to transduce its signal through the cytoplasm into the nucleus where cell cycle genes will be transcribed. The molecular pathways involved in signal transduction are highly complex, with many interacting components that are only partially understood. My goal here is to outline the best studied mitogenic signal pathway, the RAS-MAP kinase pathway, with emphasis on the following general principles: (1) phosphorylation is a universal, chemical switching mechanism used by the cell to activate its regulatory peptides, (2) protein tyrosine phosphorylation can either increase the catalytic activity of enzymes or create an attachment point for proteins that contain an SH2 domain, and (3) switching of the *RAS* gene product, $p21^{RAS}$, from an inactive GDP-bound state to an activated GTP-bound state is a com-

mon node on which multiple signal transduction pathways converge.

Many key regulatory proteins involved in signal transduction proteins contain domains called SH2 and SH3 (src homology) which form docking sites for other proteins (reviewed in (78) and (37)). SH2 domains bind to proteins through peptide motifs containing phosphotyrosine residues, whereas SH3 domains bind through short, proline-rich peptide motifs. A cytoplasmic protein called Grb2 (growth factor bound), which contains one SH2 domain and two SH3 domains, binds to the tyrosine autophosphorylation site of the activated EGF receptor dimer through its SH2 sequence (Figure 3). A second protein, SOS, binds Grb2 through the SH3 domain. SOS, a guanine nucleotide exchange factor, activates $p21^{RAS}$ at the cell membrane by catalyzing its conversion from inactive GDP-RAS to active GTP-RAS. Activation of RAS at the cell membrane initiates a cascade of signaling events wherein a chain of cytoplasmic proteins, each a protein kinase it-

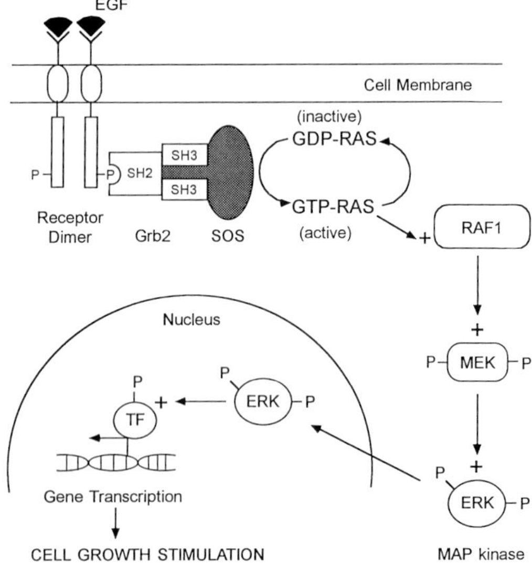

Figure 3. RAS-MAP kinase signal transduction pathway. After binding growth factor ligand (EGF), receptors dimerize and autophosphorylate via cytoplasmic tyrosine kinase domains (rectangles). Grb2-SOS complexes bind receptor at phosphorylation sites (P) via SH2 domains, then activate membrane-bound RAS. Activated RAS initiates signal transduction across the cytoplasm through non-receptor protein kinases (RAF1, MEK, ERK). Activated ERK, a MAP kinase, translocates into the nucleus to phosphorylate transcription factors (TF) that turn on growth stimulatory genes.

self, becomes activated by phosphorylation. Once activated by phosphorylation, each kinase phosphorylates, in turn, the next downstream effector protein so that the initial mitogenic stimulus at the cell membrane is propagated through the cytoplasm via this chain of non-receptor kinases to the nucleus. As shown in Figure 3, three kinases downstream of RAS are RAF1, MEK, and ERK. We do not know how *RAS* activates RAF1, only that GTP-RAS binds to RAF1 at the cell membrane where RAF1 becomes activated by phosphorylation (although not by RAS which has no kinase activity). ERK (extracellular signal regulated kinase) is a MAP kinase (mitogen activated protein kinase) that functions as relay team anchor by moving into the nucleus to activate, by phosphorylation, transcription factors that switch on cell cycle genes.

In contradistinction to tumor suppressor genes discussed earlier, signal transduction genes function normally to promote cell proliferation. How then do mutations in signal transduction genes cause tumors? *RAS* gene mutations occur frequently in human solid tumors, most often in cancer of the colon (50%), pancreas (90%), and lung (30%) (6). Mutant *RAS* genes from human tumors differ from their wild-type alleles by the presence of point mutations causing single amino acid substitutions within the encoded $p21^{RAS}$ proteins, and they induce transformation when introduced into appropriate target cells. The $p21^{RAS}$ proteins have intrinsic GTPase activity, which serves a self-regulatory function, returning the protein to a quiescent GDP-bound state after activation. Extensive characterization of mutant RAS proteins has shown that this intrinsic GTPase activity is diminished in mutant proteins. The resulting excess of activated, GTP-bound RAS within the cell transduces a continuous, growth-promoting signal. Curiously, *RAS* gene mutations have not been found in human malignant astrocytomas or PNETs, a surprising result given the frequency of RAS-activating mutations in other types of human tumors ((6), (24)). One possible explanation is that brain tumors may be caused by mutagens that do not affect *RAS* genes. Alternatively, activated GTP-RAS may not transduce a powerful growth promoting signal in neural tissues so that RAS-activating mutations may not confer a selective growth advantage to mutant cells that arise in the brain.

We know that the effect of RAS activation is dependent upon cell type. For example, activated $p21^{RAS}$ can induce differentiation or growth arrest when expressed in cells of neural crest origin ((3), (74)). In fact, the entire RAS-MAP kinase pathway appears capable of transducing both growth promoting and growth inhibiting (differentiation) signals in the same cell type. PC12, a rat pheochromocytoma cell line that differentiates into neurons *in vitro*, responds to nerve growth factor (NGF) by differentiation and to EGF by proliferation, even though both growth factors engage receptors that operate via the RAS-MAP kinase signaling pathway. One possible explanation for these divergent cellular responses lies in the quantitative differences found in certain signaling molecules during differentiation and proliferation. NGF stimulation causes persistent elevation in GTP-RAS and ERK while EGF stimulation causes only a transitory rise (reviewed in (56)). At higher cytoplasmic concentrations, ERK would be more likely to gain access to nuclear transcription factors. Although the cellular response (differentiation vs. proliferation) depends upon which transcription factors are available, the attractive feature of this model is that a cell can use transient and sustained elevations in ERK to determine different responses.

Abnormal EGF Signaling in GBM

In primary human GBMs the *EGFR* gene is amplified and overexpressed in more than 40% of cases ((49), (102)). An increase in the concentration of receptors on the cell surface could promote cell growth either by increasing ligand-receptor interaction or by favoring the formation of active receptor dimers. In addition, primary GBMs with *EGFR* gene amplification frequently contain rearranged mRNA transcripts, which create deletions in the amino-terminal, extracellular domain, and in the carboxy-terminal, cytoplasmic domain of the encoded receptor protein ((89), (14)). Insofar as these rearranged receptors have only been observed in tumors displaying amplification of both normal and abnormal *EGFR* genes, we do not know whether cell growth stimulation results simply from increased numbers of normal receptors on the cell surface or whether the rearranged receptors transduce a strong mitogenic signal by themselves. In support of an active role for rearranged receptors in signal transduction, expression of a truncated EGFR lacking the extracellular, ligand-binding domain can transform immortalized rat fibroblasts (27). Furthermore, *EGFR* constructs lacking carboxy-terminal sequences important for receptor internalization and degradation promote transformation of NIH3T3 cells in response to EGF (8). Expression of amino-terminal deletion mutants of *EGFR* in human GBM cell lines do not affect the rate of cell growth *in vitro* but do increase the tumor forming efficiency of transfected cells when implanted into nude mice (63). Although aberrant EGF signaling clearly plays an important role in promoting the growth of malignant gliomas in humans it appears to be a late event in tumor progression. *EGFR* gene amplification is restricted to end-stage GBM and is invariably associated with LOH on chromosome 10. The fact that LOH on chromosome 10 has been observed in GBMs without *EGFR* gene amplification supports the hypothesis that the latter event occurs subsequent to chromosome 10 loss during the course of astrocytoma progression (97).

HER2 (Neu), A Developmentally Regulated Growth Factor Receptor Gene, Is Mutated in Congenital Brain Tumors

Another growth factor receptor gene relevant to human glioma formation is *HER2*, also known as *ErbB-2*. The discovery of *HER2* began with the observation that when pregnant rats were exposed to the carcinogen ethylnitrosourea, brain tumors resembling glioblastomas developed in their offspring. DNA from these tumors was a potent transforming agent when transfected into NIH3T3 cells, suggesting the presence of an activated oncogene. When the transforming gene was cloned (the *Neu* oncogene), it was found to encode a receptor tyrosine kinase, p185^{Neu}, very similar in structure to EGFR (77). The oncogenic form of p185^{Neu} differed from the normal receptor only by a single amino acid substitution in the transmembrane region. Although the precise mechanism whereby this single amino acid change causes cell transformation is not known, the mutant receptors dimerize more readily and their tyrosine kinase activity increases accordingly (reviewed in (12)). In the developing rat CNS, p185^{Neu} expression is highest at a time of greatest susceptibility to the carcinogenic effect of

ethylnitrosourea and in the adult CNS, p185^{Neu} is barely detectable. These observations imply that derangements in p185^{HER2}, the human receptor, are probably more important in causing brain tumors in children than adults. The activating mutation in the rat *Neu* gene has not been found in the *HER2* gene in human tumors. However, *HER2* is amplified and/or overexpressed in a variety of human tumors, especially adenocarcinomas of the breast and ovary (88). In human gliomas, HER2 expression has been reported, with higher levels of expression present in the more malignant tumor stages (82).

A number of biologically active ligands for p185^{Neu} have been isolated from different tissue sources, each of which increases the tyrosine kinase activity of p185^{Neu}. These growth factors include heregulin (HRG) identified in human breast cancer cells, NEU differentiation factor (NDF) in transformed rat fibroblasts, NEU activation factor (NAF) in human T-cells, and several glial growth factors (GGFs) (reviewed in (12)). Sequence analysis has shown that these ligands are all splice variants derived from the same gene. The fact that the GGFs are expressed in the nervous system and stimulate proliferation of cultured Schwann cells supports the notion that defects in HER2 signaling promote glioma formation.

An Autostimulatory Feedback Loop Involving PDGF and Its Receptor Drives Glial Cell Growth

The platelet-derived growth factor (PDGF) is a potent mitogen for many types of cells, including glia. The PDGF molecule is a dimer composed of two polypeptide subunits (A and B) encoded by different genes on separate chromosomes. These two subunits are joined through disulfide bonds to form PDGF homodimers (AA or BB) or heterodimers (AB). The PDGF receptor is similar in structure to EGFR and HER2 (discussed above) and contains a cytoplasmic, tyrosine kinase domain whose activity is enhanced by ligand binding at the cell surface. There are two isoforms of the PDGF receptor (α and β), each encoded by a different gene. Since ligand binding induces receptor dimerization similar to other growth factor receptors, three PDGF receptor dimers are possible: $\alpha\alpha$, $\alpha\beta$, and $\beta\beta$. Binding studies have shown different affinities among these various growth factor and receptor isoforms, with PDGF-B capable of binding either α or β receptors and PDGF-A, only α receptors. The observation that certain transformed cells coexpress PDGF and PDGF receptors in combinations that promote avid ligand-receptor binding has led to a model of growth factor-induced transformation wherein an autocrine feedback loop continuously stimulates cell growth. That is, cells produce a growth factor for which they have their own receptor (reviewed in (100)). There is good evidence for a PDGF autostimulatory feedback loop in human gliomas (57), (64). Normal astrocytes in culture express PDGF receptors on their surfaces and respond to exogenous PDGF, but they do not express PDGF themselves. By contrast, human malignant astrocytomas simultaneously express PDGF-B subunits and PDGF β receptors—an avid ligand-receptor combination that would most likely transduce a continuous growth stimulatory signal. Moreover, dominant-negative mutants of PDGF-A, which bind with normal subunits only to form unstable or inactive heterodimers, have been shown to reverse transformation in human astrocytoma cell lines by breaking an established autocrine feedback loop (84).

VEGF Mediates Angiogenesis and Vasogenic Edema in GBM

The ability of growth factors to stimulate tumor growth is not limited to their direct mitogenic effect on tumor cells. In fact, a high mitotic rate is just one of many attributes of cancer cells, including anchorage independent growth, tissue invasiveness, migration and metastasis, and angiogenesis. Angiogenesis is essential for solid tumor growth and appears to be regulated by factors produced by tumor cells, which have a chemotactic and mitogenic effect on endothelial cells. While angiogenesis is a vast topic well beyond the scope of this chapter, the effect of one angiogenic factor, vascular endothelial growth factor (VEGF), in glioblastoma growth is an important example of the growth factor signaling theme. VEGF is not only a mitogen for endothelial cells, but also a potent vascular permeabilizing agent and a procoagulant. Immunocytochemical studies have shown that VEGF is expressed in primary GBM tumors, suggesting that VEGF may be directly responsible for endothelial cell proliferation, a

histological hallmark of GBM, and peritumoral (vasogenic) edema, invariably seen on CT and MRI scans (92). Furthermore, the procoagulant properties of VEGF may be a cause of the hypercoagulable state of many GBM patients.

Powerful functional evidence that VEGF mediates brain tumor angiopathy came from experiments showing that expression of a dominant-negative mutant of FLK1, the VEGF receptor, in mouse C6 glioblastoma cells dramatically reduced tumor growth *in vivo*. Moreover, the small tumors that did form were pale and poorly vascularized, suggesting that it was the inhibition of angiogenesis that blunted tumor growth (60). Immunocytochemical and *in situ* hybridization studies of human GBM tissue sections has shown that VEGF is produced solely by tumor cells and VEGF receptors by endothelial cells (71). This supports a paracrine mechanism of tumor angiogenesis whereby secretion of VEGF by glioblastoma cells stimulates vascular proliferation by activating cell surface receptors on neighboring endothelial cells.

Adhesion-Dependent Intracellular Signaling

The integrins comprise a family of cell surface receptors that mediate attachment to the extracellular matrix (ECM) and modulate cell-cell adhesion, cell spreading, and cytokinesis (cell locomotion) (reviewed in (10)). Most integrin receptors bind ligands that are components of the ECM (fibronectin, collagen, vitronectin). Others bind soluble ligands, like fibrinogen, or adhesion molecules on adjacent cells. Ligand binding causes integrin receptors to cluster on the cell surface, leading to the formation of a focal adhesion. It is at these focal adhesions that aggregated integrin receptors are linked to cytoskeletal proteins. Once formed, focal adhesions induce cytoskeletal changes like cell spreading and detachment from the ECM, or they convey signals across the cytoplasm into the nucleus where transcription of cell growth control genes initiate cell division. Many of the intracellular molecules that transduce integrin receptor signals also transduce growth factor receptor signals. Unlike growth factor receptors, however, the cytoplasmic domains of integrin receptors lack enzyme activity and appear to function by assembling, within the focal adhesion, cytoplasmic proteins that are catalytically active. One protein that plays a central role in integrin-mediated signal transduction is focal adhesion kinase (FAK), a tyrosine kinase whose catalytic activity is enhanced by integrin receptor engagement. Figure 4 shows some of the molecules that participate in adhesion-dependent cell signaling. When integrin receptors engage extracellular ligands, they aggregate and recruit various intracellular, cytoskeletal proteins like actin, vinculin, and talin to form a focal adhesion. Subsequently, FAK phosphorylates itself on a tyrosine residue. The proto-oncogene, SRC, a non-receptor tyrosine kinase, binds to FAK at this autophosphorylation site via its SH2 domain. SRC is then positioned to phosphorylate another tyrosine residue on FAK. This second phosphotyrosine serves as an attachment point for the Grb2/SOS complex which, in turn, activates RAS just like in growth factor signal transduction. Activated RAS is a common node from which cytoplasmic signals are passed along the MAP kinase pathway to transactivate cell growth control genes or directly to cytoskeletal

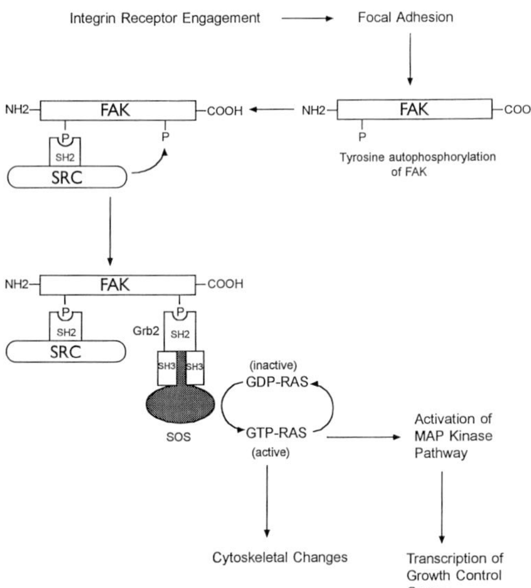

Figure 4. Adhesion-dependent signaling pathways. When integrin receptors engage extracellular matrix ligands, receptors aggregate with cytoskeletal proteins to form focal adhesions. Tyrosine autophosphorylation of FAK creates a docking site for SRC via its SH2 domain. SRC phosphorylates another tyrosine residue on FAK to create a docking site for the Grb2/SOS complex which, in turn, activates RAS. Signal transduction downstream of RAS induces cytoskeletal changes or cell proliferation.

proteins to induce changes in cell shape, motility, or attachment.

A fundamental limitation to effective glioma treatment, well-known to neurosurgeons, is the inherent invasiveness of glioma cells. Infiltration of normal brain tissue by migratory glioma cells creates neurological deficits even in low grade gliomas where tumor cells are dividing slowly. Defective adhesion-dependent signaling molecules are more likely to cause this kind of cell behavior than genes governing cell proliferation. Although there is a large body of literature about macromolecules that comprise the ECM (reviewed in (76) and (43)), far less is known about intracellular signaling events that take place after these molecules bind integrin receptors, especially in brain tumors. We do know that the composition of integrin receptor subunits is decidedly different in human GBMs compared to normal brain tissue or benign tumors like oligodendrogliomas (67). Furthermore, antibodies directed against certain integrin receptor subunits can inhibit basement membrane invasion in glioblastoma cells (68). A functional interrelationship between growth factor-dependent and adhesion-dependent signaling pathways is supported by experimental evidence that adherence of cells to the ECM is necessary for growth factors to induce cell proliferation (81) and that growth factors directly affect glioma cell motility (9).

PERSPECTIVES

In this chapter a few of the many genetic and biochemical abnormalities in gliomas have been reviewed. With our increasing knowledge about cancer biology comes a heightened awareness of the huge number of different molecules used by cells to control their growth. The human genome probably encodes 2000 different protein kinases alone, only a small percentage of which are currently identified (37). Considering the dismal prognosis for patients with malignant gliomas and the fact that earlier detection afforded by modern radiographic methods has not altered this natural history appreciably, hope for better treatment rests on improving our understanding of neural oncogenesis at the molecular level. Since the mechanisms of oncogenesis are not the same in all tissues, new cancer-causing molecules must be tested specifically in brain tumor tissues and models. To be successful, future treatment strategies must target not only the genes that govern cell proliferation, but also those that regulate cytokinesis, tissue invasiveness, and apoptosis. The complexity of the system will not make the task easy. For example, the multiple, overlapping biochemical pathways used by cells to transduce growth factor signals may thwart attempts to correct any one pathway in individual tumors. Hopefully, more effective methods of treating glioma patients need not await our complete understanding of cell growth control if we can identify a few molecules that play pivotal roles in gliomagenesis. By restoring inactive tumor suppressor genes by gene therapy or by silencing overactive oncoproteins by chemical inhibitors, we may be able to interrupt the often relentless progression of astrocytomas to end-stage GBM.

REFERENCES

1. Aaltonen, L. A., *et al.* Clues to the pathogenesis of familial colorectal cancer. *Science 260:*812–816, 1993.
2. Arap, W., Nishikawa, R., Furnari, F. B., *et al.* Replacement of the p16/CDKN2 gene suppresses human glioma cell growth. *Cancer Res. 55:*1351–1354, 1995.
3. Bar-Sagi, D., and Feramisco, J. R. Microinjection of the ras oncogene protein into PC12 cells induces morphological differentiation. *Cell 42:*841–848, 1985.
4. Bigner, S. H., Mark, J., and Bigner, D. D. Cytogenetics of human brain tumors. *Cancer Genet. Cytogenet. 47:*141–154, 1990.
5. Bigner, S. H., Mark, J., Burger, P. C., *et al.* Specific chromosomal abnormalities in malignant human gliomas. *Cancer Res. 88:*405–411, 1988.
6. Bos, J. L. ras oncogenes in human cancer: a review. *Cancer Res. 49:*4682–4689, 1989.
7. Chen, T. C., Hinton, D. R., and Apuzzo, M. L. J. Malignant progression in gliomas. In: *Benign Cerebral Gliomas*, edited by M. L. J. Apuzzo, pp. 181–188. American Association of Neurological Surgeons, Park Ridge, IL, 1995.
8. Chen, W. S., Lazar, C. S., Lund, K. A., *et al.* Functional independence of the epidermal growth factor receptor from a domain required for ligand-induced internalization and calcium regulation. *Cell 59:*33–43, 1989.
9. Chicoine, M. R., Madsen, C. L., and Silbergeld, D. L. Modification of human glioma locomotion in vitro by cytokines EGF, bFGF, PDGFbb, NGF, and TNFα. *Neurosurgery 36:*1165–1171, 1995.
10. Clark, E. A., and Brugge, J. S. Integrins and signal transduction pathways: the road taken. *Science 268:*233–239, 1995.
11. Dams, E., Van de Kelft, J. Z., Martin, J. J., *et al.* Instability of microsatellites in human gliomas. *Cancer Res. 55:*1547–1549, 1995.
12. Dougall, W. C., Quan, X., Peterson, N. C., *et al.* The neu oncogene: signal transduction pathways, transformation mechanisms and evolving therapies. *Oncogene 9:*2109–2123, 1994.
13. Eagle, L. R., Yin, X., Brothman, A. R., *et al.* Mutation of the mxi1 gene in prostate cancer. *Nature Genet. 9:*249–255, 1995.
14. Ekstrand, A. J., Sugawa, N., James, C. D., and Collins, V. P. Amplified and rearranged epidermal growth factor receptor genes in human glioblastomas reveal deletions of sequences encoding portions of the N- and/or C-terminal tails. *Proc. Natl. Acad. Sci. U.S.A. 89:*4309–4313, 1992.
15. Fearon, E. R., and Vogelstein, B. A genetic model for colorectal tumorigenesis. *Cell 61:*759–767, 1990.
16. Finlay, C. A., Hinds, P. W., and Levine, A. J. The p53 proto-oncogene can act as a suppressor of transformation. *Cell 57:*1083–1093, 1989.
17. Fishel, R., Lescoe, M. D., Rao, M. R. S., *et al.* The human mutator gene homolog MSH2 and its association with hereditary nonpolyposis colon cancer. *Cell 75:*1027–1038, 1993.
18. Fisher, D. E. Apoptosis in cancer therapy: crossing the threshold. *Cell 78:*539–542, 1994.
19. Frankel, R. H., Bayona, W., Koslow, M., and Newcomb, E. W. p53 mutations in human malignant gliomas: comparison of loss of heterozygosity with mutation frequency. *Cancer Res. 52:*1427–1433, 1992.
20. Friend, S. H., Bernards, R., Rogelj, S., *et al.* A human DNA segment with properties of the gene that predisposes to retinoblastoma and osteosarcoma. *Nature 323:*643–646, 1986.
21. Fujimoto, M., Fults, D. W., Thomas, G. A., *et al.* Loss of heterozygosity on chromosome 10 in human glioblastoma multiforme. *Genomics 4:*210–214, 1989.
22. Fults, D., Brockmeyer, D., Tullous, M. W., *et al.* p53 mutation and loss of heterozygosity on chromosomes 10 and 17 during human astrocytoma progression. *Cancer Res. 52:*674–679, 1992.
23. Fults, D., and Pedone, C. Deletion mapping of the long arm of chromosome 10 in glioblastoma multiforme. *Genes Chrom. Cancer 7:*173–177, 1993.
24. Fults, D., Petronio, J., Noblett, B. D., and Pedone, C. A. Chromosome 11p15 deletions in human malignant astrocytomas and primitive neuroectodermal tumors. *Genomics 14:*799–801, 1992.
25. Fults, D., Pedone, C. A., Thomas, G. A., and White, R. Allelotype of human malignant astrocytoma. *Cancer Res. 50:*5784–5789, 1990.
26. Giani, C., and Finocchiaro, G. Mutation rate of the CDKN2 gene in malignant gliomas. *Cancer Res. 54:*6338–6339, 1994.
27. Haley, J. D., Hsuan, J. J., and Waterfield, M. D. Analysis of mammalian fibroblast transformation by normal and mutated human EGF receptors. *Oncogene 4:*273–283, 1989.
28. Hamilton, S. R., *et al.* The molecular basis of Turcot's syndrome. *N. Engl. J. Med. 332:*839–847, 1995.
29. Hannon, G. J., and Beach, D. p15INK4B is a potential

effector of TGF-beta-induced cell cycle arrest. *Nature 371*:257–261, 1994.

30. He, J., Allen, J. R., Collins, V. P., *et al.* CDK4 amplification is an alternative mechanism to p16 gene homozygous deletion in glioma cell lines. *Cancer Res. 54*:5804–5807, 1994.

31. Heldin, C. Dimerization of cell surface receptors in signal transduction. *Cell 80*:213–223, 1995.

32. Henson, J. W., Schnitker, B. L., Correa, K. M., *et al.* The retinoblastoma gene is involved in malignant progression of astrocytomas. *Ann. Neurol. 36*:714–721, 1994.

33. Hinds, P., Finlay, C., and Levine, A. J. Mutation is required to activate the p53 gene for cooperation with the ras oncogene and transformation. *J. Virol. 63*:739–746, 1989.

34. Hinds, P. W., and Weinberg, R. A. Tumor suppressor genes. *Curr. Opin. Genet. Dev. 4*:135–141, 1994.

35. Hollstein, M., Sidransky, D., Vogelstein, B., and Harris, C. C. p53 mutations in human cancers. *Science 253*:49–53, 1991.

36. Hunter, T., and Pines, J. Cyclins and cancer II: cyclin D and CDK inhibitors come of age. *Cell 79*:573–582, 1994.

37. Hunter, T. Protein kinases and phosphatases: the yin and yang of protein phosphorylation and signaling. *Cell 80*:225–236, 1995.

38. James, C. D., Carlbom, E., Dumanski, J. P., *et al.* Clonal genomic alterations in glioma malignancy stages. *Cancer Res. 48*:5546–5551, 1988.

39. Jen, J., Harper, J. W., Bigner, S. H., *et al.* Deletion of p16 and p15 genes in brain tumors. *Cancer Res. 54*:6353–6358, 1994.

40. Jenkins, R. B., Kimmel, D. W., Moertel, C. A., *et al.* A cytogenetic study of 53 human gliomas. *Cancer Genet. Cytogenet. 39*:253–279, 1989.

41. Kamb, A., Gruis, N. A., Weaver-Feldhaus, J., *et al.* A cell cycle regulator potentially involved in genesis of many tumor types. *Science 264*:436–440, 1994.

42. Karlbom, A. E., James, C. D., Boethius, J., *et al.* Loss of heterozygosity in malignant gliomas involves at three distinct regions on chromosome 10. *Hum. Genet. 92*:169–174, 1993.

43. Lander, A. D., and Calof, A. L. Extracellular matrix in the developing nervous system, In: *Molecular Genetics of Nervous System Tumors*, edited by A. J. Levine and H. H. Schmidek, pp. 341–355. Wiley-Liss, Inc., New York, 1993.

44. Lane, D. P. p53, guardian of the genome. *Nature 358*:15–16, 1992.

45. Lane, D. P., and Crawford, L. V. T antigen is bound to a host protein in SV40-transformed cells. *Nature 278*:261–263, 1979.

46. Leach, F. S., *et al.* Mutations of a mutS homolog in hereditary nonpolyposis colorectal cancer. *Cell 75*:1215–1225, 1993.

47. Levine, A. J., Perry, M. E., Chang, A., *et al.* The 1993 Walter Hubert Lecture: The role of the p53 tumour-suppressor gene in tumorigenesis. *Br. J. Cancer 69*:409–416, 1994.

48. Liang, B. C., Ross, D. A., Greenberg, H. S., Meltzer, P. S., and Trent, J. M., Evidence of allelic imbalance of chromosome 6 in human astrocytomas. *Neurol. 44*:533–536, 1994.

49. Libermann, T. A., Nusbaum, H. R., Razon, N., *et al.* Amplification, enhanced expression, and possible rearrangement of EGF receptor gene in primary human brain tumors of glial origin. *Nature 313*:144–147, 1985.

50. Linzer, D. I. H., and Levine, A. J. Characterization of a 54K dalton cellular SV40 tumor antigen present in SV40-transformed cells and uninfected embryonal carcinoma cells. *Cell 17*:43–52, 1979.

51. Livingstone, L. R., White, A., Sprouse, J., *et al.* Altered cell cycle arrest and gene amplification potential accompany loss of wild-type p53. *Cell 70*:923–935, 1992.

52. Louis, D. N., Seizinger, B. R., and Cavenee, W. K. Molecular genetic basis of cerebral gliomas. In: *Benign Cerebral Glioma*, edited by M. L. J. Apuzzo, pp. 163–180. American Association of Neurological Surgeons, Park Ridge, IL, 1995.

53. Louis, D. N., von Deimling, A., Chung, R. Y., *et al.* Comparative study of p53 gene and protein alterations in human astrocytic tumors. *J. Neuropath. Exp. Neurol. 52*:31–38, 1993.

54. Lowe, S. W., Bodis, S., McClatchey, A., *et al.* p53 status and the efficacy of cancer therapy in vivo. *Science 266*:807–810, 1994.

55. Marshall, C. J. How does p21^{ras} transform cells? *Trends Genet. 7*:91–95, 1991.

56. Marshall, C. J. Specificity of receptor tyrosine kinase signaling: transient versus sustained extracellular signal-regulated kinas eactivation. *Cell 80*:179–185, 1995.

57. Maxwell, M., Naber, S. P., Wolfe, J. F., *et al.* Coexpression of PDGF and PDGF-receptor genes by primary human astrocytomas may contribute to their development and maintenance. *J. Clin. Invest. 86*:131–140, 1990.

58. Mercer, W. E., Shields, M. T., Amin, M., *et al.* Negative growth regulation in a glioblastoma tumor cell line that conditionally expresses human wild-type p53. *Proc. Natl. Acad. Sci. U.S.A. 87*:6166–6170, 1990.

59. Mikkelsen, T., Cairncross, J. G., and Cavenee, W. K. Genetics of the malignant progression of astrocytoma. *J. Cell. Biochem. 46*:3–8, 1991.

60. Millauer, B., Shawver, L. K., Plate, K. H., *et al.* Glioblastoma growth inhibited in vivo by a dominant-negative Flk-1 mutant. *Nature 367*:576–579, 1994.

61. Modrich, P. Mismatch repair, genetic stability, and cancer. *Science 266*:1959–1960, 1994.

62. Mori, T., *et al.* Germ-line and somatic mutations of the APC gene in patients with Turcot syndrome and analysis of APC mutations in brain tumors. *Genes Chrom. Cancer 9*:168–172, 1994.

63. Nishikawa, R., Ji, X. D., Harmon, R. C., *et al.* A mutant epidermal growth factor receptor common in human glioma confers enhanced tumorigenicity. *Proc. Natl. Acad. Sci. U.S.A. 91*:7727–7731, 1994.

64. Nister, M., Claesson-Welsh, L., Eriksson, A., *et al.* Differential expression of platelet derived growth factor receptors in human malignant glioma cell lines. *J. Biol. Chem. 266*:16755–16763, 1991.

65. Ostrowski, L. E., von Wronski, M. A., Bigner, S. H., *et al.* Expression of O6-methylguanine-DNA meth-

yltransferase in malignant human glioma cell lines. *Carcinogenesis 12:*1739–1744, 1991.

66. Parson, R., Li, G., Longley, M. J., *et al.* Hypermutability and mismatch repair deficiency in RER+ tumor cells. *Cell 75:*1227–1236, 1993.

67. Paulus, W., Baur, I., Schuppan, D., and Roggendorf, W. Characterization of integrin receptors in normal and neoplastic human brain. *Am. J. Path. 143:*154–163, 1993.

68. Paulus, W., and Tonn, J. C. Basement membrane invasion of glioma cells mediated by integrin receptors. *J. Neurosurg. 80:*515–519, 1994.

69. Peltomaki, P., *et al.* Genetic mapping of a locus predisposing to human colorectal cancer. *Science 260:* 810–812, 1993.

70. Pershouse, M. A., Stubblefield, E., Hadi, A., *et al.* Analysis of the functional role of chromosome 10 loss in human glioblastomas. *Cancer Res. 53:*5043–5050, 1993.

71. Plate, K. H., Breier, G., Weich, H. A., *et al.* Vascular endothelial growth factor and glioma angiogenesis: coordinate induction of VEGF receptors, distribution of VEGF protein and possible in vivo regulatory mechanisms. *Int. J. Cancer 59:*520–529, 1994.

72. Ransom, D. T., Ritland, S. R., Moertel, C. A., *et al.* Correlation of cytogenetic analysis and loss of heterozygosity studies in human diffuse astrocytomas and mixed oligo-astrocytomas. *Genes Chrom. Cancer 5:*357–374, 1992.

73. Rasheed, B. K. A., Fuller, G. N., Friedman, A. H., *et al.* Loss of heterozygosity for 10q loci in human gliomas. *Genes Chrom. Cancer 5:*75–82, 1992.

74. Ridley, A. J., Paterson, H. F., Noble, M., and Land, H. ras-mediated cell cycle arrest is altered by nuclear oncogenes to induce schwann cell transformation. *EMBO J. 7:*1635–1645, 1988.

75. Rubio, M., Correa, K. M., Ramesh, V., *et al.* Analysis of the neurofibromatosis 2 gene in human ependymomas and astrocytomas. *Cancer Res. 54:*45–47, 1994.

76. Rutka, J. T., Apodaca, G., Stern, R., and Rosenblum, M. The extracellular matrix of the central and peripheral nervous systems: structure and function. *J. Neurosurg. 69:*155–170, 1988.

77. Schechter, A. L., Stern, D. F., Vaidyanathan, L., *et al.* The neu oncogene: an erb-B-related gene encoding a 185,000-M_r tumour antigen. *Nature 312:*513–516, 1984.

78. Schlessinger, J. SH2/SH3 signaling proteins. *Curr. Opin. Genet. Dev. 4:*25–30, 1994.

79. Schmidt, E. E., Ichimura, K., Reifenberger, G., and Collins, V. P. CDKN2 (p16/MTS1) gene deletion or CDK4 amplification occurs in the majority of glioblastomas. *Cancer Res. 54:*6321–6324, 1994.

80. Schoenberg, B. S. Epidemiology of primary intracranial neoplasms: disease distribution and risk factors. In: *Neurobiology of Brain Tumors*, edited by M. Salcman, pp. 3–18. Williams & Wilkins, Baltimore, MD, 1991.

81. Schwartz, M. A., and Ingber, D. E. Integrating with integrins. *Mole. Biol. Cell 5:*389–393, 1994.

82. Schwechheimer, K., Laufle, R. M., Schmahl, W., *et al.* Expression of Neu/c-erbB-2 in human brain tumors. *Hum. Pathol. 25:*772–780, 1994.

83. Serrano, M., Hannon, G. J., and Beach, D. A new regulatory motif in cell-cycle control causing specific inhibition of cyclinD/CDK4. *Nature 366:*704–707, 1993.

84. Shamah, S. M., Stiles, C. D., and Guha, A. Dominant-negative mutants of platelet-derived growth factor revert the transformed phenotype of human astrocytoma cells. *Molec. Cell. Biol. 13:*7203–7212, 1993.

85. Sherr, C. J. Mammalian G1 cyclins. *Cell 73:*1059–1065, 1993.

86. Sidransky, D., Mikkelsen, T., Schwechheimer, K., *et al.* Clonal expansion of p53 mutant cells is associated with brain tumour progression. *Nature 355:* 846–847, 1992.

87. Silber, J. R., Mueller, B. A., Ewers, T. G., and Berger, M. S. Comparison of O6-methylguanine-DNA methyltransferase activity in brain tumors and adjacent normal brain. *Cancer Res. 53:*3416–3420, 1993.

88. Slamon, D. J., Godolphin, W., Jones, L. A., *et al.* Studies of the HER-2/neu proto-oncogene in human breast and ovarian cancer. *Science 244:*707–712, 1989.

89. Sugawa, N., Ekstrand, A. J., James, C. D., and Collins, V. P. Identical splicing of aberrant epidermal growth factor receptor transcripts from amplified rearranged genes in human glioblastomas. *Proc. Natl. Acad. Sci. U.S.A. 87:*8602–8606, 1990.

90. Thibodeau, S. N., Bren, G., and Schaid, D. Microsatellite instability in cancer of the proximal colon. *Science 260:*816–819, 1993.

91. Trofatter, J. A., *et al.* A novel moesin-, ezrin-, radixin-like gene is a candidate for the neurofibromatosis 2 tumor suppressor gene. *Cell 72:*791–800, 1993.

92. Tsai, J. C., Goldman, C. K., and Gillespie, G. Y. VEGF in human glioma cell lines: induced secretion by EGF, PDGF-BB and bFGF. *J. Neurosurg. 82:*864–873, 1995.

93. Ueki, K., Rubio, M., Ramesh, V., *et al.* MTS1/CDKN2 gene mutations are rare in primary human astrocytomas with allelic loss of chromosome 9p. *Hum. Mol. Genet. 3:*1841–1845, 1994.

94. van Meir, E. G., Roemer, K., Diserens, A., *et al.* Single cell monitoring of growth arrest and morphological changes induced by transfer of wild-type p53 alleles to glioblastoma cells. *Proc. Natl. Acad. Sci. U.S.A. 92:*1008–1012, 1995.

95. Vogelstein, B., and Kinzler, K. W. p53 function and dysfunction. *Cell 70:*523–526, 1992.

96. von Deimling, A., Eibl, R. H., Ohgaki, H., *et al.* p53 mutations are associated with 17p allelic loss in grade II and grade III astrocytoma. *Cancer Res. 52:*2987–2990, 1992.

97. von Deimling, A., Louis, D. N., von Ammon, K., *et al.* Association of epidermal growth factor receptor gene amplification with loss of chromosome 10 in human glioblastoma multiforme. *J. Neurosurg. 77:* 295–301, 1992.

98. von Deimling, A., Louis, D. N., von Ammon, K., *et al.* Evidence for a tumor suppressor gene on chromosome 19q associated with human astrocytomas, oligodendrogliomas and mixed gliomas. *Cancer Res. 52:*4277–4279, 1992.

99. von Deimling, A., von Ammon, K., Schoenfeld, D., *et*

al. Subsets of glioblastoma multiforme defined by molecular genetic analysis. *Brain Pathol. 3:*19–26, 1993.

100. Wagner, B. J., and Cochran, B. H. Growth factors: the PDGF paradigm, In: *Molecular Genetics of Nervous System Tumors,* edited by A. J. Levine, and H. H. Schmidek, pp. 101–122. Wiley-Liss, Inc., New York, NY, 1993.

101. Walker, D. G., Wei, D., Popovic, E. A., *et al.* Homozygous deletions of the multiple tumor suppressor gene 1 in the progression of human astrocytomas. *Cancer Res. 55:*20–23, 1995.

102. Wong, A. J., Bigner, S. H., Bigner, D. D., *et al.* Increased expression of the EGF receptor gene in malignant gliomas is invariably associated with gene amplification. *Proc. Natl. Acad. Sci. U.S.A. 84:*6899–6903, 1987.

103. Wooster, R., Cleton-Jansen, A. M., Mangion, J., *et al.* Instability of short tandem repeats (microsatellites) in human cancers. *Nature Genet. 6:*152–156, 1994.

104. Yin, Y., Tainsky, M. A., Bischoff, F. Z., *et al.* Wild-type p53 restores cell cycle control and inhibits gene amplification in cells with mutant p53 alleles. *Cell 70:*937–948, 1992.

CHAPTER 11

Molecular Effects of Ionizing Radiation

NALIN GUPTA, M.D., DENNIS F. DEEN, Ph.D.,
and PHILIP H. GUTIN, M.D.

INTRODUCTION

During the past century, medical physicists have developed a number of radiation sources for diagnostic imaging and therapy. Radiation is currently used to treat central nervous system neoplasia and arteriovenous malformations. Most patients who develop a malignant glioma or cerebral metastasis receive external-beam radiotherapy. The development and dissemination of technologies such as stereotactic radiosurgery, interstitial brachytherapy, and boron neutron capture therapy are increasing the number of patients receiving radiation therapy. The widespread use of ionizing radiation to treat neurosurgical disease and the development of novel radiation-based therapies necessitates increased understanding of molecular radiobiology by neurosurgeons.

The study of radiation biology can be divided into questions regarding its physics, chemistry, molecular biology, and cell biology: (1) the initial deposition of energy within the cell, (2) the subsequent chemical alterations of biological molecules, (3) the activation of intracellular signaling pathways following chemical changes, and (4) the consequences of these events upon cells—i.e., cell-cycle perturbations, apoptosis, cellular repair, and survival. The chemistry of many types of radiation-induced damage is known at the molecular level in some detail, and the effect of radiation upon cell growth and proliferation is fairly well described. However, until the advent of modern molecular techniques, virtually all of the intervening steps between the initial induction of damage and the cellular effect remained obscure. Molecular biology provides the tools with which to define the pathways that connect the initial effects of radiation to nuclear events such as gene expression.

This chapter will discuss the basic physics and chemistry of radiation damage in biological systems and present evidence that DNA double-strand breaks are the critical lesions in radiation-induced cell death. Some of the signal transduction pathways affected by ionizing radiation will be described, particularly those regulating the cell cycle and apoptosis. Possible mechanisms of radiation-induced oncogenesis will also be discussed.

RADIATION BIOPHYSICS

Interaction of ionizing radiation with biological material results in energy deposition unevenly within the target volume. Electromagnetic radiation—i.e., an x-ray beam—can be regarded as a wave function, as well as a stream of photons carrying discrete packets, or quanta, of energy. If the energy carried by a photon either breaks or modifies covalent bonds in intracellular molecules, biological effects may ensue. The energy of individual quanta is determined by $h\upsilon$, where h is Planck's constant and υ is the frequency of the radiation. Ionizing radiations differ from nonionizing radiations, such as heat or UV radiation, not in the total energy delivered, but in the energy of individual quanta. Most quanta of nonionizing radiations have insufficient energy to modify covalent bonds. Energy deposition raises electrons to higher energy levels and may result in ejection of electrons if the photon energy exceeds the electron binding energy. Accelerated particles, protons, and neutrons, are also used therapeutically. By virtue of their particulate nature, these radiations deposit energy in discrete volumes and set in motion other particles such as protons and α-particles.

A specific type of radiation produces biological effects only if some of its energy is absorbed by the medium through which it passes. The physical unit of absorbed dose, the Gray (Gy), is equivalent to 1 joule/kg of tissue. Different types of radiation, e.g., neutrons versus x-rays, produce dramatically different effects upon tissue. One factor that contributes to this difference is linear energy transfer (LET), the energy transferred to the medium as a function of track length. Particulate radiations, in general, impart greater energy to a medium for a given distance than do electromagnetic radiations. Consequently, proton and neutron beams are regarded as high LET radiations. Relative Biological Effectiveness (RBE) of a form of radiation relates the magnitude of its biologic effect to that of a reference type of radiation. It is calculated as the ratio of the dose of the reference radiation (usually ^{60}Co γ-rays) to the dose of the radiation being measured that produces an equivalent biological effect.

X-rays, γ-rays, and accelerated particles are all ionizing radiations. Electromagnetic radiations are considered to be ionizing if they have photon energies in excess of 124 eV. Any form of ionizing radiation, however, may interact with a vital target, e.g., DNA, creating ions and subsequent chemical modifications. This is the *direct* action of radiation. This mechanism predominates for particulate radiation (protons, neutrons, or α-particles). For example, a neutron will collide with the nucleus of an atom in the absorbing material to produce nuclear products such as recoil protons. Some authorities believe that direct action causes most biologically significant damage (100). Others believe the interaction of a photon with orbital electrons of the absorbing intracellular medium, water in biological samples, is most important. This interaction ejects fast electrons from outer shells. Multiple ionizations occur along the tracks of these electrons. These ions generate free radicals that damage intracellular molecules. This *indirect* action of radiation is the predominant one for x-rays and γ-rays (Fig. 1). Using free radical scavengers such as dimethyl sulfoxide,

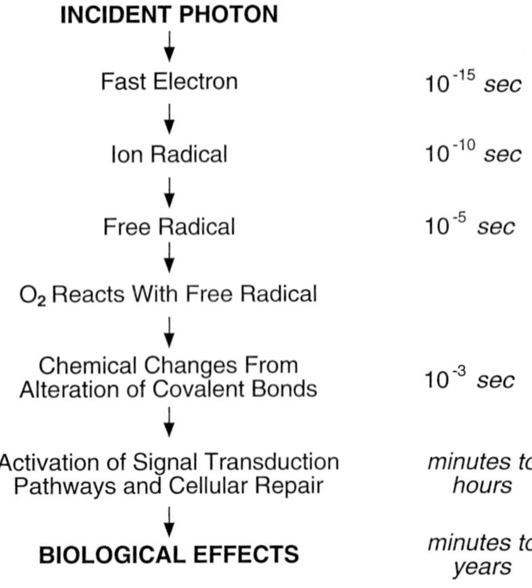

Figure 1. The course of events leading from the initial ionization event of ionizing radiation to final biological effects. The resistance of hypoxic cells to ionizing radiation reflects the absence of molecular oxygen (O$_2$). O$_2$ "fixes" the production of damage by reactions that convert free radicals to stable species. (Adapted from Hall, E. J. *Radiobiology for the Radiologist*. 4th ed. J. B. Lippincott, Philadelphia, 1994.)

Ward estimated that 65% of single-strand breaks (SSB) in chromosomal DNA are formed from OH free radicals (206). The time course of these early events is extremely rapid. The initial ionization occurs in 10^{-15} seconds. Ion radicals and free radicals exist for only 10^{-10} to 10^{-5} seconds. Cell death resulting from radiation-induced chemical alterations may not occur for hours or days, and genetic changes may not be apparent for generations. For more information, the reader is referred to Hall's excellent text (66) for a review of radiation biology and Spinks and Woods' text for a detailed description of radiation chemistry (186).

DNA AS THE TARGET FOR IONIZING RADIATION

One of the dogmas of radiation biology stipulates that damage to DNA is the critical determinant of radiation-induced cell death. Although radiation produces ionizations randomly throughout the cell, damage to other cellular components, such as proteins, mRNA, and lipids, is thought to be relatively insignificant because many copies of these components exist and damaged molecules are rapidly replaced by new synthesis. Ionizing radiation damage to the plasma membrane, however, can activate a cascade of signaling pathways that alter gene transcription and induce cell death in some cell types.

Early experiments used ionizing particles with a limited range to selectively irradiate the nucleus or the cytoplasm (131) and assessed survival as an endpoint. Cells whose cytoplasm was selectively irradiated tolerated ten times the radiation dose tolerated by cells that received mainly nuclear irradiation. This suggested that damage to a nuclear target has a far greater impact on cell survival than damage to cytoplasm. In other experiments using more convincing methodology, cells that incorporated a radioactive DNA precursor, ^{125}I-iododeoxyuridine, were two orders of magnitude more sensitive to decay events than cells treated with a compound (^{125}I-labeled concavalin A) that localizes to the cell membrane (210). Furthermore, sensitization to ionizing radiation occurs after cells incorporate halogenated pyrimidines in their DNA (190).

Later studies showed that the major types of lesions caused by ionizing radiations such as x-rays and γ-rays are DNA base damage, DNA-DNA or DNA-protein crosslinks, and scissions of the DNA phosphodiester backbone leading to

SSB or double-strand breaks (DSB) (54, 79, 171, 201). Lesions are characterized as being simple—i.e., with no damage to neighboring groups, or complex—where combinations of lesions or multiple lesions exist (205, 208). These represent only broad categories of lesions since the exact chemical changes are extremely diverse. It is unlikely that these different types of damage are repaired with equal efficiency or fidelity. The challenge is to identify and study the lesions that lead to biologically significant effects. Often, determination of the significance of the lesion is limited by the inability to quantitate the degree of damage.

DNA DSB are the type of injury most critical to radiation-induced cell death. DSB are formed either by cooperation of two SSB or a single event that injures both strands. The latter creates a *local multiply damaged site* (205, 207) and is the more important type of lesion. Assays used to measure DNA DSB are listed in Table 1 and are discussed in several reviews (79, 28, 215). Using different methodologies, these assays measure the degree of DNA fragmentation that occurs after ionizing radiation. They demonstrate a strong correlation between DNA DSB and cell killing. Nonrejoined DNA breaks, as measured by alkaline sucrose gradients, correlate well with cell killing (148, 172). In certain yeast strains unable to repair DNA DSB, there

TABLE 1
Assays Used to Measure DNA DSB[a]

Assay	Technical Principle	Disadvantages
Comet	DSB allow for greater migration of DNA from individual cells in thin agarose gels	Technically difficult with cell-to-cell heterogeneity requiring many measurements
DNA precipitation	DNA fragments have different solubility	Poor reproducibility
End tailing	Site of strand break labeled by radionuclides	Poor reproducibility
Halo	Damaged chromatin rewinds less when PI concentration is increased	Time-consuming, difficult to quantify, and majority of lesions detected are SSB
Neutral filter elution	Larger fragments of DNA elute slowly through a filter membrane	Variations in DNA conformation, cell cycle phase and pH affect results
PFGE	Mobility of high molecular weight DNA in agarose gel is determined by DNA relaxation and reorientation rates	DNA conformation alters results
Sucrose velocity sedimentation	Larger DNA fragments sediment further in a sucrose gradient	Genomic DNA causes anomalous results

Adapted from Whitaker, S. J., Powell, S. N., and McMillan, T. J. Eur. J. Cancer, *27:*922–928, 1991.
[a] DSB, double strand breaks; PFGE, pulsed-field gel electrophoresis; PI, propidium iodide; SSB, single strand breaks.

TABLE 2
Phenotypes Observed with Homozygous Defects in the AT Gene

Progressive cerebellar degeneration (especially of Purkinje
  cells)
Immunological defects:
  Thymic atrophy
  Diminished T cell response
  Recurrent infections
Sensitivity to ionizing radiation
  Increased cell killing
  Increase in specific chromosomal aberrations
  Cell cycle checkpoint abnormalities
  Inappropriate apoptosis
Neoplasia
  Expansion of clonal lymphocyte populations
  Increase in lymphoid leukemias and lymphomas
Telangiectasia of bulbar conjunctive, ear, face and hands
Premature aging

Adapted from Harnden, D. G. Int. J. Radiat. Biol. *66:*S13–
19, 1994.

is a direct relationship between unrepaired DSB and cell killing. These strains are particularly vulnerable to radiation (55). Restriction enzymes electroporated into cells cause DNA DSB, elevation of p53 levels, and cell cycle perturbations similar to those seen after irradiation (142). This was not observed after treatment with other agents that damage DNA but do not produce DSB. Finally, the incidence of chromosomal aberrations correlates very well with radiation dose (1, 38, 130, 141, 192).

Other lesions are not as important. DNA SSB increase in proportion to radiation dose and are caused by hydroxyl radicals (91, 123, 124). The induction of SSB, however, does not correlate with cell killing (207, 209). DNA-protein crosslinks (DPC) result from covalent bonding of DNA to nuclear matrix proteins (26, 219). DPC do not contribute to radiation-induced cell killing. DPC do occur during the normal growth of unirradiated cells, but they are cleared efficiently (144). Radiation produces only 150 DPC per Gy in hamster V79 cells (169). Under hypoxic conditions where radioresistance is observed, the number of DPC is increased (52). Damaged bases are removed from eukaryotic cells by two mechanisms: nucleotide excision repair (NER), which is best suited for repair of UV-induced damage (30), and base excision repair (BER), which efficiently repairs x-ray-induced base damage (204). As with DPC, experimental evidence shows no correlation between the amount of base damage and 1)

hypoxic protection, 2) hyperthermic enhancement of radiation-induced cell killing, or 3) cellular radiosensitivity (156, 166).

PRIMARY MOLECULAR EVENTS

The cellular events caused by ionizing radiation are collectively referred to as the radiation stress response, akin to the stress responses that follow heat shock, hypoxia, or nutrient depletion (211). The initial deposition of energy in living cells produces chemical changes within a nanosecond. These chemical changes quickly activate cellular enzymes and second messengers (68, 69). These enzymes and second messengers eventually modulate the expression of early response genes, mostly transcription factors, that cause secondary effects by inducing or repressing the expression of other genes. The immediate responses can be divided into 1) DNA repair, 2) activation of tyrosine kinase signal transduction pathways, and 3) induction of the early response genes. These events are studied with assays that measure the appropriate endpoints—i.e., DNA DSB, tyrosine kinase activity, and protein and mRNA expression, respectively.

DNA Repair

Clonogenic assays have shown that cells can recover from radiation-induced damage if progression through the cell cycle is inhibited (105, 159). This phenomenon is called potentially lethal damage repair (PLDR); its kinetics are determined by measuring repair of DNA DSB. PLDR has two phases: one is very rapid ($t_{1/2}$ of 2–20 minutes), and a subsequent one is quite slow ($t_{1/2}$ of 1–3 hours) (75, 78, 80, 105). The vast majority of DNA DSB are rejoined during the fast phase of PLDR (Fig. 2). It is likely that the initial phase is completed by constitutively active enzymes such as DNA ligase or polymerase. "Rejoining" does not imply that DNA double-stranded helices are being repaired accurately. Improperly rejoined DNA DSB result in chromosomal aberrations and mutations. All of the current assays for DNA DSB, however, are based upon differences in the size of DNA molecules and measure total rejoining rather than the fidelity of this process. The proteins that identify radiation-induced DNA template changes and control the rapid and slow phases of repair are unknown.

A) Dose Response

B) Repair Kinetics

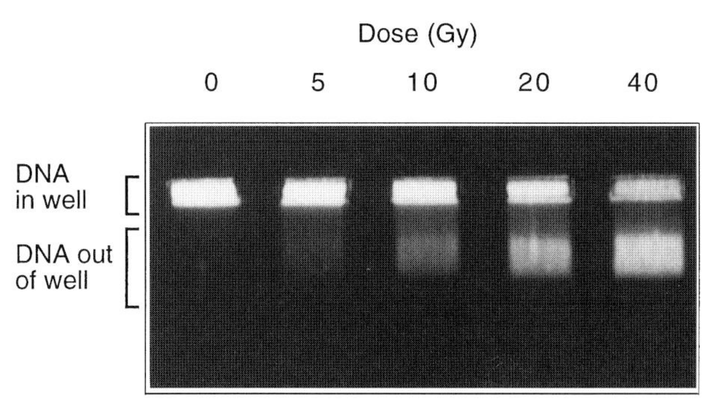

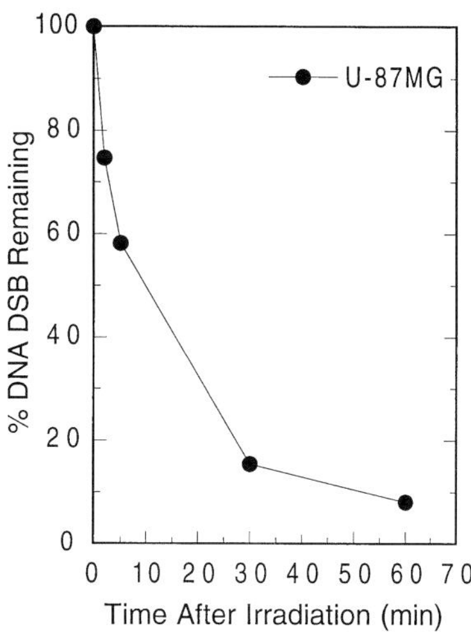

Figure 2. A) The results of a pulsed field gel electrophoresis (PFGE) experiment are shown. DNA extracted from cells treated with increasing doses of radiation is loaded into wells at the top of the gel and run under electrophoretic conditions (from top to bottom) that allow the separation of large molecular weight fragments. A clear dose response is seen with larger amounts of DNA migrating out of the well with higher doses. The gel is a standard ethidium bromide stained agarose gel photographed under UV light. B) A plot of DNA repair kinetics obtained by quantifying the amount of DNA that migrates out of a well when dose is kept constant (30 Gy) but repair time is varied from 0 time to 60 minutes. There is an initial fast component of repair followed by a slower component. (Photograph and data for plot provided by J. Wang, Ph.D., UCSF).

Cytoplasmic Signal Transduction Pathways

Cytoplasmic signaling pathways are also involved in the cellular response to ionizing radiation. These pathways are normally activated by transmembrane events, i.e., an extracellular growth factor binds to a transmembrane receptor that activates associated intracellular molecules. Intermediate components of the pathway transmit and amplify the signal. The final components enter the nucleus to effect expression or repression of specific genes. Several signal transduction pathways are well characterized. One contains protein kinase C (PKC), which regulates expression of the *c-jun* proto-oncogene, a transcription factor. The PKC pathway is likely involved in the radiation stress response (68, 69). Phorbol ester depletion of PKC or H7 inhibition of kinase activity abolishes the induction of c-JUN and EGR-1 expression that follows irradiation. Peak PKC activity occurs only 30 seconds after irradiation and returns to baseline after 1 minute. Significant gene expres-

sion and protein translation are unlikely to occur in this interval.

Uckun and colleagues, using human B-lymphocytes to study early signal transduction events after irradiation (195, 196), have demonstrated that tyrosine kinase activity is required for radiation-induced apoptosis and activation of a PKC pathway. Tyrosine kinase inhibitors (genistein and herbimycin) prevented activation of PKC following irradiation. Other kinase pathways are involved in the response to ionizing radiation (87, 88). A member of the Src family of tyrosine kinases, $p56/p53^{lyn}$, is activated and associated with a cell-cycle protein, CDC2, following irradiation. Since $p56/p53^{lyn}$ is a cytoplasmic protein, this suggests that some radiation-induced cell-cycle perturbations may be caused, or at least modified, by purely cytoplasmic events.

Early Response Genes

Many early response genes code for transcription factors. Transcription factors are proteins that function by regulating the expression of other genes. This process is mediated by a protein domain that binds to specific DNA sequences, usually upstream of the regulated genes. A second domain interacts with elements of the RNA transcriptional machinery, such as RNA polymerase II, resulting in increased transcription.

Expression of the JUN transcription factor is induced by ionizing and ultraviolet irradiation (37, 182). JUN and another protein, FOS, form a heterodimer, AP-1, that regulates the expression of a large number of genes (35, 157). At baseline, the activity of AP-1 is prevented by a repressor protein. Following irradiation, the repressor protein disassociates from AP-1 and transcriptional activation occurs (67). The AP-1 repressor, in effect, keeps a set of genes "poised" for transcription once the appropriate stimulus—i.e., irradiation—arises. Other transcription factors induced after ionizing radiation include NF-κB, EGR-1, and p53 (17, 68, 83, 195). The function of the NF-κB and EGR-1 transcription factors following ionizing radiation is unclear.

Boothman and colleagues used two-dimensional gel electrophoresis to identify eight major polypeptides, called XIPs or x-ray-induced proteins, whose levels in U1-Mel malignant melanoma cells were increased five- to tenfold following ionizing radiation (16). Because induction of these proteins is delayed until 4 to 5 hours after irradiation, XIPs may be involved in the slow phase of DNA repair (120). The identity and function of the XIPs are unknown.

SECONDARY EVENTS

Cell Cycle Checkpoints

Basic Principles

The cell cycle is the basic plan that virtually all eukaryotic cells follow in order to reproduce. The period of DNA replication, the S phase, and mitosis, the M phase, are separated by two gap phases, named G_1 and G_2 (Fig. 3). Although important cellular changes occur during G_1 and G_2, they are preliminary to more important events in S and M phases. During the past 15 years, many of the biochemical mechanisms that account for the precise sequence and timing of cell-cycle events have been identified. Foremost among these is a family of cyclin-depen-

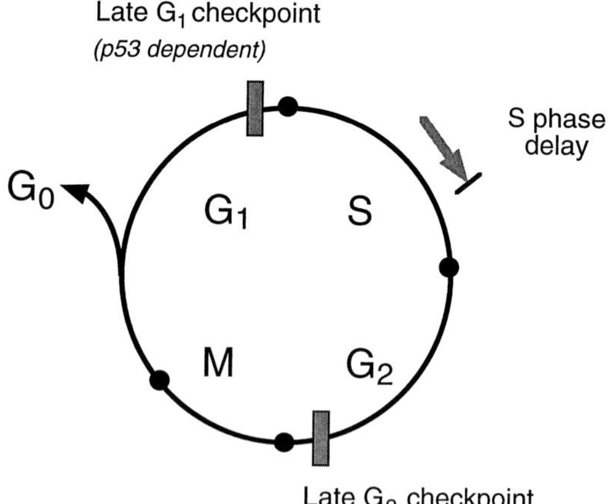

Figure 3. A schematic representation of the cell cycle. The sites where cells commonly arrest in response to ionizing radiation are indicated. In general, the duration of G_1 varies the most between cells of different tissue types while the durations of S, G_2 and M phases are similar for many somatic mammalian cells.

dent protein kinases (CDKs). At various points in the cell cycle, such as entry into mitosis or S phase, the activity of kinases initiates a cascade of events that drives cell-cycle progression. Interpretation of cell-cycle physiology is greatly complicated in eukaryotes by the involvement of associated proteins, such as cyclins, required for proper activity of these kinases. The CDK/cyclin complex is the focal point of the cell cycle. In simple eukaryotes (e.g., yeast), there is only one CDK (called CDC2), whereas in humans there are at least six. There is such conservation of CDK function that human CDC2 protein can replace its equivalent yeast protein (98). Many regulatory pathways converge at the CDKs to produce a dynamic cell cycle responsive to a wide variety of external and internal stimuli. Abnormalities in the control of the cell cycle underlie tumorigenesis (43, 49, 71, 77, 82, 128, 136). This section describes the effect of ionizing radiation on the cell cycle.

Cytokinetic Events After Irradiation

Ionizing radiation (99, 132, 147, 149, 151, 220, 223) interrupts cell-cycle progression from late G_1 into S phase, during S phase, and from late G_2 into M phase (Fig. 3). In a series of classic experiments, Robert Painter, by measuring the percentage of mitotic HeLa cells (the mitotic index) at a number of time points, demonstrated an 8-hour delay in cell division following a 5 Gy dose of ionizing radiation (149) and later showed that this was due to a reduction in the rate of DNA synthesis (147). Terasima and Tolmach found that the delay in division was influenced by the phase of the cell cycle in which irradiation occurred. It was longest for cells in G_2, shortest for cells in G_1, and intermediate for cells in S (191). Leeper subsequently showed that the duration of the G_2 "arrest" was dose-dependent (99). G_1 arrest in some cell types may represent an irreversible block to progression (39).

The point in the cell cycle where arrest occurs is variable and can be modified pharmacologically. Cells whose DNA is damaged by nitrogen mustard usually arrest in G_2 (94, 133). When treated with both nitrogen mustard and caffeine, however, cells continue into mitosis.

Cell-Cycle Checkpoints in Yeast

Much of our understanding of the eukaryotic cell cycle has come from the study of budding yeast, Saccharomyces cerevisiae. S. cerevisiae reproduces by budding at the onset of DNA synthesis. By examining the size of the bud, the approximate position of individual cells in the cell cycle can be assessed. Analyzing live mammalian cells for their position in the cell cycle remains technically difficult.

Normal yeast cells arrest in G_2 following irradiation. Arrest is evident in budded cells that fail to enter mitosis. Those that repair DNA damage progress into M phase after a delay and remain viable. Weinert and Hartwell (214) first attributed delay in cell-cycle progression following ionizing radiation to a specific gene. They screened several radiation-sensitive yeast mutants, designated *rad*, for failure to delay in G_2 following irradiation. Assuming that G_2 delay permits repair before progression into M phase, they reasoned that cells defective for a G_2 delay should be more sensitive to DNA damage. One mutant, *rad^9*, that failed to arrest in G_2 was identified (32). Further characterization of this mutant confirmed that the absence of a G_2 delay led to increased radiation sensitivity and showed that pharmacological induction of a 4-hour G_2 delay increased survival dramatically. Weinert and Hartwell coined the term "checkpoint" to designate a decision point in the cell cycle where specific proteins that monitor cell-cycle progression respond to cell damage

by delaying the cell cycle to provide time for repair.

Murray postulated that components of this control system consists of 1) a sensor to detect damage, 2) a signaling pathway to communicate this information, and 3) a component of the cell-cycle machinery to effect arrest at a precise point, i.e., the checkpoint (137). A large number of genes involved in the response to stimuli, such as unreplicated DNA, damaged DNA, and improper spindle assembly, have been identified in yeast. Much of this work suggests that cellular damage or dysfunction is assessed and repaired during delays at G_2.

G_2 Cell-Cycle Proteins in Mammalian Cells Affected by Ionizing Radiation

Activity of CDC2, the mammalian G_2/M CDK, is required for cells to progress from G_2 into M phase. CDC2 activity is modulated, in turn, by other kinases (128). The total amount of CDC2 protein remains the same throughout the cell cycle, but its association with cyclin B and phosphorylation of critical residues determines the timing of its activity. Rapid dephosphorylation of tyrosine residues at positions 14 and 15 on CDC2 causes activation of the entire CDC2-cyclin B1 complex. Histones and nuclear laminins may be the substrates of this kinase complex. Phosphorylation of these proteins leads to mitotic events such as chromosome condensation and disappearance of the nuclear membrane. Rapid degradation of cyclin B1 then triggers movement from metaphase into anaphase. Mutations of cyclin B1 that interfere with protein degradation effectively arrest cells at the metaphase/anaphase boundary.

The normal biochemistry of the cell cycle is altered by ionizing radiation (113). HeLa cells blocked pharmacologically at the G_1/S boundary and then released into drug-free media remain synchronized for enough time to study cell-cycle phase-specific events. Cells irradiated shortly after release into S phase progress slowly through S phase and demonstrate a prolonged G_2 delay (138). During this delay, cyclin B1 mRNA levels remain low. If cells are irradiated in early G_2, cyclin B1 mRNA levels rise, but protein levels remain low. This indicates that radiation regulates cyclin B levels at both the mRNA and protein level, depending upon the cell cycle phase where irradiation occurs. CDC2 phosphorylation of histone H1 (a measure of its kinase activity) *in vitro* is inhibited rapidly after irradiation (18). There is some evidence that the duration of G_2 delay correlates with increased survival (118, 187). It thus appears that the cell-cycle delay after irradiation permits DNA repair to occur before mitosis.

p53

Structure and Function

The p53 protein was first discovered as a cellular protein that co-precipitated with the SV-40 virus large T-antigen (93). T-antigen and analogous proteins from other viruses disrupt normal cell cycle controls by binding to and inactivating proteins such as p53 that prevent excessive proliferation. p53 is a tumor suppressor gene whose loss or inactivation by mutation can result in tumorigenesis (101, 198, 200). p53 is the most commonly mutated gene in human cancer (64). Knockout mice lacking both copies of the p53 gene are normal at birth but develop tumors, primarily lymphomas and sarcomas, before they reach 6 months of age (42).

The p53 protein is a transcription factor. Loss of regulation of p53-dependent gene expression contributes to cancer initiation and/or progression. Wild-type p53 can also repress transcription by binding to specific DNA sequences. The p53 protein has at least four domains: an amino terminal domain, a core domain, an oligomerization domain, and a carboxy-terminal domain (160). The amino domain contains the site of interaction with transcriptional machinery, the transactivation domain. This site is bound by the cellular protein MDM2 and the adenovirus E1b protein (103). Both of these proteins interfere with the ability of p53 to activate transcription. Excess MDM2 can function as an oncogene by interfering with p53 function (127, 145). Whether this domain is essential for p53 function is unclear. In some studies, the function of the p53 transactivation domain was required for p53-dependent growth suppression (161). In others, p53-dependent apoptosis occurred in the absence of protein or RNA synthesis (21).

The core domain is required for sequence-specific binding of DNA. The 20-base-pair consensus binding site consists of two copies of a 10-bp sequence separated by up to 13 bp (47, 56). The mutations in the core domain commonly found in human tumors block p53's suppression of proliferation by precluding its binding to specific DNA sites (161). The crystal structure of this domain is known and should provide important information about p53 protein-DNA interactions (28). p53 also can bind to DNA in a nonspecific manner and suppress a variety of promoters containing TATA elements (106, 111, 116, 168, 177, 180, 193, 194).

The oligomerization domain is required for p53 to form the tetramer required for efficient binding to DNA sequences. Mutations in this domain interfere with the ability of p53 molecules to form tetramers. When one allele in a cell contains a mutation in this domain and the other is wild-type, p53 function is lost as p53 complexes containing both wild-type and mutant proteins are inactive. Such p53 mutants are "dominant-negative" since only one mutant allele results in a mutant phenotype. This is in contrast with most tumor suppressors that require inactivation of both alleles before a mutant phenotype is produced.

The carboxy-terminal is involved in the non-specific association of p53 to free DNA ends (4, 143). This DNA binding of p53 may be involved in p53 induction by ionizing radiation. Because this carboxy terminus can be deleted without an effect upon growth suppression, it is likely that p53 has multiple functions (161).

p53 and the G_1 Checkpoint

Early studies showing that p53 was a substrate of and associated with CDC2 hinted at the relationship between p53 and the cell cycle (11, 125). A role for p53 in cellular radiation response was first suggested by Kastan's demonstration using immunoprecipitation and flow cytometry that p53 protein levels rise in myeloid leukemia cells (wild-type for p53) after ionizing radiation (83). This response is rapid (1 hour after irradiation) and occurs after relatively low radiation doses (105 cGy). Some cells in G_1 fail to progress into S phase following a 208-cGy radiation dose. Kastan's results provide additional evidence that p53 is involved in the progression of cells from G_1 into S phase (83, 104). Indeed, p53 may connect recognition of DNA damage to the growth arrest at G_1 first described by Little (104).

Experimental evidence from yeast (described above) suggests that a delay in cell-cycle progression before the start of a critical process, such as DNA synthesis or mitosis, allows time for repair of DNA damage (213, 214). If this applies to mammalian cells, two predictions can be made. First, delay at the G_1 checkpoint must be temporary, eventually followed by progression to S phase. Second, cells with wild-type p53 and G_1 delay should manifest enhanced repair, less "fixed" DNA damage, and increased clonogenic survival. There is as yet no definitive proof that the G_1 delay in mammalian cells leads to increased repair of DNA damage (132, 135). Because G_2 delay and radiosensitivity are genetically separate in fission yeast, this might pertain for the G_1 checkpoint in mammalian cells (7).

A number of studies have found that the presence of wild-type p53 is correlated with either unchanged or increased cell killing after irradiation (3, 18, 19, 97). This is not the result expected if the G_1 checkpoint served a protective function. The activation of the G_1 checkpoint in normal human fibroblasts (wild-type p53) leads to a prolonged, and presumably permanent, G_1 arrest that resembles senescence (39). This clearly suggests that in certain situations, the function of the G_1 checkpoint is not to allow repair before entry into S phase but to prevent the growth of damaged cells. Furthermore, these findings have implications for targeting cell cycle events with cancer therapy. If the G_1 arrest proves to be a generalized phenomenon, it may represent a desirable endpoint in the treatment of malignant cells.

p53 Regulated Genes

Identification of p53 as a transcription factor induced by irradiation begs the question: which genes are controlled by p53? Identification of p53 regulated genes should increase understanding of p53's function and identify therapeutic opportunities. Two genes regulated by p53 (*WAF1/CIP1* and *GADD45*) are involved in pathways activated by DNA damage. p53 also regulates expression of genes encoding other proteins, such as P-glycoprotein (responsible for the multidrug resistance phenotype) and some growth factors (FGF and EGF) (36, 61, 197).

Using subtractive hybridization, a p53-inducible gene, *WAF1* or *CIP1*, that suppressed tumor growth *in vitro* was identified (48, 65, 70). This gene has at least one p53 binding site upstream of the coding sequence. The protein encoded by the gene, a phosphatase-designated p21$^{WAF1/}$

CIP1 or just *WAF1/CIP1*, is a potent inhibitor of several CDKs and delays progression through the cell cycle (217). *WAF1/CIP1* induction follows the induction of p53 by ionizing radiation and precedes a G_1 arrest (46). This constitutes a direct link between p53 induction and a well defined cell-cycle event (Fig. 4). There are likely to be many other pathways that control cell cycle inhibitors such as *WAF1/CIP1*.

The *GADD* (Growth Arrest and DNA Damage-inducible) genes were isolated by virtue of the increase in their mRNA that follows DNA damage or other stimuli that produce growth arrest (53). One of these genes, *GADD45*, is strongly induced after x-irradiation (155). Using a variety of cell lines, including those from patients with ataxia telanglectasia (AT), Kastan and colleagues determined that *GADD45* is not induced in cells lacking the AT and/or p53 genes (84). These results strongly suggest a linear connection leading from the AT protein to p53 to *GADD45*. DNA binding assays have confirmed that p53 binds to a putative p53 consensus site within an intron of the *GADD45* gene.

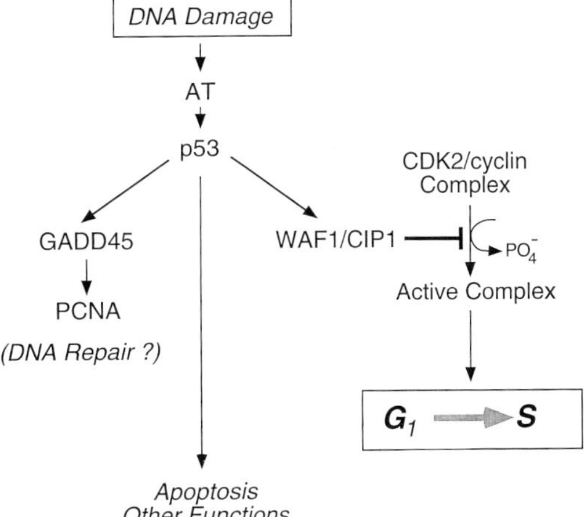

Figure 4. A proposed model of a signal transduction pathway leading from DNA damage, via p53, to a variety of responses. The exact response observed, i.e., apoptosis or cell cycle arrest, is often dependent upon the cell type studied and the exact nature and extent of DNA damage. There are probably many other components that regulate the proteins depicted, as well as other pathway that are, as yet, undiscovered. As an example, the AT protein is involved in other cellular functions besides cell cycle control but the pathways leading to them are unknown.

GADD45 is involved in nucleotide excision repair (NER). NER is the identification, removal, and replacement of a damaged nucleotide using information of the complementary strand (30, 176). This process requires at least 17 polypeptides and is best characterized in the removal of UV-induced base damage. Three human diseases arise from defects in NER: xeroderma pigmentosa, Cockayne's syndrome, and trichothiodystrophy. The cellular protein, proliferating cell nuclear antigen (PCNA), is involved in both DNA replication and repair (112, 162, 163). PCNA associates with DNA polymerases δ and ϵ and is required for NER (184). *GADD45* associates with PCNA and, when added in excess to an *in vitro* assay, promotes NER (185). These findings establish a connection between the p53/GADD45 pathway and DNA NER. A complicating finding from other studies is that *WAF1/CIP1*, the CDK inhibitor, inhibits DNA replication through an interaction with PCNA without affecting PCNA-dependent repair of DNA (25, 102, 183, 203, 218, 225). The degree of overlap between the NER and DNA DSB repair following ionizing radiation is unknown.

Apoptosis

Apoptosis is a form of cell death with morphological and biochemical features that differ from those of acute necrosis (85, 167, 216). Necrosis is characterized by cell swelling, cell lysis, and often an inflammatory response. In apoptosis, there is cell shrinkage, chromatin condensation, nuclear blebbing, nonrandom DNA fragmentation, and rapid phagocytosis by macrophages. Apoptosis differs from other types of cell death by requiring newly synthesized proteins.

Information about apoptosis is changing established views regarding radiation-induced cell killing. In older studies, dead, irradiated cells were described as having undergone either a "reproductive" death or an "interphase" death. Reproductive death is the inability of a single cell to produce a colony of at least 50 cells. This is usually measured by the standard clonogenic assay. It is attributed to the formation of chromosomal aberrations that prevent successful mitoses (9, 164, 165). Interphase death refers to impairment of cellular function and loss of cell integrity prior to mitosis. It resembles apoptosis.

Apoptosis in C. elegans

The clearest experimental evidence for the genetic basis of apoptosis comes from studies in the nematode Caenorhabditis elegans. In this organism, a precisely defined number of cells (exactly 131) normally undergo cell death during development. A pair of genes, *ced-3* and *ced-4*, is required for cell death to occur. If either one of these genes is mutated, the cells that usually undergo apoptosis fail to do so (224). Conversely, another gene, *ced-9*, limits apoptosis. Its absence leads to the death of many cells that otherwise survive (72). *ced-3* is homologous to the mammalian gene encoding interleukin-1 β-converting enzyme (ICE). Overexpression of either *ced-3* or murine ICE in a rodent cell line induces apoptosis. *ced-9* is homologous to the human oncogene bcl-2 that prevents apoptosis (73). Thus, apoptosis is genetically conserved in divergent organisms. During development, when cell proliferation is maximal, apoptosis eliminates superfluous cells and those that might interfere with further growth and differentiation. Cells in which apoptosis is prevented by the action of certain oncogenes (such as *bcl-2*) may generate tumors.

p53 and Apoptosis

p53 functions as a tumor suppressor by inducing apoptosis in deviant cells. Transfection of cells in culture with wild-type p53 blocks their proliferation (5, 40, 121) and induces apoptosis in leukemia and colon cancer cell lines (181, 222). In knockout mice homozygous for a p53 deletion, the absence of p53 protects thymocytes against apoptosis engendered by ionizing radiation but not by phorbol esters (that mimic T-cell receptor engagement) or glucocorticoids (29, 109). Fifty percent of wild-type thymocytes lost viability after 2.5 Gy, while only 20% of cells lacking p53 lost viability after a much higher dose of radiation (20 Gy). These data support the hypothesis that p53 is a member of a pathway that links the detection of cellular damage, such as DNA DSB, to prevention of proliferation by inducing apoptosis.

The occurrence of apoptosis seems to depend upon the cell type involved. In an experiment using p53-null or p53-heterozygous knockout mice, expression of a mutated form of the SV40 large T antigen that binds the Rb tumor suppressor protein but not p53 produced aggressive choroid-plexus tumors in the null mice (189).

This is not surprising given that two tumor suppressor proteins are either nonfunctional (Rb) or absent (p53). In p53 wild-type mice, however, the choroid-plexus epithelial cells were frequently apoptotic, indicating elimination of excessively proliferating epithelial cells. Focal tumors that arose in p53-heterozygous mice had lost the remaining p53 allele and demonstrated decreased levels of apoptosis. The differential responses of different tumor types to various forms of therapy may reflect different tendencies to undergo apoptosis (51).

GENETIC BASIS OF RADIOSENSITIVITY

Ataxia-Telangiectasia

Genetic Features

Ataxia telangiectasia is an autosomal recessive disease with a varied and complex phenotype that includes increased sensitivity to radiation (Table 2). Initial cell-fusion experiments using cells derived from AT patients identified four genetic complementation groups (A, C, D, and E) (81, 134). Linkage analysis of 31 families mapped AT group A to chromosome 11q22-23. Studies suggesting that only one AT locus (117) exists were validated by the cloning of the gene responsible for AT, designated ATM (or AT mutated) (178). ATM was mutated in families belonging to all complementation groups, suggesting that mutations in this gene alone are responsible for the observed phenotypes. Analysis of the ATM cDNA sequence reveals similarity to the lipid kinase domain of the 100-kD catalytic subunit of the phosphatidylinositol-3′ (PI-3) kinases and other signal transducers. The PI-3 kinases are activated by mitogenic growth factors and insulin (41). Whether AT is a member of a PI-3 kinase pathway is unknown. The paradox of four complementation groups from a single AT locus may be explained by 1) various alleles of the gene producing various groups, 2) varying expression of mutants, 3) differing genetic backgrounds in patients, or 4) unknown downstream events.

Radiosensitivity

AT cells are particularly vulnerable to a variety of agents that cause DNA damage (119). It was proposed that cell-cycle perturbations (outlined below) are responsible for increased radi-osensitivity, but delaying cell-cycle progression of AT cells does not increase survival (34). Although the initial numbers of DNA strand breaks following radiation are similar, more chromosomal breaks are created in AT cells than in normal cells (74, 152–154). AT cells also have increased rates of intrachromosomal recombination (122). The relative instability of DNA in AT may underlie the observed deficiencies of the nervous and immune systems.

Cell-Cycle Perturbations

AT cells fail to heed cell-cycle checkpoints. The cell-cycle phase when irradiation occurs is critical (8). When irradiated in G_1, AT cells fail to arrest at the late G_1 checkpoint and enter S phase (139, 175). Cells already in S phase do not delay but continue to synthesize DNA; this feature of AT cells is termed radioresistant DNA synthesis (8, 76, 96, 150). Cells irradiated in G_2 do not arrest at the G_2/M checkpoint but proceed into mitosis (8, 179). Cells irradiated in G_1 or S accumulate at the G_2/M boundary and subsequently lose viability.

The G_1 checkpoint defect in AT cells involves the p53 protein (Fig. 4) (14, 84, 86, 100). Expression of p53 and other proteins regulated by p53 (such as *GADD45*, *WAF1/CIP1* and *MDM2*) is delayed and reduced in a radiation dose-dependent manner in AT cells (22). Interestingly, induction of p53 in AT cells by agents such as mimosine and aphidicolin that affect cell-cycle progression without causing DNA damage is normal (95). These results argue that the AT protein is involved in a signal transduction pathway, probably proximal to p53, linking radiation-induced DNA damage and cell-cycle delay.

Proteins Involved in DNA Repair

Genes involved in repair of DNA DSB have been identified by studying rodent cell lines that are radiosensitive and/or immunodeficient. They fall into three complementation groups named XRCC 4, 5, and 7.

Ku Autoantigen

The Ku autoantigen (126) is a circulating antigen found in human autoimmunity diseases such as lupus (170). Ku protein is a heterodimer (composed of 70 and 86 kD subunits) that can bind to free DNA double-stranded ends (15, 146). The XRCC 5 phenotype is caused by a deficiency of the 86 kD component of the Ku protein. Ku recognizes DNA DSB and binds to the free DNA ends. This creates a specific site for the 350 kD catalytic component of an enzyme complex named DNA-activating protein kinase, or DNA-PK (44, 188). DNA-PK, a serine-threonine kinase, is active only when bound to free double-stranded DNA ends (23, 63). Although *in vivo* DNA-PK substrates are unknown, *in vitro* experiments show that nuclear transcription factors and RNA polymerase II are phosphorylated by the active complex (44, 63).

SCID Defect

The SCID (Severe Combined ImmunoDeficient) mouse (hamster complementation group XRCC 7) is unable to join the free DNA of coding strands during the T cell receptor and immunoglobulin gene recombination events that occur in immature lymphocytes. Interestingly, noncoding and signal sequences are joined normally (12, 13, 114). These mice lack both B and T cell immunity as they are unable to generate antibodies and T cell receptors. Even though cells from SCID mice demonstrate some DNA DSB rejoining, their radiosensitivity probably reflects an overall deficiency in the repair of biologically relevant DSB (10, 20, 90). Efforts to isolate the gene involved in SCID began with complementation studies in which introduction of normal genetic material reversed the SCID phenotype (6, 92).

It appears that a mutation in the catalytic component of DNA-PK, p350, is responsible for the SCID defect. Kirchgessner and colleagues demonstrated that a portion of chromosome 8 is sufficient to complement the SCID defect (89). A parental SCID cell line was fused with irradiated human cells containing fragments of human chromosomes. Mouse/human hybrids were screened for radiation resistance. The radiation-resistant hybrids were those that contained the chromosome fragment 8q11.1-8q11.2. Complementation also reversed the defect in DNA recombination. Efforts to isolate the SCID gene product have identified a p350 protein in radiation-resistant hybrids that is absent from radiation-sensitive hybrids. Proof that p350 is the SCID gene product awaits the cloning of the gene and demonstration of the ability of the wild-type gene to restore normal function in SCID cells.

The mutant phenotypes of the XRCC 5 and 7 (SCID) complementation groups are caused by defective Ku and DNA-PK proteins, respectively. The cause of the defect in XRCC4 is presently unknown although the phenotype is similar to XRCC5 and 7 and can be complemented by human chromosome 5 (58–60).

RADIATION INDUCED ONCOGENESIS

Radiation-induced DNA damage, if inadequately repaired, could result in gene mutations, deletions, or dysregulation that are tumorigenic. Oncogenesis requires several genetic changes before the full malignant phenotype appears (27, 199). The order of appearance, rapidity of appearance, and exact type of genetic changes may vary between tumor types and even within the same tumor type.

The epidemiology of radiation-induced tumors is highly suggestive. Atomic bomb survivors in Japan have increased incidences of cancer (62, 140, 174). Israeli youths who received an average dose of 1.4 Gy of x-rays for tinea capitis had a sevenfold increase in nervous system tumors, most of which were meningiomas (173). The brevity of survival makes it difficult to determine whether radiation treatment of malignant tumors, such as glioblastoma and metastasis, causes tumors. Some patients, especially children, have developed second tumors after irradiation (31). The effect of radiation upon the phenotype of recurrent tumors, including their resistance to subsequent therapy, is not known.

Mechanisms of Tumor Initiation

Genetic alterations can be grouped into gain-of-function or loss-of-function mutations. Some cellular genes, when expressed at a high level (gain-of-function) can accelerate cellular proliferation. The gene products are usually members of signaling pathways (e.g., RAS, growth factor receptors) or transcription factors (e.g., FOS, JUN, NF-κB) (45, 50). With other genes, designated tumor suppressor genes, inactivation of both copies (loss-of-function) allows increased cell proliferation. *Rb1* (retinoblastoma), *APC*, *MCC*, and *DCC* (colorectal cancer), *BRCA*-1 (breast and ovarian cancer), and *p53* are examples.

The type of DNA alterations—i.e., base substitutions or deletions—caused by ionizing radiation determine whether gene expression is affected. Studies of radiation-induced mutations have used selectable genes such as the X-linked *HPRT* locus or cell lines hemizygous for the autosomal *APRT* locus to detect mutations in a single gene. Since loss of the *HPRT/APRT* enzyme allows growth in special media, cells mutated at this locus can be selected easily. Although base pair changes are caused by radiation, most radiation-induced alterations of DNA are deletions. These deletions are often large: 12 of 19 mutants isolated after x-irradiation had DNA deletions in excess of 10 kb (202). Restriction enzymes electroporated into cells to induce DNA DSB evoke cellular changes that mimic those which follow x-irradiation (2, 129). Inducing DSB with restriction enzymes and selecting for APRT mutations identified deletions in *APRT* ranging in size from 1 to 36 bp (158). Sequencing the *APRT* locus of the isolated mutants revealed that illegitimate recombination (13) was the predominant mechanism producing the deletions. These studies suggest that if deletions are the major form of x-ray induced damage, loss-of-function mutations should predominate in radiation-induced tumors (33).

Genomic Instability

Cytogenetic analysis of malignant tumors has revealed myriad chromosome abnormalities. It is uncertain whether this genomic instability causes tumor progression, if it is a consequence of this process, or both. Loss of wild-type p53 predisposes cells to gene amplification (107, 221). These findings suggest that cells mutant for p53 should demonstrate greater genetic variation. X-irradiation causes chromosomal aberrations that appear many generations after the initial DNA damage (24, 115). Tumor progression may result from mutually reinforcing chromosomal aberration and cellular damage.

Knockout mice lacking p53 spontaneously develop tumors at high rates. Without p53, cells lack the ability to detect and respond to DNA damage by apoptosis. Without a G_1 checkpoint, cells fix DNA damage during DNA replication and thus perpetuate mutations.

CONCLUSION

The response of cells to ionizing radiation is being dissected at both biochemical and genetic levels. In particular, understanding the role of p53 in linking DNA damage to changes in the cell cycle holds promise for the identification of new targets for therapies of neurological disorders (212).

Acknowledgments

The authors thank Angel Islas, Charles Limoli, John Murnane, and Jingli Wang for critically reviewing this manuscript and offering helpful suggestions.

REFERENCES

1. Abella Columna, E., Giaccia, A. J., Evans, J. W., *et al.* Analysis of restriction enzyme-induced chromosomal aberrations by fluorescence in situ hybridization. Environ. Mol. Mutagen. *22:*26–33, 1993.
2. Ager, D. D., Phillips, J. W., Columna, E. A., *et al.* Analysis of restriction enzyme-induced DNA double-strand breaks in Chinese hamster ovary cells by pulsed-field gel electrophoresis: implications for chromosome damage. Radiat. Res. *128:*150–156, 1991.
3. Arlett, C. F., Green, M. H., Priestley, A., *et al.* Comparative human cellular radiosensitivity: I. The effect of SV40 transformation and immortalisation on the gamma-irradiation survival of skin derived fibroblasts from normal individuals and from ataxia-telangiectasia patients and heterozygotes. Int. J. Radiat. Biol. *54:*911–928, 1988.
4. Bakalkin, G., Yakovleva, T., Selivanova, G., *et al.* p53 binds single-stranded DNA ends and catalyzes DNA renaturation and strand transfer. Proc. Natl. Acad. Sci. U.S.A. *91:*413–417, 1994.
5. Baker, S. J., Markowitz, S., Fearon, E. R., *et al.* Suppression of human colorectal carcinoma cell growth by wild-type p53. Science *249:*912–915, 1990.
6. Banga, S. S., Hall, K. T., Sandhu, A. K., *et al.* Complementation of V(D)J recombination defect and X-ray sensitivity of SCID mouse cells by human chromosome 8. Mutat. Res. *315:*239–247, 1994.
7. Barbet, N. C., and Carr, A. M. Fission yeast wee1 protein kinase is not required for DNA damage-dependent mitotic arrest. Nature *364:*824–827, 1993.
8. Beamish, H., and Lavin, M. F. Radiosensitivity in ataxia-telangiectasia: anomalies in radiation-induced cell cycle delay. Int. J. Radiat. Biol. *65:*175–184, 1994.
9. Bedford, J. S., Mitchell, J. B., Griggs, H. G., *et al.* Radiation-induced cellular reproductive death and chromosome aberrations. Radiat. Res. *76:*573–586, 1978.
10. Biedermann, K. A., Sun, J. R., Giaccia, A. J., *et al.* SCID mutation in mice confers hypersensitivity to ionizing radiation and a deficiency in DNA double-strand break repair. Proc. Natl. Acad. Sci. U.S.A. *88:*1394–1397, 1991.
11. Bischoff, J. R., Friedman, P. N., Marshak, D. R., *et al.* Human p53 is phosphorylated by p60-cdc2 and

cyclin B-cdc2. Proc. Natl. Acad. Sci. U.S.A. *87:* 4766–4770, 1990.

12. Blackwell, T. K., and Alt, F. W. Molecular characterization of the lymphoid V(D)J recombination activity. J. Biol. Chem. *264:*10327–10330, 1989.

13. Blackwell, T. K., Malynn, B. A., Pollock, R. R., *et al.* Isolation of SCID pre-B cells that rearrange kappa light chain genes: formation of normal signal and abnormal coding joins. EMBO J. *8:*735–742, 1989.

14. Blattner, C., Knebel, A., Radler-Pohl, A., *et al.* DNA damaging agents and growth factors induce changes in the program of expressed gene products through common routes. Environ. Mol. Mutagen. *24:*3–10, 1994.

15. Blier, P. R., Griffith, A. J., Craft, J., *et al.* Binding of Ku protein to DNA. Measurement of affinity for ends and demonstration of binding to nicks. J. Biol. Chem. *268:*7594–7601, 1993.

16. Boothman, D. A., Bouvard, I., and Hughes, E. N. Identification and characterization of x-ray-induced proteins in human cells. Cancer Res. *49:*2871–2878, 1989.

17. Brach, M. A., Hass, R., Sherman, M. L., *et al.* Ionizing radiation induces expression and binding activity of the nuclear factor kappa B. J. Clin. Invest. *88:*691–695, 1991.

18. Brachman, D. G., Beckett, M., Graves, D., *et al.* p53 mutation does not correlate with radiosensitivity in 24 head and neck cancer cell lines. Cancer Res. *53:*3667–3669, 1993.

19. Bristow, R. G., Jang, A., Peacock, J., *et al.* Mutant p53 increases radioresistance in rat embryo fibroblasts simultaneously transfected with HPV16-E7 and/or activated H-ras. Oncogene *9:*1527–1536, 1994.

20. Budach, W., Hartford, A., Gioioso, D., *et al.* Tumors arising in SCID mice share enhanced radiation sensitivity of SCID normal tissues. Cancer Res. *52:* 6292–6296, 1992.

21. Caelles, C., Helmberg, A., and Karin, M. p53-dependent apoptosis in the absence of transcriptional activation of p53-target genes. Nature *370:*220–223, 1994.

22. Canman, C. E., Wolff, A. C., Chen, C. Y., *et al.* The p53-dependent G1 cell cycle checkpoint pathway and ataxia-telangiectasia. Cancer Res. *54:*5054–5058, 1994.

23. Carter, T., Vancurova, I., Sun, I., *et al.* A DNA-activated protein kinase from HeLa cell nuclei. Mol. Cell. Biol. *10:*6460–6471, 1990.

24. Chang, W. P., and Little, J. B. Persistently elevated frequency of spontaneous mutations in progeny of CHO clones surviving x-irradiation: association with delayed reproductive death phenotype. Mutat. Res. *270:*191–199, 1992.

25. Chen, J., Jackson, P. K., Kirschner, M. W., *et al.* Separate domains of p21 involved in the inhibition of Cdk kinase and PCNA. Nature *374:*386–388, 1995.

26. Chiu, S. M., Xue, L. Y., Friedman, L. R., *et al.* Copper ion-mediated sensitization of nuclear matrix attachment sites to ionizing radiation. Biochemistry *32:* 6214–6219, 1993.

27. Cho, K. R., and Vogelstein, B. Suppressor gene alterations in the colorectal adenoma-carcinoma sequence. J. Cell. Biochem. (Suppl.) *16G:*137–141, 1992.

28. Cho, Y., Gorina, S., Jeffrey, P. D., *et al.* Crystal structure of a p53 tumor suppressor-DNA complex: understanding tumorigenic mutations. Science *265:* 346–355, 1994.

29. Clarke, A. R., Purdie, C. A., Harrison, D. J., *et al.* Thymocyte apoptosis induced by p53-dependent and independent pathways. Nature *362:*849–852, 1993.

30. Cleaver, J. E. It was a very good year for DNA repair. Cell *76:*1–4, 1994.

31. Cohen, M. E., and Duffner, P. K. Long-term consequences of CNS treatment for childhood cancer, Part I: Pathologic consequences and potential for oncogenesis. Pediatr. Neurol. *7:*157–163, 1991.

32. Cox, B. S., and Parry, J. M. The isolation, genetics and survival characteristics of ultraviolet light sensitive mutants in yeast. Mutat. Res. *6:*37–55, 1968.

33. Cox, R. Molecular mechanisms of radiation oncogenesis. Int. J. Radiat. Biol. *65:*57–64, 1994.

34. Cox, R., Masson, W. K., Weichselbaum, R. R., *et al.* The repair of potentially lethal damage in ataxia telangiectasia fibroblasts. Int. J. Radiat. Biol. *39:* 357–365, 1981.

35. Curran, T., and Franza, B. R., Jr. Fos and Jun: the AP-1 connection. Cell *55:*395–397, 1988.

36. Deb, S. P., Munoz, R. M., Brown, D. R., *et al.* Wild-type human p53 activates the human epidermal growth factor receptor promoter. Oncogene *9:*1341–1349, 1994.

37. Devary, Y., Gottlieb, R. A., Lau, L. F., *et al.* Rapid and preferential activation of the c-jun gene during the mammalian UV response. Mol. Cell. Biol. *11:* 2804–2811, 1991.

38. Dewey, W. C., Miller, H. H., and Leeper, D. B. Chromosomal aberrations and mortality of X-irradiated mammalian cells: Emphasis on repair. Proc. Natl. Acad. Sci. U.S.A. *68:*667–671, 1971.

39. Di Leonardo, A., Linke, S. P., Clarkin, K., *et al.* DNA damage triggers a prolonged p53-dependent G1 arrest and long-term induction of Cip1 in normal human fibroblasts. Genes Dev. *8:*2540–2551, 1994.

40. Diller, L., Kassel, J., Nelson, C. E., *et al.* p53 functions as a cell cycle control protein in osteosarcomas. Mol. Cell. Biol. *10:*5772–5781, 1990.

41. Divecha, N., and Irvine, R. F. Phospholipid signaling. Cell *80:*269–278, 1995.

42. Donehower, L. A., Harvey, M., Slagle, B. L., *et al.* Mice deficient for p53 are developmentally normal but susceptible to tumors. Nature *356:*215–221, 1992.

43. Draetta, G. F. Mammalian G1 cyclins. Curr. Opin. Cell Biol. *6:*842–846, 1994.

44. Dvir, A., Peterson, S. R., Knuth, M. W., *et al.* Ku autoantigen is the regulatory component of a template-associated protein kinase that phosphorylates RNA polymerase II. Proc. Natl. Acad. Sci. U.S.A. *89:*11920–11924, 1992.

45. Egan, S. E., and Weinberg, R. A. The pathway to signal achievement. Nature *365:*781–783, 1993.

46. el-Deiry, W. S., Harper, J. W., O'Connor, P. M., *et al.* WAF1/CIP1 is induced in p53-mediated G1 arrest and apoptosis. Cancer Res. *54:*1169–1174, 1994.

47. el-Deiry, W. S., Kern, S. E., Pietenpol, J. A., *et al.* Definition of a consensus binding site for p53. Nat. Genet. *1:*45–49, 1992.

48. el-Deiry, W. S., Tokino, T., Velculescu, V. E., *et al.* WAF1, a potential mediator of p53 tumor suppression. Cell *75:*817–825, 1993.

49. Elledge, S. J., and Harper, J. W. Cdk inhibitors: on the threshold of checkpoints and development. Curr. Opin. Cell Biol. *6:*847–852, 1994.

50. Fantl, W. J., Johnson, D. E., and Williams, L. T. Signalling by receptor tyrosine kinases. Annu. Rev. Biochem. *62:*453–481, 1993.

51. Fisher, D. E. Apoptosis in cancer therapy: crossing the threshold. Cell *78:*539–542, 1994.

52. Fornace, A. J., Jr., and Little, J. B. DNA crosslinking induced by x-rays and chemical agents. Biochim. Biophys. Acta. *477:*343–355, 1977.

53. Fornace, A. J., Jr., Nebert, D. W., Hollander, M. C., *et al.* Mammalian genes coordinately regulated by growth arrest signals and DNA-damaging agents. Mol. Cell. Biol. *9:*4196–4203, 1989.

54. Frankenberg-Schwager, M. Induction, repair and biological relevance of radiation-induced DNA lesions in eukaryotic cells. Radiat. Environ. Biophys. *29:*273–292, 1990.

55. Frankenberg-Schwager, M., and Frankenberg, D. DNA double-strand breaks: their repair and relationship to cell killing in yeast. Int. J. Radiat. Biol. *58:*569–575, 1990.

56. Funk, W. D., Pak, D. T., Karas, R. H., *et al.* A transcriptionally active DNA-binding site for human p53 protein complexes. Mol. Cell. Biol. *12:*2866–2871, 1992.

57. Gatti, R. A., Berkel, I., Boder, E., *et al.* Localization of an ataxia-telangiectasia gene to chromosome 11q22-23. Nature *336:*577–580, 1988.

58. Giaccia, A. J., Denko, N., MacLaren, R., *et al.* Human chromosome 5 complements the DNA double-strand break-repair deficiency and gamma-ray sensitivity of the XR-1 hamster variant. Am. J. Hum. Genet. *47:*459–469, 1990.

59. Giaccia, A. J., MacLaren, R. A., Denko, N., *et al.* Increased sensitivity to killing by restriction enzymes in the XR-1 DNA double-strand break repair-deficient mutant. Mutat. Res. *236:*67–76, 1990.

60. Giaccia, A. J., Richardson, E., Denko, N., *et al.* Genetic analysis of XR-1 mutation in hamster and human hybrids. Somat. Cell. Mol. Genet. *15:*71–77, 1989.

61. Goldsmith, M. E., Gudas, J. M., Schneider, E., *et al.* Wild type p53 stimulates expression from the human multidrug resistance promoter in a p53-negative cell line. J. Biol. Chem. *270:*1894–1898, 1995.

62. Goodman, M. T., Mabuchi, K., Morita, M., *et al.* Cancer incidence in Hiroshima and Nagasaki, Japan, 1958–1987. Eur. J. Cancer *30A:*801–807, 1994.

63. Gottlieb, T. M., and Jackson, S. P. The DNA-dependent protein kinase: requirement for DNA ends and association with Ku antigen. Cell *72:*131–142, 1993.

64. Greenblatt, M. S., Bennett, W. P., Hollstein, M., *et al.* Mutations in the p53 tumor suppressor gene: clues to cancer etiology and molecular pathogenesis. Cancer Res. *54:*4855–4878, 1994.

65. Kamb, A. Cell-cycle regulators and cancer. Trends Genet. *11:*136–140, 1995.

66. Kastan, M. B., Onyekwere, O., Sidransky, D., *et al.* Participation of p53 protein in the cellular response to DNA damage. Cancer Res. *51:*6304–6311, 1991.

67. Kastan, M. B., Zhan, Q., el-Deiry, W. S., *et al.* A mammalian cell cycle checkpoint pathway utilizing p53 and GADD45 is defective in ataxia-telangiectasia. Cell *71:*587–597, 1992.

68. Kerr, J. F., Wyllie, A. H., and Currie, A. R. Apoptosis: a basic biological phenomenon with wide-ranging implications in tissue kinetics. Br. J. Cancer *26:*239–257, 1972.

69. Khanna, K. K., and Lavin, M. F. Ionizing radiation and UV induction of p53 protein by different pathways in ataxia-telangiectasia cells. Oncogene *8:*3307–3312, 1993.

70. Kharbanda, S., Saleem, A., Shafman, T., *et al.* Activation of the pp90^{rsk} and mitogen-activated serine/threonine protein kinases by ionizing radiation. Proc. Natl. Acad. Sci. U.S.A. *91:*5416–5420, 1994.

71. Kharbanda, S., Yuan, Z. M., Rubin, E., *et al.* Activation of Src-like p56/p53^{lyn} tyrosine kinase by ionizing radiation. J. Biol. Chem. *269:*20739–20743, 1994.

72. Kirchgessner, C. U., Patil, C. K., Evans, J. W., *et al.* DNA-dependent kinase (p350) as a candidate gene for the murine SCID defect. Science *267:*1178–1183, 1995.

73. Kirchgessner, C. U., Tosto, L. M., Biedermann, K. A., *et al.* Complementation of the radiosensitive phenotype in severe combined immunodeficient mice by human chromosome 8. Cancer Res. *53:*6011–6016, 1993.

74. Krisch, R. E., Flick, M. B., and Trumbore, C. N. Radiation chemical mechanisms of single- and double-strand break formation in irradiated SV40 DNA. Radiat. Res. *126:*251–259, 1991.

75. Kurimasa, A., Nagata, Y., Shimizu, M., *et al.* A human gene that restores the DNA-repair defect in SCID mice is located on 8p11.1 → q11.1. Hum. Genet. *93:*21–26, 1994.

76. Lane, D. P., and Crawford, L. V. T antigen is bound to a host protein in SV40-transformed cells. Nature *278:*261–263, 1979.

77. Lau, C. C., and Pardee, A. B. Mechanism by which caffeine potentiates lethality of nitrogen mustard. Proc. Natl. Acad. Sci. U.S.A. *79:*2942–2946, 1982.

78. Lavin, M. F., Khanna, K. K., Beamish, H., *et al.* Defect in radiation signal transduction in ataxia-telangiectasia. Int. J. Radiat. Biol. *66:*S151–156, 1994.

79. Lavin, M. F., and Schroeder, A. L. Damage-resistant DNA synthesis in eukaryotes. Mutat. Res. *193:*193–206, 1988.

80. Lee, J. M., and Bernstein, A. p53 mutations increase resistance to ionizing radiation. Proc. Natl. Acad. Sci. U.S.A. *90:*5742–5746, 1993.

81. Lee, M. G., and Nurse, P. Complementation used to clone a human homologue of the fission yeast cell cycle control gene cdc2. Nature *327:*31–35, 1987.

82. Leeper, D. B., Schneiderman, M. H., and Dewey,

W. C. Radiation-induced division delay in synchronized Chinese hamster ovary cells in monolayer culture. Radiat. Res. *50:*401–417, 1972.

83. Lett, J. T. Damage to DNA and chromatin structure from ionizing radiations, and the radiation sensitivities of mammalian cells. Prog. Nucleic Acid. Res. Mol. Biol. *39:*305–352, 1990.

84. Levine, A. J., Momand, J., and Finlay, C. A. The p53 tumour suppressor gene. Nature *351:*453–456, 1991.

85. Li, R., Waga, S., Hannon, G. J., *et al.* Differential effects by the p21 CDK inhibitor on PCNA-dependent DNA replication and repair. Nature *371:*534–537, 1994.

86. Lin, J., Chen, J., Elenbaas, B., *et al.* Several hydrophobic amino acids in the p53 amino-terminal domain are required for transcriptional activation, binding to mdm-2 and the adenovirus 5 E1B 55-kD protein. Genes Dev. *8:*1235–1246, 1994.

87. Little, J. B. Delayed initiation of DNA synthesis in irradiated human diploid cells. Nature *218:*1064–1065, 1968.

88. Little, J. B. Repair of sublethal and potentially lethal radiation damage in plateau phase cultures of human cells. Nature *224:*804–806, 1969.

89. Liu, X., Miller, C. W., Koeffler, P. H., *et al.* The p53 activation domain binds the TATA box-binding polypeptide in Holo-TFIID, and a neighboring p53 domain inhibits transcription. Mol. Cell. Biol. *13:*3291–3300, 1993.

90. Livingstone, L. R., White, A., Sprouse, J., *et al.* Altered cell cycle arrest and gene amplification potential accompany loss of wild-type p53. Cell *70:*923–935, 1992.

91. Lock, R. B., and Ross, W. E. Possible role for p34^{cdc2} kinase in etoposide-induced cell death of Chinese hamster ovary cells. Cancer Res. *50:*3767–3771, 1990.

92. Lowe, S. W., Schmitt, E. M., Smith, S. W., *et al.* p53 is required for radiation-induced apoptosis in mouse thymocytes. Nature *362:*847–849, 1993.

93. Lu, X., and Lane, D. P. Differential induction of transcriptionally active p53 following UV or ionizing radiation: Defects in chromosome instability syndromes? Cell *75:*765–778, 1993.

94. Mack, D. H., Vartikar, J., Pipas, J. M., *et al.* Specific repression of TATA-mediated but not initiator-mediated transcription by wild-type p53. Nature *363:*281–283, 1993.

95. Madsen, P., and Celis, J. E. S-phase patterns of cyclin (PCNA) antigen staining resemble topographical patterns of DNA synthesis. A role for cyclin in DNA replication? FEBS Lett. *193:*5–11, 1985.

96. Maity, A., McKenna, W. G., and Muschel, R. J. The molecular basis for cell cycle delays following ionizing radiation: a review. Radiother. Oncol. *31:*1–13, 1994.

97. Malynn, B. A., Blackwell, T. K., Fulop, G. M., *et al.* The SCID defect affects the final step of the immunoglobulin VDJ recombinase mechanism. Cell *54:*453–460, 1988.

98. Marder, B. A., and Morgan, W. F. Delayed chromosomal instability induced by DNA damage. Mol. Cell. Biol. *13:*6667–6677, 1993.

99. Martin, D. W., Munoz, R. M., Subler, M. A., *et al.* p53 binds to the TATA-binding protein-TATA complex. J. Biol. Chem. *268:*13062–13067, 1993.

100. McConville, C. M., Byrd, P. J., Ambrose, H. J., *et al.* Genetic and physical mapping of the ataxia-telangiectasia locus on chromosome 11q22-q23. Int. J. Radiat. Biol. *66:*S45–56, 1994.

101. McKenna, W. G., Iliakis, G., Weiss, M. C., *et al.* Increased G2 delay in radiation-resistant cells obtained by transformation of primary rat embryo cells with the oncogenes H-ras and V-myc. Radiat. Res. *125:*283–287, 1991.

102. McKinnon, P. J. Ataxia-telangiectasia: an inherited disorder of ionizing-radiation sensitivity in man. Hum. Genet. *75:*197–208, 1987.

103. McLauglin, P. W., Schea, R., McKeever, P. E., *et al.* Radiobiological effects and changes in gene expression in central nervous system in response to ionizing radiation. In: *Molecular Genetics of Nervous System Tumors*, edited by A. J. Levine and H. H. Schmidek, pp. 163–177, Wiley-Liss, New York, 1993.

104. Mercer, W. E., Shields, M. T., Amin, M., *et al.* Negative growth regulation in a glioblastoma tumor cell line that conditionally expresses human wild-type p53. Proc. Natl. Acad. Sci. U.S.A. *87:*6166–6170, 1990.

105. Meyn, M. S. High spontaneous intrachromosomal recombination rates in ataxia-telangiectasia. Science *260:*1327–1330, 1993.

106. Milligan, J. R., Aguilera, J. A., and Ward, J. F. Variation of single-strand break yield with scavenger concentration for plasmid DNA irradiated in aqueous solution. Radiat. Res. *133:*151–157, 1993.

107. Milligan, J. R., and Ward, J. F. Yield of single-strand breaks due to attack on DNA by scavenger-derived radicals. Radiat. Res. *137:*295–299, 1994.

108. Milner, J., Cook, A., and Mason, J. p53 is associated with p34^{cdc2} in transformed cells. EMBO J. *9:*2885–2889, 1990.

109. Mimori, T., Akizuki, M., Yamagata, H., *et al.* Characterization of a high molecular weight acidic nuclear protein recognized by autoantibodies in sera from patients with polymyositis-scleroderma overlap. J. Clin. Invest. *68:*611–620, 1981.

110. Momand, J., Zambetti, G. P., Olson, D. C., *et al.* The Mdm-2 oncogene product forms a complex with the p53 protein and inhibits p53-mediated transactivation. Cell *69:*1237–1245, 1992.

111. Morgan, D. O. Principles of CDK regulation. Nature *374:*131–134, 1995.

112. Morgan, W. F., Ager, D., Chung, H. W., *et al.* The cytogenetic effects of restriction endonucleases following their introduction into cells by electroporation. Prog. Clin. Biol. Res. *340B:*355–361, 1990.

113. Painter, R. B. The direct effect of X-irradiation on HeLa S3 deoxyribonucleic acid synthesis. Radiat. Res. *16:*846–859, 1962.

114. Painter, R. B. The role of DNA damage and repair in cell killing induced by ionizing radiation. In: *Radiation Biology in Cancer Research*, edited by R. E. Meyn and H. R. Withers, Raven Press, New York, 1980.

115. Painter, R. B., and Robertson, J. S. Effect of irradia-

tion and theory of role of mitotic delay on the time course of labeling of HeLa S3 cells with tritiated thymidine. Radiat. Res. *11:*206–217, 1959.

116. Painter, R. B., and Young, B. R. Radiosensitivity in ataxia-telangiectasia: a new explanation. Proc. Natl. Acad. Sci. U.S.A. *77:*7315–7317, 1980.

117. Painter, R. B., and Young, B. R. X-ray-induced inhibition of DNA synthesis in Chinese hamster ovary, human HeLa, and mouse L cells. Radiat. Res. *64:* 648–656, 1975.

118. Pandita, T. K., and Hittelman, W. N. The contribution of DNA and chromosome repair deficiencies to the radiosensitivity of ataxia-telangiectasia. Radiat. Res. *131:*214–223, 1992.

119. Pandita, T. K., and Hittelman, W. N. Increased initial levels of chromosome damage and heterogeneous chromosome repair in ataxia telangiectasia heterozygote cells. Mutat. Res. *310:*1–13, 1994.

120. Pandita, T. K., and Hittelman, W. N. Initial chromosome damage but not DNA damage is greater in ataxia telangiectasia cells. Radiat. Res. *130:*94–103, 1992.

121. Papathanasiou, M. A., Kerr, N. C. K., Robbins, J. H., *et al.* Induction by ionizing radiation of the gadd45 gene in cultured human cells: Lack of mediation by protein kinase C. Mol. Cell. Biol. *11:*1009–1016, 1991.

122. Paterson, M. C., and Smith, P. J. Ataxia telangiectasia: an inherited human disorder involving hypersensitivity to ionizing radiation and related DNA-damaging chemicals. Annu. Rev. Genet. *13:*291–318, 1979.

123. Pennypacker, K. R., Hong, J. S., and McMillian, M. K. Pharmacological regulation of AP-1 transcription factor DNA binding activity. FASEB J. *8:*475–478, 1994.

124. Phillips, J. W., and Morgan, W. F. Illegitimate recombination induced by DNA double-strand breaks in a mammalian chromosome. Mol. Cell. Biol. *14:*5794–5803, 1994.

125. Phillips, R. A., and Tolmach, L. J. Repair of potentially lethal damage in x-irradiated HeLa cells. Radiat. Res. *29:*413–432, 1966.

126. Picksley, S. M., and Lane, D. P. p53 and Rb: their cellular roles. Curr. Opin. Cell Biol. *6:*853–858, 1994.

127. Pietenpol, J. A., Tokino, T., Thiagalingam, S., *et al.* Sequence-specific transcriptional activation is essential for growth suppression by p53. Proc. Natl. Acad. Sci. U.S.A. *91:*1998–2002, 1994.

128. Prelich, G., Kostura, M., Marshak, D. R., *et al.* The cell-cycle regulated proliferating cell nuclear antigen is required for SV40 DNA replication in vitro. Nature *326:*471–475, 1987.

129. Prelich, G., Tan, C. K., Kostura, M., *et al.* Functional identity of proliferating cell nuclear antigen and a DNA polymerase-delta auxiliary protein. Nature *326:*517–520, 1987.

130. Puck, T. T. Action of radiation on mammalian cells. III. Relationship between reproductive death and induction of chromosome anomalies by X-irradiation of euploid human cells in vitro. Proc. Natl. Acad. Sci. U.S.A. *44:*772–780, 1958.

131. Puck, T. T., and Marcus, P. I. Action of x-rays on mammalian cells. J. Exp. Med. *103:*653–666, 1956.

132. Radford, I. R. Effect of radiomodifying agents on the ratios of X-ray-induced lesions in cellular DNA: use in lethal lesion determination. Int. J. Radiat. Biol. Relat. Stud. Phys. Chem. Med. *49:*621–637, 1986.

133. Raff, M. C. Social controls on cell survival and cell death. Nature *356:*397–400, 1992.

134. Ragimov, N., Krauskopf, A., Navot, N., *et al.* Wild-type but not mutant p53 can repress transcription initiation in vitro by interfering with the binding of basal transcription factors to the TATA motif. Oncogene *8:*1183–1193, 1993.

135. Ramakrishnan, N., Chiu, S. M., and Oteinick, N. L. Yield of DNA-protein cross-links in gamma-irradiated Chinese hamster cells. Cancer Res. *47:*2032–2035, 1987.

136. Reeves, W. H., Satoh, M., Wang, J., *et al.* Systemic lupus erythematosus. Antibodies to DNA, DNA-binding proteins, and histones. Rheum. Dis. Clin. North. Am. *20:*1–28, 1994.

137. Riley, P. A. Free radicals in biology: oxidative stress and the effects of ionizing radiation. Int. J. Radiat. Biol. *65:*27–33, 1994.

138. Ritter, M. A., Cleaver, J. E., and Tobias, C. A. High-LET radiations induce a large proportion of non-rejoining DNA breaks. Nature *266:*653–655, 1977.

139. Ron, E., Modan, B., Boice, J. D., Jr., *et al.* Tumors of the brain and nervous system after radiotherapy in childhood. N. Engl. J. Med. *319:*1033–1039, 1988.

140. Ron, E., Preston, D. L., Mabuchi, K., *et al.* Cancer incidence in atomic bomb survivors. Part IV: Comparison of cancer incidence and mortality. Radiat. Res. *137:*S98–112, 1994.

141. Rudolph, N. S., and Latt, S. A. Flow cytometric analysis of X-ray sensitivity in ataxia telangiectasia. Mutat. Res. *211:*31–41, 1989.

142. Sancar, A. Mechanisms of DNA excision repair. Science *266:*1954–1956, 1994.

143. Sang, B. C., Chen, J. Y., Minna, J., *et al.* Distinct regions of p53 have a differential role in transcriptional activation and repression functions. Oncogene *9:*853–859, 1994.

144. Savitsky, K., Bar-Shira, A., Gilad, S., *et al.* A single ataxia-telangiectasia gene with a product similar to PI-3 kinase. Science *268:*1749–1753, 1995.

145. Scott, D., and Zampetti-Bosseler, F. Cell cycle dependence of mitotic delay in X-irradiated normal and ataxia telangiectasia fibroblasts. Int. J. Radiat. Biol. *42:*679–683, 1982.

146. Seto, E., Usheva, A., Zambetti, G. P., *et al.* Wild-type p53 binds to the TATA-binding protein and represses transcription. Proc. Natl. Acad. Sci. U.S.A. *89:*12028–12032, 1992.

147. Shaw, P., Bovey, R., Tardy, S., *et al.* Induction of apoptosis by wild-type p53 in a human colon tumor-derived cell line. Proc. Natl. Acad. Sci. U.S.A. *89:*4495–4499, 1992.

148. Sherman, M. L., Datta, R., Hallahan, D. E., *et al.* Ionizing radiation regulates expression of the c-jun protooncogene. Proc. Natl. Acad. Sci. U.S.A. *87:*5663–5666, 1990.

149. Shivji, M. K., Grey, S. J., Strausfeld, U. P., *et al.* Cip1 inhibits DNA replication but not PCNA-dependent

nucleotide excision-repair. Curr. Biol. *4:*1062–1068, 1994.

150. Shivji, M. K. K., Kenny, M. K., and Wood, R. D. Proliferating cell nuclear antigen is required for DNA excision repair. Cell *69:*367–374, 1992.

151. Smith, M. L., Chen, I. T., Zhan, Q., *et al.* Interaction of the p53-regulated protein Gadd45 with proliferating cell nuclear antigen. Science *266:*1376–1380, 1994.

152. Spinks, J. W. T., and Woods, R. J. *An Introduction to Radiation Chemistry.* 3rd ed. Wiley, New York, 1990.

153. Su, L. N., and Little, J. B. Prolonged cell cycle delay in radioresistant human cell lines transfected with activated ras oncogene and/or Simian Virus 40 T-antigen. Radiat. Res. *133:*73–79, 1993.

154. Suwa, A., Hirakata, M., Takeda, Y., *et al.* DNA-dependent protein kinase (Ku protein-p350 complex) assembles on double-stranded DNA. Proc. Natl. Acad. Sci. U.S.A. *91:*6904–6908, 1994.

155. Symonds, H., Krall, L., Remington, L., *et al.* p53-dependent apoptosis suppresses tumor growth and progression in vivo. Cell *78:*703–711, 1994.

156. Szybalski, W. X-ray sensitization by halopyrimidines. Cancer Chemother. Rep. *58:*539–557, 1974.

157. Terasima, T., and Tolmach, L. J. Variations in several responses of HeLa cells to X-irradiation during the division cycle. Biophys. J. *3:*11–33, 1963.

158. Thacker, J. The study of responses to 'model' DNA breaks induced by restriction endonucleases in cells and cell-free systems: achievements and difficulties. Int. J. Radiat. Biol. *66:*591–596, 1994.

159. Thut, C. J., Chen, J. L., Klemm, R., *et al.* p53 transcriptional activation mediated by coactivators TAFII40 and TAFII60. Science *267:*100–104, 1995.

160. Truant, R., Xiao, H., Ingles, C. J., *et al.* Direct interaction between the transcriptional activation domain of human p53 and the TATA box-binding protein. J. Biol. Chem. *268:*2284–2287, 1993.

161. Uckun, F. M., Schieven, G. L., Tuel-Ahlgren, L. M., *et al.* Tyrosine phosphorylation is a mandatory proximal step in radiation-induced activation of the protein kinase C signaling pathway in human B-lymphocyte precursors. Proc. Natl. Acad. Sci. U.S.A. *90:*252–256, 1993.

162. Uckun, F. M., Tuel-Ahlgren, L., Song, C. W., *et al.* Ionizing radiation stimulates unidentified tyrosine-specific protein kinases in human B-lymphocyte precursors, triggering apoptosis and clonogenic cell death. Proc. Natl. Acad. Sci. U.S.A. *89:*9005–9009, 1992.

163. Ueba, T., Nosaka, T., Takahashi, J. A., *et al.* Transcriptional regulation of basic fibroblast growth factor gene by p53 in human glioblastoma and hepatocellular carcinoma cells. Proc. Natl. Acad. Sci. U.S.A. *91:*9009–9013, 1994.

164. Ullrich, S. J., Anderson, C. W., Mercer, W. E., *et al.* The p53 tumor suppressor protein, a modulator of cell proliferation. J. Biol. Chem. *267:*15259–15262, 1992.

165. Vogelstein, B., and Kinzler, K. W. The multistep nature of cancer. Trends Genet. *9:*138–141, 1993.

166. Vogelstein, B., and Kinzler, K. W. p53 function and dysfunction. Cell *70:*523–526, 1992.

167. von Sonntag, C. Radiation chemistry in the 1990s: pressing questions relating to the areas of radiation biology and environmental research. Int. J. Radiat. Biol. *65:*19–26, 1994.

168. Vrieling, H., Simons, J. W., Arwert, F., *et al.* Mutations induced by X-rays at the HPRT locus in cultured Chinese hamster cells are mostly large deletions. Mutat. Res. *144:*281–286, 1985.

169. Waga, S., Hannon, G. J., Beach, D., *et al.* The p21 inhibitor of cyclin-dependent kinases controls DNA replication by interaction with PCNA. Nature *369:*574–578, 1994.

170. Wallace, S. S. DNA damages processed by base excision repair: biological consequences. Int. J. Radiat. Biol. *66:*579–589, 1994.

171. Ward, J. F. Biochemistry of DNA lesions. Radiat. Res. *104:*S103–111, 1985.

172. Ward, J. F. Mechanisms of radiation action on DNA in model systems—their relevance to cellular DNA. In: *The Early Effects of Radiation on DNA,* edited by E. M. Fielden and P. O. O'Neill, Springer-Verlag, Berlin, 1991.

173. Ward, J. F. Radiation mutagenesis: the initial DNA lesions responsible. Radiat. Res. *142:*362–368, 1995.

174. Ward, J. F. The yield of DNA double-strand breaks produced intracellularly by ionizing radiation: a review. Int. J. Radiat. Biol. *57:*1141–1150, 1990.

175. Ward, J. F., Blakely, W. F., and Joner, E. I. Mammalian cells are not killed by DNA single-strand breaks caused by hydroxyl radicals from hydrogen peroxide. Radiat. Res. *103:*383–392, 1985.

176. Warters, R. L., Hofer, K. G., Harris, C. R., *et al.* Radionuclide toxicity in cultured mammalian cells: elucidation of the primary site of radiation damage. Curr. Top. Radiat. Res. Q. *12:*389–407, 1978.

177. Weichselbaum, R. R., Hallahan, D., Fuks, Z., *et al.* Radiation induction of immediate early genes: effectors of the radiation-stress response. Int. J. Radiat. Oncol. Biol. Phys. *30:*229–234, 1994.

178. Weichselbaum, R. R., Hallahan, D. E., Beckett, M. A., *et al.* Gene therapy targeted by radiation preferentially radiosensitizes tumor cells. Cancer Res. *54:*4266–4269, 1994.

179. Weinert, T., and Hartwell, L. Control of G2 delay by the RAD9 gene of Saccharomyces cerevisiae. J. Cell. Sci. Suppl. *12:*145–148, 1989.

180. Weinert, T. A., and Hartwell, L. H. The RAD9 gene controls the cell cycle response to DNA damage in Saccharomyces cerevisiae. Science *241:*317–322, 1988.

181. Whitaker, S. J., Powell, S. N., and McMillan, T. J. Molecular assays of radiation-induced DNA damage. Eur. J. Cancer *27:*922–928, 1991.

182. Wyllie, A. H., Kerr, J. F., and Currie, A. R. Cell death: the significance of apoptosis. Int. Rev. Cytol. *68:*251–306, 1980.

183. Xiong, Y., Hannon, G. J., Zhang, H., *et al.* p21 is a universal inhibitor of cyclin kinases. Nature *366:*701–704, 1993.

184. Xiong, Y., Zhang, H., and Beach, D. D type cyclins associate with multiple protein kinases and the

DNA replication and repair factor PCNA. Cell *71:* 505–514, 1992.

185. Xue, L. Y., Friedman, L. R., Oleinick, N. L., *et al.* Induction of DNA damage in gamma-irradiated nuclei stripped of nuclear protein classes: differential modulation of double-strand break and DNA-protein crosslink formation. Int. J. Radiat. Biol. *66:*11–21, 1994.

186. Yamada, M., and Puck, T. T. Action of radiation on mammalian cells. IV. Reversible mitotic lag in the S3 HeLa cell produced by low doses of X-rays. Proc. Natl. Acad. Sci. U.S.A. *47:*1181–1191, 1961.

187. Yin, Y., Tainsky, M. A., Bischoff, F. Z., *et al.* Wild-type p53 restores cell cycle control and inhibits gene amplification in cells with mutant p53 alleles. Cell *70:*937–948, 1992.

188. Yonish-Rouach, E., Resnitzky, D., Lotem, J., *et al.* Wild-type p53 induces apoptosis of myeloid leukaemic cells that is inhibited by interleukin-6. Nature *352:*345–347, 1991.

189. Yu, C. K., and Sinclair, W. K. Mitotic delay and chromosomal aberrations induced by X-rays in synchromized Chinese hamster cells in vitro. J. Natl. Cancer Inst. *39:*619–632, 1967.

190. Yuan, J. Y., and Horvitz, H. R. The Caenorhabditis elegans genes ced-3 and ced-4 act cell autonomously to cause programmed cell death. Dev. Biol. *138:*33–41, 1990.

191. Zhang, H., Xiong, Y., and Beach, D. Proliferating cell nuclear antigen and p21 are components of multiple cell cycle kinase complexes. Mol. Cell. Biol. *4:*897–906, 1993.

CHAPTER 12

Molecular Basis of Chemotherapy for Brain Tumors

STEPHEN H. PETERSDORF, M.D., MITCHEL S. BERGER, M.D.

Nearly 17,000 patients were diagnosed with primary malignant brain tumors in 1995. This diagnosis carried an extremely poor prognosis, particularly for adults. The vast majority of patients die of this malignancy within a few years. Surgical resection and radiotherapy are the primary modalities of treatment for most brain tumors, particularly high-grade astrocytomas. While improvements in surgical technique and radiation therapy have changed the outcome for some patients, the overall prognosis remains extremely poor. Despite *in vitro* data suggesting the potential effectiveness of chemotherapy against brain tumors, the addition of chemotherapy produces only modest benefit (40). Adjuvant chemotherapy for primary glioblastoma multiforme is not well supported and is often reserved for recurrent disease. There is, however, support for adjuvant chemotherapy for particular histologies, such as anaplastic astrocytomas (43) and anaplastic oligodendrogliomas (15).

Nitrosoureas, introduced more than 20 years ago, were the first agents to demonstrate *in vitro* cytotoxicity against brain tumors. They remain the most effective drugs for primary brain tumors. The mechanism of action of these alkylating agents and the cellular responses to them are well understood. Although *in vitro* data predict substantial activity against brain tumors, the clinical results continue to be disappointing (50). Over the past 20 years, there have been few advances in the chemotherapy of brain tumors. New methods of administration and multidrug combinations have not significantly im-

proved patient outcome. Analysis of the causes of these poor results begins with consideration of the main determinants of drug efficacy: 1) concentration of the drug delivered to the tumor; 2) cytotoxicity of the drug; 3) absence of intrinsic and acquired drug resistance. Multiple factors, many unique to malignant gliomas, adversely affect these determinants and limit the effectiveness of chemotherapy for brain tumors. The relative importance of these factors varies with histology and other differences among patients. For example, in glioblastoma multiforme, intrinsic cellular resistance to chemotherapy is more limiting than the blood brain barrier might be disrupted enough to permit adequate drug delivery. Conversely, anaplastic astrocytomas with less disruption of the blood-brain barrier are more responsive to chemotherapy because of less intrinsic resistance to drugs. Improved understanding of the molecular basis of the cytotoxic effects of chemotherapy and the mechanisms of tumor cell resistance may lead to opportunities for improvement in therapy for patients with brain tumors.

DRUG TRANSPORT IN BRAIN TUMORS

The blood-brain barrier has long been considered the most important factor precluding effective chemotherapy for brain tumors. The blood-brain barrier results from the tight intracellular junctions of brain capillary endothelium. These prevent egress of large, water-soluble, or protein-bound molecules from capillaries into normal brain parenchyma. Many of the drugs used for systemic solid tumors are excluded by the barrier (28). The blood-brain barrier may be disrupted by either penetration of the tumor into the brain parenchyma or inflammation surrounding the tumor. Disruption of the blood-brain barrier is demonstrated by contrast enhancement on computerized tomography (CT) or magnetic resonance imaging (MRI) scans. To circumvent barrier delivery issues, lipid-soluble agents such as the nitrosoureas that readily cross the blood-brain barrier and are cytotoxic *in vitro* have been used clinically. The minimal effect of these drugs brings into question the importance of the barrier vs. other factors influencing *in vivo* efficacy (72).

The delivery of chemotherapy to brain tumors is also affected by several local factors. Neovascularization produces heterogeneity of local blood flow within the tumor. Underperfusion of the center of tumors limits delivery of drugs there (7).

ACTIVE CHEMOTHERAPEUTIC AGENTS IN BRAIN TUMORS

Few chemotherapeutic agents are active against brain tumors. Most of these drugs given alone have response rates of less than 30%. Alkylating agents are the mainstay of treatment because cytotoxic concentrations in the brain are achievable. The most commonly used agents are listed in Table 1.

Other drugs, such as vincristine, 6-thioguanine, and 5-fluorouracil (5-FU) that have little antitumor effect when used alone, are included in combination regimens to potentiate the activity of the more commonly used agents. Most of these agents are small and lipophilic.

Alkylating Agents Used in Brain Tumors

Alkylating agents form covalent bonds with electron-rich atoms in DNA, RNA, and pro-

TABLE 1
Single Agents Currently Used for the Treatment of Malignant Brain Tumors

Lomustine (CCNU)
Carmustine (BCNU)
Procarbazine
Cyclophosphamide
Temozolomide
Cisplatin
Carboplatin
Etoposide
Hydroxyurea

teins. There are several types: nitrogen mustards, nitrosoureas, azridines, and alkyl sulfonates. In DNA, the most frequent target, alkylating agents (or their metabolites) react with amino, carboxyl, and phosphate groups. Alkylating agents also bind to small molecules such as amino acids and glutathione.

The alkylation of DNA has several effects. These include crosslinking of DNA by the reaction of the bifunctional drug molecule with two bases on the same or opposite strands (intra- or interstrand crosslinking). Bifunctional alkylating agents usually produce interstrand crosslinking of DNA. This disrupts the DNA template, inhibits DNA synthesis, and kills the cell. The alkylating agents preferentially react with specific nitrogen bases. Nitrogen mustards react with the N^7 position of guanylic acid, whereas the nitrosoureas preferentially alkylate the O^6 position of guanylic acid.

Other effects of alkylation include DNA mutations, monoadduct formation, and strand breakage. These interfere with cellular replication of DNA, transcription of DNA into RNA, and translation of mRNA into protein. Cytotoxicity is the most common result, but mutagenesis, teratogenesis, and carcinogenesis can also occur.

Nitrosoureas

The nitrosoureas preferred for brain tumors are carmustine (BCNU) and lomustine (CCNU) (Fig. 1). Newer nitrosoureas such as ACNU, which is more water soluble than BCNU or CCNU, are under investigation in clinical trials. All of these agents are lipid soluble and cross the blood-brain barrier into the central nervous system. Decomposition of carmustine or lomustine leads to two active compounds. The first is chloroethyl diazohydroxide. Its alkylating activity resides in a chloroethyl carbonium ion. The second is an isocyanate that reacts with amino acids to form carbamoylated proteins. Cytotoxicity arises when these carbamoylated proteins attack the guanine residues of DNA, leading to

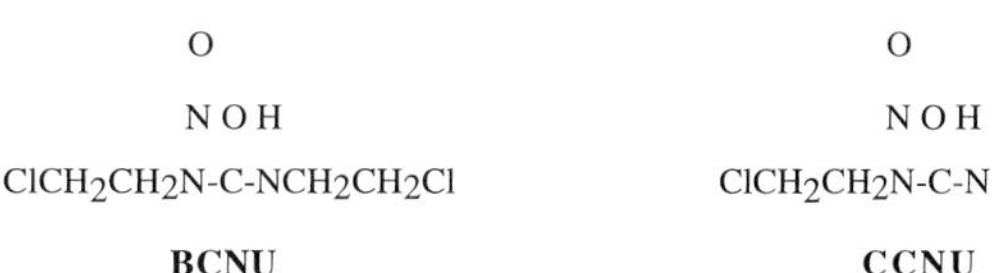

Figure 1. Nitrosourea structure.

chlorethyl adducts (31). This produces an unstable intermediate that forms interstrand DNA and DNA-protein crosslinks (18).

Classic Alkylating Agents: Mechlorethamine (Nitrogen Mustard) and Cyclophosphamide

Nitrogen mustard and cyclophosphamide are classic alkylating agents. Both produce highly reactive carbonium ions for alkylation. These agents act independently of the cell cycle; they kill both resting and dividing cells.

Cyclophosphamide is activated by the hepatic cytochrome P-450 microsomal system. Activation yields two intermediates, aldophosphamide and 4-hydroxycyclophosphamide, which in turn form two active intracellular alkylators, acrolein and phosphoramide mustard (17). The phosphoramide mustard is cytotoxic; acrolein is not. The active metabolites prevent cell division by crosslinking DNA strands so as to disrupt the DNA template for replication and transcription. DNA-protein adducts and single-strand breaks are also formed. These disrupt normal cellular processes.

Mechlorethamine is a bifunctional alkylator. It alkylates the N^7 guanine leading to abnormal base pairing of guanine with thymidine. This causes DNA miscoding, cleavage of the imidazole ring of guanine, depurination of DNA, resulting in single-strand breakage and crosslinking of DNA by guanine-guanine pairs. DNA crosslinking is the most important cytotoxic action of mechlorethamine. The cytotoxic effects are not cell cycle specific. Cytotoxicity is greater in rapidly proliferating cells than in quiescent ones. This may account for the fact that this agent, although active *in vitro*, is ineffective against malignant gliomas that contain many cells in gap 0 (G_0).

Platinum Compounds Used in Brain Tumors

The platinum compounds have significant activity in a wide variety of tumors, including brain tumors. In glioma cell lines, cisplatin is active at relatively low concentrations (2). Similar to the alkylating agents, the platinum compounds disrupt DNA structure by forming crosslinks. Cisplatin was the first inorganic compound to be used in the treatment of human malignancies. Cisplatin and carboplatin are the drugs currently in clinical use (Fig. 2).

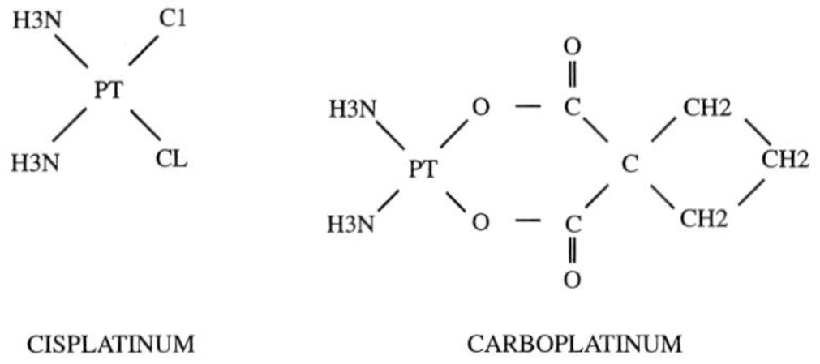

H3N   Cl
PT
H3N   CL
CISPLATINUM

H3N   O — C   O   CH2
PT   C   CH2
H3N   O — C   CH2
CARBOPLATINUM

Figure 2. Platinum compounds in clinical use.

Cisplatin becomes cytotoxic when the chloride concentration is low. In thin cells, where the concentration of chloride is low, the chloride atoms are replaced by water molecules that can react with DNA, RNA, or protein molecules. Both interstrand and intrastrand guanine-platinum-guanine adducts are formed. Cytotoxicity results from the formation of DNA crosslinks. Over 90% of the adducts are intrastrand rather than interstrand. Like those produced by traditional alkylators, intrastrand cisplatin-DNA adducts greatly distort DNA and disrupt replication and transcription (60).

Methylating Agents Used in Brain Tumors

Methylating agents are often called "nonclassical alkylating agents." Unlike the classic alkylators that have bifunctional capacity, these agents have monofunctional capacity. Methylation of individual nucleic acid bases produces single-strand DNA breaks which inhibit DNA and RNA synthesis. Two methylating agents, procarbazine and temozolomide, are currently used for brain tumors.

Procarbazine

Procarbazine requires metabolic activation to be effective. Metabolism by the hepatic cytochrome P-450 enzyme system yields alkyl diazonium intermediates with methylating activity. Methylation produces monofunctional alkylation of DNA (48). DNA replication and RNA synthesis are impaired by processes that resemble those of classical bifunctional alkylating agents. In experimental laboratory models, however, procarbazine does not demonstrate cross-resistance with alkylating agents. Unlike other alkylating agents that lack cell cycle specificity, procarbazine is cytotoxic primarily in S and G2 phases of the cell cycle.

Temozolomide

Temozolomide is a new oral agent showing promise in early clinical trials (52, 75). It is a derivative of imidazotetrazine. It has excellent tissue distribution in the brain. Temozolomide forms *N*-monomethyl triazenoimidazol carboxamide (MTIC), a potent methylating agent. Unlike decarbazine, temozolomide does not require metabolic activation to form MTIC (71). Like procarbazine, temozolomide methylates DNA and forms monoadducts affecting DNA replication.

Miscellaneous Agents Used for the Chemotherapy of Brain Tumors

A number of drugs, the size or mechanism of action of which would not predict efficacy in the brain, have proven beneficial for brain tumors. Such drugs as vincristine, etoposide, and hydroxyurea are used in multiple drug combinations.

Vincristine

Vincristine is isolated from the periwinkle plant, *Vinca rosea*. Vincristine binds to tubulin, a protein that polymerizes to form microtubules. This inhibits formation of microtubules and thus of the mitotic spindle. Although vincristine kills cells in all phases of the cell cycle, cells in late S phase are the most sensitive. It is highly protein bound and does not readily penetrate the central nervous system. Vincristine is not used as a single agent but is often combined with CCNU and procarbazine.

Etoposide (VP-16)

Etoposide is an epipodophyllotoxin that inhibits topoisomerase II. Topoisomerase II is an enzyme that alters the three-dimensional arrangement of DNA. It mediates the passage of one double-strand DNA segment through another DNA segment. Etoposide does not intercalate between DNA strands as do other topoisomerase II inhibitors such as doxorubicin. Rather, etoposide, by trapping the enzyme-DNA complex, stabilizes the DNA double-strand break. Maximum cell killing occurs in S and G2 phases and prevents cells from progressing beyond G2 (61). This agent is currently being tested in high-dose regimens.

Hydroxyurea

Hydroxyurea is a component of many chemotherapy regimens for malignant brain tumors. It diffuses passively into cells and blocks ribonucleotide reductase. This inhibits DNA synthesis without interfering with RNA or protein synthesis by blocking the conversion of ribonucleotides to deoxyribonucleotides. Hydroxyurea also blocks the incorporation of thymidine into DNA (41).

Results of Chemotherapy

The only drug commonly used as a single agent for the treatment of brain tumors is BCNU. It produces partial responses in up to 30% of patients with relapsed high-grade gliomas. The benefit of BCNU in the adjuvant setting after surgery and radiotherapy is small. The sentinel study suggesting a benefit for adjuvant BCNU was BTCG 7201, in which patients treated with BCNU after radiation had a median survival of 51 weeks compared to 36 weeks for patients who received radiotherapy alone (77). The addition of other agents such as cisplatin to BCNU has not improved on the BTCG 7201 results, although clinical trials of this combination continue (54).

Combination chemotherapy has also been employed for malignant gliomas in both the relapsed and adjuvant settings. Besides cisplatin and BCNU, the combinations used most often include PCV (procarbazine, CCNU, and vincristine), cyclophosphamide and vincristine, and a six-drug regimen (CCNU, 6-thioguanine, dibromodulcitol, procarbazine, hydroxyurea, 5-FU). For patients with recurrent disease, the benefit of these regimens is limited (62).

The role of adjuvant chemotherapy for high-grade gliomas remains controversial. Fine's meta-analysis of randomized trials between 1975 and 1989 (21) showed a statistically significant survival advantage for patients treated with chemotherapy and radiotherapy (10.1 and 8.6% increase in survival at 1 and 2 years, respectively; $p = .002$). The patients who derived the most benefit were those with anaplastic astrocytomas. This potential benefit of adjuvant chemotherapy for patients with anaplastic astrocytomas was further confirmed by Levin in the NCOG trial 6G61 (43). Patients with anaplastic astrocytomas lived 151 weeks with PCV therapy compared to 82 weeks with BCNU alone. Adjuvant chemotherapy is also beneficial for anaplastic oligodendrogliomas. Eighteen of 24 patients in a phase II study responded to PCV, and 38% had a complete response. A phase III trial is underway (15).

DRUG RESISTANCE IN BRAIN TUMORS

Cellular resistance to chemotherapeutic agents is a major barrier to their efficacy. Drug resistance is a complex phenomenon that may be either innate to brain tumor cells or acquired as a response to chemotherapy. Resistance results from reduction of the intracellular concentration of the drug either by decreasing drug uptake or increasing drug efflux, by repairing drug-induced damage, or by increasing drug deactivation.

Each of these mechanisms contributes to the drug resistance seen in brain tumors (57). Attempts to overcome resistance through novel delivery systems, high-dose therapy, or pharmacological manipulation of the cellular repair process may improve the outcome of patients with high-grade gliomas.

Resistance to Nitrosoureas

The effectiveness of nitrosoureas against gliomas reflects their rapid diffusion into tumor tissue and their toxicity to tumor cells. Several mechanisms inhibit the *in vivo* activity of nitrosoureas against brain tumors. These include enhanced DNA repair and interference with alkylation.

One site of DNA alkylation by nitrosoureas is the O^6 position of guanine. Repair of the interstrand crosslinks formed by the nitrosoureas is mediated by O^6-alkylguanine-DNA alkyltransferase (O^6-AGAT). This enzyme rapidly removes the alkyl group from the O^6 position of guanine (34). Cells that have measurable O^6-AGAT activity demonstrate methyl excision repair MER(+) activity. Schold (69) found that 10 of 15 xenograft cell lines from human brain tumors are MER(+). Resistance to BCNU in glioma samples and their derived cell lines has been correlated with O^6-AGAT activity (9). Conversely, cells that are MER(−) are more sensitive to the chloronitrosoureas. O^6-alkylguanine-DNA alkyltransferase activity occurs in varying degrees in brain tumors (8). Frosina assayed 27 brain tumor specimens for AGAT activity (26). Meningiomas had the highest activity followed by sarcomas, glioblastomas, astrocytomas, oligodendrogliomas, and lymphomas. This correlates with the sensitivity to chemotherapy of each of these tumors. This enzyme also decreases the cytotoxicity of other unrelated agents such as the platinum compounds and procarbazine (63).

As the importance of O^6-AGAT activity is understood, means of decreasing the activity of O^6-AGAT in order to enhance the cytotoxicity of nitrosoureas have been studied in the laboratory. One strategy involves depletion of O^6-AGAT by introducing alkylguanines or methylating agents. Such approaches have elevated the cytotoxicity of the nitrosoureas in resistant glioma cell lines. The substituted guanines, O^6-methyl guanine and O^6-benzyl guanine, may saturate O^6-AGAT, thereby minimizing its effect on the nitrosourea. The methylating agent streptozotocin may also produce sufficient O^6-methylguanine to saturate the O^6-AGAT enzyme, but only at toxic doses (47). The combination of O^6-benzylguanine and BCNU produces tumor regression in athymic nude mice with glioblastoma multiforme or medulloblastoma much more commonly than does BCNU alone (25). The clinical utility of this strategy remains to be studied, although it is quite likely that only a few tumors depend exclusively on this particular resistance mechanism (10).

Another important mechanism of resistance involves the inactivation of alkylating agents with glutathione or glutathione *S*-transferase. Glutathione inactivates electrophilic molecules such as hydroxyl radicals and alkylating agents (64). Alkylating agents can be inactivated by nonenzymatic conjugation of a thiol group with the alkylating moiety. This same reaction is catalyzed by glutathione *S*-transferase (GST). There are several isoenzymes with substrate specificities that may differ between individual alkylating agents. For example, GST μ isoenzymes inactivate BCNU better than do the π or α classes (70). The observation that high doses of glutathione decrease nitrosourea-induced cytotoxicity *in vitro* suggests that this mechanism of resistance may be important (4). Whether depletion of glutathione improves cytotoxicity in patients remains to be tested.

Resistance to Platinum Compounds

Although the platinum compounds lack cross-resistance with nitrosoureas (2), the mechanisms of resistance to each are similar. These include decreased uptake of the drug into resistant cells, inactivation of the drug by thiols such as glutathione, and enhanced repair of DNA.

Several investigators have shown that decreased intracellular uptake of drugs may contribute to resistance (5). Intracellular uptake of platinum may occur by passive diffusion or by active transport. However, increase in efflux of the platinum out of the cells has not been demonstrated. The mechanism of decreasing uptake of platinum by the cells has not yet been elucidated. Changes in the cellular membrane that could alter drug uptake have not been identified (45).

Resistance to cisplatin is also mediated by glutathione and glutathione S-transferase. Platinum-resistant cell lines have elevated glutathione levels, and depletion of glutathione levels decreases platinum resistance. For example, depletion of glutathione by buthionine sulfoxime overcomes platinum resistance and appears to enhance the cytotoxicity of platinum (65). Increased expression of glutathione S-transferase has been demonstrated in resistant ovarian and squamous cell tumor lines. The isoenzyme of glutathione transferase that appears to cause cisplatin resistance is GST π (66, 76).

Resistance to platinum agents has also been correlated with levels of another sulfhydryl-containing protein, metallothionein. Metallothionein binds and facilitates clearance of heavy metals, such as platinum and zinc. Exposure of cells to high concentrations of heavy metals induces transcription of the metallothionein gene. Evidence that metallothionein causes cisplatin resistance includes the 10-fold increase in metallothionein and the four-fold increase in resistance to cisplatin that follow transfection of mouse C127 cells with the human metallothionein gene. The sulfhydryl group of metallothionein also nonspecifically inactivates other alkylating agents such as melphalan and chlorambucil (38).

As with alkylating agents, enhanced DNA repair contributes to cisplatin resistance. Methyl excision repair by O^6-AGAT plays a minor role (24). Cells deficient in nucleotide excision repair, such as those of patients with Fanconi's anemia, are very sensitive to the platinum compounds (58). Other repair mechanisms may be involved. Increased levels of dihydrofolate reductase, thymidate synthetase, and DNA polymerases α and β occur in cisplatin-resistant ovarian carcinoma cells (68). How these changes produce resistance is yet to be defined. In addition, topoisomerase II may play a role in the repair process (27). Inhibition of topoisomerase II by various agents may decrease the DNA repair process and improve cytotoxicity of the platinum compounds. For example, novobiocin, among its multiple activities, impairs DNA repair by inhibiting topoisomerase II. Ali-Osman *et al.* have shown that inhibition of topoisomerase II by novobiocin decreases DNA repair and enhances the cytotoxicity of both nitrosoureas and cisplatin in human glioblastoma cell lines (3).

Another method of overcoming resistance to the platinum compounds uses intracarotid administration of cisplatin to increase drug delivery. This approach does improve efficacy, but, unfortunately is more toxic. Other methods of increasing the intracellular concentration of platinum have been studied. Anguidine enhances cisplatin cytotoxicity by improving drug uptake (35). Anguidine itself has some anti-glioma activity. Cytosine arabinoside inhibits DNA repair and in combination improves cisplatin cytotoxicity (73). Clinical trials of this combination are under way. Actinomycin D is the only known inhibitor of metallothionein synthesis; finally, analogs of platinum that do not engender cross-resistance to platinum, such as tetraplatin, may be useful in cisplatin-resistant brain tumors.

Resistance to Vincristine and Etoposide

Resistance to both vincristine and etoposide arises from increased DNA repair. In a majority of cell lines, resistance to vincristine results from mutations of the α- or β-subunits of the tubulin heterodimer which reduce binding of the vinca alkaloids. Inhibition of DNA repair can block the development of resistance to etoposide (33), and reduction in topoisomerase II concentrations can enhance resistance to VP-16 (59). However, for both vincristine and etoposide, expression of the multidrug resistance phenotype (MDR) is the most important—and intensively investigated—mechanism of resistance.

Multidrug Resistance

This simultaneous development of resistance to multiple unrelated chemotherapeutic agents after exposure to a single drug may be important in brain tumors. Overexpression of the MDR-1 gene and its product, P-glycoprotein (PgP), and overexpression of the multidrug resistance-associated protein (MRP) gene and its product, an ATP-binding protein, underlie this phenomenon.

The MDR-1 gene encodes a 1280 amino acid transmembrane glycoprotein. P-170 is an ATP-dependent pump that transports a wide variety of structurally unrelated agents out of the cells. Expression of P-170 glycoprotein occurs in both normal and neoplastic cells. High expression of MDR-1 mRNA and protein have been detected in brain capillary endothelial cells. In addition, expression of MDR-1 occurs in adrenal cortex, kidney, colon, and liver and may help form the blood-brain barrier (32, 53). Tumors from these tissues likely retain expression of the MDR-1 gene (23). Chemotherapeutic drugs transported from cells by PgP include vincristine, vinblastine, etoposide, teniposide, doxorubicin, mitoxantrone, taxol, and actinomycin D (39).

PgP is present in normal brain capillary endothelium. Immunohistochemical techniques have identified P-glycoprotein in 2 of 22 glioblastomas and 1 of 1 meningeal sarcoma but not in 14 anaplastic gliomas, two gliosarcomas, and three low-grade gliomas (32). In the 22 glioblastoma samples evaluated, P-glycoprotein was seen in the vascular endothelial cells in 17 samples. Hybridization studies revealed increased MDR-1 gene expression in 6 of 12 pediatric primitive neuroectodermal tumors and up to a three-fold increase in 8 of 32 gliomas (20).

The clinical importance of MDR-1 expression in brain tumors is poorly defined (32). Excepting vincristine and possibly etoposide, the drugs affected by MDR have limited activity against gliomas. Methods to reverse MDR function are being evaluated in both laboratory and clinical studies. Calcium channel blockers block drug efflux by binding to the PgP. Other agents capable of reversing P-glycoprotein multidrug resistance include quinine, cyclosporine, progesterone, and tamoxifen. The clinical benefit of many MDR-reversing agents is limited by their toxicity. The search for less toxic agents capable of inhibiting MDR function is ongoing.

The multidrug resistance-associated protein (MRP) is a 190-kD membrane-associated ATP-binding glycoprotein that also contributes to multidrug resistance. MRP was initially identified in cells that were resistant to doxorubicin but did not express P-glycoprotein. This second protein was heralded by cells that possessed cross-resistance to vincristine, etoposide, and other chemotherapeutic agents but did not contain P-glycoprotein. MRP pumps drugs from the nucleus into the cytoplasm, preventing them from reaching intranuclear targets (16). Glioma cell lines with high MRP mRNA levels have increased resistance to agents such as etoposide (1). One study found low levels of MRP expression in 12 of 15 brain tumor specimens (20). Therefore, it appears that MRP expression is more common than MDR expression in gliomas. The clinical importance of MRP expression is yet to be determined.

The mechanisms of drug resistance in brain tumors are complex. Our current understanding is summarized in Table 2. A variety of strategies for improving the efficacy of conventional chemotherapy have been studied. Many of these trials evaluate protocols designed to combat chloroethylnitrosourea resistance. For example, one six-drug combination was planned to enhance lomustine (CCNU) effectiveness (42). Patients received 6-TG, procarbazine, and dibromodulcitol (DBD) prior to CCNU followed by 5-FU and hydroxyurea 14 days later to diminish anticipated cell division. The rationale for this combination came from *in vitro* studies that have demonstrated that 6-thioguanine enhances nitrosourea cytotoxicity by adding an alkylating target, 6-thioguanine, into DNA. This increases the DNA crosslinks formed by nitrosoureas (11). Procarbazine increases the cytotoxicity of BCNU- and CCNU-induced crosslinks by methylation. DBD alkylates DNA and produces DNA-DNA crosslinks and DNA monoadducts. This agent has little independent activity against brain tumors, but pretreatment of cells with DBD for 4 hours enhances nitrosourea activity (44). In a trial of this six-drug combination, 61% of patients with glioblastoma multiforme had partial response or stable disease. Patients who had previously failed nitrosourea had minimal benefit. Therefore, despite the *in vitro* rationale for such an approach, little

TABLE 2
Mechanisms of Drug Resistance to Commonly Used Drugs in Brain Tumors

Drug	Mechanism
BCNU/CCNU	Increased O^6-alkylguanine-DNA alkytransferase
	Increased glutathione S-transferase
Cisplatinum	Increased O^6-alkylguanine-DNA alkyltransferase?
	Increased glutathione S-transferase
	Increased glutathione
	Increased metallothionein
	Decreased transport
	Increased DNA polymerase, DHFR?
Procarbazine	Increased O^6-alkylguanine-DNA alkyltransferase
	Increased glutathione S-transferase
	Increased glutathione
	Increased metallothionein
Cyclophosphamide	Increased O^6-alkylguanine-DNA alkyltransferase?
	Increased glutathione S-transferase
	Increased glutathione
Vincristine	Increased MDR, MRP
Etoposide	Increased MDR, MRP
	Altered topoisomerase II activity

clinical benefit was apparent in patients with established nitrosourea resistance.

Increased delivery of drugs to the tumor might counteract cell resistance. Three methods have been studied: 1) blood-brain barrier disruption, 2) implanted drug polymers, and 3) high-dose chemotherapy with stem cell support.

The effect of the blood-brain barrier on drug delivery to brain tumors remains controversial (72). Tumors are heterogenous: centrally the barrier is disrupted but peripherally, where neoplastic cells infiltrate normal brain parenchyma, the barrier may be intact. Manipulation with mannitol has been shown to disrupt the blood-brain barrier. The clinical benefit of pharmacological barrier modification is limited by the rapid diffusion of drugs into surrounding brain tissue. This "sump effect" precludes attaining adequate tumor concentration of drugs for a sufficient time. Enhancement of blood-brain barrier disruption must be accompanied by a decreased sump effect. Increased delivery to the brain around tumors is one means, but this requires drugs cytotoxic to tumor cells but not to normal brain.

Most clinical studies disrupt the blood-brain barrier with hyperosmolar mannitol. Published trials vary with regard to the duration of mannitol infusion, documentation of the extent of disruption of the blood-brain barrier, and the chemotherapeutic agents used for treatment (Table 3).

The two largest studies achieved a median survival of 17.5 months for patients with glioblastoma following barrier modification and cyclophosphamide and methotrexate treatment; in these studies 74% of tumors sampled had evidence of necrosis. In another study that employed the same treatment following radiotherapy, 54% of tumors had necrosis, but there was no correlation between necrosis and survival. Thirty-seven patients with high-grade gliomas had a median survival of 22 months from the time of initiation of therapy. Although barrier modification did result in blindness, stroke, seizures, and death in the two largest studies, most

TABLE 3
Trials Using Blood-Brain Barrier Disruption

Author	n	Agents Used	Deaths	Seizure	Neurological Deterioration
Bonastelle *et al.* (12)	18	5-FU/adriamycin	1	2	4
Fauchon *et al.* (19)	16	CNDP, adriamycin/bleo/ara-C	1	2	5
Neuwalt *et al.* (51)	38	Cyclophosphamide/methotrexate	0	21	22
Gumerlock *et al.* (30)	37	Cyclophosphamide/methotrexate	1	16	11

patients had a stable Karnofsky score after treatment. Other agents that modify the blood-brain barrier through different mechanisms, e.g., the bradykinin analogue RmP 2, are under study.

Another approach that could enhance delivery of antineoplastic agents is the implantation of drug-impregnated biodegradable polymers. Drug release from polymers as they degrade provides homogeneously high local concentrations of drugs for prolonged periods. Interstitial implantation circumvents the problems of heterogeneous delivery and exclusion of large charged drugs posed by the blood-brain barrier.

Wafers of BCNU-impregnated biodegradable polymers produce high local concentrations of BCNU in tumors and adjacent brain in animals (29). Recently, polymer wafers have also been used to deliver 4-hydroxycyclophosphamide (4-HC) (37); 20% saturation with 4-HC had minimal toxicity and maximal efficacy. Rats with 9L tumors treated with 4-HC wafers had a median survival of 77 days compared to 21 days for those receiving BCNU wafers. Other agents, including Taxol, are being investigated (78).

Two clinical trials of BCNU-impregnated wafers have been completed. In a phase I-II trial, BCNU-impregnated polymer wafers were implanted in 21 patients with recurrent malignant gliomas. No adverse effects were reported, and 38% of patients lived more than a year after implantation (13). A subsequent multicenter randomized, placebo-controlled phase III trial placed polymer wafers in the surgical bed following reoperation for recurrent malignant gliomas (14). The 110 patients receiving BCNU polymers had a median survival of 31 weeks compared to 23 weeks for the 112 patients who received placebo polymers ($p = .006$). Again there were no clinically apparent adverse effects. These studies strongly suggest the clinical utility of such polymers in the treatment, but studies comparing the technique with standard intravenous administration are needed.

A third approach to drug resistance in brain tumors uses high-dose chemotherapy and stem cell support. For many solid tumors, increasing the dose of chemotherapeutic agents improves the response rate. The efficacy of alkylating agents, in particular, is highly dependent on dose. *In vitro*, increasing the concentration of these drugs overcomes drug resistance. *In vivo*, it increases penetration of the blood-brain barrier by creating a steeper concentration gradient.

Yet, dose-limiting myelosuppression limits the increase in dose of the alkylating agents. However, limits placed on dose by marrow suppression can be circumvented by replacing bone marrow or peripheral blood stem cells injured by high-dose alkylating agents. Contamination of the replacement marrow with brain tumor cells is extremely unlikely to occur (55).

Most high-dose regimens for both systemic tumors and gliomas use alkylating agents. Nitrosoureas, other alkylators such as thiotepa or cyclophosphamide, and the topoisomerase II inhibitor drug, etoposide, have been used in high-dose schemes for astrocytomas. Trials using these agents were initially performed in patients with refractory or recurrent disease.

The initial trials used high-dose BCNU and were notable for significant toxicity, including pulmonary dysfunction and myelosuppression. In one study using BCNU at a dose of 1,050–1200 mg/m^2 with 5-FU (49), 9 of 11 patients responded, 2 patients had a complete response, and 2 died from sepsis. These favorable results in this heavily pretreated and refractory population suggested that high-dose therapy could overcome resistance in a population that had failed conventional therapy. More recently, small phase II trials have investigated this approach in the adjuvant setting.

In a subsequent larger trial, BCNU in a single dose of 600–1400 mg/m^2 was used in 28 patients with high-grade gliomas. Marrow replacement was required in 18 patients. Nine patients died of treatment-related causes, and another nine had significant neurological toxicity. Despite this toxicity, 8 of 24 evaluable patients had an objective response, and four remained alive more than 15 months after transplant (74). In a similar study, 27 patients with progressive disease received 1,050, 1200, or 1350 mg/m^2 BCNU in divided doses over 3 days (56). Twelve of the 27 patients had an objective response. Two of these patients remained free of progression 84 and 60 months after treatment. Three of the nine patients who received this protocol as adjuvant treatment remained alive 70, 48, and 27 months after bone marrow transplant. However, the median survival was only 4 months for this heavily pretreated population. Fatal toxicity occurred in 17%, and 14% had severe interstitial pneumonitis.

TABLE 4
Adjuvant High-Dose Chemotherapy Regimens for Malignant Gliomas

Author	No. of Patients	Drug	Toxic Deaths	Response	Med. Survival (mo)	1 Year Survival (%)
Mbidde *et al.* (46)	22	BCNU	3/22	NR	17	59
Phillips *et al.* (56)	9	BCNU	0	NR	16	55
Wolff *et al.* (79)	18	BCNU	4/18	NR	17.5	NR
Johnson *et al.* (36)	25	BCNU	4/25	64%	26	78
Ascensao *et al.* (6)	7	Thiotepa	0	65%	NR	NR

These trials encouraged use of dose-intensive chemotherapy as part of adjuvant therapy. Nine patients treated in an adjuvant setting with the 3-day protocol just mentioned had a median survival of 16 months, a 1-year survival of 55%, and no toxic deaths. In another study, 25 patients with high-grade unresectable gliomas were treated with BCNU at 350 mg/m^2/day for 3 days within 3 weeks of surgery (36). This was followed by whole brain irradiation. Ten patients had a complete response, and the median survival for all patients was 26 months, significantly better than that of historical controls. Four died from treatment-related toxicity. Three other studies (see Table 4) used similar doses of BCNU and had lower response rates. Other small studies have used different alkylating agents. Four of seven patients treated after resection and before radiotherapy with high-dose thiotepa had evidence of response (6). Encephalopathy was less common in these adjuvant studies than in those treating recurrent disease. Delivery of radiotherapy after rather than before the chemotherapy may be responsible.

In the pediatric population, high-dose chemotherapy with stem cell support has been used for other CNS tumors, including medulloblastoma, ependymomas, and peripheral neuroectodermal tumors. Many of the studies in children use other agents such as busulfan, thiotepa, and etoposide. Results in children are slightly more promising than these in adults (22), but this approach is not yet accepted as standard therapy.

SUMMARY

Relatively little progress has occurred in the treatment of gliomas over the past 20 years. While surgery and radiation therapy comprise the standard treatment for most patients with malignant glial tumors, chemotherapy appears to be beneficial only for those patients with anaplastic astrocytomas and anaplastic oligodendrogliomas. The clinical effectiveness of both BCNU and newer agents is surprisingly poor when compared with the apparent sensitivity of glioma cell lines to these drugs *in vitro*. Improved understanding of the mechanisms of resistance may improve the results with chemotherapy. Subverting resistance mechanisms dependent upon O^6-alkylguanine-DNA alkyltransferase, glutathione *S*-transferase, metallothionein, and the multiple drug resistance genes is an appealing strategy. Study of the molecular mechanisms involved in drug resistance, and the development of clinical strategies to alter them, are just beginning, but initial results suggest great promise of improved clinical outcomes in the future.

Acknowledgments

This work was supported in part by the American Cancer Society Professor of Clinical Oncology Grant No. 071 and NIH-NINCDS T32 NS07289 (M. S. Berger).

REFERENCES

1. Abe, T., Hasegawa, S., Taniguchi, K., *et al.* Possible involvement of multidrug-resistance-associated protein (MRP) gene expression in spontaneous drug resistance to vincristine, etoposide and adriamycin in human glioma cells. Int. J. Cancer *58:*860–864, 1994.
2. Aida, T., and Bodell, W. J. Cellular resistance to chloroethylnitrosoureas, nitrogen mustard, and cis-diamminedichloroplatinum (II) in human glial-derived cell lines. Cancer Res. *47:*1361–1366, 1987.
3. Ali-Osman, F., Berger, M. S., Rajagopal, S., *et al.* Topoisomerase II inhibition and altered kinetics of formation and repair of nitrosourea and cisplatin-induced DNA interstrand cross-links and cytotoxicity in human glioblastoma cells. Cancer Res. *53:*5663–5668, 1993.
4. Ali-Osman, F., Caughlan, J., and Gray, G. S. Decreased DNA interstrand cross-linking and cytotoxicity induced in human brain tumor cells by 1,3-bis(2-chlo-

roethyl)-1-nitrosourea after in vitro reaction with glutathione. Cancer Res. *49:*5954–5958, 1989.

5. Andrews, P. A., Murphy, M. P., and Howell, S. B. Cis-diamminedichloroplatinum (II) accumulation in sensitive and resistant human ovarian cancer cells. Cancer Res. *48:*68–71, 1988.

6. Ascensao, J., Ahmed, T., Feldman, E., *et al.* High dose thiotepa with autologous bone marrow transplantation (ABMT) and localized radiotherapy for patients with astrocytoma grade III/IV (glioma): a promising approach. Proc. Am. Soc. Clin. Oncol. *8:*90, 1989.

7. Blasberg, R. G., and Groothuis, D. R. Chemotherapy of brain tumors: physiological and pharmacokinetic considerations. Semin. Oncol. *13:*70–82, 1986.

8. Bobola, M. S., Berger, M. S., and Silber, J. R. Contribution of O^6-methylguanine-DNA methyltransferase to monofunctional alkylating agent resistance in human brain tumor-derived cell lines. Mol. Carcinog. *13:*70–80, 1995.

9. Bobola, M. S., Berger, M. S., and Silber, J. R. Contribution of O^6-methylguanine-DNA methyltransferase to resistance to 1,3-bis(2-chloroethyl)-1-nitrosourea in human brain tumor-derived cell lines. Mol. Carcinog. *13:*81–88, 1995.

10. Bobola, M. S., Tseng, S.-H., Blank, A., *et al.* Role of O^6-methylguanine-DNA methyltransferase in resistance of human brain tumor cell lines to the clinically relevant methylating agents temozolomide and streptozotocin. Clin. Cancer Res. *2:*735–741, 1996.

11. Bodell, W. J., Morgan, W. F., Rasmussen, J., *et al.* Potentiation of 1,3-bis (2-chloroethyl)-1-nitrosourea (BCNU)-induced cytotoxicity in 9L cells by pretreatment with 6-thioguanine. Biochem. Pharmacol. *34:* 515–520, 1985.

12. Bonastelle, C. T., Kori, S. H., and Rekate, H. Intracarotid chemotherapy of glioblastoma after induced blood-brain barrier disruption. AJNR Am. J. Neuroradiol. *4:*810–812, 1983.

13. Brem, H., Mahaley, M. S., Jr., Vick, N. A., *et al.* Interstitial chemotherapy with drug polymer implants for the treatment of recurrent gliomas. J. Neurosurg. *74:*441–446, 1991.

14. Brem, H., Piantadosi, S., Burger, P. C., *et al.* Placebo-controlled trial of safety and efficacy of intraoperative controlled delivery by biodegradable polymers of chemotherapy for recurrent gliomas. Lancet *345:* 1008–1012, 1995.

15. Cairncross, G., Macdonald, D., Ludwin, S., *et al.* Chemotherapy for anaplastic oligodendroglioma. J. Clin. Oncol. *12:*2013–2021, 1994.

16. Cole, S. P., Bhardwaj, G., Gerlach, J. H., *et al.* Overexpression of a transporter gene in a multidrug-resistant human lung cancer cell line. Science *258:* 1650–1654, 1992.

17. Colvin, M., Padgett, C. A., and Fenselau, C. A biologically active metabolite of cyclophosphamide. Cancer Res. *33:*915–918, 1973.

18. Erickson, L. C., Bradley, M. O., Ducore, J. M., *et al.* DNA crosslinking cytotoxicity in normal and transformed human cells treated with antitumor nitrosoureas. Proc. Natl. Acad. Sci. U.S.A. *77:*467–471, 1980.

19. Fauchon, F., Chiras, J., Poisson, M., *et al.* Intra-arterial chemotherapy by cisplatin and cytarabine after temporary disruption of the blood-brain barrier for the treatment of malignant gliomas in adults. J. Neuroradiol. *13:*151–162, 1986.

20. Feun, L. G., Savaraj, N., and Landy, H. J. Drug resistance in brain tumors. J. Neurol. Oncol. *20:*165–176, 1994.

21. Fine, H. A., Dear, K. B. G., Loeffler, J. S., *et al.* Meta-analysis of radiation therapy with and without adjuvant chemotherapy for malignant gliomas in adults. Cancer *71:*2585–2597, 1993.

22. Finlay, J. L., August, C., Packer, R., *et al.* High dose multi-agent chemotherapy followed by bone marrow 'rescue' for malignant astrocytomas of childhood and adolescence. J. Neurooncol. *9:*239–248, 1990.

23. Fojo, A. T., Ueda, K., Slamon, D. J., *et al.* Expression of a multidrug-resistance gene in human tumors and tissues. Proc. Natl. Acad. Sci. U.S.A. *84:*265–269, 1987.

24. Fravel, H. N., and Roberts, J. J. Excision repair of cis-diamminedichloroplatinum (II)-induced damage to DNA of Chinese hamster ovary cells. Cancer Res. *39:*1793–1796, 1979.

25. Friedman, H. S., Dolan, M. E., Moschel, R. C., *et al.* Enhancement of nitrosourea activity in medulloblastoma and glioblastoma multiforme. J. Natl. Cancer Inst. *84:*1926–1931, 1992.

26. Frosina, G., Rossi, O., Arena, G., *et al.* O^6-alkylguanine-DNA alkyltransferase activity in human brain tumors. Cancer Lett. *55:*153–158, 1990.

27. Gedick, C. M., and Collins, A. R. Comparison of effects of fostriecin, novobiocin, and camptothecin, inhibitors of DNA topoisomerases, on DNA replication and repair in human cells. Nucleic Acids Res. *18:*1007–1013, 1990.

28. Greig, N. H. Optimizing drug delivery to brain tumors. Cancer Treat. Rev. *14:*1–28, 1987.

29. Grossman, S. A., Reinhard, C., Colvin, O. M., *et al.* The intracerebral distribution of BCNU delivered by surgical implanted biodegradable polymers. J. Neurosurg. *76:*640–547, 1992.

30. Gumerlock, M. K., Belshe, B. D., Madse, R., *et al.* Osmotic blood-brain barrier disruption and chemotherapy in the treatment of high grade malignant glioma: patient series and literature review. J. Neurooncol. *12:*33–46, 1992.

31. Heal, J. M., Fox, P. A., and Schein, P. S. Effect of carbamoylation on the repair of nitrosourea-induced DNA alkylation damage in L1210 cells. Cancer Res. *39:*82–29, 1979.

32. Henson, J. W., Cordon-Cardo, C., and Posner, J. B. P-glycoprotein expression in brain tumors. J. Neurooncol. *14:*37–43, 1992.

33. Hill, B. T., and Bellamy, A. S. Establishment of an etoposide-resistant human epithelial tumor cell line in vitro: characterization of patterns of cross-resistance and drug sensitivities. Int. J. Cancer *33:*599–608, 1984.

34. Hotta, T., Saito, Y., Fujita, H., *et al.* O^6-alkylguanine-DNA alkyltransferase activity of human malignant glioma and its clinical implications. J. Neurooncol. *21:*135–140, 1994.

35. Hromas, R. A., and Yung, W. K. Anguidine potentiates cis-platinum in human brain tumor cells. J. Neurooncol. *3:*343–348, 1986.

36. Johnson, D. B., Thompson, J. M., Corwin, J. A., *et al.* Prolongation of survival for high-grade malignant gliomas with adjuvant high-dose BCNU and autologous bone marrow transplantation. J. Clin. Oncol. *5:*783–789, 1987.

37. Judy, K. D., Olivi, A., Buahin, K. G., *et al.* Effectiveness of controlled release of a cyclophosphamide derivative with polymers against rat gliomas. J. Neurosurg. *82:*481–486, 1995.

38. Kelley, S. L., Basu, A., Teicher, B. A., *et al.* Overexpression of metallothionein confers resistance to anticancer drugs. Science *241*(4874):1813–1815, 1988.

39. Lehnert, M. Multidrug resistance in human cancer. J. Neurooncol. *22:*239–243, 1994.

40. Lesser, G. J., and Grossman, S. A. The chemotherapy of adult primary brain tumors. Cancer Treat. Rev. *19:*261–281, 1993.

41. Levin, V. A. The place of hydroxyurea in the treatment of primary brain tumors. Semin. Oncol. *19*(suppl.):34–39, 1992.

42. Levin, V. A., and Prados, M. D. Treatment of recurrent gliomas and metastatic brain tumor with a polydrug protocol designed to combat nitrosourea resistance. J. Clin. Oncol. *10:*766–771, 1992.

43. Levin, V. A., Silver, P., Hannigan, J., *et al.* Superiority of post-radiotherapy adjuvant chemotherapy with CCNU, procarbazine, and vincristine (PCV) over BCNU for anaplastic gliomas: NCOG 6G61 final report. Int. J. Radiat. Oncol. Biol. Phys. *18:*321–324, 1990.

44. Levin, V. A., and Wheeler, K. T. Chemotherapeutic approaches to brain tumors. Experimental observations with dianhydrogalactitol and dibromodulcitol. Cancer Chemother. Pharmacol. *8:*125–131, 1982.

45. Mann, S. C., Andrews, P. A., and Howell, S. B. Comparison of lipid content, surface membrane fluidity, and temperature dependence of cis-diamminedichloroplatinum (II) accumulation in sensitive and resistant human ovarian cancer cells. Anticancer Res. *8:*1211–1215, 1988.

46. Mbidde, E. K., Selby, P. J., Perren, T. J., *et al.* High dose BCNU chemotherapy with autologous bone marrow transplantation and full dose radiotherapy for grade IV astrocytoma. Br. J. Cancer *58:*779–782, 1988.

47. Micetich, K. C., Futscher, B., Koch, D., *et al.* Phase I study of streptozocin- and carmustine-sequenced administration in patients with advanced cancer. J. Natl. Cancer Inst. *84:*256–260, 1992.

48. Moloney, S. J., Wiebkin, P., Cummings, S. W., *et al.* Metabolic activation of the terminal N-methyl group of N-isopropyl-alpha-(2-methylhydrazino)-p-toluamide hydrochloride (procarbazine). Carcinogenesis *6:*397–401, 1985.

49. Mortimer, J. E., Hewlett, J. S., and Bay, J. High dose BCNU with autologous bone marrow rescue in the treatment of recurrent malignant gliomas. J. Neurooncol. *1:*269–274, 1983.

50. Moynihan, T. J., and Grossman, S. A. The role of chemotherapy in the treatment of primary tumor of the central nervous system. Cancer Invest. *12:*88–97, 1994.

51. Neuwalt, E. A., Howieson, J., Frenkel, E. P., *et al.* Therapeutic efficacy of multiagent chemotherapy with drug delivery enhancement by blood-brain barrier modification in glioblastoma. Neurosurgery *19:*573–582, 1986.

52. O'Reily, S. M., Newlands, E. S., Glaser, M. G., *et al.* Temozolamide: a new oral cytotoxic chemotherapeutic agent with promising activity against primary brain tumors. Eur. J. Cancer *29A:*940–942, 1993.

53. Pastan, I., and Gottesman, M. Multiple-drug resistance in human cancer. N. Engl. J. Med. *316:*1388–1393, 1987.

54. Petersdorf, S., Upchurch, C., Eyre, H., *et al.* A phase II study of external beam radiation and chemotherapy with cisplatin/BCNU followed by BCNU alone for the treatment of incompletely resected high grade brain tumors: preliminary results of a Southwest Oncology Group (SWOG) Study (SWOG 9016) (Abstract). Proc. Am. Soc. Clin. Oncol. *12:*176, 1993.

55. Petersdorf, S. H., and Livingston, R. B. High dose chemotherapy for the treatment of malignant brain tumors. J. Neurooncol. *20:*155–163, 1994.

56. Phillips, G. L., Wolff, S. N., Fay, J. W., *et al.* Intensive 1,3-bis(2-chloroethyl)-1-nitrosourea (BCNU) monochemotherapy and autologous marrow transplantation for malignant glioma. J. Clin. Oncol. *4:*639–645, 1986.

57. Phillips, P. C. Antineoplastic drug resistance in brain tumors. Neurol. Clin. *9:*383–404, 1991.

58. Poll, E. H., Arwert, F., Kortbeek, H. T., *et al.* Fanconi anemia cells are not uniformly deficient in unhooking of DNA interstrand crosslinks, induced by mitomycin C or 8-methoxypsoralen plus UVA. Hum. Genet. *68:*228–234, 1984.

59. Pommier, Y., Kerrigan, D., Schwartz, R. D., *et al.* Altered DNA topoisomerase II activity in Chinese hamster cells resistant to topoisomerase II inhibitors. Cancer Res. *46:*3075–3081, 1986.

60. Rice, J. A., Crothers, D. M., Pinto, A. L., *et al.* The major adduct of the antitumor drug cis-diamminedichloroplatinum (II) with DNA bends the duplex by approximately equal to 40 degrees toward the major groove. Proc. Natl. Acad. Sci. U.S.A. *85:*4158–4161, 1988.

61. Ross, W., Rowe, T., Glisson, B., *et al.* Role of topoisomerase II in mediating epipodophyllotoxin induced SNA cleavage. Cancer Res. *44:*5857–5860, 1984.

62. Rostomily, R., Spence, A., Duong, D., *et al.* Multimodality management of recurrent adult malignant gliomas: results of a phase II multiagent chemotherapy study and analysis of cytoreductive surgery. Neurosurgery *35:*378–388, 1994.

63. Russell, S. J., Yun-Wei, M. S., Waber, P. G., *et al.* P53 mutations, O^6-alkylguanine DNA alkyltransferase activity, and sensitivity to procarbazine in human brain tumors. Cancer *75:*1339–1342, 1995.

64. Russo, A., Carmichael, J., Friedman, N., *et al.* The roles of intracellular glutathione in antineoplastic chemotherapy. Int. J. Radiat. Oncol. Biol. Phys. *12:*1347–1354, 1986.

65. Russo, A., DeGraff, W., Friedman, N., *et al.* Selective modulation of glutathione levels in human normal versus tumor cells and subsequent differential response to chemotherapy drugs. Cancer Res. *46*(6):2845–2846, 1986.

66. Saburi, Y., Makagawa, M., Ono, M., *et al.* Increased expression of glutathione s-transferase gene in cis-diamminedichloroplatinum(II)-resistant variants of a Chinese hamster ovary cell line. Cancer Res. *49:* 7020–7025, 1989.

67. Sariban, E., Kohn, K. W., Zlotogorski, C., *et al.* DNA cross-linking responses of human malignant glioma cell strains to chloroethylnitrosoureas, cisplatin, and diaziquone. Cancer Res. *47:*3988–3994, 1987.

68. Scanlon, K. J., and Kashani-Sabet, M. Elevated expression of thymidylate synthase cycle genes in cisplatin-resistant human ovarian carcinoma A2780 cells. Proc. Natl. Acad. Sci. U.S.A. *85:*650–653, 1988.

69. Schold, S. C., Brent, T. P., Von Hofe, *et al.* O^6-alkyl-guanine-DNA-alkyltransferase and sensitivity to procarbazine in human brain-tumor xenografts. J. Neurosurg. *70:*573–577, 1989.

70. Smith, M. T., Evans, C. G., Doane-Setzer, P., *et al.* Denitrosation of 1,3-bis(2-chloroenthyl)-1-nitrosourea by class mu glutathione transferases and its role in cellular resistance in rat brain tumor cells. Cancer Res. *49:*2621–2625, 1989.

71. Stevens, Hickman, J. A., Langdon, S. P., *et al.* Antitumor activity and pharmacokinetics in mice of 8-carbamoyl-3-methyl-imidazo[5,1-d]-1,2,3,5-tetrazin-4 (3)-one (CCRG 81045;M& B39831), a novel drug with potential as an alternative to decarbazine. Cancer Res. *47:*5846–5852, 1987.

72. Stewart, D. J. A critique of the role of the blood-brain barrier in the chemotherapy of human brain tumors. J. Neurooncol. *20:*121–139, 1994.

73. Stewart, D. J., Hugenholtz, H., DaSilva, V., *et al.* Cytosine arabinoside plus cisplatin and other drugs as chemotherapy for gliomas. Semin. Oncol. *14*(2 suppl. 1):110–115, 1987.

74. Takvorian, T., Parker, L. M., Hochberg, F. H., *et al.* Autologous bone-marrow transplantation: host effects of high-dose BCNU. J. Clin. Oncol. *1:*611–620, 1983.

75. Taylor, S. A. New agents in the treatment of primary brain tumors. J. Neurooncol. *20:*141–153, 1994.

76. Teicher, B. A., Holden, S. A., Kelley, M. J., *et al.* Characterization of a human squamous carcinoma cell line resistant to cis-diamminedichloroplatinum(II). Cancer Res. *47:*388–393, 1990.

77. Walker, M. D., Green, S. B., Byar, D. P., *et al.* Randomized comparisons of radiotherapy and nitrosoureas for the treatment of malignant glioma after surgery. N. Engl. J. Med. *303:*1323–2329, 1980.

78. Walter, K. A., Cahan, M. A., Gur, A., *et al.* Interstitial taxol delivered from a biodegradable polymer implant against experimental malignant glioma. Cancer Res. *54:*2207–2212, 1994.

79. Wolff, S. N., Phillips, G. L., and Herzig, G. P. High-dose carmustine with autologous bone marrow transplantation for the adjuvant treatment of high-grade gliomas of the central nervous system. Cancer Treat. Rep. *71:*183–185, 1987.

CHAPTER 13

Immune Response Against Malignant Astrocytic Tumors and Related Therapy

PIERRE-YVES DIETRICH, M.D., NICOLAS de TRIBOLET, M.D.

INTRODUCTION

Despite aggressive multimodality therapy, the prognosis of patients with malignant astrocytomas remains poor. In glioblastoma, the median survival after surgery and adjuvant radiotherapy is less than 1 year, and few patients are still alive 2 years after their diagnosis (48, 96, 158). The relative ineffectiveness of current therapy warrants an intense search for other treatment strategies. Immunotherapy is one approach that has been vigorously used in the last 3 decades. At first glance, this approach may appear a strange one, considering the long-held belief that the CNS is an immunologically privileged site (89). However, substantial evidence indicates that immune responses mediated by various cell types occur within the CNS and that the manipulation of the immune system is a promising strategy for gliomas.

In this chapter, the 10-year history of clinical research with interleukin-2 (IL-2) and *in vitro* amplified immune cells will be presented. Recent advances in fundamental immunology, current knowledge of the complex interaction between tumor cells and host immune system, lessons from other tumors such as melanoma, and mechanisms by which gliomas may escape immune surveillance will be reviewed and used as background to introduce some of the promising immunological treatment strategies currently under investigation for glioma.

CLINICAL IMMUNOTHERAPY

Rationale and IL-2 in Monotherapy

In 1970, the theory of immunosurveillance was elaborated: cells undergoing malignant transformation are recognized as foreign by immune cells and destroyed (42). If this hypothesis is true, then tumor growth within an immunocompetent host implies dysfunction of immunosurveillance. The discovery of IL-2 and its dramatic *in vitro* immunostimulatory properties suggested an *in vivo* role for immune surveillance. First identified in the supernatant of T cells in culture and, therefore, named T-cell growth factor in 1976 (194), IL-2 is a pleiotropic cytokine that amplifies the immune response. Mainly produced by T cells, IL-2 stimulates the proliferation and differentiation of T and B lymphocytes, increases the cytotoxicity of T lymphocytes and NK cells, activates monocytes and eosinophils (probably by way of secondary IL-5 secretion from T-cells), enhances antibody-dependent cell cytotoxicity (ADCC), and upregulates adhesion molecules (*e.g.,* ICAM-1, LFA-3) that recruit immune effector cells during inflammation. The various IL-2 effects are mediated either directly by the IL-2 specific receptor (189) or indirectly by the secondary release of numerous cytokines (*e.g.,* IFN-γ, IL-5, GM-CSF, M-CSF, TNF-α, IL-6, or IL-1β) from lymphocytes, macrophages, eosinophils, and other cell types. Some of these cytokines contribute to the side effects and the antitumor effect of IL-2.

IL-2 given systemically induces a response in 15–30% of patients with metastatic melanoma or renal cell carcinoma; approximately 5% are complete responders (134, 164, 232). More equivocal results are seen in patients with lymphoma and leukemia (79). Despite the low percentages, these responses are the first clinical proof that manipulation of the immune system is an effective way to treat cancer.

In vitro, treatment of glioma cells with IL-2 produced variable results: Some glioma cell lines were inhibited, but others were stimulated (25). Clinically, the intravenous administration of IL-2 to patients with a glioma is limited by the exacerbation of peritumoral edema by IL-2-induced capillary leakage. Therefore, glioma patients were treated with intracavitary or intracerebroventricular injections of IL-2. Low doses (10,000 IU/injection) were relatively well tolerated, but higher doses (50,000 IU) increased edema (184). Only marginal antitumoral effects were observed. Secondary release of other cytokines likely contributes to IL-2 induced edema. Indeed, the intraventricular administration of IL-2 induces increases of TNF-α, IL-6, IL1-β, IFN-γ, and IL-2R (165).

LAK Cells (lymphokine activated killers)

The hypothesis that IL-2 is antineoplastic by its activation of immune cells prompted efforts to amplify this effect by adoptive immunotherapy. In adoptive immunotherapy, peripheral blood lymphocytes are harvested, transformed into LAK cells *in vitro* by IL-2, and then administered to the patient. Mainly derived from a natural killer (NK) cell subset, LAK cells are large granular lymphocytes with cytolytic activity against Daudi (a NK-cell resistant tumor line) cells, most tumor cell lines, and fresh tumors. The combination of adoptive transfer of LAK cells and intravenous IL-2 produced regression of a variety of advanced metastatic cancers in animal models. Unfortunately, LAK cells do not improve the results obtained with IL-2 alone in human tumors (145, 216). In gliomas, LAK cells and IL-2 were injected into the tumor cavity either immediately after resection or later through an Ommaya reservoir. In the most carefully conducted trials, the results were disappointing. Clinical responses were the exception; all patients had adverse effects, and many experienced early worsening of their neurological deficits. The median duration of survival after immunotherapy was only a few weeks (as with standard salvage therapy) (17, 163, 185).

TIL (Tumor-Infiltrating Lymphocytes)

The poor efficacy of LAK cells may reflect the lack of specificity of their cytotoxicity. This lack of specificity results from the choice of nonspecific resting precursors in peripheral blood for stimulation by IL-2. Rosenberg hypothesized that because tumor-infiltrating lymphocyte (TIL) are in close contact with tumor cells and are, thus, likely to have been preactivated *in vivo* (44, 231). Using methods similar to those for developing LAK cells, TIL may be extracted from tumor cultured *in vitro* with IL-2 to stimulate preactivated T cells and then returned to patients in conjunction with IL-2. However, the low number of T cells within gliomas, as well as their numerous proliferative and functional abnormalities (see below) (234), may render this approach ineffective. Encouraging data has been obtained in murine brain tumors (239), although the usefulness of TIL in human gliomas has yet to be determined. The disappointing results obtained in more accessible tumors (*e.g.*, melanoma) suggest that this strategy has little promise.

To further enhance the specific antitumor effect of immune cells, antigen-sensitized cytolytic lymphocytes (CTL) have been developed. In one model (123, 124), the splenocytes of rats immunized *in vivo* with RT2 anaplastic astrocytoma cells were restimulated *in vitro* with irradiated RT2 plus IL-2. This procedure should generate T cells with specific cytotoxicity against RT2 tumor cells. The intravenous administration of these RT2-sensitized splenocytes caused rejection of RT2 intracerebral tumors in rats and prolonged survival, compared with that of rats treated with LAK cells and IL-2. This approach has not yet been attempted in humans.

Bifunctional Monoclonal Antibodies

Produced by sophisticated fusion of B-cell hybridomas, a bifunctional antibody links an F(ab′) fragment with tumor antigen specificity with an F(ab′) fragment specific for a surface molecule of an immune effector cell (*e.g.*, CD3 on T cells or CD16 on NK cells) (Fig. 1). It can recognize two unique antigenic structures and may be very useful in bringing effector immune

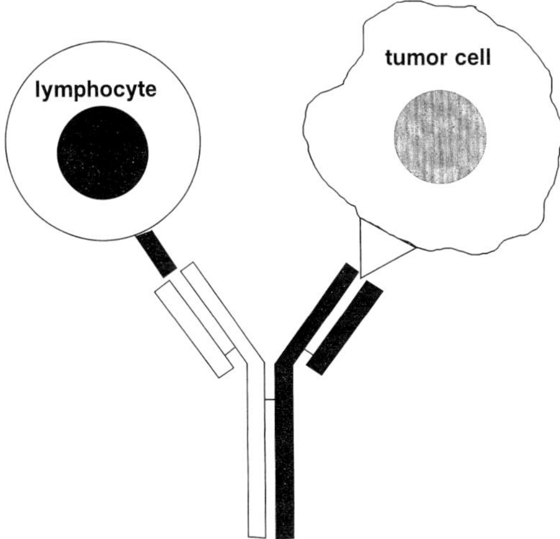

Figure 1. Bifunctional antibodies. Also termed bispecific antibodies, they are produced by fusion of two B-cell hybridomas. They recognize one antigenic structure on the surface of tumor cells and another on immune effector cells.

cells into close interaction with tumor cells by an antibody bridge (140, 273). The cure of human Hodgkin's disease grafted into immunodeficient mice using bispecific monoclonal antibodies in conjunction with blood lymphocytes has been reported (222). Bifunctional antibodies have been developed for gliomas. They simultaneously recognize the CD3 complex on T cells and a human glioma-associated antigen and markedly enhance the *in vitro* cytolytic activity of glioma patients' LAK cells against the human glioma cell line U251MG (204). Based on these *in vitro* data, a clinical study was conducted to evaluate the therapeutical potential of these bifunctional antibodies in glioma patients (204, 206). Ten glioma patients received LAK cells preincubated with bifunctional antibody, and the results were compared with those from 10 patients treated with LAK cells alone. No recurrence was seen in the 10–18 months of follow-up in the LAK-plus-bifunctional antibody group, but further follow-up has not been reported. Additional study will determine whether the lack of absolute specificity of bifunctional antibodies is a serious limitation, whether a therapeutical effect can be achieved without major adverse effects, and whether the human antiantibody response against xenogeneic antibodies can be circumvented.

HOW GLIOMA CELLS SHOULD INTERACT WITH IMMUNE SYSTEM

Results obtained with IL-2 alone or in association with immune cells suggest that the nonspecific stimulation of the immune system may be an effective way to treat some cancer patients. However, in most studies, relatively few patients benefit, and treatment-related toxicity has been severe. More specific stimulation of the T cells involved in tumor cell recognition that avoids the unnecessary and probably counterproductive activation of the entire immune system may diminish toxicity. Selective stimulation of the immune system may increase efficacy while decreasing toxicity.

Antigen Presentation and Major Histocompatibility Complex (MHC)

Self and foreign proteins are continuously presented to immune cells. In contrast with immunoglobulins that recognize antigens in their native structure, T cells recognize antigenic peptides presented by MHC molecules. MHC molecules are a set of polymorphic genes encoding class I and class II cell surface glycoproteins (1, 36). Class I molecules, consisting of a polymorphic transmembrane heavy chain and a soluble subunit termed β2-microglobulin, bind and present peptides of 8–10 amino acids to CD8+ T lymphocytes (193). Class II molecules, transmembrane heterodimers composed of α and β chains, present larger peptides (14–22 residues) to CD4+ T cells (236). Before being presented to T cells, antigens are processed intracellularly by division into peptides. This antigen processing differs for class I and class II associated antigens (Fig. 2) (115). MHC class I antigens are unfolded and degraded by proteasomes. Proteasomes are 2000-kD cytosolic structures that account for about 1% of protein in mammalian cells (114). They contain two major components, a 20S particle that is proteolytic and a 19S part that contains several ATPases. IFN-γ enhances antigen presentation by inducing the expression of three β subunits of proteasomes. These newly synthesized subunits replace pre-existing homologous subunits in proteasomes. The resulting proteasomes cleave antigen peptides preferentially after hydrophobic and basic residues. Thus, IFN-γ favors production of antigenic peptides with hydrophobic or basic carboxyl-termini. Such

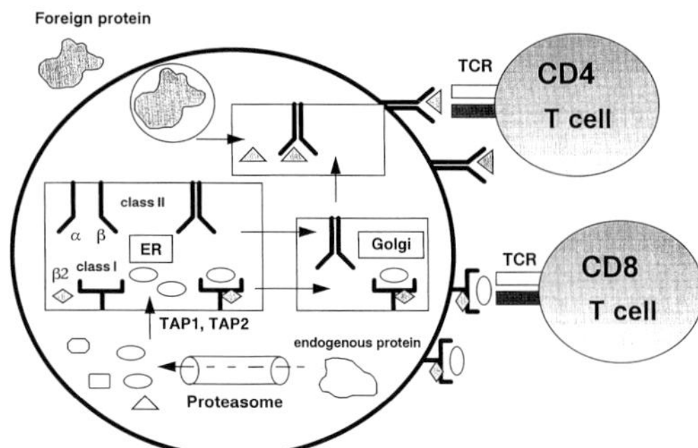

Figure 2. Antigen processing and presentation. The intracellular pathway of antigenic proteins presented by class I or class II molecules is schematically illustrated (see text). ER, endoplasmic reticulum; TAP, peptide transporter; TCR, T-cell receptor.

peptides are preferentially transported into the endoplasmic reticulum and bind tightly to MHC class I receptors.

The majority of peptides processed by proteasomes are rapidly hydrolyzed into amino acids by cytosolic exopeptidases. A minority of these peptides are of a size suitable for transport into the endoplasmic reticulum (ER) by peptide transporters called TAP molecules. A TAP molecule is a heterodimeric protein formed of two homologous polypeptides encoded by the TAP-1 and TAP-2 genes located in the MHC class II region (254). Mutant cell lines not expressing this transporter and knockout mice lacking TAP-1 and/or TAP-2 genes do not present antigen to CD8+ T cells and have reduced levels of surface class I MHC molecules. In humans, a genetic defect in TAP has been linked to an inherited immune deficiency (71).

MHC class II-associated antigens follow a different pathway. Most are derived from exogenous proteins (202). Exogenous antigens are endocytosed by cells and digested during passage through intracellular compartments (endosomes, lysosomes). α and β chains of class II molecules assemble in the ER and then reach the trans-Golgi reticulum via the Golgi apparatus. Thus, MHC class II molecules bind proteolyzed peptides at a site that varies with cell type and antigen presented (275) (Fig. 3). MHC class II molecules bearing peptides are transported to the cell surface in a manner currently unknown. A rare inherited disease, MHC class II deficiency results from a defect in one of the two transcription factors (*i.e.*, CIITA or the het-

erodimer RFX) regulating MHC class II gene expression (170, 223, 249, 250).

Excepting germ and placental cells, all cells express class I molecules and may be able to present antigenic peptides to CD8+ cells. In contrast, expression of class II molecules is limited to a few cell types, whose main function is antigen presentation (46). The monocytes, macrophages, B lymphocytes, and dendritic cells involved are called antigen-presenting cells (APC). Dendritic cells (DC) originate from bone marrow progenitors and are distributed to nearly all tissues of the body (229). Langerhans cells in the skin, interdigitating DC in the thymus and lymph nodes, and interstitial DCs in the heart, kidney, gut, and lung have a dendritic morphology. They contain CD1a, MHC class II molecules, accessory molecules (*e.g.*, B7, CD58 or LFA2, CD54 or ICAm-1; see below) in the delivery of a second signal to T cells, and intracytoplasmic Birbeck granules (146, 156). GM-CSF markedly increases the capacity of DC to present antigen. DC may be generated *in vitro* from blood progenitors stimulated by GM-CSF and either TNF-a or IL-4 (45, 209, 229).

Within the CNS, astrocytes may express MHC class I and II molecules and present antigens. Studies of cultured astrocytes suggest that MHC expression is inducible rather than constitutive (69, 142, 277, 286). For example, expression of MHC class I and II molecules on the surface of cultured astrocytes is increased after incubation with IFN-γ. Some murine and human astrocytes treated with IFN-8 present foreign antigens to class I- and class II-re-

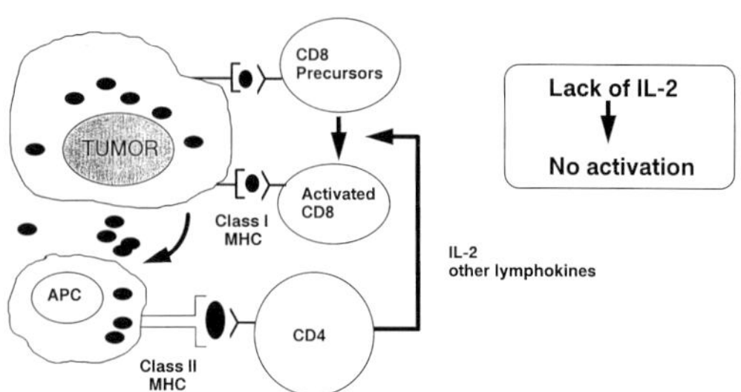

Figure 3. Ideal presentation of tumor antigens to both CD4 and CD8 T cells. An adequate antitumor immune response requires activation of both helper and cytolytic T lymphocytes. The secretion of cytokines such as IL-2 or INF-γ is critical to activation of resting CD8 T lymphocytes. Some antigens may have both MHC class I and class II epitopes.

stricted human CTL (69) but fail to stimulate T-cell proliferation and activation (277). Interestingly, *in vivo* expression of class II molecules is present in about 40% of gliomas while expression of MHC class I molecules is very rare (63, 151, 195). Some human glioblastoma cell lines activate T cells in an antigen-specific, MHC class II-dependent manner (69). Even though some normal and neoplastic glial cells may possess the intracellular machinery for antigen presentation, the importance of this function is unknown.

Other CNS cells may function as APC. Microglia originate from bone marrow and are a type of DC (281, 285). Smooth muscle cells of precapillary arterioles and capillary pericytes of normal brain express class II molecules, and IFN-γ, TNF-α, and IL-1 induce the expression of adhesion molecules and MHC molecules on the surface of brain endothelial cells (89, 90, 214). The perivascular location of pericytes, smooth muscle cells, and endothelial cells make them good candidates for APCs. The presence of lymphatic connections among deep cervical lymph nodes draining the brain supports this possibility (68). Microglia and other perivascular cells may migrate to cervical lymph nodes and elicit an immune response (afferent way), just as Langerhans cells or DC cells migrate from skin, cardiac, or renal transplants to regional lymph nodes and the spleen (11, 18, 152, 169).

Antigen Recognition by T Cells

Two molecules are involved in antigen recognition: antibodies and the T-cell receptors (TCR) of T lymphocytes. More than 80% of peripheral blood lymphocytes are T lymphocytes expressing either α/β TCR (95% of T cells) or γ/δ TCR (2–5%) on their surface (181, 215, 252). Mature α/β T lymphocytes recognize antigenic peptides presented by MHC molecules through their heterodimeric α/β TCR. The noncovalently linked CD3 molecular complex is involved in intracellular signal transduction (56) (Fig. 4).

Each TCR α and β chain contains a variable and a constant region. Variable regions determine antigen specificity. A huge range of TCR specificities is needed to match the myriad antigenic determinants that an organism's immune system might encounter (57, 154, 162). During T-cell differentiation, unique variable-region

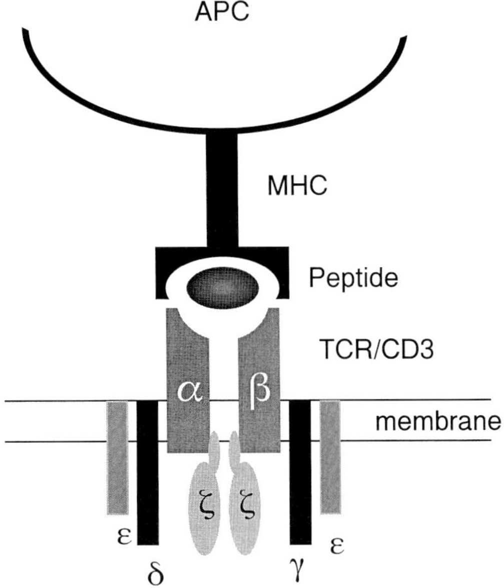

Figure 4. Peptide recognition by TCR/CD3 complex.

genes are created by recombination of variable (V), diversity (D), and joining (J) segments for the β locus and of V and J segments for the α locus. This random joining of segments generates *combinatorial diversity* (Fig. 5). In humans, 63 Vβ and more than 65 Vα gene segments have been identified and classified into 25 and 32 subfamilies, respectively, based on similarities in the nucleotide sequences of their coding regions (95, 230). Thirteen Jβ and sixty-one Jα gene segments have also been identified (278). TCR diversity also arises from shortening of V, D, or J segments (nibbling) and adding encoded nucleotides to the N regions interspersed between these gene segments during recombination (*junctional diversity*) (70) (Fig. 6). Corresponding to the hypervariable regions of Ig molecules, N regions (also termed CDR3) are essential for binding to the antigenic peptide presented by a MHC molecule. Expression of unique rearranged TCR gene products thus determines the specificity of a given T cell (57, 177). Finally, the random combination of the α and β chains encoded by these genes further increases the diversity of the TCR complement.

The crucial role of T cells in antigen recognition warrants study of the cytolytic activity of TIL. Similar to LAK cells generated from PBL *in vitro*, TIL isolated from various tumors acquire lytic activity. They lyse autologous tumor

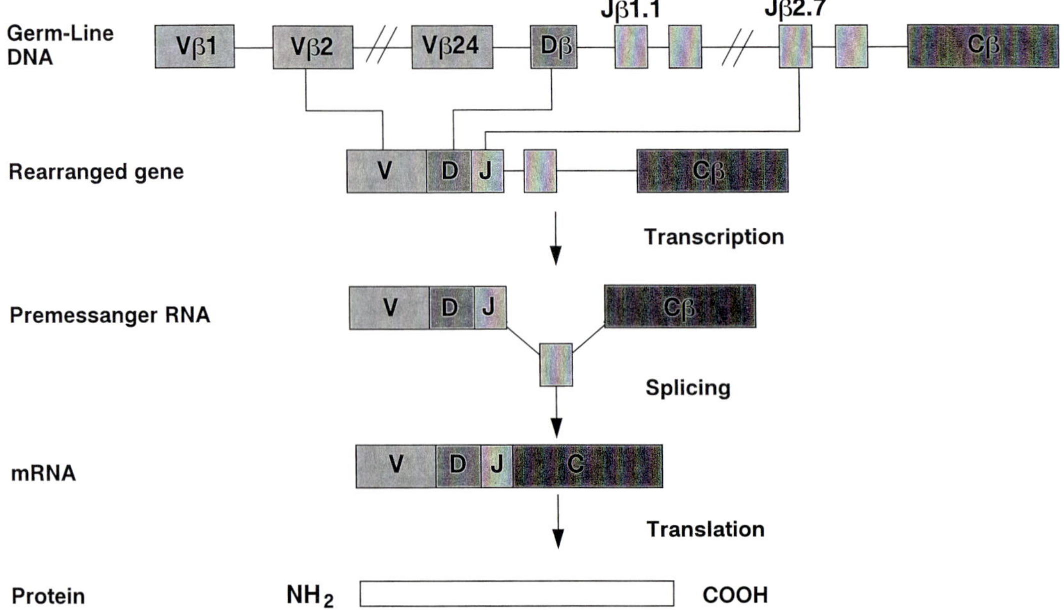

Figure 5. Gene rearrangement generating β chain *combinatorial diversity*. Similar mechanisms occur for α chain.

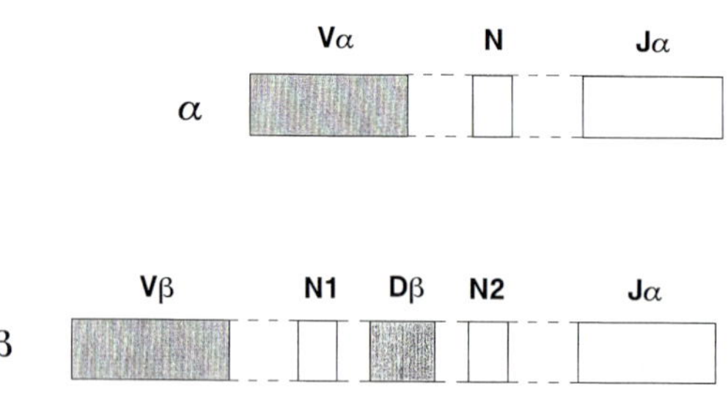

Figure 6. *Junctional diversity.*

cells, but this lysis is nonspecific, as allogeneic tumor cells and NK- or LAK-target cells are also killed (K562, Daudi). However, the *in vitro* generation of CTL lines or CTL clones exhibiting an MHC-restricted cytotoxicity directed specifically against autologous tumor cells indicates that tumor-specific antigenic peptides exist. CTL clones have been derived mainly from melanoma (24, 264) and have been used as biological reagents to identify tumor-specific antigens, such as MAGE (see below) (188, 190, 234, 242). They are usually obtained from mixed lymphocyte-tumor cell cultures (MLTC) containing T cells, autologous and allogeneic tumor cells, and APC in the presence of IL-2. A CTL clone is grown from a few TIL cells selected from the highly heterogeneous cellular

population of a given tumor. Multiple genetic alterations occur during the first *in vitro* passages. Some lymphocytes expand slowly or not at all; others proliferate rapidly. This produces a distribution of TCR that differs from that *in vivo* (Dietrich, unpublished data).

Analysis of the molecular structures of TCR produced by TIL permit verification that a specific antitumor T-cell immune response occurs *in vivo*. Antigen-driven expansion of a given T-cell clone can be identified by PCR-based methods that reveal identical TCR transcripts in a subpopulation of T cells (26, 59, 74, 75, 88, 111, 211, 212). Using these methods, T-cell clonal expansion has been observed in melanoma, renal cell carcinoma, head and neck cancer, and chronic lymphatic leukemia (43, 91, 94, 110, 172, 173). This molecular approach does not assess the functional activity of detected clonal expansions. However, the recent demonstration in melanoma and RCC that T-cell clones detected by TCR molecular analysis are cytolytic against autologous tumor cells in a MHC-restricted fashion suggests that such clones are potentially useful. Nitta and coworkers reported that most gliomas show preferential expression of Vα7 and Vβ13 genes in TIL and limited use of TCR Vα and Vβ gene segments

(81, 205). Sequencing of amplified TCR Vα7 and Vβ13 transcripts showed that these overexpressed transcripts corresponded to clonal T-cell expansions (80). Identical clones were expanded in several different patients who shared the same HLA haplotype, as well as in one with a different HLA haplotype. If confirmed, these data suggest that *in vivo* clonal expansion of glioma-specific T cells occurs in the tumor, supporting the hypothesis that the antigen recognized may be very commonly expressed in gliomas. This molecular approach must be combined with a more classical cellular approach to define the function of these Vβ12 T-cell clones and to characterize the recognized glioma antigen.

Tumor Antigens

Generation of a specific immune response against a tumor requires antigens on tumor cells that can be recognized by immune cells. Tumor-specific transplantation antigens (TSTA) have long been recognized on experimental tumors. TSTA are antigens, expressed on tumor cells, that can be recognized and rejected after being grafted into syngeneic mice (21, 143). While experimental tumors artificially induced by oncogenic viruses (141), ultraviolet irradiation (147), or chemical carcinogens (*e.g.*, methylcholanthrene) (15, 221) are highly immunogenic, TSTA have been difficult to demonstrate in spontaneously occurring tumors.

The first gene encoding a human *tumor-specific antigen* recognized by CTL was MAGE-1 (melanoma-antigen) (272) (Fig. 7). The normal function of the MAGE-1 gene product is not known. The encoded antigenic peptide is a nonamer presented by the HLA-A1 molecule (267). Additional antigens (designated MAGE-1, -2, and -3) have been found on a breast tumor, non-small cell lung tumor, head and neck carcinoma, and glioma cells (31, 32, 107, 271).

Other antigens elicit CTL responses in melanoma, including a series of recently defined *differentiation antigenic peptides*. These peptides are derived from tyrosinase, Melan-A (also called MART-1), gp 100, and gp 75 (14, 37, 65, 138). Melanoma differentiation antigens are expressed on both neoplastic and normal melanocytes and also in contrast to tumor-specific antigens; they are not expressed in other types of tumor. Certain peptides derived from these antigens are shared by a high proportion of HLA-A2 melanomas. These common immunogenic epitopes are thus potential targets for immunotherapy (138). Unfortunately, the therapeutic usefulness of differentiation antigens in glioma may be limited by toxicity to normal brain, as these antigens are also expressed in the retina, inner ear, and brain. However, because the level of expression of such antigens is much higher in tumor cells than in normal cells, a therapeutic window might exist (213).

Peptides derived from mutated human protooncogenes or peptides encoded by chimeric genes resulting from chromosomal translocations (*e.g.*, fusion protein *bcr-abl* in chronic myeloid leukemia) may be able to elicit T-cell immunity (53, 54, 93, 104, 148). These proteins, structurally altered during neoplastic transformation, may be the best candidates for inducing a specific antitumor immune response. *In vitro* responses to mutated forms of *ras* oncogene have been demonstrated in murine and human systems (101, 109, 136). Immunization of mice with vaccinia virus expressing mutant *ras* protein allows generation of CTL that could lyse targets cells carrying the mutated, but not the normal, *ras* gene (246). Similarly, a tumor-specific antigen may be the product of a tumor suppressor gene; specific cytotoxic T-cell clones have been generated *in vitro* against mutated p53 protein (125, 253, 282). Of gliomas, 40–60% have mutations in p53, frequently in association with a loss of portions of the short arm of chromosome 17, and 30% of malignant glioma have amplification of a mutated EGF receptor gene (161). Whether the altered pro-

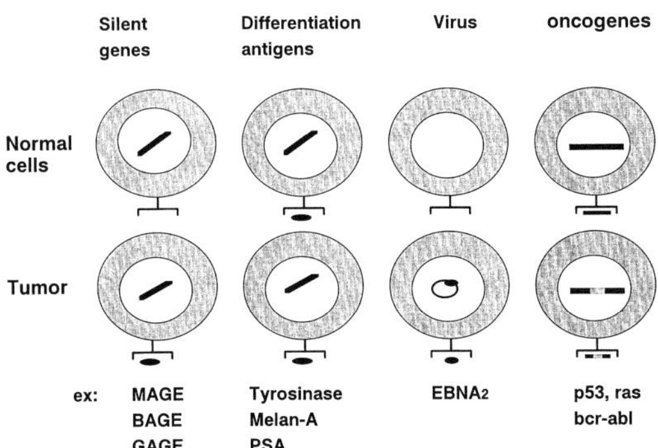

Figure 7. Schematic representation of tumor antigens into four major categories.

teins from these mutated genes can serve as targets for glioma immunotherapy is unknown.

Adhesion Molecules

Adhesion molecules are transmembrane receptors, such as integrins, cadherins, selectins, CD44, and some members of the immunoglobulin supergene family (218). The expression of diverse adhesion molecules on glioma cells, TIL, and endothelial cells within brain tumors permits study of the cellular and molecular basis of the interactions between glioma cells and immune cells (63). Because a detailed description of all adhesion molecules involved in interactions among cells and between cells and extracellular matrix in gliomas is beyond the scope of this review, only a few examples that demonstrate the biological significance of these molecules will be discussed.

Intercellular adhesion molecule-1 (ICAM-1) is a member of the immunoglobulin supergene family. Although weakly expressed or absent from low-grade astrocytomas and absent from normal brain, ICAM-1 is strongly expressed by high-grade glioma cells *in vivo* (150). The natural ligand of ICAM-1 is lymphocyte function-associated antigen (LFA-1), which is present on the surface of TIL in gliomas. The interaction between ICAM-1 and LFA-1 results in efficient binding between glioma cells and immune cells and is necessary for efficient killing of tumor cells by LAK cells and T cells. Monoclonal antibodies against ICAM-1 and LFA-1 inhibit the binding of TIL or LAK cells to human glioblastoma cells (63). In addition, melanoma cells shed ICAM-1 from their surface, and soluble ICAM-1 abrogates the cytotoxicity mediated by NK cells and T-cell clones (22, 23). LFA-3 and CD44 are two other adhesion molecules expressed by glioblastoma cells (149). LFA-3 is the ligand for the lymphocyte CD2 molecule. CD44 is a broadly distributed cell surface glycoprotein implicated in lymphocyte homing, T-cell activation (128), and adhesion to hyaluronate, a major component of the extracellular matrix (19). Several CD44 isoforms are generated by differential mRNA splicing and by cell type-specific glycosylation. Overexpression of certain isoforms has been associated with metastasis in a range of human tumors (178). CD44 is strongly expressed in glioblastoma and weakly expressed in other CNS tumors and normal brain. More importantly, glioblastomas express novel splice variants (159).

Intratumoral endothelial cells also express ICAM-1 (63). ICAM-1 and other adhesion molecules could cause arrest of circulating lymphocytes that occurs within tumors (13). Whether this contributes to the lymphoid infiltration observed in high-grade glioma is unknown. ICAM-1 expression by glioblastoma and endothelial cells leads lymphocytes into the tumor tissue. TNF-α, IL1-β, or INF-γ enhances ICAM-1 expression, but other secreted cytokines do not (244, 274). Endothelial cells also express vascular cell adhesion molecule-1 (VCAM-1) and endothelial-leukocyte adhesion molecule-1 (ELAM-1). The role of ELAM-1 in gliomas is unknown. ELAM-1 normally induces adherence of neutrophils and monocytes to vascular endothelium, but these cells rarely infiltrate glioblastomas. VCAM-1 is linked to very late antigen (VLA)-4 on melanoma cells, glioblastoma cells, and lymphoctyes. This interaction may also contribute to lymphocyte infiltration into gliomas. Expression of adhesion molecules is inducible and often transient.

HOW GLIOMAS ESCAPE IMMUNE SURVEILLANCE

As discussed above, although T cells recognize tumor-associated peptides as foreign, these peptides fail to induce immune response sufficient to prevent tumor development and growth *in vivo*. Possible reasons for this failure can be classified as defects in antigen presentation or defects in T-cell function.

Defect in Antigen Presentation

Adequate immune response requires correct expression of MHC class I and/or class II molecules on the surface of tumor cells and/or APC (Fig. 3). Many mechanisms may block expression of MHC class I molecules such that cancer cells avoid being killed by T cells (30, 62, 67, 78, 225, 237). In virally infected cells, for example, virus proteins (*e.g.*, E3 glycoprotein of adenovirus, H301 of cytomegalovirus) bind to class I heavy chain or β2-microglobulin, causing the class I MHC complex to be retained in the endoplasmic reticulum (4, 41, 72, 208). Downregulation of MHC class I molecules may also reflect inhibition of transcription of the heavy chain or β-2-microglobulin gene (76,

153). However, normal levels of heavy chain and β-2 microglobulin RNAs are observed in some cancers devoid of class I MHC surface molecules, usually because inadequate TAP-1 or TAP-2 expression diminishes an active transport of peptides into ER. As described above, the absence of peptide in the MHC peptide groove interrupts progression of class I molecules toward the Golgi apparatus. Although this mechanism was delineated in a virus-associated cancer, human cervical carcinoma (66), and could represent a way commonly used by viruses to escape inactivation by T cells (103, 120), it also occurs in lung, colon, and mammary carcinomas not caused by viruses (66). In gliomas, low expression of MHC class I molecules results from the absence of MHC class I molecules on the surface of normal astrocytes, rather than from malignant transformation (69, 142, 227, 286). The mechanisms suppressing expression of MHC class I molecules in glial cells and whether it is possible to induce expression of these molecules are unknown.

Antigen presentation to CD4+ T cells can be accomplished either by tumor cells themselves or by APC in or about the tumor. The 40% of gliomas expressing MHC class II molecule *in vivo* generally coexpress ICAM-1; glioma cells may thus be able to elicit CD4 T-cell response *in vivo*, as they do *in vitro* (69, 277). The expression of MHC class II molecules on glioma cells' surface is strongly inducible *in vitro* by IFN-γ. This cytokine, secreted by glioma cells, monocytes, and other CNS APC, may involve MHC class II expression. The fluctuating secretion of cytokines may explain the variability in MHC class II expression. Although not specifically studied in astrocytes or glioma cells, CIITA transcription factor, whose expression is controlled by IFN-γ, is a likely mediator of this process, as it is in other cell types (170).

In contrast, other cytokines, such as TGF-β2, may downregulate expression of class II molecules. As already discussed, microglia, pericytes, and endothelial cells function as APC. The expression of class II molecules on their surfaces is also regulated by a complex network of positive and negative signals triggered by different cytokines. Whether immunosuppressive factors, such as TGFβ2, produced by glioma cells modify their APC abilities is unknown.

Defect in T-cell Functions

A majority of high-grade astrocytomas are infiltrated by lymphocytes, mostly CD8 cells; B cells, NK cells, and CD4+ T cells are encountered less frequently (148, 210). The intensity of infiltration is variable. It is highest in the tumor periphery and perivascular regions. Although suggested in some studies (38), T-lymphocyte infiltration does not connote a favorable prognosis in gliomas (233, 240). Several deficiencies of immune function have been identified in patients with gliomas. These include an abnormal delayed hypersensitivity to antigens, such as *Mycobacterium*, tuberculosis, or *Candida albicans*; a low count of circulating T cells; a depressed proliferative response to mitogens, such as phytohemagglutinin, concanavalin A or phorbol ester; a decreased antibody response to tetanus toxoid, influenza virus or other antigens, probably related to failure of CD4 T cells to function as helper cells for immunoglobulin secretion; and a deficient antibody-mediated and T-cell cytotoxicity *in vitro* (39, 40, 83, 175, 187, 235, 283, 288). A number of different mechanisms may contribute to the reduced T-cell unresponsiveness of glioma patients: abnormalities in IL-2 production and IL-2 receptor expression, the lack of S chain within the CD3 complex and its consequence in signal transduction, the alterations in NF-kB/Rel proteins, the alteration of peptides presented by MHC molecules, and the immunosuppressive agents secreted by glioma cells themselves.

IL2-Receptor Abnormalities

Ex vivo, glioma TIL lose their ability to proliferate in culture after a few weeks as IL-2R expression declines even when IL-2 is added to culture medium (242). Moreover, the *in vitro* production of IL-2 by lectin-stimulated T cells obtained from glioma patients is less than that obtained from normal individuals, and the addition of recombinant IL-2 does not restore their impaired proliferation (84). Such data implicate defective IL-2R expression by T cells from patients with gliomas. IL-2 exerts its biological effects through specific binding to its receptor. The IL-2R is a complex structure with low, intermediate, or high affinity for its ligand, depending on its composition. Lymphocytes expressing either α or $\beta\gamma$ chains have low or intermediate affinity, respectively, and require high IL-2 concentrations to be saturated. Activated T cells and a small subset of NK cells express the 3 α, β, and γ chains and require very low concentrations of IL-2 to be activated (259) (Fig. 8). T cells obtained from glioma patients do not express the α chain (p55) after appropriate antigenic stimulation and, therefore, fail to assemble high-affinity IL-2R (82). The molecular basis of this failure of p55 expression is unknown. These T cells express normal levels of p55 mRNA and adequately glycosylated p55 protein. The failure of glioma T cells to express α chain is a crucial defect, because the proliferation and activation of T cells are dependent on expression of the heterotrimeric $\alpha\beta\gamma$ IL2-R. The γ chain is a subunit common to IL-2, IL-4, IL-7, IL-9, and IL-15 receptors. It determines whether T cells expand clonally or remain quiescent (34).

Abnormalities in T-Cell Signal Transduction

Binding of the HLA-peptide complex by TCR induces a cascade of intracellular signals that ends in the cell nucleus (7, 47, 132, 251, 280) (Fig. 9). Blockade of this signaling pathway may prevent T cells from efficiently responding to an otherwise adequate signal from an antigen. Several abnormalities in T-cell signaling have been recently described in cancer patients. One abnormality is the lack of CD3 S chain and p56[Ick] PTK in T lymphocytes infiltrating tumors (191, 268). One or two CD3 S chains are replaced by one or two γ chains of the receptor for immunoglobulin E. This impairs mobilization of intracellular calcium in response to activation signals and markedly diminishes the antitumor effects mediated by T

cells (168, 245). Both CD4 and CD8 T cells are affected. First described in mice bearing colon carcinoma (MCA-38) or renal cell carcinoma (Renca), this abnormality has been demonstrated with human tumors. Western blot and immunohistology reveal a marked decrease in TCR S chain and p56[Ick] expression in the TILs of 10/11 cases of renal cell carcinoma (RCC) (97) and in all 14 cases of colorectal cancers analyzed (201). TILs are more severely affected than PBL, suggesting that a factor within the tumor microenvironment may be responsible. The recent observation that macrophages at certain stages of activation are able to induce the loss of S chain strengthens this thesis (5). The systemic alteration of T cells may facilitate metastasis. Whether CD3 S chains are absent in the T lymphocytes of high-grade astrocytoma is unknown.

A second alteration in downstream signaling events involves kB enhancer-binding proteins, NF-kB1 (p50), RelA (p65), and c-Rel. They regulate expression of many genes associated with T-cell activation such as IFN-γ, IL-2, and IL-2R α chain. In resting T cells, p65 is associated with its inhibitor in cytoplasm, whereas p50 is located in the nucleus. Activation of T lymphocytes disassociates p65 from its inhibitor (termed 1kBα), permitting its translocation into the nucleus. In the nucleus, p65 binds to p50 to form an active heterodimer transcription factor (p50/p65). In TIL isolated from animal and human RCC, p65 does not translocate into the nucleus, and there is no induction of a normal NF-kB complex (p50/p65) (112, 160). Persistent repression of several genes, including IL-2 and IL-2R α chain, results (137). Whether such a molecular event occurs in T lymphocytes infiltrating glioma has not been investigated. In particular, whether the downregulation of IL2-R α chain observed in lymphocytes is related to failure to translocate p65 to the nucleus is unknown. NF-kB abnormalities may be one of a number of defects in signaling. The release of p65 from its inhibitor involves phosphorylation of the inhibitor by protein kinase C (PKC). Cells missing CD3 S chains, p56[Ick], and p59fyn are unable to activate PKC. Thus the lack of early events in T-cell signaling may hinder the phosphorylation of IkB and, thus, the binding of p50 with p65 in the nucleus.

T-cell signaling may also be impaired by alterations of the peptide presented by the MHC

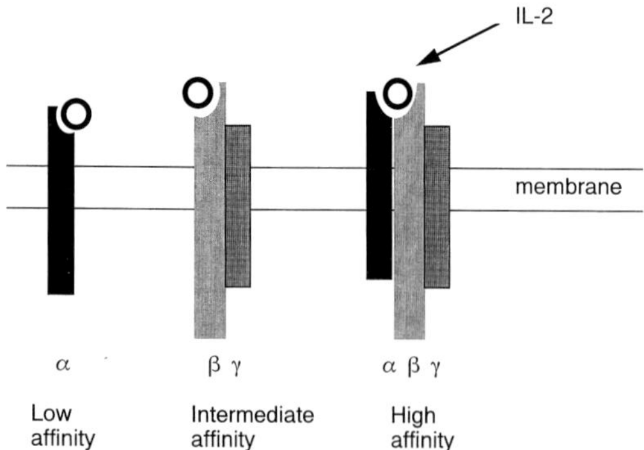

Figure 8. Interleukin-2 receptor (IL-2R). IL-2R is an heterotrimeric and transmembrane molecule, whose affinity for IL-2 is related to its composition.

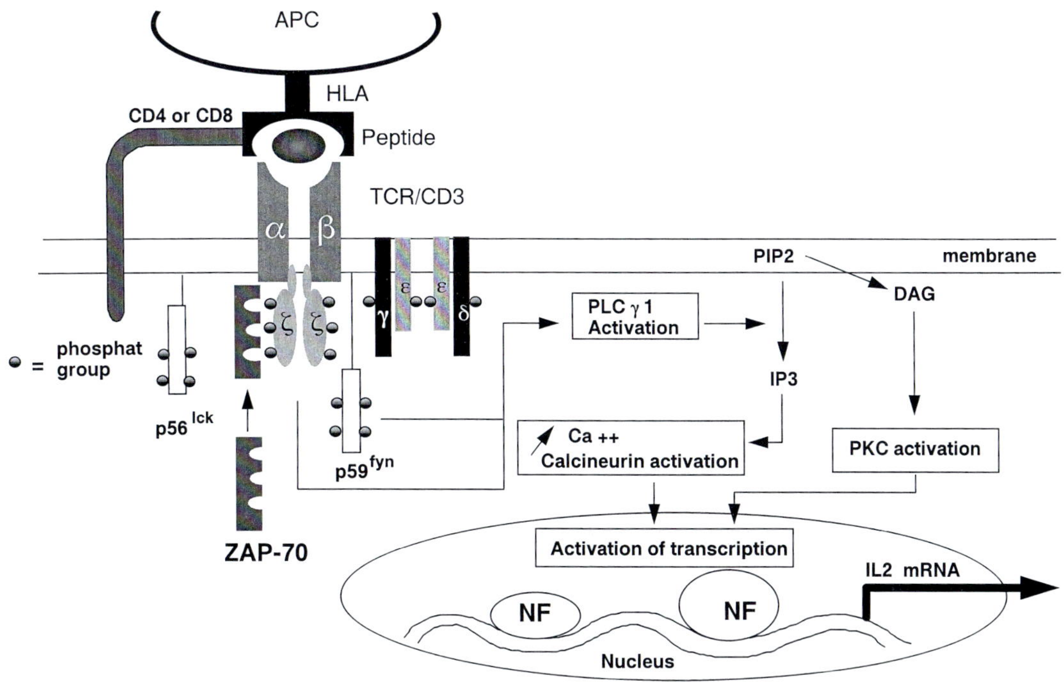

Figure 9. Intracellular steps leading to T-cell activation. Binding of an HLA-peptide complex to TCR activates a series of protein tyrosine kinases (PTK). Belonging to the *src* family, p56[lck] is a membrane-bound PTK that interacts with the cytoplasmic domain of CD4 or CD8 α chain. The phosphorylation of p56[lck] tyrosine residues favors alignment of p56[lck] and CD3 S chains and subsequent phosphorylation of tyrosine ARAM (antigen recognition activation motif) or TAM (tyrosine-based activation motif) domains of S chains. Another member of the *src* family, p59[fyn], associates with the S chain and functions in a similar manner. Phosphorylation of S chains recruits cytoplasmic ZAP-70, a 70 PTK of the *syk* family not constitutively localized in the cell membrane. This tyrosine phosphorylation cascade activates phospholipase Cγl (PLC γl), which in turn induces hydrolysis of phosphatidylinositol 4,5-diphosphate (PIP2) into phosphatidylinositol 2, 4,5-triphosphate (IP3) and diacylglycerol (DAG). DAG activates protein kinase C (PKC), which leads to change in the activity of specific nuclear transcription factors (NF). On the other hand, IP3 increases levels of free intracytoplasmic calcium and consequently activates the calcineurin. Calcineurin, a serine phosphatase that is inhibited by cyclosporin A, aligns the cytoplasmic subunit of the transcription factor NF-AT with its nuclear subunit so as to induce transcription of IL-2 gene. IL-2 transcription can be enhanced by other factors, such as Oct1, NFKB, and AP-1, a dimeric of *fos* and *jun*. NFkB regulates expression of the IL-2R α chain.

molecule. Minor modifications may affect either the interaction between peptide and MHC molecule (*e.g.*, amino acids at positions 2 and 9 are implicated in interaction with class I molecules) or suppress recognition by TCR (207, 279) (Fig. 10). Subtle amino acid substitutions can yield analog-mutated peptides that can still interact with the TCR but do not deliver a fully stimulatory signal. T cells stimulated *in vitro* by such peptides become anergic to subsequent stimulation with the nonmutated peptide. *In vitro* models have shown that anergy correlates with a unique pattern of TCR S chain phosphorylation and a subsequent lack of association

with ZAP-70 (87, 122, 131, 144, 174, 176, 247, 248). Hepatitis B virus and HIV-1 virus may exploit such mechanisms to evade immune attack (26, 144). The contribution of this phenomenon to the escape from immune surveillance by cancer cells is still hypothetical. Cancer progression may be at least partly related to subtle residue changes in one or several tumor peptides. For example, the substitution of an arginine by a glycine at position 3 of a 9 amino acid peptide derived from human papillomavirus (HPV 16) is detected in 30% of invasive cervical cancer associated with HLA-B7 haplotype, a genotype associated with poor prognosis (86).

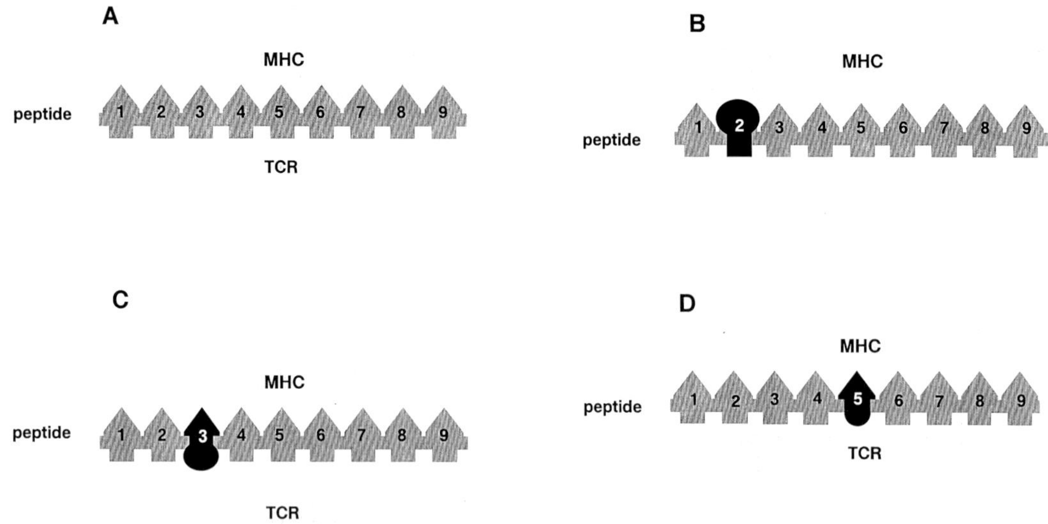

Figure 10. Consequences of peptide alterations. Panel *A* depicts presentation of a normal 9 residue peptide by an MHC class I molecule and its recognition by TCR. In panel *B*, the substitution of a different amino acid at position 2 abrogates the binding with the MHC molecule, as does substitution of an amino acid at position 9. The substitution of an amino acid at position 3, shown in panel *C*, inhibits recognition of the peptide by TCR. Finally, peptides with substitution of amino acids not critical for MHC or TCR binding (panel *D*), may still interact with MHC molecule and TCR but are unable to elicit a secondary signal. Such subtle alterations may induce the most serious effects on T-cell functions, since T cells stimulated by such peptides become anergic to subsequent stimulation by the nonmutated peptide.

Immunosuppressive Factors

Soluble factors produced by gliomas hinder the immune response. For example, the addition of glioma cyst fluid or supernatant from glioblastoma cell lines or fresh glioma explants inhibit several lymphocyte functions (see above). T lymphocytes from normal individuals exhibit similar immunological abnormalities when cultured with glioma supernatant (85). These findings imply the existence of soluble suppressor factors derived from gliomas. Candidates include TGF-β, IL-10, and 2GF-1 (Fig. 11).

* TGF-β

TGF-β was first identified in the supernatant of a human glioblastoma cell line able to suppress T-cell growth (99). Initially called glioblastoma cell-derived T-cell suppressor factor (G-Tsf), it was renamed TGF-β2 after purification and cloning revealed sequence homology with TGF-β1.

In fact, three TGF-β isoforms have been identified so far. They are encoded by genes

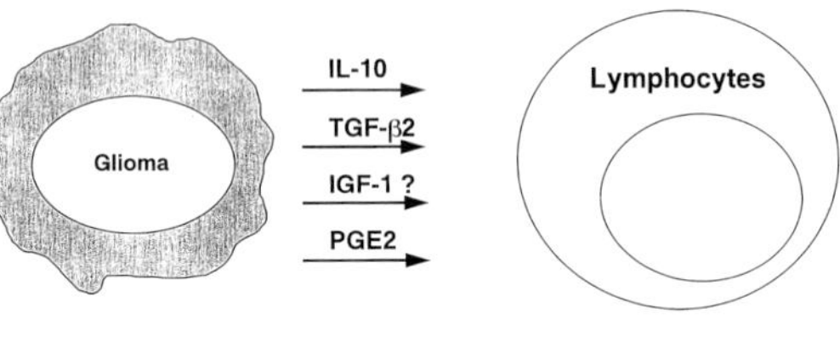

Figure 11. Immunosuppressive factors produced by glioma cells. The cytokines produced by glioma cells blocked T-cell responsiveness in a paracrine fashion.

located on chromosomes 19 (TGF-β), 1 (TGF-β2), and 14 (TGF-β3). TGF-β are secreted as large inactive precursors that are cleaved to active TGF-β by proteases such as plasmin or cathepsin (33). Murine astrocytes in culture express mRNA of all three TGF-β isoforms and secrete TGF-β2 in its inactive form. In contrast, glioblastoma cell lines also synthesize all three TGF-β isoform transcripts but secrete TGF-β2 in its *active cleaved* form (29, 64). A study using protease inhibitors demonstrated that

TGF-β2-mediated T-cell suppression requires proteases produced by glioma cells (127). *In vivo*, TGF-β1, TGF-β2, and TGF-β3 transcripts are found in a majority of gliomas and meningiomas, but not in brain metastases or normal brain (29, 182). TGF-β immunoreactivity was detected in glioblastoma in a heterogeneous pattern; it was strong in perivascular areas devoid of macrophages that expressed TNFα/IL-6 and IL-2R+ lymphocytes and weak in areas containing these cells (182, 244).

The active TGF-β2 secreted by glioma cells inhibits NK and LAK cell activity, B-cell proliferation and differentiation, and the secretion of function of numerous cytokines (IFN-γ, TNF-α, TNF-β, IL-1, IL-2, IL-3, IL-6, and GM-CSF). Moreover, TGF-β2 strongly inhibits T-cell growth by activating TGF-β bound to the membrane of T cells (139, 182). Finally, TGF-β2 downregulates MHC class II molecules on glioma cells *in vitro* (290), thus decreasing the cells' ability to present antigens (69). These properties suggest that TGF-β2 contributes substantially to the escape of gliomas escape from immune surveillance. Antisense TGF-β2 phosphorothioate oligonucleotides inhibit TGF-β2 secretion by glioblastoma cell lines and reverse the suppressive effects of TGF-2 upon the proliferative and cytotoxic functions of autologous lymphocytes in glioma patients (133).

* IL-10

IL-10 is a newly identified cytokine with a broad spectrum of biological activity that includes crucial immunosuppressive effects. Located on chromosome 1q, the human IL-10 gene was cloned because of its homology to the mouse gene. Both genes exhibit strong DNA sequence homology with the BCRF1 open reading frame of Epstein-Barr virus (EBV). BCRF1 could provide a selective advantage to the virus by inhibiting cell-mediated antiviral immune responses (196).

Two types of T helper cells are involved in cell-mediated and antibody immune responses. Th1 cells produce IL-2, IFN-γ, and TNF-α and strongly activate cell-mediated responses, whereas Th2 cells produce IL-4, IL-5, IL-6, IL-10, and IL-13 and stimulate B cells to generate an antibody response. INF-γ inhibits the proliferation of Th2 clones, while IL-4 and IL-10 inhibit that of Th1 clones. This dichotomy partially explains the commonly observed mutual exclusion of these two types of immune response *in vivo* (228). Predominantly produced by T cells, IL-10 exerts numerous biological effects through binding to its widely expressed receptor (167). *In vitro*, IL-10 inhibits antigen-dependent and mitogen-dependent proliferation of T cells, inhibits phagocytic activity, nitric oxide production, and secretion of IFN-γ, IL-1, IL-6, IL-8, IL-12, G-CSF, and GM-CSF by activated monocytes, and suppresses MHC class II molecule expression and antigen presentation by macrophages (196).

Whether such mechanisms are involved *in vivo* in gliomas' avoidance of immune surveillance is unknown. IL-10 mRNA is found, however, in a high proportion of glioblastomas (186, 203). Tumors expressing IL-10 expression express neither IFN-γ nor GM-CSF. Furthermore, the discovery of IL-10 (15–200 pg/ml) in the peripheral blood of four patients with brain tumors suggests its potential to impair Th1-mediated immune responses systemically (129). However, because IL-10 mRNA was also detected in normal brain, more precise definition of the role of IL-10 in immune suppression by gliomas awaits further study.

* IGF-1

Insulin-like growth factor-1 and insulin-like growth factor-2 are polypeptides with crucial roles in normal growth and development during fetal, neonatal, and pubertal stages. Interacting with a common IGF-I receptor, they are growth factors for fibroblasts, epithelial cells, smooth muscle cells, osteoclasts, and bone marrow stem cells. Their vital role in development is evident in the profound fetal growth retardation of IGF-1 or IGF-1R knockout mice (166). In addition, IGF-1 or IGF-2 is a tumorigenic growth factor in breast cancer, osteosarcoma, rhabdomysarcoma, and Wilms tumor (157). IGF-1 may be an immunostimulant cytokine, as it stimulates both repopulation of the atrophied thymus of diabetic rats (27) and lymphopoiesis (58). These observations, however, are inconsistent with the restoration of immune response that follow treatment of rat glioblastoma cells with antisense IGF-1mRNA (see below) (269, 270).

** Others*

The secretion of prostaglandin E_2 (PGE$_2$) by glioblastoma has been demonstrated both *in vitro* and *in vivo* (100, 241). PGE$_2$ profoundly suppresses the production of IL-2 and IFN-γ by Th1 cells, while it enhances antibody-mediated immune responses (217). Thus, together with IL-10 and TGF-β, PGE$_2$ may contribute to the defect in cellular immunity observed in gliomas.

IL-1α, IL-1β and the IL-1 receptor are produced by a significant proportion of high-grade astrocytomas (108, 255). IL-1 from glial cells might induce secondary release of other cytokines (IL-6, IL-8, MCP-1) and increase production of adhesion molecules such as ICAM-1 or VCAM from tumor and endothelial cells. The recent description of an IL-1-receptor antagonist produced by a glioma is also intriguing (256). Whether IL-1 is involved in tumor growth in an autocrine or a paracrine manner, whether IL-1 actually initiates an immune response *in vivo*, and whether such effects are inhibited by an IL-1 receptor antagonist produced by glioma cells is unknown.

Absence of Costimulatory Signals: the Example of B7

A subgroup of surface molecules called costimulatory molecules does not initiate T-cell clonal expansion but rather facilitates generation and amplification of the T-cell immune response after stimulation by an antigen. Antigen-specific T-cell clonal activation and expansion require two signals. The first signal, which confers the antigen specificity, arises from the interaction between the MHC-peptide complex and the TCR. The second signal, which is nonspecific, enables lymphokine secretion, T-cell clonal expansion and enhancement of effector functions. The absence of a second signal results in the unresponsiveness of T cells, a state termed anergy (Fig. 12). The B7-CD28 interaction determines whether a cell is reactive or anergic (117, 135). The two cloned B7 molecules, B7-1 and B7-2, are members of the Ig supergene family containing two Ig-like domains (12, 102, 119). Both are located on chromosome 3q. Their expression on B cells and APC is enhanced by IFN-γ. The differences in the expression of B7-1 and B7-2 after B-cell activation suggests that they have complementary costimulatory functions. Activation of B

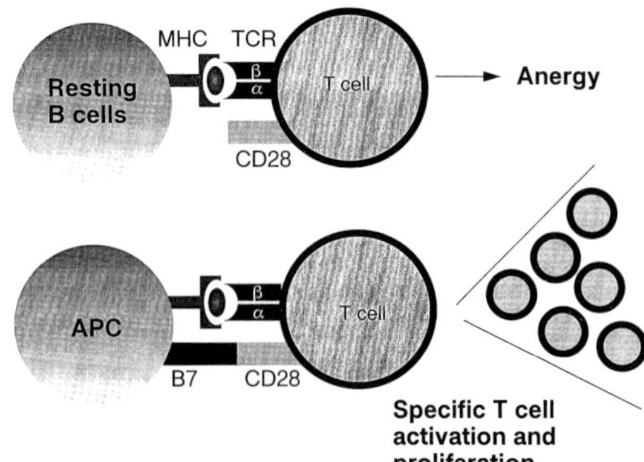

Figure 12. A b7-mediated costimulatory signal.

cells, which express either B7-1 or B7-2 in the resting state, induces the expression of B7-2 within 24 hours; CD28 may be the T-cell B7 receptor. B7-1 appears later (35). CD28 is a homodimeric glycoprotein belonging to the 1g supergene family. Its expression is restricted to T cells and plasma cells. A molecule highly homologous to CD28 has been cloned and called CTLA-4 (284). Both CD28 and CTLA-4 may bind both B7-1 and B7-2 (Fig. 13).

The expression of B7 molecules within the CNS is poorly studied. As for other tumors, B7 is not found on the surface of glioma cells. On the other hand, some macrophages within or around these tumors express B7 molecules (Tada, unpublished data). The induction by cytokines, such as IFN-γ, of B7 expression in glioma cells or macrophages and the role of B7/CD28 molecules in determining T-cell activation or anergy in gliomas have not been established.

RESTORATION OF AN APPROPRIATE IMMUNE RESPONSE

Tumor immune surveillance involves a complex web of interaction between tumor cells and immune cells that occurs with or without the help of APC. These interactions are mediated by cytokines. Defects in these interactions underlie tumor cell escape from immune surveillance. Enhancement of immune mechanisms may overcome these deficiencies and be of therapeutic value for gliomas.

Antigen-based Vaccination Strategies

Tumor antigens have been used as immunogens in vaccination studies. Several different

APC - T lymphocyte interactions

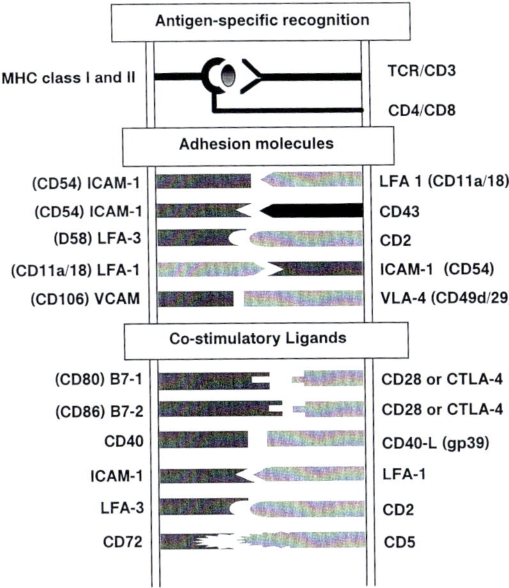

Figure 13. Interactions between APC and T cell. Three types of interaction are required to induce a T-cell response. First, intercellular contact is mediated by *adhesion molecules* and their respective ligands. Some molecules are lineage-restricted (CD2 is exclusively expressed on T cells), but others may be expressed on both cell types involved in the interaction (ICAM-1 and LFA-1 are both expressed on T cells and APC). Second, the antigen-specific signal is delivered by the interaction between MHC-peptide complex and TCR. Third, costimulatory molecules, such as B7-CD28 and CD40-CD40L and the adhesion molecules ICAM-1/LFA-1 (expressed on glioma cells and TIL), assist in cytokine production, cellular proliferation, and effector function.

tumor peptides and full-length proteins have been used to vaccinate patients with melanoma. Although such antigens may occasionally elicit a specific immune response, in general, free peptides are poor inducers of cytotoxic T-cell responses *in vivo*. A variety of alternative approaches are being considered. Incorporation of tumor antigens in liposomes is a clever strategy, as lipopeptide conjugates are readily engulfed by APC, and, after being in lysosomes, generate an efficient T-cell response (73, 118, 200). Dendritic cells generated from hematopoietic progenitors are also being used (46, 130). Dendritic cells pulsed with the appropriate peptides can induce a cytotoxic T-cell response against HIV,

p53, and an idiotype of lymphoma in mice (98, 199, 258, 287).

Specific adoptive immunotherapy consists of *in vitro* expansion of T cells recognizing a tumor-specific antigen and reinfusion of the cells into tumor-bearing patients. Such therapy is highly efficient in treating *cytomegalovirus* infections occurring during the course of bone marrow transplants (226). Because no tumor antigen has been clearly identified in gliomas, such approaches are not yet applicable.

Genetically Modified Tumor Cells as a Tumor Vaccine

Lessons from Tumors Other Than Glioma

The progression of a cancer may reflect defects in immune surveillance. Tumor cells can be genetically modified to increase their interactions with immune cells and, thus, restore a strong and specific immune response against them. Examples of candidate genes and their effects are as follows: IFN-γ increases expression of MHC class I and II molecules expression, B7 delivers the obligatory costimulatory signal, GM-CSF improves APC abilities, and IL-2 induces a global immune activation (Fig. 11). Tumor cells transfected with these genes could be used as immunogens. When injected subcutaneously, they might induce an immune response. Many different cytokine genes have been transfected into tumor cells in various animal models.

The tumorigenicity of transfected tumor cells injected into syngeneic animals can be compared to that of the parental (nontransfected) tumor cells. In a series of experiments using animal models, tumor cells transfected with several genes—IL-2, IFN-γ, IL-4, IL-3, IL-6, IL-7, TNF-α, IL-12, GM-CSF, and B7 (3, 10, 16, 20, 28, 50–52, 60, 61, 77, 92, 105, 106, 116,

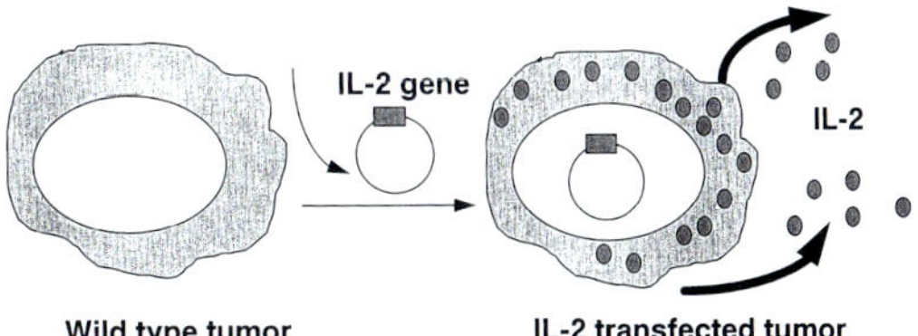

Figure 14. Tumor cell transfection by IL-2 gene. Tumor cells are engineered to produce IL-2 and to enhance the immune response against transfected tumor cells and, hopefully, wild-type tumor.

121, 179, 183, 197, 219, 220, 257, 261–263, 266, 276)—were rejected by host immune response, but corresponding parental cells grew well. In marked contrast to cytokines, the transfection of TGF-β promotes the growth of immunogenic tumors that otherwise are rejected (49, 265).

Tumors generated from cells engineered to express IL-2, IFN-γ, IL-4, IL-6, IL-7, TNF-α, GM-CSF, or B7 genes prevent tumor growth after subsequent challenge with wild-type tumor cells (10, 16, 28, 77, 105, 106, 183, 197, 220, 257). In some models, transfected tumor cells suppressed growth from wild-type tumor cells when the tumor cell types were injected simultaneously.

In some cases, transfected tumor cells have induced regression of pre-existing tumors from wild-cell types. T cells transfected with IL-2, GM-CSF, γ-IFN, IL-6, or B7 are effective in some models but only against small tumor burdens (61, 77, 179, 219, 220). Few studies have demonstrated that the immune response induced by tumors from transfected cells is tumor-specific (51, 77, 105, 106, 270) or that immunological memory is established.

In a rat model of glioma, however, the injection of IL-2 secreting tumor cells fails to evoke an immune response sufficient to induce tumor regression, even though the IL-2 transduced tumor cells produced high levels of IL-2. This unexpected result may reflect the paucity of high-affinity IL-2 receptors on glioma lymphocytes (82). On the other hand, it may reflect a nonlinear dependence of efficacy on IL-2 production: in a melanoma model testing cells genetically engineered to produce IL-2, the best immunizations were achieved with vaccines producing intermediate amounts of IL-2; vaccines producing low or high levels of IL-2 were ineffective (243). The amount of cytokine produced by transfected tumor cells may be a crucial variable in tumor vaccine strategy.

IL-7 is a growth factor for T cells that function independently of IL-2. It enhances the generation of LAK cells and cytotoxic T lymphocytes (CTL) (2). The immunoregulatory effect of tumor cells engineered to produce IL-7 has been analyzed in a murine glioma (ependymoblastoma) model (6). IL-7 transfected glioma cells were rejected by a CD8 T cell-mediated immune response in proportion to the level of IL-7 produced. The antitumor effect observed was tumor specific. IL-7 may be a good candidate cytokine for us in such vaccination (121).

** Antisense Anti-IGF-1*

IGF-1 and IGF-2 are involved in the normal growth and differentiation of the CNS. IGFs are expressed in the developing brain of rodents and humans (55) and in fetal astrocytes in culture. IGF-1-receptor is found in normal human and rat brain tissue. IGF-1 stimulates *in vitro* growth of fetal brain cells (155), increases the expression of cytoskeletal proteins, and promotes the proliferation and differentiation of normal rat oligodendroglia. IGF-2 is abundantly expressed in the human adult brain (238). IGF-1 is expressed in a variety of tumors (157). Neuroblastoma cells produce IGF-1 and IGF-2 peptides, which stimulate growth in an autocrine manner.

Rat C6 glioma cells express glial fibrillary acidic protein (GFAP), IGF-1, and IGF-1R. C6 glioma cells lose tumorigenicity when transfected with an episome-based vector containing DNA antisense to IGF-1 (270). An intense mononuclear infiltrate, predominantly CD8 T cells, occurs at the site of injection of transfected glioma cells. The subcutaneous injection of C6 cells transfected with IGF-1 antisense prevented the development of tumors from nontransfected (parental) C6 cells. Pre-existing parental C6 tumors in the brain regress after injection of transfected cells into the flank. Mixing experiments demonstrated the specificity of the antitumor immune response: IGF-1 antisense-transfected cells prevented the development of tumors from parental C6 glioma cells, but they did not prevent the growth of B104 neuroblastoma cells. These data suggest that the inhibition of IGF-1 expression restores an adequate and specific immune response. The duration of this antitumor immune response and the consequences of depleting CD8 T cells have not been studied. The dramatic immunological effects of antisense IGF-1 are surprising, considering IGF-1's immunostimulatory ability (27, 58). Blocking the effects of both IGF-1 and IGF-2 with an antisense RNA to IGF-1 *receptor* produces similar results (224, 270). This approach should be applicable to all human glioma that produce IGF-1. Data available offer conflicting views of the prevalence of IGF-1 in human gliomas. One study reported that 20–50% of tumor cells of grade III/IV astrocytomas express IGF-1 protein (Trojan, unpublished data). Another, however, failed to detect IGF-1 in none of 12 glioma explants analyzed by specific radioimmunoassay. IGF-2 was detected in about one third (113).

* IL-4

IL-4 is a cytokine produced by CD4 T cells. It activates B cells, enhances IgE production by activated B lymphocytes, increases T-cell proliferation and cytotoxicity, and stimulates eosinophil proliferation and differentiation. IL-4 also suppresses proliferation of tumor cell lines from lung cancer, gastric cancer, renal cell carcinoma, and multiple myeloma (227, 260). Vaccines of murine tumor cells transfected with IL-4 have potent antitumor effects *in vivo*. The presence of the antitumoral effect in nude mice suggests the IL-4 effect does not require T cells (262). The ability of IL-4 to mediate an antitumor response against human glioma in a nude mouse model has been studied. Human glioma cells (U87) injected subcutaneously with IL-4 producing plasmocytoma cells (LT-1) recruited eosinophils and inhibited tumor growth (289). Intracerebral injection of U87 and LT-1 cells prolonged the survival, compared to that observed when U87 and IL-4 negative plasmacytoma cells were used. However, in these experiments, a direct antiproliferative effect mediated by IL-4 can not be totally excluded. This approach is not a vaccination strategy but a means of obtaining persistent local delivery of IL-4 and an *in vivo* antitumor effect within the CNS. The independence from T-cell function of this antitumor effect could be an advantage in glioma patients who show several T-cell abnormalities.

In Vitro Studies

Liposomal transfection of IFN-γ into human glioma cells increases LAK-mediated cytotoxicity. Abrogation of this effect by anti-ICAM-1 monoclonal antibodies but not by anti-MHC class I and II monoclonal antibodies suggests that ICAM-1-LFA-1 is involved (192). No *in vivo* data have been reported. TGF-β2 likely contributes to the T-cell immunosuppression of glioma patients. Preventing expression of TGF-β2 may restore normal immune responsiveness. TGF-β2 phosphorothioate-antisense oligodeoxynucleotides enhance the proliferation of autologous lymphocytes and their *in*

vitro tumor cytotoxicity (133). *In vivo* studies are needed.

* Transfection of Oncogenes and Tumor Suppressor Genes with Subsequent Immunological Effects

Cytokine expression can be modified by transfecting glioma cells with tumor suppressor genes involved in glial tumorigenesis. Wild type p53 represses the expression of genes such as p53 having a TATA-box promotor sequence (171). In contrast, mutant p53 protein increases secretion of TGF-β2 and VEGF, an important glioma angiogenic factor. Since p53 alteration is an early event in gliomal tumorigenesis replacing the p53 gene mutated in gliomas with the wild type gene may have favorable immunological and antiangiogenic consequences.

The c-*myc* gene belongs to the MYC family of proteins critical to cellular proliferation, transformation, and apoptosis. The c-*myc* protein inhibits progression of the glioma cell cycle toward S phase and induces apoptosis of tumor cells (9). In *in vivo* models (rat 9L and C6 gliomas), coinjection of the c-*myc* gene linked to a viral promoter with glioma cells prevents formation of either subcutaneous or brain tumors. The inhibitory effect is restricted to the glioma cell line injected, strongly suggesting that a specific immune response occurs (8).

CONCLUSION

Remarkable insights into the molecular interaction between tumor cells and immune cell promise the development of new immune strategies for gliomas. Identification of a specific glioma antigen is key. Detection of identical expanded T-cell clones in numerous different gliomas suggests that such an antigen exists. Discovery of a tumor-specific antigenic protein expressed exclusively at the surface of glioma cells, or the identification of an oncogene or tumor suppressor gene product differentially expressed by normal and tumoral astrocytes would be helpful.

One of the more promising immune approaches is the use of genetically modified glioma cells as immunogens. The immunogenic effects of different genes (IL-2, IFN-γ, B7, GM-CSF, or antisense antiTGF-β) transfected into glioma cells alone or in combination will be compared in animal models to determine the best candidates for human therapy. Another approach stereotactically injects glioma cells engineered to deliver cytokines directly into the tumor. Sustained production of a cytokine and promotion of its diffusion throughout the glioma are challenges to be addressed. These and other approaches will proceed to clinical benefit only as further understanding of glioma immunobiology is achieved.

REFERENCES

1. Accolla, R. S., Adorini, L., Sartoris, S., *et al.* MHC: orchestrating the immune response. Immunol. Today *16*(1):8–11, 1995.
2. Alderson, M. R., Sassenfeld, H. M., and Widmer, M. B. Interleukin-7 enhances cytolytic T lymphocyte generation and induces lymphokine-activated killer cells from human peripheral blood. J. Exp. Med. *172*:577–587, 1990.
3. Amato, I. A stimulating new approach to cancer treatment. Science *259*:310–311, 1993.
4. Andersson, M. L., Paabo, S., Nilsson, T., *et al.* Impaired intracellular transport of class I MHC antigens as a possible means for adenoviruses to evade immune surveillance. Cell *43*(1):215–222, 1985.
5. Aoe, T., Okamoto, Y., Saito, T. Activated macrophages induce structural abnormalities of the T cell receptor-CD3 complex. J. Exp. Med. *181*(5):1881–1886, 1995.
6. Aoki, T., Tashiro, K., Miyatake, S. L., *et al.* Expression of murine interleukin 7 in a murine glioma cell line results in reduced tumorigenicity in vivo. Proc. Natl. Acad. Sci. U.S.A. *89*:3850–3854, 1992.
7. Appleby, M. W., Gross, J. A., Cooke, M. P., *et al.* Defective T cell receptor signaling in mice lacking the thymic isoform of p59^{fyn}. Cell *70*:751–763, 1992.
8. Asai, A., Miyagi, Y., Hashimoto, H., *et al.* Modification of tumor immunogenicity of rat glioma cells by s-Myc expression: eradication of rat gliomas in vivo. Cell Growth Differ. *5*:1153–1158, 1994.
9. Asai, A., Miyagi, Y., Sugiyama, A., *et al.* The s-Myc protein having the ability to induce apoptosis is selectively expressed in rat embryo chondrocytes. Oncogene *9*:2345–2352, 1994.
10. Asher, A. L., Mule, J. J., Kasid, A., *et al.* Murine tumor cells transduced with the gene for tumor necrosis factor-α. J. Immunol. *146*:3227–3234, 1991.
11. Austyn, J. M., and Larsen, C. P. Migration patterns of dendritic leukocytes: implications for transplantation. Transplantation *49*(1):1–7, 1990.
12. Azuma, M., Ito, D., Yagita, H., *et al.* B70 antigen is a second ligand for CTLA-4 and CD28. Nature *366*:76–79, 1993.
13. Baadsgaard, O., Fischer, G. J., Voorhees, J. J., *et al.* Interactions of epidermal cells and T cells in inflammatory skin diseases. J. Am. Acad. Dermatol. *23*:1312–1316, 1990.
14. Bakker, A. B. H., Schreurs, M. W. J., de Boer, A. J., *et al.* Melanocyte lineage-specific antigen gp 100 is recognized by melanoma-derived tumor-infiltrating lymphocytes. J. Exp. Med. *179*(3):1005–1009, 1994.
15. Baldwin, R. W. Immunity to methylcholanthrene-induced tumors in inbred rats following atrophy and regression of the implanted tumors. Br. J. Cancer *9*:652–657, 1955.
16. Bannerji, R., Arroyo, C. D., Cordon-Cardo, C., *et al.* The role of IL-2 secreted from genetically modified tumor cells in the establishment of antitumor immunity. J. Immunol. *152*:2324–2332, 1994.
17. Barba, D., Saris, S. C., Holder, C., *et al.* Intratumoral LAK cells and interleukin-2 therapy of human gliomas. J. Neurosurg. *70*:175–182, 1989.
18. Barker, C. F., and Billingham, R. E. The role of regional lymphatics in the skin homograft response. Transplantation *5*:962–966, 1967.
19. Bartolazzi, A., Peach, R., Aruffo, A., *et al.* Interaction between CD44 and hyaluronate is directly implicated in the regulation of tumor development. J. Exp. Med. *180*:53–66, 1994.
20. Baskar, S., Ostrand-Rosenberg, S., Nabavi, N., *et al.* Constitutive expression of B7 restores immunogenicity of tumor cells expressing truncated MHC class II molecules. Proc. Natl. Acad. Sci. U.S.A. *90*:5687–5690, 1993.
21. Basombrio, M. A.: Search for common antigenicities among twenty-five sarcomas induced by methylcholanthrene. Cancer Res. *30*:2458–2462, 1970.
22. Becker, J. C., Dummer, R., Hartmann, A. A., *et al.* Shedding of ICAM-1 from human melanoma cell lines induced by IFN-gamma and tumor necrosis facto-alpha. Functional consequences on cell-mediated cytotoxicity. J. Immunol. *147*(12):4398–4401, 1991.
23. Becker, J. C., Termeer, C., Schmidt, R. E., *et al.* Soluble intercellular adhesion molecule-1 inhibits MHC-restricted specific T cell/tumor interaction. J. Immunol. *151*(12):7224–7232, 1993.
24. Belldegrun, A., Muul, L. M., Rosenberg, S. A. Interleukin 2 expanded tumor-infiltrating lymphocytes in human renal cell cancer: isolation, characterization, and antitumor activity. Cancer Res. *48*:206–214, 1988.
25. Benveniste, E. N., Tozawa, H., Gasson, J. C., *et al.* Response of human glioblastoma cell sot recombinant interleukin-2. J. Neuroimmunol. *17*:301–314, 1988.
26. Bertoletti, A., Sette, A., Chisari, F. V., *et al.* Natural variants of cytotoxic epitopes are T-cell receptor antagonists for antiviral cytotoxic T-cells. Nature *369*:407–410, 1994.
27. Kinz, K., Joller, P., Froesh, P., *et al.* Repopulation of the atrophied thymus in diabetic rats by insulin-like growth factor. I. Proc. Natl. Acad. Sci. U.S.A. *87*:3690–3604, 1990.
28. Blankenstein, T., Qin, Z., Uberla, K., *et al.* Tumor suppression after tumor cell targeted tumor necrosis-α gene transfer. J. Exp. Med. *173*:1047–1052, 1991.
29. Bodmer, S., Strommer, K., Frei, K., *et al.* Immunosuppression and transforming growth factor β in glioblastoma. Preferential production of transforming growth factor-beta 2. J. Immunol. *143*(10):3222–3229, 1989.

30. Bodmer, W. F., Browning, M. J., Krausa, P., *et al.* Tumor escape from immune response by variation in HLA expression and other mechanisms. Ann. N. Y. Acad. Sci. *690:*42–49, 1993.

31. Boon, T. Toward a genetic analysis of tumor rejection antigens. Adv. Cancer Res. *58:*177–210, 1992.

32. Boon, T., Cerottini, J. C., Van den Eynde, *et al.* Tumor antigens recognized by T lymphocytes. Annu. Rev. Immunol. *12:*337–365, 1994.

33. Border, W. A., and Noble, N. A. Transforming growth factor β in tissue fibrosis. N. Engl. J. Med. *331*(19): 1286–1292, 1994.

34. Boussiotis, V. A., Barber, D. L., Nakarai, T., *et al.* Prevention of T cell anergy by signaling through the ν chain of the IL-2 receptor. Science *266:*1039–1042, 1994.

35. Boussiotis, V. A., Freeman, G. J., Gribben, J. G., *et al.* Activated human B lymphocytes express three CTLA-4 counterreceptors that costimulate T-cell activation. Proc. Natl. Acad. Sci. U.S.A. *90:*11059–11063, 1993.

36. Braciale, T. J., and Braciale, V. L. Antigen presentation: structural themes and functional variations. Immunol. Today *12*(4):124–129, 1991.

37. Brichard, V., Van Pel, A., Wölfel, T., *et al.* The tyrosinase gene codes for an antigen recognized by autologous cytolytic T lymphocytes on HLA-A2 melanomas. J. Exp. Med. *178:*489–495, 1993.

38. Brooks, W. H., Maresbery, W. R., Gupta, G. D., *et al.* Relationship of lymphocyte invasion and survival of brain tumor patients. Ann. Neurol. *4:*219–224, 1978.

39. Brooks, W. H., Roszman, T. L., Mahaley, M. S., *et al.* Immunobiology of primary intracranial tumors. II. Analysis of lymphocyte subpopulations in patients with primary brain tumors. Clin. Exp. Immunol. *29:*61–66, 1977.

40. Brooks, W. H., Roszman, T. L., and Rogers, A. S. Impairment of rosette-forming T lymphocytes in patients with primary intracranial tumors. Cancer *37:*1869–1873, 1976.

41. Browne, H., Smith, G., Beck, S., *et al.* A complex between the MHC class I homologue encoded by human cytomegalovirus and β2-microglobulin. Nature *347:*770–772, 1990.

42. Burnet, F. M. The concept of immunological surveillance. Prog. Exp. Tumor Res. *13:*1–27, 1970.

43. Caignard, A., Dietrich, P. Y., Morand, V., *et al.* Evidence for T-cell clonal expansion in patients with squamous cell carcinoma of the head and neck. Cancer Res. *54:*1292–1297, 1994.

44. Cameron, R. B., Spiess, P. J., and Rosenberg, S. A. Synergistic antitumor activity of tumor-infiltrating lymphocytes interleukin 2, and local tumor irradiation: studies on the mechanism of action. J. Exp. Med. *171:*249–263, 1990.

45. Caux, C., Dezutter-Dambuyant, C., Schmitt, D., *et al.* GM-CSF and TNF-α cooperate in the generation of dendritic langerhans cells. Nature *360:*258–261, 1992.

46. Cauz, C., Liu, Y. J., and Banchereau, J. Recent advances in the study of dendritic cells and follicular dendritic cells. Immunol. Today *16*(1):2–4, 1995.

47. Chan, A. C., Iwashima, M., Turck, C. W., *et al.* ZAP-70 kd protein-tyrosine kinase that associates with the TCR S chain. Cell *72:*649–662, 1992.

48. Chang, C. H., Horton, J., Schoenfeld, D., *et al.* Comparison of postoperative radiotherapy and combined postoperative radiotherapy and chemotherapy in the multidisciplinary management of malignant gliomas: a joint radiation therapy oncology group and Eastern Cooperative Oncology Group Study. Cancer *52:*997–1007, 1983.

49. Chang, H. L., Gillett, N., Figari, I., *et al.* Increased transforming growth factor β expression inhibits cell proliferation in vitro, yet increases tumorigenicity and tumor growth of Meth A sarcoma cells. Cancer Res. *53:*4391–4398, 1993.

50. Chen, L., Ashe, S., Brady, W., *et al.* Costimulation of antitumor immunity by the B7 counterreceptor for the T lymphocyte molecules CD28 and CTLA4. Cell *71:*1093–1102, 1992.

51. Chen, L., Linsley, P. S., Hellström, K. E. Costimulation of T cells for tumor immunity. Immunol. Today *14*(10):483–486, 1993.

52. Chen, L., McGowan, P., Ashe, S., *et al.* Tumor immunogenicity determines the effect of B7 costimulation on T cell-mediated tumor immunity. J. Exp. Med. *179:*523–532, 1994.

53. Chen, L., Thomas, E. K., Hu, S. L., *et al.* Human papillomavirus type 16 nucleoprotein E7 is a tumor rejection antigen. Proc. Natl. Acad. Sci. U.S.A. *88:*110–114, 1991.

54. Chen, W., Peace, D. J., Rovira, D. K., *et al.* T cell immunity to the joining region of p210 bcr-abl protein. Proc. Natl. Acad. Sci. U.S.A. *89:*1468–1472, 1992.

55. Chernausek, S. D. Insulin-like growth factor-I (IGF-I) production by astroglial cells: regulation and importance for epidermal growth factor-induced cell replication. J. Neurosci. Res. *34:*189–197, 1993.

56. Chien, Y. H., and Davis, M. M. How ab T-cell receptors see peptide/MHC complexes. Immunol. Today *14:*597–601, 1993.

57. Chothia, C., Boswell, D. R., and Lesk, A. M. The outline structure of the T-cell alpha/beta receptor. EMBO J. *7:*3745–3755, 1988.

58. Clark, R., Strasser, J., McCabe, S., *et al.* Insulin-like growth factor-1 stimulation of lymphopoiesis. J. Clin. Invest. *92:*540–548, 1993.

59. Cochet, M., Pannetier, C., Regnault, A., *et al.* Molecular detection and in vivo analysis of the specific T cell response to a protein antigen. Eur. J. Immunol. *22*(10):2639–2647, 1992.

60. Colombo, M. P., Ferrari, G., Stoppacciaro, A., *et al.* Granulocyte-colony stimulating factor gene suppresses tumorigenicity of a murine adenocarcinoma in vivo. J. Exp. Med. *173:*889–897, 1991.

61. Connor, J., Bannerji, R., Saito, S., *et al.* Regression of bladder tumors in mice treated with interleukin-2 gene modified tumor cells. J. Exp. Med. *177:*1127–1134, 1993.

62. Connor, M. E., and Stern, P. L. Loss of MHC class-I expression in cervical carcinomas. Int. J. Cancer *46*(6):1029–1034, 1990.

63. Couldwell, W. T., de Tribolet, N., Antel, J. P., *et al.* Adhesion molecules and malignant gliomas: impli-

cations for tumorigenesis. J. Neurosurg. *76:*782–791, 1992.

64. Couldwell, W. T., Yong, V. W., Dore-Duffy, P., *et al.* Production of soluble autocrine inhibitory factors by human glioma cell lines. J. Neurol. Sci. *110:* 178–185, 1992.

65. Coulie, P. G., Brichard, V., Van Pel, A., *et al.* A new gene coding for a differentiation antigen recognized by autologous cytolytic T lymphocytes on HLA-A2 melanomas. J. Exp. Med. *180:*35–42, 1994.

66. Cromme, F. V., Airey, J., Heemels, M. T., *et al.* Loss of transporter protein, encoded by the TAP-1 gene, is highly correlated with loss of HLA expression in cervical carcinomas. J. Exp. Med. *179:*335–340, 1994.

67. Cromme, F. V., Meijer, C. J., Snijders, P. J., *et al.* Analysis of MHC class I and II expression in relation of presence of HPV genotypes in premalignant and malignant cervical lesions. Br. J. Cancer *67*(6): 1372–1380, 1993.

68. Cserr, H. F., and Knopf, P. M. Cervical lymphatics, the blood-brain barrier and the immunoreactivity of the brain: a new view. Immunol. Today *13*(12): 507–512, 1992.

69. Däubener, W., Zennati, S. S., Wernet, P., *et al.* Human glioblastoma cell line 86HG39 activates T cells in an antigen specific major histocompatibility complex class II-dependent manner. J. Neuroimmunol. *41:*21–28, 1992.

70. Davis, M. M., and Bjorkman, P. J. T-cell antigen receptor genes and T-cell recognition. Nature *334:* 395–402, 1988.

71. De la Salle, H., Hanau, D., Fricker, D., *et al.* Homozygous human TAP peptide transporter mutation in HLA class I deficiency. Science *265:*237–241, 1994.

72. Del Val, M., Hengel, H., Häcker, H., *et al.* Cytomegalovirus prevents antigen presentation by blocking the transport of peptide-loaded major histocompatibility complex class I molecules into the medial-Golgi compartment. J. Exp. Med. *176*(3):729–738, 1992.

73. Deres, K., Schild, H., Wiesmuller, K. H., *et al.* In vivo priming of virus-specific cytotoxic T lymphocytes with synthetic lipopeptide vaccine. Nature *342:*561–564, 1989.

74. Dietrich, P. Y., Caignard, A., Diu, A., *et al.* Analysis of T cell receptor variability in transplanted patients with human cutaneous acute graft versus host disease. Blood *80:*2419–2424, 1992.

75. Dietrich, P. Y., Caignard, A., Lim, A., *et al.* In vivo T-cell clonal amplification in human acute graft versus host disease. Blood *84:*2815–2820, 1994.

76. Doyle, A., Martin, W. J., Funa, K., *et al.* Markedly decreased expression of class I histocompatibility antigens, proteins, and mRNA in human small-cell lung cancer. J. Exp. Med. *161*(5):1135–1151, 1985.

77. Dranoff, G., Jaffee, E., Lazenby, A., *et al.* Vaccination with irradiated tumor cells engineered to secrete murine granulocyte-macrophage colony-stimulating factor stimulates potent, specific, and long-lasting anti-tumor immunity. Proc. Natl. Acad. Sci. U.S.A. *90:*3539–3543, 1993.

78. D'Urso, C. M., Wang, Z., Cao, Y., *et al.* Lack of HLA class I expression by cultured melanoma cells FO-1 due to a defect in β2m gene expression. J. Clin. Invest. *87*(1):284–292, 1991.

79. Dutcher, J. P., and Wiernik, P. H. The role of recombinant interleukin-2 in therapy for hematologic malignancies. Semin. Oncol. *20*(6)(suppl. 9):33–40, 1993.

80. Ebato, M., Nitta, T., Yagita, H., *et al.* Shared amino acid sequences in the NDβN and Nα regions of the T cell receptors of tumor-infiltrating lymphocytes within malignant glioma. Eur. J. Immunol. *24:*2987–2992, 1994.

81. Ebato, M., Nitta, T., Yagita, H., *et al.* Skewed distribution of TCR Va 7-bearing T cells within tumor infiltrating lymphocytes of HLA-A24(9) positive patients with malignant glioma. Immunol. Lett. *39:* 53–64, 1994.

82. Elliott, L., Brooks, W., and Roszman, T. Inability of mitogen-activated lymphocytes obtained from patients with malignant intracranial tumors to express high affinity interleukin-2 receptors. J. Clin. Invest. *86*(1):80–86, 1990.

83. Elliott, L. H., Brooks, W. H., and Roszman, T. L. Activation of immunoregulatory lymphocytes obtained from patients with malignant gliomas. J. Neurosurg. *67:*231–236, 1987.

84. Elliott, L. H., Brooks, W. H., and Roszman, T. L. Role of interleukin-2 and IL-2 receptor expression in the proliferative defect observed in mitogen-stimulated lymphocytes from patients with gliomas. J. Natl. Cancer Inst. *78*(5):919–922, 1987.

85. Elliott, L. H., Brooks, W. H., and Roszman, T. L. Suppression of high affinity IL-2 receptors on mitogen activated lymphocytes by glioma-derived suppressor factor. J. Neurooncol. *14*(1):1–7, 1992.

86. Ellis, J. R. M., Keating, P. J., Baird, J., *et al.* The association of an HPV16 oncogene variant with HLA-B7 has implications for vaccine design in cervical cancer. Nature Med. *1*(5):464–470, 1995.

87. Evavold, B. D., Sloan-Lancaster, J., and Allen, P. M. Tickling the TCR: selective T-cell functions stimulated by altered peptide ligands. Immunol. Today *14*(12):602–609, 1993.

88. Even, J., Lim, A., Puisieux, I., *et al.* T-cell repertoire in healthy and diseased human tissues analysed by T-cell receptor b-chain CDR3 size determination: evidence for oligoclonal expansions in tumors and inflammatory diseases. Res. Immunol. *146:*65–80, 1995.

89. Fabry, Z., Raine, C. S., and Hart, M. N. Nervous tissue as an immune compartment: the dialect of the immune response in the CNS. Immunol. Today *15:* 218–224, 1994.

90. Fabry, Z., Waldschmidt, M. M., Hendrickson, D., *et al.* Adhesion molecules on murine brain microvascular endothelial cells: expression and regulation of ICAM-1 and Lgp 55. J. Neuroimmunol. *36:*1–11, 1992.

91. Farace, F., Kremer, F., Dietrich, P. Y., *et al.* T-cell repertoire in patients with B-chronic lymphocytic leukemia: evidence for in vivo T cell clonal expansions. J. Immunol. *153:*4281–4290, 1994.

92. Fearon, E. R., Pardoll, D. M., Itaya, T., *et al.* Interleukin-2 production by tumor cells bypasses T helper

function in the generation of an antitumor response. Cell *60:*397–403, 1990.

93. Feltkamp, M. C. W., Smits, H. L., Vierboom, M. P. M., *et al.* Vaccination with cytotoxic lymphocyte epitope protects against a tumor induced by human papillomavirus type 16-transformed cells. Eur. J. Immunol. *23:*2242–2249, 1993.

94. Ferradini, L., Mackensen, A., Genevee, C., *et al.* Analysis of T cell receptor variability in tumor-infiltrating lymphocytes from a human regression melanoma. Evidence for in situ T cell clonal expansion. J. Clin. Invest. *91*(3):1183–1190, 1993.

95. Ferradini, L., Roman-Roman, S., Azocar, J., *et al.* Analysis of T-cell receptor alpha/beta variability in lymphocytes infiltrating a melanoma metastasis. Cancer Res. *52:*4649–4654, 1992.

96. Fine, H. A., Dear, K. G. B., Loeffler, J. S., *et al.* Meta-analysis of radiation therapy with and without adjuvant chemotherapy for malignant gliomas in adults. Cancer *71:*2585–2597, 1993.

97. Finke, J. H., Zea, A. H., Stanley, J., *et al.* Loss of T-cell receptor S chain and p56^lck in T-cells infiltrating human renal cell carcinoma. Cancer Res. *53:*5613–5616, 1993.

98. Flamand, V., Sornasse, T., Thielemans, K., *et al.* Murine dendritic cells pulsed in vitro with tumor antigen induce tumor resistance in vivo. Eur. J. Immunol. *24:*605–610, 1994.

99. Fontana, A., Hengartner, H., de Tribolet, N., *et al.* Glioblastoma cells release interleukin-1 and factors inhibiting interleukin-2-mediated effects. J. Immunol. *132:*1837–1844, 1984.

100. Fontana, A., Kristensen, F., Dubs, R., *et al.* Production of prostaglandin and interleukin-1 like factor by culture astrocytes in C6 glioma cells. J. Immunol. *129:*2413–2419, 1982.

101. Fossum, B., Gedde-Dahl, T., Hansen, T., *et al.* Overlapping epitopes encompassing a point mutation (12 gly-arg) in p21 ras can be recognized by HLA-DR, -DP, and -DQ restricted T cells. Eur. J. Immunol. *23:*2687–2691, 1993.

102. Freeman, G. J., Gribben, J. G., Boussiotis, V. A., *et al.* Cloning of B7-2: a CTLA-4 counter-receptor that costimulates human T cell proliferation. Science *262:*844–845, 1993.

103. Früh, K., Ahn, K., Djaballah, H., *et al.* A viral inhibitor of peptide transporters for antigen presentation. Nature *375:*415–418, 1995.

104. Gambacorti-Passerini, C., Grignani, F., Arienti, F., *et al.* Human CD4 lymphocytes specifically recognize a peptide representing the fusion region of the hybrid protein pml/RARa present in acute promyelocytic leukemia cells. Blood *81:*1369–1375, 1993.

105. Gansbacher, B., Bannerji, R., Daniels, B., *et al.* Retroviral vector-mediated γ-interferon gene transfer into tumor cells generates potent and long lasting antitumor immunity. Cancer Res. *50:*7820–7825, 1990.

106. Gansbacher, B., Zier, K., Daniels, B., *et al.* Interleukin-2 gene transfer into tumor cells abrogates tumorigenicity and induces protective immunity. J. Exp. Med. *172:*1217–1224, 1990.

107. Gaugler, B., Van Den Eynde, B., Van der Bruggen, P., *et al.* Human gene MAGE-3 codes for an antigen recognized on a melanoma by autologous cytolytic T lymphocytes. J. Exp. Med. *179:*921–930, 1994.

108. Gauthier, T., Hamou, M. F., Monod, L., *et al.* Expression and release of interleukin-1 by human glioblastoma cells in vitro and in vivo. Acta Neurochir. *121:*199–205, 1993.

109. Gedde-Dahl, T. I., Fossum, B., Eriksen, J. A., *et al.* T cell clones specific for p21 ras-derived peptides: characterization of their fine specificity and HLA restriction. Eur. J. Immunol. *23:*754–760, 1993.

110. Genevee, C., Dietrich, P. Y., Robache, S., *et al.* In vivo local expansion of clonal T cell subpopulations in renal cell carcinoma. Cancer Res. *55:*685–590, 1995.

111. Genevee, C., Diu, A., Nierat, J., *et al.* An experimentally validated panel of sub-family-specific oligonucleotide primers (Vα1-w29/Vβ1-w24) for the study of human T cell receptor variable V gene segment usage by polymerase chain reaction. Eur. J. Immunol. *22:*1261–1269, 1992.

112. Ghosh, P., Sica, A., Young, H. A., *et al.* Alterations in NFkB/Rel family proteins in splenic T-cells from tumor-bearing mice and reversal following therapy. Cancer Res. *54:*2969–2972, 1994.

113. Glick, R. P., Unterman, T. G., Van der Woude, M., *et al.* Insulin and insulin-like growth factors in central nervous system tumors. Part V. Production of insulin-like growth factors I and II in vivo. J. Neurosurg. *77:*445–450, 1992.

114. Goldberg, A. L. Functions of the proteasome: the lysis at the end of the tunnel. Science *268:*522–523, 1995.

115. Goldberg, A. L., and Rock, K. L. Proteolysis, proteasomes and antigen presentation. Nature *357:*275–279, 1992.

116. Golumbek, P. T., Lazenby, A. J., Levitsky, H. I., *et al.* Treatment of established renal cancer by tumor cells engineered to secrete interleukin-4. Science *254:*713–716, 1991.

117. Guinan, E. C., Gribben, J. G., Boussiotis, V. A., *et al.* Pivotal role of the B7:CD28 pathway in transplantation tolerance and tumor immunity. Blood *84*(10): 3261–3282, 1994.

118. Harding, C. V., Collins, D. S., Slot, J. W., *et al.* Liposome-encapsulated antigens are processed in lysosomes, recycled, and presented to T cells. Cell *64:*393–401, 1991.

119. Hathcock, K. S., Laszlo, G., Dickler, H. B., *et al.* Identification of an alternative CTLA-4 ligand costimulatory for T cell activation. Science *262:*905–911, 1993.

120. Hill, A., Jugovic, P., York, I., *et al.* Herpes simplex virus turns off the TAP to evade host immunity. Nature *375:*411–415, 1995.

121. Hock, H., Dorsch, M., and Diamanstein, T. Interleukin-7 induces CD4+ T cell-dependent tumor rejection. J. Exp. Med. *174:*1291–1298, 1991.

122. Hogquist, K. A., Jameson, S. C., Heath, W. R., *et al.* T cell receptor antagonist peptides induce positive selection. Cell *76:* 17–27, 1994.

123. Holladay, F. P., Heitz, T., Chen, Y. L., *et al.* Successful treatment of a malignant rat glioma with cytotoxic T lymphocytes. Neurosurgery *31:*528–533, 1992.

124. Holladay, F. P., Heitz, T., and Wood, G. W. Antitumor activity against established intracerebral gliomas exhibited by cytotoxic T lymphocytes, but not lymphokine-activated killer cells. J. Neurosurg. *77:* 757–762, 1992.

125. Houbier, J. G. A., Nijman, H. W., van der Burg, S. H., *et al.* In-vitro induction of human cytotoxic T lymphocyte responses against peptides of mutant and wild type p53. Eur. J. Immunol. *23:*2072–2077, 1993.

126. Houghton, A. N. Cancer antigens: immune recognition of self and altered peptides. J. Exp. Med. *180:* 1–4, 1994.

127. Huber, D., Philipp, J., and Fontana, A. Protease inhibitors interfere with the transforming growth factor-β-dependent but not the transforming factor-β-independent pathway of tumor cell-mediated immunosuppression. J. Immunol. *148*(1):277–284, 1992.

128. Huet, S., Groux, H., Caillou, B., *et al.* CD44 contributes to T cell activation. J. Immunol. *143:*798–803, 1989.

129. Huettner, C., Paulus, W., and Roggendorf, W. Messenger RNA expression of the immunosuppressive cytokine IL-10 in human gliomas. Am. J. Pathol. *146*(2):317–322, 1995.

130. Inaba, K., Inaba, M., Romani, N., *et al.* Generation of large numbers of dendritic cells from mouse bone marrow cultures supplemented with granulocyte/macrophage colon-stimulating factor. J. Exp. Med. *176:*1693–1702, 1992.

131. Isakov, N., Wange, R. L., Burgess, W. H., *et al.* ZAP-70 binding specificity to T cell receptor tyrosine-based activation motifs: the tandem SH2 domains of ZAP-70 bind distinct tyrosine-based activation motifs with varying affinity. J. Exp. Med. *181:*375–380, 1995.

132. Iwashima, M., Irving, B. A., Van Oers, N. S. C., *et al.* Sequential interactions of the TCR with two distinct cytoplasmic tyrosine kinases. Science *263:*1136–1139, 1994.

133. Jachimczak, P., Bogdahn, U., Schneider, J., *et al.* The effect of TGF-β2-specific phosphorothiote-antisense oligodeoxynucleotides in reversing immunosuppression in malignant glioma. J. Neurosurg. *78:* 944–951, 1993.

134. Jones, M., Philip, T., Palmer, P., *et al.* The impact of interleukin-2 alone on survival in renal cancer: a multivariate analysis. Cancer Biother. *8*(4):275–288, 1993.

135. June, C. H., Bluestone, J. A., Nadler, L. M., *et al.* The B7 and CD29 receptor families. Immunol. Today *15*(7):321–325, 1994.

136. Jung, S., and Schluesener, H. J. Human T lymphocytes recognize a peptide of single point-mutated, oncogenic ras proteins. J. Exp. Med. *173:*273–276, 1991.

137. Kang, S. M., Tran, A. C., Grilli, M., *et al.* NF-kB subunit regulation in nontransformed CD4+ T lymphocytes. Science *256:*1452–1456, 1992.

138. Kawakami, Y., Eliyahu, S., Sakaguchi, K., *et al.* Identification of the immunodominant peptides of the MART-1 human melanoma antigen recognized by the majority of HLA-A2-restricted tumor infiltrating lymphocytes. J. Exp. Med. *180:*347–352, 1994.

139. Kehrl, J. H., Wakefield, L. M., Roberts, A. B., *et al.* Production of transforming growth factor β by human T lymphocytes and its potential role in the regulation of T cell growth. J. Exp. Med. *163*(5): 1037–1050, 1986.

140. Kerr, L., Huntoon, C., Donohue, J., *et al.* Heteroconjugate antibody-directed killing of autologous human renal carcinoma cells by in vitro-activated lymphocytes. J. Immunol. *144:*4060–4067, 1990.

141. Khera, K. S., Ashkenasi, A., Rapp, F., *et al.* Immunity in hamsters to cells transformed in vitro and in vivo by SV40. Tests for antigenic relationship among the papovaviruses. J. Immunol. *91:*604–613, 1963.

142. Kim, S. U., Moretto, G., and Shin, D. H. Expression of 1a antigens on the surface of human oligodendrocytes and astrocytes in culture. J. Neuroimmunol. *10:*141–149, 1985.

143. Klein, G., Sjogren, H. O., Klein, E., *et al.* Demonstration of resistance against methylcholanthrene-induced sarcomas in the primary autochthonous host. Cancer Res. *20:*1516–1572, 1960.

144. Klenerman, P., Rowland-Jones, S., McAdam, S., *et al.* Cytotoxic T-cell activity antagonized by naturally occurring HIC-1 gag variants. Nature *369:*403–407, 1994.

145. Koretz, M. J., Lawson, D. H., York, R. M., *et al.* Randomized study of interleukin 2 (IL-2) alone vs. IL-2 plus lymphokine-activated killer cells for treatment of melanoma and renal cell cancer. Arch. Surg. *126:*898–903, 1991.

146. Kosco-Vilbois, M. H., Gray, D., Scheidegger, D., *et al.* Follicular dendritic cells help resting B cells to become effective antigen-presenting cells: induction of B7/BB1 and upregulation of major histocompatibility complex class II molecules. J. Exp. Med. *178:*2055–2066, 1993.

147. Kripke, M. L. Antigenicity of murine skin tumors induced by ultraviolet light. J. Natl. Cancer Inst. *53:*1333–1336, 1974.

148. Kuppner, M. C., Hamou, M. F., and de Tribolet, N. Immunohistological and functional analyses of lymphoid infiltrated in human glioblastomas. Cancer Res. *48:*6926–6932, 1988.

149. Kuppner, M. C., Van Meir, E., Gauthier, T., *et al.* Differential expression of the CD44 molecule in human brain tumours. Int. J. Cancer *50:*572–577, 1992.

150. Kuppner, M. C., Van Meir, E., Hamou, M. F., *et al.* Cytokine regulation of intercellular adhesion molecule-1 (ICAM-1) expression on human glioblastoma cells. Clin. Exp. Immunol. *81:*142–148, 1990.

151. Lampson, L. A., and Hichey,W. F. Monoclonal antibody analysis of MHC expression in human brain biopsies: tissue ranging from histologically normal to that showing different levels of glial tumor involvement. J. Immunol. *136:*4054–4062, 1986.

152. Larsen, C. P., Steinmann, R. M., Witmer-Plack, M., *et al.* Migration and maturation of Langerhans cells in skin transplants and explants. J. Exp. Med. *172*(5): 1483–1493, 1990.

153. Lassam, N., and Jay, G. Suppression of MHC class I RNA in highly oncogenic cells occurs at the level

of transcriptional initiation. J. Immunol. *143*(11): 3792–3797, 1989.

154. Lefranc, M. P. Organization of the human T-cell receptor genes. Eur. Cytokine Netw. *1*(3):121–130, 1990.

155. Lenoir, D., and Honegger, P. Insulin-like growth factor I (IGF I) stimulates DNA synthesis in fetal rat brain cell culture. Brain Res. *283:*205–213, 1983.

156. Lenz, A., Heine, M., Schuler, G., *et al.* Human and murine dermis contain dendritic cells: isolation by means of a novel method and phenotypical and functional characterization. J. Clin. Invest. *92:* 2587–2596, 1993.

157. LeRoith, D., Baserga, R., Helman, L., *et al.* Insulin-like growth factors and cancer. Ann. Intern. Med. *122:*54–59, 1995.

158. Lesser, G. J., and Grossman, S. The chemotherapy of high-grade astrocytomas. Semin. Oncol. *21*(2): 220–235, 1994.

159. Li, H., Hamou, M. F., de Tribolet, N., *et al.* Variant CE44 adhesion molecules are expressed in human brain metastases but not in glioblastomas. Cancer Res. *53:*5345–5349, 1993.

160. Li, X., Liu, J., Park, J. K., *et al.* T cells from renal cell carcinoma patients exhibit an abnormal pattern of kB-specific DNA-binding activity: a preliminary report. Cancer Res. *54:*5424–5429, 1994.

161. Libermann, T. A., Nusbaum, H. R., Razon, N., *et al.* Amplification, enhanced expression and possible rearrangement of EGF receptor gene in primary human brain tumours of glial origin. Nature *313:* 144–147, 1985.

162. Lieber, M. R. The mechanism of V(D)J recombination: a balance of diversity, specificity, and stability. Cell *70:*873–876, 1992.

163. Lillehei, K. O., Mitchell, D. H., Johnson, S. D., *et al.* Long-term follow-up with patients with recurrent gliomas treated with adjuvant adoptive immunotherapy. Neurosurgery *10:*89–94, 1991.

164. Lissoni, P., Barni, S., Ardizzola, A., *et al.* Prognostic factors of the clinical response to subcutaneous immunotherapy with interleukin-2 alone in patients with metastatic renal cell carcinoma. Oncology *51:* 59–62, 1994.

165. List, J., Moser, R. P., Steuer, M., *et al.* Cytokine responses to intraventricular injection of interleukin 2 into patients with leptomeningeal carcinomatosis: rapid induction of tumor necrosis factor alpha, interleukin 1 beta, interleukin 6, gamma-interferon, and soluble interleukin 2 receptor (MR 55,000 protein). Cancer Res. *52*(5):1123–1128, 1992.

166. Liu, J. P., Baker, J., Perkins, A. S., *et al.* Mice carrying null mutations of the gene encoding insulin-like growth factor I (IGF-I) and type 1 IGF receptor. Cell *75:*59–72, 1993.

167. Liu, Y., Wei, S. H., Ho, A. S., *et al.* Expression cloning and characterization of a human IL-10 receptor. J. Immunol. *152:*1821–1829, 1994.

168. Loeffler, C. M., Smyth, M. J., Longo, D. L., *et al.* Immunoregulation in cancer-bearing hosts: downregulation of gene expression and cytotoxic function in CD8+ T cells. J. Immunol. *149:*949–956, 1992.

169. Macatonia, S. E., Knight, S. C., Edwards, A. J., *et*

al. Localization of antigen on lymph node dendritic cells after exposure to the contact sensitizer fluorescein isothiocyanate. J. Exp. Med. *166:*1654–1667, 1987.

170. Mach, B. MHC class II regulation: lessons from a disease. N. Engl. J. Med. *332:*120–122, 1995.

171. Mack, D. H., Vartilar, J., Pipas, J. M., *et al.* Specific repression of TATA-mediated but not initiator-mediated transcription by wild-type p53. Nature *363:* 281–283, 1993.

172. Mackensen, A., Carcelain, G., Viel, S., *et al.* Direct evidence to support the immunosurveillance concept in a human regressive melanoma. J. Clin. Invest. *93*(4):1397–1402, 1994.

173. Mackensen, A., Ferradini, L., Carcelain, G., *et al.* Evidence for in situ amplification of cytotoxic T-lymphocytes with antitumor activity in a human regressive melanoma. Cancer Res. *53*(15):3569–3573, 1993.

174. Madrenas, J., Wange, R. L., Wang, J. L., *et al.* S Phosphorylation without ZAP-70 activation induced by TCR antagonists or partial agonists. Science *267:*515–518, 1995.

175. Mahaley, M. S., Brooks, W. H., Roszman, T. L., *et al.* Immunobiology of primary intracranial tumors. Part I. Studies of the cellular and humoral general immune competence of brain-tumor patients. J. Neurosurg. *46:*467–476, 1977.

176. Marx, J. The T cell receptor begins to reveal its many facets. Science *267:*459–460, 1995.

177. Matis, L. A. The molecular basis of T cell specificity. Annu. Rev. Immunol. *8:*65–82, 1990.

178. Matsumara, Y., and Tarin, D. Significance of CD44 gene products for cancer diagnosis and disease evaluation. Lancet *340:*1053–1058, 1992.

179. Matulonis, U. A., Dosio, C., Lamont, C., *et al.* Role of B7-1 in mediating an immune response to myeloid leukemia cells. Blood *85*(9):2507–2515, 1995.

180. Maudsley, D. J., and Pound, J. D.: Modulation of MHC antigen expression by viruses and oncogenes. Immunol. Today *12*(12):429–431, 1991.

181. Mauer, S. C., Fitzgerald, K. A., Hussey, R. E., *et al.* Clonotypic structures involved in antigen-specific human T cell function. J. Exp. Med. *157:*705–719, 1983.

182. Maxwell, M., Galanopoulos, T., Neville-Golden, J., *et al.* Effect of the expression of transforming growth factor-β2 in primary human glioblastomas on immunosuppression and loss of immune surveillance. J. Neurosurg. *76:*799–804, 1992.

183. McBride, W. H., Thacker, J. D., Comora, S., *et al.* Genetic modification of a murine fibrosarcoma to produce interleukin-7 stimulates host cell infiltration and tumor immunity. Cancer Res. *52:*3931–3937, 1992.

184. Merchant, R. E., McVicar, D. W., Merchant, L. H., *et al.* Treatment of recurrent malignant glioma by repeated intracerebral injections of human recombinant interleukin-2 alone or in combination with systemic interferon-alpha. Results of a phase I clinical trial. J. Neurooncol. *12*(1):75–83, 1992.

185. Merchant, R. E., Merchant, L. H., and Cook, S. H. Intralesional infusion of lymphokine-activated killer (LAK) cells in recombinant interleukin-2

(rIL-2) for the treatment of patients with malignant brain tumor. Neurosurgery 23:725–732, 1988.

186. Merlo, A., Juretic, A., Zuber, M., et al. Cytokine gene expression in primary brain tumours, metastases and meningiomas suggests specific transcription patterns. Eur. J. Cancer 29A(15):2118–2125, 1993.

187. Miescher, S., Whiteside, T. L., Carrel, S., et al. Functional properties of tumor infiltrating and blood lymphocytes in patients with solid tumors: effects of tumor cells and their supernatants on proliferative responses of lymphocytes. J. Immunol. 136: 1899–1907, 1986.

188. Miescher, S., Whiteside, T. L., de Tribolet, N., et al. In situ characterization, clonogenic potential, and antitumor cytolytic activity of T lymphocytes infiltrating human brain cancers. J. Neurosurg. 68:438–448, 1988.

189. Minami, Y., Kono, T., Myazaki, T., et al. The IL-2 receptor complex: its structure, function, and target genes. Annu. Rev. Immunol. 11:245–267, 1993.

190. Miyatake, S., Kikuchi, H., Iwasaki, K., et al. Specific cytotoxic activity of T lymphocyte clones derived from a patient with gliosarcoma. J. Neurosurg. 69(5):751–759, 1988.

191. Mizoguchi, H., O'Shea, J. J., Longo, D. L., et al. Alterations in signal transduction molecules in T lymphocytes from tumor-bearing mice. Science 258: 1795–1797, 1992.

192. Mizuno, M., Yoshida, J., Takaoka, T., et al. Liposomal transfection of human γ-interferon gene into human glioma cells and adoptive immunotherapy using lymphokine-activated killer cells. J. Neurosurg. 80:510–514, 1994.

193. Monaco, J. J. A molecular model of MHC class-I-restricted antigen processing. Immunol. Today 13(5):173–178, 1992.

194. Morgan, D. A., Ruscetti, F. W., and Gallo, R.: Selective in vitro growth of T lymphocytes from normal human bone marrows. Science 193:1007–1010, 1976.

195. Morioka, T., Baba, T., Black, K. L., et al. Immunophenotypic analysis of infiltrating leukocytes and microglia in an experimental rat glioma. Acta Neuropathol. 83:590–597, 1992.

196. Mosmann, T. R. Properties and functions of interleukin-10. Adv. Immunol. 56:1–26, 1994.

197. Mullen, C. A., Coale, M., Levy, A. T., et al. Fibrosarcoma cells transduced with the IL-6 gene exhibit reduced tumorigenicity, increased immunogenicity and decreased metastatic potential. Cancer Res. 52: 6020–6024, 1992.

198. Murray, R. J., Kurilla, M. G., Brooks, J. M., et al. Identification of target antigens for the human cytotoxic T cell response to Epstein-Barr virus (EBV): implications for the immune control of EBV positive malignancies. J. Exp. Med. 176:157–168, 1992.

199. Nair, S., Babu, J. S., Dunham, R. G., et al. Induction of primary, antiviral cytotoxic and proliferative responses with antigen administered via dendritic cells. J. Virol. 67:4062–4069, 1993.

200. Nair, S., Zhou, F., Reddy, R., et al. Soluble proteins delivered to dendritic cells via pH-sensitive liposomes induce primary cytotoxic T lymphocyte responses in vitro. J. Exp. Med. 175:609–612, 1992.

201. Nakagomi, H., Petersson, M., Magnusson, I., et al. Decreased expression of the signal-transducing zeta chains in tumor-infiltrating T cells and NK cells of patients with colorectal carcinoma. Cancer Res. 53(23):5610–5612, 1993.

202. Neefjes, J. J., and Ploegh, H. L. Intracellular transport of MHC class II molecules. Immunol. Today 13(5): 179–184, 1992.

203. Nitta, T., Hishii, M., Sato, K., et al. Selective expression of interleukin-10 gene within glioblastoma multiforme. Brain Res. 649(1–2):122–128, 1994.

204. Nitta, T., Sato, K., Okumura, K., et al. Induction of cytotoxicity in human T cells coated with anti-glioma × anti-CD3 bispecific antibody against human glioma cells. J. Neurosurg. 72(3):476–481, 1990.

205. Nitta, T., Sato, K., Okumura, K., et al. An analysis of T-cell receptor variable region genes in tumor infiltrating lymphocytes within malignant tumors. Int. J. Cancer 49:545–550, 1991.

206. Nitta, T., Sato, K., Yagita, H., et al. Preliminary trail of specific targeting therapy against malignant glioma. Lancet 335:368–371, 1990.

207. Nolan, G. P., Ghosh, S., Liou, H. C., et al. DNA binding and IkB inhibition of the cloned p65 subunit of NF-kB, a rel-related peptide. Cell 64:961–969, 1991.

208. Paabo, S., Sverinsson, L., Andersson, M., et al. Adenovirus proteins and MHC expression. Adv. Cancer Res. 52:151–163, 1989.

209. Paglia, P., Girolomoni, G., Robbiati, F., et al. Immortalized dendritic cell line fully competent in antigen presentation initiates primary T cell responses in vivo. J. Exp. Med. 178:1893–1201, 1993.

210. Paine, J. T., Hajime, H., Yamasaki, J., et al. Immunohistochemical analysis of infiltrating lymphocytes in central nervous system tumors. Neurosurgery 18:766–772, 1986.

211. Pannetier, C., Cochet, M., Darche, S., et al. The sizes of the CDR3 hypervariable regions of the murine T-cell receptor β chains vary as a function of the recombined germ-line segments. Proc. Natl. Acad. Sci. U.S.A. 90(9):4319–4323, 1993.

212. Pannetier, C., Even, J., and Kourilsky, P. T cell repertoire diversity and clonal expansions in normal and clinical samples. Immunol. Today 16(4):176–180, 1995.

213. Pardoll, D. M. Tumour antigens: a new look for the 1990s. Nature 369:357–358, 1994.

214. Pardridge, W. M., Yang, J., Buciak, J., et al. Human brain microvascular DR-antigen. J. Neurosci. Res. 23(3):337–341, 1989.

215. Penninger, J. M., Wen, T., Timms, E., et al. Spontaneous resistance to acute T-cell leukemias in TCRVγ1.1Jγ4Cγ4 transgenic mice. Nature 375: 241–244, 1995.

216. Phillips, J. H., and Lanier, L. L. Dissection of the lymphokine-activated killer phenomenon: relative contribution of peripheral blood natural killer cells and lymphocytes to cytolysis. J. Exp. Med. 164: 814–825, 1986.

217. Phipps, R. P., Stein, S. H., and Roper, R. L. A new

view of prostaglandin E regulation of the immune response. Immunol. Today *12:*349–352, 1991.

218. Pignatelli, M., and Vessey, C. J. Adhesion molecules: novel molecular tools in tumor pathology. Hum. Pathol. *25(9):*849–856, 1994.

219. Porgador, A., Bannerji, R., Watanabe, Y., *et al.* Antimetastatic vaccination of tumor-bearing mice with two types of IFN-γ gene inserted tumor cells. J. Immunol. *150:*1458–1470, 1993.

220. Porgador, A., Tzehoval, E., Katz, A., *et al.* Interleukin-6 gene transfection into Lewis lung carcinoma tumor cells suppresses the malignant phenotype and confers immunotherapeutic competence against parental metastatic cells. Cancer Res. *52:*3679–3686, 1992.

221. Prehn, R. T., and Main, J. M. Immunity to methylcholanthrene-induced sarcomas. J. Natl. Cancer Inst. *18:*769–777, 1957.

222. Reener, C., Jung, W., Sahin, U., *et al.* Cure of xenografted human tumors by bispecific monoclonal antibodies and human T cells. Science *264:*833–835, 1994.

223. Reith, W., Siegrist, C. A., Durand, B., *et al.* Function of major histocompatibility complex class II promoters requires cooperative binding between factors RFX and NF-Y. Proc. Natl. Acad. Sci. U.S.A. *91:*554–558, 1994.

224. Resnicoff, M., Sell, C., Rubini, M., *et al.* Rat glioblastoma cells expressing an antisense RNA to the insulin-like growth factor-1 (IGF-1) receptor are nontumorigenic and induce regression of wild-type tumors. Cancer Res. *54:*2218–2222, 1994.

225. Restifo, N. P., Esquivel, F., Kawakami, Y., *et al.* Identification of human cancers deficient in antigen processing. J. Exp. Med. *177(2):*265–272, 1993.

226. Riddel, S. R., Watanabe, K. S., Goodrich, J. M., *et al.* Restoration of viral immunity in immunodeficient humans by the adoptive transfer of T cell clones. Science *257(5067):*238–241, 1992.

227. Romagnani, S. Regulatory role of IL-4 and other cytokines in the function and the development of human T-cell clones. Res. Immunol. *144:(8):*625–628, 1993.

228. Romagnani, S. Human TH1 and TH2 subset: <<eppur si muove>>. Eur. Cytokine Netw. *5:* 7–12, 1994.

229. Romani, N., Gruner, S., Brang, D., *et al.* Proliferating dendritic cell progenitors in human blood. J. Exp. Med. *180:*83–93, 1994.

230. Roman-Roman, S., Ferradini, L., Azocar, J., *et al.* Studies on the human T cell receptor alpha/beta variable region genes. I. Identification of 7 additional V alpha subfamilies and 14 J alpha gene segments. Eur. J. Immunol. *21:*927–933, 1991.

231. Rosenberg, S. A., Spiess, P., and Lafreniere, R. A. A new approach to the adoptive immunotherapy of cancer with tumor-infiltrating lymphocytes. Science *233:*1318–1321, 1986.

232. Rosenberg, S. A., Yang, J. C., Topalian, S. L., *et al.* Treatment of 283 consecutive patients with metastatic melanoma or renal cell carcinoma using highdose bolus interleukin-2. J.A.M.A. *271:*907–913, 1994.

233. Rossi, M. L., Hughes, J. T., Esiri, M. M., *et al.* Immunohistological study of mononuclear cell infiltrate in malignant glioma. Acta Neuropathol. *74:*269–277, 1987.

234. Roszman, T., Elliott, L., and Brooks, W. Modulation of T-cell function by gliomas. Immunol. Today *12(10):*370–374, 1991.

235. Roszman, T. L., Brooks, W. H., and Elliot, L. H. Immunobiology of primary intracranial tumors. VI. suppressor cell function and lectin-binding lymphocyte subpopulations in patients with cerebral tumors. Cancer *50:*1273–1279, 1982.

236. Rudensky, A. Y., Preston-Hurlburt, P., Hong, S. C., *et al.* Sequence analysis of peptides bound to MHC class II molecules. Nature *353:*622–627, 1991.

237. Ruiz-Cabello, F., Klein, E., and Garrido, F. MHC antigens on human tumors. Immunol. Lett. *29(3):* 181–189, 1991.

238. Sandberg, A. C., Engberg, C., Lake, M., *et al.* The expression of insulin-like growth factor I and insulin-like growth factor II genes in the human fetal and adult brain and in gliomas. Neurosci. Lett. *93:*114–119, 1988.

239. Saris, S. C., Spiess, P., and Lieberman. Treatment of murine primary brain tumors with systemic interleukin-2 and tumor-infiltrating lymphocytes. J. Neurosurg. *76:*513–519, 1992.

240. Savrou, D., Anzil, A. P., and Weidenbach, W. Immunofluorescence study of lymphocytic infiltration in gliomas: identification of T lymphocytes. J. Neurol. Sci. *33:*275–282, 1977.

241. Sawamura, Y., Diserens, A. C., and de Tribolet, N. In vitro prostaglandin E2 production by glioblastoma cells and its effect on interleukin-2 activation of oncolytic lymphocytes. J. Neurooncol. *9:*125–130, 1990.

242. Sawamura, Y., Hosokawa, M., Kuppner, M. C., *et al.* Antitumor activity and surface phenotypes of human glioma-infiltrating lymphocytes after in vitro expansion in the presence of interleukin-2. Cancer Res. *49:*1843–1849, 1989.

243. Schmidt, W., Schweighoffer, T., Herbst, E., *et al.* Cancer vaccines: the interleukin 2 dosage effect. Proc. Natl. Acad. Sci. U.S.A. *92:*4711–4714, 1995.

244. Schneider, J., Hofman, F. M., Apuzzo, M. L., *et al.* Cytokines and immunoregulatory molecules in malignant glial neoplasms. J. Neurosurg. *77:*265–273, 1992.

245. Shores, E. W., Huang, K., Tran, T., *et al.* Role of TCR S chain in T cell development and selection. Science *266:*1047–1050, 1994.

246. Skipper, J., and Stauss, H. J. Identification of two cytotoxic T lymphocyte-recognized epitopes in the Ras protein. J. Exp. Med. *177:*1493–1498, 1993.

247. Sloan-Lancaster, J., Evavold, B. D., and Allen, P. M. Induction of T-cell anergy by altered T-cell-receptor ligand on live antigen-presenting cells. Nature *363:*156–159, 1993.

248. Sloan-Lancaster, J., Shaw, A. S., Rothbard, J. B., *et al.* Partial T cell signaling: altered phospho-S and lack of Zap70 recruitment in APL-induced T cell anergy. Cell *79:*913–922, 1994.

249. Steimle, V., Otten, L. A., Zufferey, M., *et al.* Complementation cloning of an MHC class II transactivator mutated in hereditary MHC class II deficiency (or

bare lymphocyte syndrome). Cell *75:*135–146, 1993.

250. Steimle, V., Siegrist, C. A., Mottet, A., *et al.* Regulation of MHC class II expression by interferon-gamma mediated by the transactivator gene CIITA. Science *265:*106–109, 1994.

251. Straus, D. B., and Weiss, A. Genetic evidence for the involvement of the Ick tyrosine kinase in signal transduction through the T cell antigen receptor. Cell *70:*585–593, 1992.

252. Strominger, J. L. The gamma/delta T cell receptor and class 1b MHC-related proteins: enigmatic molecules of immune recognition. Cell *57:*895–898, 1989.

253. Stuber, G., Leder, G. H., Storkus, W. J., *et al.* Identification of wild type and mutant p53 peptides binding to HLA-A2 assessed by a peptide loading-deficient cell line assay and a novel major histocompatibility complex class I peptide binding assay. Eur. J. Immunol. *24:*765–768, 1994.

254. Suh, W. K., Cohen-Doyle, M. F., Fruh, K., *et al.* Interaction of MHC class I molecules with the transporter associated with antigen processing. Science *264:*1322–1325, 1994.

255. Tada, M., Diserens, A. C., Desbaillet, I., *et al.* Analysis of cytokine receptor messenger RNA expression in human glioblastoma cells and normal astrocytes by reverse-transcription polymerase chain reaction. J. Neurosurg. *80:*1063–1073, 1994.

256. Tada, M., Diserens, A. C., Desbaillet, I., *et al.* Production of interleukin-1 receptor antagonist by human glioblastoma cells in vitro and in vivo. J. Neuroimmunol. *50:*187–194, 1994.

257. Tahara, H., Zeh, H. J., Storkus, W. J., *et al.* Fibroblasts genetically engineered to secrete interleukin 12 can suppress tumor growth and induce antitumor immunity to a murine melanoma in vivo. Cancer Res. *54:*182–189, 1994.

258. Takahashi, H., Nakagawa, Y., Yokomuro, K., *et al.* Induction of CD8+ cytotoxic T lymphocytes by immunization with syngeneic irradiated HIV-1 envelope derived peptide-pulsed dendritic cells. Int. Immunol. *5:*849–857, 1993.

259. Taniguchi, T., and Yasuhiro, M. The IL-2/IL-2 receptor system: a current overview. Cell *73:*5–8, 1993.

260. Tepper, R. I. The anti-tumor and pro-inflammatory actions of IL-4. Res. Immunol. *144*(8):633–637, 1993.

261. Tepper, R. I., Coffmann, R. L., and Leder, P. An eosinophil-dependent mechanism for the antitumor effect of IL-4. Science *257:*548–551, 1992.

262. Tepper, R. I., and Mule, J. J. Experimental and clinical studies of cytokine gene-modified tumor cells. Hum. Gene Ther. *5:*153–164, 1994.

263. Tepper, R. I., Pattengale, P. K., and Leder, P. Murine interleukin-4 displays potent antitumor activity in vivo. Cell *57:*503–512, 1989.

264. Topalian, S. L., Muul, L. M., Solomon, D., *et al.* Expansion of human tumor infiltrating lymphocytes for use in immunotherapy trials. J. Immunol. Meth. *102:*127–141, 1987.

265. Torre-Amione, G., Beauchamp, R. D., Koeppen, H., *et al.* A highly immunogenic tumor transfected with a murine transforming growth factor β1 cDNA escapes immune surveillance. Proc. Natl. Acad. Sci. U.S.A. *87:*1486–1490, 1990.

266. Townsend, S., and Allison, J. Tumor rejection after direct costimulation of CD8+ T cells by B7-transfected melanoma cells. Science *259:*368–370, 1993.

267. Traversari, C., Van der Bruggen, P., Luescher, I. F., *et al.* A nonapeptide encoded by human gene MAGE-1 is recognized on HLA-A1 by CTL directed against tumor antigen MZ2-E. J. Exp. Med. *176:*1453–1457, 1992.

268. Travis, J. Do tumor-altered T cells depress immune responses? Cancer Res. *258:*1732–1733, 1992.

269. Trojan, J., Blossey, B. K., Jonson, T. R., *et al.* Loss of tumorigenicity of rat glioblastoma directed by episome-based antisense cDNA transcription of insulin-like growth factor 1. Proc. Natl. Acad. Sci. U.S.A. *89:*4874–4878, 1992.

270. Trojan, J., Johnson, T. R., Rudin, S. D., *et al.* Treatment and prevention of rat glioblastoma by immunogenic C6 cells expressing antisense insulin-like growth factor I RNA. Science *259:*94–96, 1993.

271. Van der Bruggen, P., Bastin, J., Gajewski, T., *et al.* A peptide encoded by human gene MAGE-3 and presented by HLA-A2 induces cytolytic T lymphocytes that recognize tumor cells expressing MAGE-3. Eur. J. Immunol. *24:*3038–3043, 1994.

272. Van der Bruggen, P., Traversari, C., Van der Eynde, B., *et al.* A gene encoding an antigen recognized by cytoltyic T lymphocytes on a human melanoma. Science *254:*1643–1647, 1991.

273. Van Duk, J., Zegveld, S. T., Fleuren, G. J., *et al.* Localization of monoclonal antibody G250 and bispecific monoclonal antibody CD3/G250 in human renal-cell carcinoma xenografts: relative effects of size and affinity. Int. J. Cancer *48:*738–743, 1991.

274. Van Meir, E. Cytokines and tumors of the central nervous system. Glia in press, 1995.

275. Wade, W. F., Davoust, J., Salamero, J., *et al.* Structural compartmentalization of MHC class II signaling function. Immunol. Today *14*(11):539–546, 1993.

276. Watanabe, Y., Kuribayashi, K., Miyatake, S., *et al.* Exogenous expression of mouse interferon γ cDNA in mouse neuroblastoma C1300 cells results in reduced tumorigenicity by augmented anti-tumor immunity. Proc. Natl. Acad. Sci. U.S.A. *86:*9456–9460, 1989.

277. Weber, F., Meinl, E., Aloisi, F., *et al.* Human astrocytes are only partially competent antigen presenting cells: possible implications for lesion development in multiple sclerosis. Brain *117:*59–69, 1994.

278. Wei, S., Charmley, P., Robinson, M. A., *et al.* The extent of the human germline T cell receptor V beta gene segment repertoire. Immunogenetics *40:*27–36, 1994.

279. Weiss, A., Koretzky, G., Schatzman, R., *et al.* Functional activation of the T-cell antigen receptor induces tyrosine phosphorylation of phospholipase C-γ1. Proc. Natl. Acad. Sci. U.S.A. *88:*5484–5488, 1991.

280. Weiss, A., and Littman, D. R. Signal transduction by lymphocyte antigen receptors. Cell *76:*263–274, 1994.

281. Williams, K., Bar-Or, A., Ulverstad, E., *et al.* Biology of adult human microglia in culture: comparisons with peripheral blood monocytes and astrocytes. J. Neuropathol. Exp. Neurol. *51:*538–549, 1992.

282. Wong, A. J., Zoltick, P. W., and Moscatello, D. K. The molecular biology and molecular genetics of astrocytic neoplasm. Semin. Oncol. *21*(2):139–148, 1994.

283. Wood, G. W., and Morantz, R. A. In vitro reversal of depressed T-lymphocyte function in the peripheral blood of brain tumor patients. J. Natl. Cancer Inst. *68:*27–33, 1982.

284. Wu, Y., Guo, Y., and Liu, Y. A major costimulatory molecule on antigen-presenting cells, CTLA4 ligand A, is distinct from B7. J. Exp. Med. *178:* 1789–1793, 1993.

285. Wucherpfennig, K. W. Autoimmunity in the central nervous system: mechanisms of antigen presentation and recognition. Clin. Immunol. Immunopathol. *72*(3):293–306, 1994.

286. Yamada, M., Kakimoto, K., Shinbori, T., *et al.* Accessory function of human glioma cells for the induction of CD3-mediated T cell proliferation: a potential role of glial cells in T cell activation in the central nervous system. J. Neuroimmunol. *38:*263–273, 1992.

287. Yanuck, M., Carbone, D. P., Pendleton, C. C., *et al.* A mutant p53 tumor suppressor protein is a target for peptide-induced CD8+ cytotoxic T-cells. Cancer Res. *53:*3257–3261, 1993.

288. Young, H. F., Sakalas, R., and Kaplan, A. M. Inhibition of cell mediated immunity in patients with brain tumors. Surg. Neurol. *5*(1):19–23, 1976.

289. Yu, J. S., Wei, M. X., Chiocca, E. A., *et al.* Treatment of glioma by engineered interleukin 4-secreting cells. Cancer Res. *53:*3125–3128, 1993.

290. Zuber, P., Kuppner, M. C., and de Tribolet, N. Transforming growth factor-β2 down-regulates HLA-DR antigen expression on human malignant glioma cells. Eur. J. Immunol. *18:*1623–1626, 1988.

CHAPTER 14

Gene Transfer Technology and Its Application to Brain Tumor Therapy

E. ANTONIO CHIOCCA, M.D., Ph.D., GRIFFITH R. HARSH IV, M.D.

INTRODUCTION

The genetics and biology of vectors currently available for gene therapy were discussed in Chapter 3. In this chapter, current applications of gene therapy to animal models of brain tumors and their translation into human clinical trials will be reviewed. The use of any novel approach with curative intent must have strong scientific and clinical justification. Current treatments for gliomas, the most common type of primary brain tumors, include surgery, radiation therapy delivered focally or regionally, and chemotherapy. Failures in therapy of gliomas result from tumor recurrence, either locally or at a distance, or from treatment-related toxicity.

Possible reasons for tumor recurrence include failure to extirpate all tumor cells within the main tumor mass and failure to eradicate tumor cells that have migrated away from the main tumor mass; a new or different grade of tumor may develop from glial cells in the region of a previously treated tumor or from progression of a relatively benign tumor to one of more malignant histology (possibly as a consequence of spontaneous, radiation- or drug-induced mutations in proto-oncogenes or tumor suppressor genes).

Toxicity to normal neural tissue results from the lack of anatomical selectivity of surgery and radiosurgery for tumors and the narrow therapeutic indices of radiotherapy and chemotherapy. This toxicity precludes the more aggressive use of current brain tumor therapies needed to eradicate all tumor cells.

Gene transfer technology has the potential to avoid the narrow therapeutic indices that limit other therapies by achieving tumor-specific expression of anticancer genes (33, 34, 42, 68). Although gene therapy possesses tremendous potential, and this potential has prompted intense investigation, meaningful translation of gene therapy into the clinic has not yet been achieved. This chapter will review recent experimental results from a variety of gene therapy strategies for gliomas, discuss current efforts to move promising modalities into the clinic, and suggest future directions for this nascent field.

THERAPEUTIC GENES

Several types of genes have been shown to control tumor growth in animal models of brain tumors (Table 1). The experimental strategy consists of inoculating the tumor with a replication-deficient or replication-compromised virus (the "vector") bearing the therapeutic gene (3, 37, 58). One of the limitations of this strategy is that the gene is not expressed in all of the tumor cells; the antitumor effect of the therapeutic gene thus must extend to nontransduced, as well as transduced, neoplastic cells (10). Furthermore, with currently available promoter and enhancer elements, gene expression is usually transient (days to weeks); therapeutic genes encoding products that are cytotoxic rather than cytostatic are thus preferred.

Prodrug-activating Genes

Expression of a gene whose product activates a prodrug into a cytotoxic metabolite within tumor cells should improve the metabolite's therapeutic index. Higher levels of active drug should be achieved within the tumor with less toxicity to normal tissue. Two general strategies have been pursued: 1) transfer and expression of a gene encoding a prodrug-activating capability that is not normally present within mammalian cells. Examples effective against experimental brain tumors include the *Escherichia coli guanine phosphoribosyl transferase* (gpt) gene that activates 6-thioxanthine (44, 62), the *E. coli* cytosine deaminase gene, which activates 5-fluorocytosine (26), and the herpes simplex thymidine kinase (HSV-TK) gene that activates ganciclovir (42, 43); and 2) supplementing the action of an active mammalian prodrug-activating enzyme by transfer and expression of a gene encoding a different enzyme with similar activating capability. Examples effective against experimental brain tumors include the rat CYP2B1 gene responsible for activating cyclophosphamide/ifosfamide (7, 8, 69, 70) and the *E. coli* gpt gene that activates 6-thioguanine (62). The *E. coli* gpt gene can both activate a prodrug not normally active in mammalian cells (6-thioxanthine) and supplement the action of a mammalian enzyme (HGPRT) in activating the prodrug, 6-thioguanine. Although this list is relatively short, numerous other enzyme-prodrug

TABLE 1
Therapeutic Transgenes for Brain Tumors

Prodrug-activating enzyme genes
    Genes providing a new activating capability
        E. coli gpt activating 6-thioxanthine
        E. coli cytosine deaminase activating 5-fluorocytosine
        HSV thymidine kinase activating ganciclovir and BvUDR
    Genes supplementing a pre-existent capability
        E. coli gpt activating 6-thioguanine
        Rat CYP2B1 activating cyclophosphamide and ifosfamide
Immune-enhancing genes
    Cytokines expressed within tumors
        IL-2, IL-4, γ-IFN, GM-CSF
    Antisense for cytokines
        TGF-β1, IGF-1
    Cytokines expressed in tumor cell vaccines
        GM-CSF
    Dominant mutants of angiogenesis genes
        Angiogenic factors and their receptors (bFGF, VEGF, TGFα, TGFβ, PF4)
Tumor suppressor and apoptosis genes
    p53, ICE

---

combinations have been proposed and await testing in brain tumor models (12).

The thymidine kinase (TK)/ganciclovir (GCV) gene therapy paradigm (42) has been studied in multiple animal models of brain tumor using genetically engineered cells (20, 60), retroviral vectors (13, 27, 52, 61), adenoviral vectors (9), and herpes simplex virus vectors (4, 37) to deliver the TK gene. The HSV-TK enzyme phosphorylates ganciclovir, as well as ganciclovir analogs (such as BvUDR), which are used as nucleotides in DNA synthesis. During subsequent DNA replication, these "false" nucleotides induce premature termination of DNA synthesis and, ultimately, cell death (18).

A variation of this approach combines gene transfer with radiotherapy. The incorporated "false" nucleotide, particularly that produced by TK from BvUDR, can sensitize DNA to radiation (32). Use of a radiation-inducible promoter provides a "switch" that will turn on TK gene expression when the cell is irradiated. The TK enzyme activates BvUDR, which, when incorporated, enhances the radiosensitivity of the tumor cell's DNA (32).

Selective killing of tumor cells by such approaches results from the vector, the activated drug, or both vector and drug targeting dividing cells while sparing neurons and other postmitotic or slowly dividing cells in the brain. Retrovirus and some of the herpes simplex virus vectors mediate transgene expression exclusively in dividing cells (3, 37), whereas adenovirus vectors do so in both mitotic and postmitotic cells (3, 5, 47). Prodrugs that act selectively on dividing cells include ganciclovir, 6-thioxanthine, 6-thioguanine, and 5-fluorocytosine. However, all but ganciclovir also affect RNA synthesis and thus might be toxic to quiescent, as well as dividing cells. Cyclophosphamide and ifosfamide produce covalent intrastrand and interstrand crosslinks in DNA, regardless of the phase of the cell cycle (11); deleterious effects are manifest primarily during subsequent cell division. The transient nature of gene expression is usually not limiting, inasmuch as the prodrug is administered within 14 days of vector transduction. Nevertheless, long-term expression of an anticancer gene within a tumor is desirable as it might permit tumor cell killing if the neoplasm recurs.

Diffusion of a chemotherapeutic metabolite from the site of prodrug activation should compensate for the failure to achieve expression of the transgene in all tumor cells. For instance, conversion of ganciclovir to its phosphorylated derivatives has been associated with a bystander effect in which the activated ganciclovir kills neighboring tumor cells, even if they do not express the TK gene (13, 42). In cell cultures, this killing of cells not expressing the transgene has been shown to depend on the formation of gap junctions between cells which permit diffusion of phosphorylated ganciclovir from cell to cell (19, 22, 35, 39). However, other hypotheses regarding the basis of the bystander effect *in vivo* have been proposed: 1) transduction of and injury to tumor endothelial cells (53); 2) endocytosis of apoptotic tumor vesicles (23); and 3) immune recognition of the tumor cell expressing a foreign transgene (1, 63). A possible immune mechanism involves MHC1-presentation of the foreign antigen (lacZ or TK) and induction of a cytotoxic T-cell response against it and other tumor-specific antigens. A T-cell response directed against tumor-specific antigens other than the antigen encoded by the transgene could kill adjacent tumor cells even if they do not express the transgene antigen. In addition, a cytotoxic T-cell response generates cytokines and toxic substances that might injure adjacent tumor cells. Although each of these hypothetical mechanisms may contribute to the bystander effect, verification and quantification of the importance of each have not been achieved experimentally.

Immune-enhancing Genes

The rapid progress in molecular immunology has identified cytokines, receptors, and cofactors contributing to the rejection of neoplasms and has dissected the molecular events responsible for the immune response against tumor cells. Expression of a number of different cytokines in brain tumors has been achieved either by grafting genetically engineered cells into tumors or by transducing tumor cells *in vivo* with retroviral and adenoviral vectors. Cytokines thus expressed in tumor cells include interleukin-2 (64), interleukin-4 (68, 70–72), granulocyte macrophage-colony stimulating factor (GM-CSF) (14, 73), γ-interferon (64), and antisense transforming growth factor-β1 (TGF-β1) (21). Many other molecules that exert antitumor effects are potential candidates for gene therapy of brain tumor models. These include interleukin-1, interleukin-3, interleukin-6, interleukin-7, interleukin-12, tumor necrosis factor-α, JE, IP-10, foreign major histocompatibility complex proteins, and B7 (15). Laboratory evaluation of various vector-gene combinations is clearly warranted.

A related immunological approach attempts vaccination against brain tumor formation. Tumor cells are genetically altered in culture with vectors that encode a cytokine, lethally irradiated, and then implanted subcutaneously in animals. The ability of the immune response evoked to protect against a subsequent challenge of tumor cells is then evaluated. As discussed by Dranoff *et al.* (14), a potential problem with experiments evaluating this strategy has been the use of tumor cell lines that are inherently immunogenic by virtue of repeated passage in tissue culture. In one study, nonimmunogenic tumor cells transduced by a retrovirus vector carrying the GM-CSF gene were used to vaccinate rats. The vaccination protected the animals from subsequent intracerebral tumor challenges but produced minimal effects against established intracerebral tumors (73). Such vaccination might best be used to protect against tumor recurrence.

In another study, expression of antisense insulin-like growth factor-I (IGF-1) induced regression of intracerebral rat C6 glioma tumors in the BDX strain of rats (65). This regression was mediated by cytotoxic T cells. Protective immunity against further C6 tumor challenges was also induced. However, the cell line employed for these studies was originally derived from an outbred rat strain (2), and differences in minor antigens between BDX rats and the tumor cells could possibly influence this immune response.

The selectivity of an immune response results from recognition of tumor-specific antigens by cytotoxic T lymphocytes and the local production of cytokines and toxic metabolites. It is unknown whether cytotoxic T cell-mediated killing of tumor cells that express the transgene produces bystander toxicity to nonexpressing tumor cells. For instance, when interleukin-4 is generated intratumorally either by cell lines (72) or by retrovirus vectors (70), eosinophils infiltrate the tumor mass to attack tumor cells even if they are not expressing interleukin-4.

Angiogenesis Genes

The process of tumor neovascularization offers another target for gene therapy. The recent molecular characterization of receptors and ligands that stimulate and modulate the ingrowth of blood vessels into tumors has prompted attempts to disrupt these processes. Angiogenic factors and their corresponding receptors that may contribute to tumor growth include basic fibroblast growth factor (FGF) and its receptor, vascular endothelial growth factor (VEGF) and its receptors (VEGF-R1 or flk-1 and VEGF-R2 or flk-2), TGF-α and the epidermal growth factor (EGF) receptors, TGF-β and its receptor, and human platelet factor 4 (PF4) and its receptor (36).

At least three reports have provided evidence that genetic methods can be used to disrupt angiogenesis in brain tumors. When a dominant mutant of the flk (VEGF-R2) receptor was introduced by a retroviral vector into C6 glioma cells in a nude mouse, tumor involution was observed (40). Using a different strategy, Saleh et al. (56) selected C6 glioma cells stably transfected with an antisense VEGF cDNA. These cells produced much less VEGF and in nude mice were much less tumorigenic than were parenteral cells because blood vessel formation was inhibited. In another study, expression of antisense bFGF cDNA correlated with reduced proliferation of C6 cells in culture. Because *in vivo* experiments were not performed, the vascularity of the tumors from parental C6 cells was not compared with that of tumors from C6 cells expressing antisense bFGF (54). Taken in conjunction, these experiments show that gene therapy strategies using either antisense or dominant negative mutants can inhibit tumor growth. So far, the VEGF/flk receptor pair has been most effectively targeted.

The selectivity of antiangiogenesis strategies for tumors arises from at least two sources: 1) the molecules targeted (such as VEGF/flk receptor) are common in blood vessels within brain tumors but not in those of normal brain (57); and 2) inhibition of angiogenesis primarily affects rapidly dividing cells (such as tumor cells) that require plentiful nutrients and thus abundant vascularity. It is unclear whether the inability to deliver antiangiogenesis genes to all tumor cells or all tumor endothelial cells will significantly compromise antiangiogenesis gene

therapy because the experiments described above were performed on stably transfected cell lines rather than on tumors *in vivo*. Perhaps intra-arterial injection of adenovirus or herpes virus vectors bearing antiangiogenesis genes will provide an effective *in vivo* method of delivery (46). It is also unclear whether blocking a particular angiogenic pathway (for instance, VEGF/flk) will select for angiogenesis and growth of tumors that are dependent on another pathway (for example, bFGF/FGFR). Nevertheless, disruption of angiogenesis remains a potentially promising therapeutic approach.

Tumor Suppressor and Apoptosis Genes

Because tumorigenesis appears to involve defects in genes that control progression through the cell cycle and DNA repair (30), strategies to replace these defective genes are being developed. The most impressive results thus far have been achieved with adenovirus vectors injected into established tumors at a relatively high ratio of vector to tumor cell. Because this approach has not been studied extensively in experimental brain tumors, results of studies using other tumor models will be reviewed.

Replacement of defective p53 genes has been described in several tumor models, including medulloblastoma, lung cancer, head and neck squamous cell carcinoma, and prostate cancer. Recent work has shown that p53 is involved in both the induction of the arrest at cell-cycle checkpoints (primarily G1/S) that permits repair of DNA damage and in the promotion of apoptosis of cells that are not able to achieve such repair. p53 works through multiple mechanisms: 1) transcriptional induction of p21, an inhibitor of cyclin-dependent kinase (CDK), needed for cell-cycle progression (16, 17, 30); 2) transcriptional induction of Gadd45 (59) and regulatory interactions with ERCC3 and other factors involved in repair of DNA damage and nucleotide excision (59, 66, 67); and 3) induction of apoptosis when DNA repair cannot be accomplished (30). A defective p53 gene allows cells to proceed through the cell cycle and to propagate replicative errors in cellular DNA. In the overwhelming majority of cases, these errors are fatal to the cell, but sometimes these errors lead to uncontrolled cell proliferation and tumorigenesis. In such tumors, replacement of the defective p53 gene should correct the molecular defect underlying tumor development.

Two studies have attempted to replace the p53 gene in experimental brain tumor cells in culture. In the first, an HSV amplicon was used to deliver a wild-type p53 gene into DAOY cells, a medulloblastoma line bearing a mutant p53 gene (55). Findings suggestive of correction of the genetic defect included increased expression of a gene regulated by p53 and loss of immunocytochemical staining for cyclin E, a protein that accumulates when the parenteral DAOY cells fail to arrest at G1/S. In the second, an adenoviral vector was used to deliver a wild-type p53 gene into six glioblastoma cell lines which either expressed a wild-type ($n = 3$) or a mutant ($n = 3$) p53 gene (24). Different effects were observed after gene transfer: the growth of wild-type p53 cell was inhibited; cells with the mutant p53 underwent apoptotic death. Although both of these strategies appear promising in cell culture, their effects *in vivo* have not been confirmed.

Although transfer of other transgenes involved in DNA repair and control of the cell cycle of brain tumor cells has not been reported, transfer of a gene linked to apoptosis has been shown to cause regression of experimental brain tumors (75). As in the p53 gene-transfer experiments, the ability to transfer these genes into all tumor cells has not been demonstrated.

CLINICAL TRIALS

Phase I/II trials of gene therapy of human brain tumors have been conducted at several institutions in the United States, including the National Institutes of Health. These trials, sponsored by Genetic Therapy Inc. (Gaithersburg, MD), employed cell lines that produce a retrovirus containing the TK gene which confers chemosensitivity to ganciclovir. Institutions in other countries (France, Germany, and Canada) are also actively pursuing the TK-ganciclovir strategy. Three surgical protocols have been used: 1) stereotactic injection of producer cells at multiple sites within a glioblastoma, 2) injection of producer cells through an Ommaya reservoir into a resection cavity, and 3) free-hand injections of producer cells within a tumor bed at the time of surgical resection. Patients with recurrent glioblastomas that had failed other treatments were eligible for these trials. Prelim-

inary results have been presented at scientific meetings, but no published reports of the outcomes of these studies have appeared. One abstract reported that transgene expression was identified in only 0.17% of tumor cells (51). Adverse effects included intracerebral hemorrhages in 2 of 19 patients. A multi-institutional phase III study has been initiated to evaluate therapeutic efficacy.

At Massachusetts General Hospital, a phase I/II trial is under way using retrovirus producer cells provided by Somatix Therapy Corporation (Alameda, CA). This trial was designed to study the safety and mechanism of the antitumor effect of the TK ganciclovir paradigm in humans. A dose escalation scheme is used to determine the maximally tolerated dose of vector-producing cells. At the time of biopsy of a recurrent malignant glioma, vector-producing cells are injected into the tumor mass. Seven days later the tumor is resected *en bloc*, and TK gene transfer is evaluated by immunocytochemistry (49). The anatomical extent of TK gene transfer within human tumor is measured using an antibody raised against TK. In a second group of patients, tumor cell killing is evaluated by injecting vector-producing cells and then 7 days later administering ganciclovir for 14 days. An *en bloc* resection of tumor is then performed, and the extent of tumor cell killing is measured. Finally, a more extensive therapeutic trial will be performed in which stereotactic administration of producer cells at multiple sites within and about the tumor in a dose-escalation scheme is followed by ganciclovir treatment. This clinical design will permit measurement of *in vivo* gene transfer in humans and correlation of the extent of gene expression with therapeutic effects.

CONCLUSIONS

The field of gene transfer is in its infancy. Because questions related to extent of gene delivery, amount of prodrug conversion *in situ*, and effects on the immune response can only be answered in the context of human clinical trials, phase I and II studies exploring safety and mechanism are warranted. However, claims regarding the curative potential of this novel therapy are premature, and phase III trials require further justification. Problems that remain to be addressed before gene transfer can be used as an effective anticancer treatment, as well as potential solutions, are as follows:

1. Inefficient delivery of vector and prodrug. The interaction between molecular engineering and molecular biology might help address this problem (28). For instance, pharmacological disruption of the blood-tumor barrier may increase the distribution of the vector (50). Convection induced by prolonged infusion and implantation of polymers containing prodrug may be of value (6).
2. Inefficient gene transduction within tumor cells. More efficient gene transfer vectors, regulatable cell-specific enhancer and promoter elements, and agents to enhance vector uptake and transgene localization to the nucleus hold promise (48).
3. Inefficient prodrug conversion. The engineering of "super" enzymes that can convert prodrugs more efficiently or the use of multiple prodrug-converting enzymes might circumvent this limitation.
4. Development of tumor cell resistance. Use of multiple gene therapies in combination might solve this problem. Alternative approaches involve the use of antisense RNA or ribozyme molecules designed to block production of the factors involved in tumor cell resistance.

As the molecular genetic basis of neurological diseases are elucidated, opportunities for treating these diseases with gene transfer therapy will increasingly become available. Neurosurgeons should provide the scientific and clinical leadership in translating gene transfer technology into clinical neurogenetic surgery.

REFERENCES

1. Barba, D., Hardin, J., Sadelain, M., *et al.* Development of anti-tumor immunity following thymidine kinase-mediated killing of experimental brain tumors. Proc. Natl. Acad. Sci. U.S.A. *91:*4348–4352, 1994.
2. Benda, P., Someda, K., Messer, J., *et al.* Morphological and immunochemical studies of rat glial tumors and clonal strains propagated in culture. J. Neurosurg. *34:*310–323, 1971.
3. Boviatsis, E. J., Chase, M., Wei, M. X., *et al.* Gene transfer into experimental brain tumors mediated by adenovirus, herpes simplex virus (HSV), and retrovirus vectors. Hum. Gene Ther. *5:*183–191, 1994.
4. Boviatsis, E. J., Park, J. S., Sena-Esteves, M., *et al.* Long-term survival of rats harboring brain tumors treated with ganciclovir and a herpes simplex virus vector that maintains an intact thymidine kinase gene. Cancer Res. *54:*5745–5751, 1994.
5. Boviatsis, E. J., Scharf, J. M., Chase, M., *et al.* Antitumor activity and reporter gene transfer into rat brain neoplasms inculated with herpes simplex virus vectors defective in thymidine kinase or ribonucleotide reductase. Gene Ther. *1:*323–331, 1994.
6. Brem, H., Mahaley, M. S., Jr., Vick, N. A., *et al.* Interstitial chemotherapy with drug polymer implants for the treatment of recurrent gliomas. J. Neurosurg. *74:*441–446, 1991.
7. Chen, L., and Waxman, D. J. Intratumoral activation and enhanced chemotherapeutic effect of oxazaphosphorines following cytochrome P450 gene transfer: development of a combined chemotherapy/cancer gene therapy strategy. Cancer Res. *55:*581–589, 1995.
8. Chen, L., Waxman, D. J., Chen, D., *et al.* Sensitization of human breast cancer cells to cyclophosphamide and ifosfamide by transfer of a liver cytochrome P450 gene. Cancer Res. *56:*1331–1340, 1996.
9. Chen, S. H., Shine, H. D., Goodman, J. C., *et al.* Gene therapy for brain tumors: regression of experimental gliomas by using adenovirus-mediated gene transfer in vivo. Proc. Natl. Acad. Sci. U.S.A. *91:*3054–3057, 1994.
10. Chiocca, E. A., Andersen, J. K., Takamiya, Y., *et al.* Virus-mediated genetic treatment, of rodent gliomas. In: *Gene Therapeutics*, edited by J. A. Wolff, pp. 245–262 Birkhauser Publishers, Boston, 1994.
11. Colvin, O. M. Alkylating agents and platinum compounds. In: *Cancer Medicine*, edited by J. F. Holland et al., pp. 733–734. Lea & Febiger, Philadelphia, 1993.
12. Connors, T. A. The choice of prodrugs for gene directed enzyme prodrug therapy of cancer. Gene Ther. *2:*702–709, 1995.
13. Culver, K. W., Ram, Z., Wallbridge, S., *et al.* In vivo gene transfer with retroviral vector-producer cells for treatment of experimental brain tumors. Science *256:*1550–1552, 1992.
14. Dranoff, G., Jaffee, E., Lazenby, A., *et al.* Vaccination with irradiated tumor cells engineered to secrete murine granulocyte-macrophage colony-stimulating factor stimulates potent, specific, and long-lasting anti-tumor immunity. Proc. Natl. Acad. Sci. U.S.A. *90:*3539–3543, 1993.
15. Dranoff, G., and Mulligan, R. C. Gene transfer as cancer therapy. Adv. Immunol. *58:*417–454, 1995.
16. Dulic, V., Kaufmann, W. K., Wilson, S. J., *et al.* p53-dependent inhibition of cyclin-dependent kinase activities in human fibroblasts during radiation-induced G1 arrest. Cell *76:*1013–1023, 1994.
17. El-Deiry, W. S., Harper, J. W., O'Connor, P. M., *et al.* WAF1/CIP1 is induced in p53-mediated G1 arrest and apoptosis. Cancer Res. *54:*1169–1174, 1994.
18. Elion, G. B. The biochemistry and mechanism of action of acyclovir. J. Antimicrob. Chemother. *12*(suppl. B):9–17, 1983.
19. Elshami, A. A., Saavedra, A., Zhang, H., *et al.* Gap junctions play a role in the bystander effect of the herpes simplex virus thymidine kinase/ganciclovir system in vitro. Gene Ther. *3:*85–92, 1996.
20. Ezzeddine, Z. D., Martuza, R. L., Platika, D., *et al.*

Selective killing of glioma cells in culture and in vivo by retrovirus transfer of the herpes simplex virus thymidine kinase gene. New Biol. *3:*608–614, 1991.

21. Fakhrai, H., Dorigo, O., Shawler, D. L., *et al.* Eradication of established intracranial rat gliomas by transforming growth factor beta antisense gene therapy. Proc. Natl. Acad. Sci. U.S.A. *93:*2909–2914, 1996.

22. Fick, J., Barker, F. G., Dazin, P., *et al.* The extent of heterocellular communication mediated by gap junctions is predictive of bystander tumor cytotoxicity *in vitro.* Proc. Natl. Acad. Sci. U.S.A. *92:* 11071–11075, 1995.

23. Freeman, S. M., Abboud, C. N., Whartenby, K. A., *et al.* The "bystander effect": tumor regression when a fraction of the tumor mass is genetically modified. Cancer Res. *53:*5247–5283, 1993.

24. Gomez-Manzano, C., Fueyo, J., Kyritsis, A. P., *et al.* Adenovirus-mediated transfer of the p53 gene produces rapid and generalized death of human glioma cells via apoptosis. Cancer Res. *56:*694–699, 1996.

25. Hartwell, L. H., and Kastan, M. B. Cell cycle control and cancer. Science *266:*1821–1828, 1994.

26. Huber, B. E., Austin, E. A., Goode, S. S., *et al.* In vivo antitumor activity of 5-fluorocytosine on human colorectal carcinoma cells genetically modified to express cytosine deaminase. Cancer Res. *53:*4619, 1993.

27. Huber, B. E., Richards, C. A., and Krenitsky, T. A. Retroviral-mediated gene therapy for the treatment of hepatocellular carcinoma: an innovative approach for cancer therapy. Proc. Natl. Acad. Sci. U.S.A. *88:*8039–8043, 1991.

28. Jain, R. Delivery of molecular medicine to solid tumors. Science *271:*1079–1080, 1996.

29. Kashani-Sabet, M., and Scanlon, K. J. Application of ribozymes to cancer gene therapy. In: *The Internet Book of Gene Therapy: Cancer Therapeutics,* edited by R. E. Sobol, K. J. Scanlon, pp. 91–102. Appleton & Lange, Stamford, CT, 1995.

30. Kastan, M. B., Onyekwere, O., Sidranski, D., *et al.* Participation of p53 protein in the cellular response to DNA damage. Cancer Res. *51:*6304–6311, 1991.

31. Kastan, M. B., Zhan, Q., El-Deiry, W. S., *et al.* A mammalian cell cycle checkpoint pathway utilizing p53 and GADD45 is defective in ataxia-telangiectasia. Cell *71:*587–597, 1992.

32. Kim, K. J., Kim, S. H., Brown, S. L., *et al.* Selective enhancement by an antiviral agent of the radiation-induced cell killing of human glioma cells transduced with HSV-tk gene. Cancer Res. *54:*6053–6056, 1994.

33. Kramm, C., Breakefield, X. O., and Chiocca, E. A. Genetic strategies against brain tumors. In: *The Internet Book of Gene Therapy: Cancer Gene Therapeutics,* edited by R. Sobol and K. Scanlon, pp. 235–246. Appleton & Lange, Stamford, CT, 1995.

34. Kramm, C. M., Sena-Esteves, M., Barnett, F. H., *et al.* Gene therapy for brain tumors (Review). Brain Pathol. *5:*345–381, 1995.

35. Li Bi, W., Parysek, L. M., Warnick, R., *et al.* In vitro evidence that metabolic cooperation is responsible for the bystander effect observed with HSVtk retroviral gene therapy. Hum. Gene Ther. *4:*725–731, 1993.

36. Maione, T. E., Gray, G. S., Hunt, A. J., *et al.* Inhibition of tumor growth in mice by an analogue of platelet factor 4 that lacks affinity for heparin and retains potent angiostatic activity. Cancer Res. *51:* 2077–2083, 1991.

37. Martuza, R. L., Malick, A., Markert, J. M., *et al.* Experimental therapy of human glioma by means of a genetically engineered virus mutant. Science *252:* 854–856, 1991.

38. Mercola, D., and Cohen, J. S. Antisense approaches to cancer gene therapy In: *The Internet Book of Gene Therapy: Cancer Therapeutics,* edited by R. E. Sobol and K. J. Scanlon, pp. 77–89. Appleton & Lange, Stamford, CT, 1995.

39. Mesnil, M., Piccoli, C., Tiraby, G., *et al.* Bystander killing of cancer cells by herpes simplex virus thymidine kinase gene is mediated by Connexins. Proc. Natl. Acad. Sci. U.S.A. *93:*1831–1835, 1996.

40. Milauer, B., Shawyer, L. K., Plate, K. H., *et al.* Glioblastoma growth inhibited in vivo by a dominant-negative Flk-1 mutant. Nature *367:*576–578, 1994.

41. Mineta, T., Rabkin, S. D., Yazaki, T., *et al.* Attenuated multi-mutated herpes simplex virus-1 for the treatment of malignant gliomas. Nature Med. *1:*938–943, 1995.

42. Moolten, F. L. Tumor chemosensitivity conferred by inserted thymidine kinase genes: paradigm for a prospective cancer control strategy. Cancer Res. *46:*5276–5281, 1986.

43. Moolten, F. L., Wells, J. M., Heyman, R. A., *et al.* Lymphoma regression induced by ganciclovir in mice bearing a herpes thymidine kinase transgene. Hum. Gene Ther. *1:*125–134, 1991.

44. Mroz, P. J., and Moolten, F. L. Retrovirally transduced Escherichia coli gpt genes combine selectability with chemosensitivity capable of mediating tumor eradication. Hum. Gene Ther. *4:*589–595, 1993.

45. Mullen, C. A., Kilstrup, M., and Blaese, R. M. Transfer of the bacterial gene for cytosine deaminase to mammalian cells confers lethal sensitivity to 5-fluorocytosine: a negative selection system. Proc. Natl. Acad. Sci. U.S.A. *59:*33–37, 1992.

46. Nabel, E. G., Yang, Z., Plautz, G., *et al.* Recombinant fibroblast growth factor-1 promotes intimal hyperplasia and angiogenesis in arteries in vivo. Nature *362:*844–846, 1993.

47. Nilaver, G., Muldoon, L. L., Kroll, R. A., *et al.* Delivery of herpesvirus and adenovirus to nude rat intracerebral tumors after osmotic blood-brain barrier disruption. Proc. Natl. Acad. Sci. U.S.A. *92:* 9829–9833, 1995.

48. Paulus, W., Baur, I., Boyce, F. M., *et al.* Self-contained, tetracycline-regulated retroviral vector system for gene delivery to mammalian cells. J. Virol. *70:*62–67, 1996.

49. Rainov, N. G., Kramm, C. K., Aboody-Gutterman, K., *et al.* Retrovirus-mediated gene therapy of experimental brain neoplasms using the HSV-TK/ganciclovir paradigm. Cancer Gene Ther. *3:*99–106, 1996.

50. Rainov, N. G., Zimmer, C., Chase, M., *et al.* Selective intra-arterial delivery of viral and microcrystalline particles to experimental brain tumors. Hum. Gene Ther. *6:*1543–1552, 1995.

51. Ram, Z., Culver, K., Oshiro, E., *et al.* Summary of results and conclusions of the gene therapy of malignant brain tumors: a clinical study (abstract). J. Neurosurg. *82:*343A, 1995.

52. Ram, Z., Culver, K. W., Walbridge, S., *et al.* In situ retroviral-mediated gene transfer for the treatment of brain tumors in rats. Cancer Res. *53:*83–88, 1993.

53. Ram, Z., Walbridge, S., Shawker, T., *et al.* The effect of thymidine kinase transduction and ganciclovir therapy on tumor vasculature and growth of 9L gliomas in rats. J. Neurosurg. *81:*256–260, 1994.

54. Redekop, G. J., and Nuas, C. C. G. Transfection with bFGF sense and antisense cDNA resulting in modification of malignant glioma growth. J. Neurosurg. *82:*83–90, 1995.

55. Rosenfeld, M. R., Meneses, P., Dalmau, J., *et al.* Gene transfer of wild-type p53 results in restoration of tumor suppressor function in a medulloblastoma cell line. Neurology:1533–1539, 1995.

56. Saleh, M., Stacker, S. A., and Wilks, A. F. Inhibition of growth of C6 glioma cells in vivo by expression of antisense vascular endothelial growth factor sequence. Cancer Res. *56:*393–401, 1996.

57. Samoto, K., Ikezaki, K., Ono, M., *et al.* Expression of vascular endothelial growth factor and its possible relation with neovascularization in human brain tumors. Cancer Res. *55:*1189–1193, 1995.

58. Short, M. P., Choi, B. C., Lee, J. K., *et al.* Gene delivery to glioma cells in rat brain by grafting of a retrovirus packaging cell line. J. Neurosci. Res. *27:*427–439, 1990.

59. Smith, M. L., Chen, I. T., Zhan, Q., *et al.* Interaction of the p53-regulated protein Gadd45 with proliferating cell nuclear antigen. Science *266:*1376–1380, 1994.

60. Takamiya, Y., Short, M. P., Ezzeddine, Z. D., *et al.* Gene therapy of malignant brain tumors: a rat glioma line bearing the herpes simplex virus type 1-thymidine kinase gene and wild type retrovirus kills other tumor cells. J. Neurosci. Res. *33:*493–500, 1992.

61. Takamiya, Y., Short, M. P., Moolten, F. L., *et al.* An experimental model of retrovirus gene therapy for malignant brain tumors. J. Neurosurg. *79:*104–110, 1993.

62. Tamiya, T., Ono, Y., Wei, M. X., *et al.* The Escherichia coli gpt gene sensitizes rat glioma cells to killing by 6-thioxanthine or 6-thioguanine. Cancer Gene Ther., in press, 1996.

63. Tapscott, S. J., Miller, A. D., Olson, J. M., *et al.* Gene therapy of rat 9L gliosarcoma tumors by transduction with selectable genes does not require drug selection. Proc. Natl. Acad. Sci. U.S.A. *91:*8185–8189, 1994.

64. Tjuvajev, J., Gansbacher, B., Desai, R., *et al.* RG-2 glioma growth attenuation and severe brain edema caused by local production of interleukin-2 and interferon-gamma. Cancer Res. *155:*1902–1910, 1995.

65. Trojan, J., Johnson, T. R., Rudin, S. D., *et al.* Treatment and prevention of rat glioblastoma by immunogenic C6 cells expressing antisense insulin-like growth factor I RNA. Science *259:*94–97, 1993.

66. Wang, X. W., Forrester, K., Yeh, H., *et al.* Hepatitis B virus protein X inhibits p53 sequence-specific DNA binding, transcriptional activity, and association with transcription factor ERCC3. Proc. Natl. Acad. Sci. U.S.A. *91:*2230–2234, 1994.

67. Wang, X. W., Yeh, H., Schaeffer, L., *et al.* p53 modulation of TFIIH-associated nucleotide excision repair activity. Nat. Genet. *10:*188–195, 1995.

68. Wei, M. X., Tamiya, T., Breakefield, X. O., *et al.* Virus vector mediated transfer of drug-sensitivity genes for experimental brain tumor therapy. In: *Viral Vectors: Gene Therapy and Neuroscience Applications,* edited by M. G. Kaplitt and A. D. Loewy, pp. 239–259. Academic Press, San Diego, CA, 1995.

69. Wei, M. X., Tamiya, T., Chase, M., *et al.* Experimental tumor therapy in mice with the cyclophosphamide-activating cytochrome P450 2B1 gene. Hum. Gene Ther. *5:*969–978, 1994.

70. Wei, M. X., Tamiya, T., Hurford, R. K., *et al.* Enhancement of interleukin 4-mediated tumor regression in athymic mice by in situ retroviral gene transfer. Hum. Gene Ther. *6:*439–445, 1995.

71. Wei, M. X., Tamiya, T., Rhee, R. J., *et al.* Diffusible cytotoxic metabolites contribute to the in vitro bystander effect associated with cyclophosphamide/cytochrome P450 2B1 gene therapy. Clin. Cancer Res. *1:*1171–1177, 1995.

72. Yu, J., Wei, M. X., Chiocca, E. A., *et al.* Treatment of human glioma by engineered interleukin-4 secreting cells. Cancer Res. *53:*3125–3128, 1993.

73. Yu, J. S., Herrlinger, U., Kramm, C. K., *et al.* Gene therapy for brain tumors by vaccination with granulocyte-macrophage colony-stimulating factor-transduced tumor cells, submitted for publication, 1996.

PART IV

Molecular Basis of Cerebrovascular Disease

CHAPTER 15

Molecular Events in Cerebral Ischemia

ANDREAS SPULER, M.D., WILLIAM K.M. TAN, Ph.D., and
FREDRIC B. MEYER, M.D.

INTRODUCTION

The complex pathophysiology of ischemic brain injury has been elucidated in increasing detail in recent years (see refs. 1–5 for review). This chapter will focus on recent data investigating the consequences of energy failure on gene expression and structural cell death. The oxygen requirements of the human brain are ten times higher than its contribution to body weight (6). Since neurons possess limited stores of ATP or of substrates metabolizable to ATP (7), the mammalian brain depends on the near continuous delivery of glucose and oxygen. To perform the complicated tasks of information processing, neurons actively maintain ion gradients across the cell membrane and intracellular compartments. Regulation of these gradients and the process of chemical signal transmission are highly energy-consuming.

There are many variables effecting the molecular events that transpire during ischemia. First, during ischemia the initial precipitating insult is energy failure. Energy failure subsequently results in the accumulation of lactic acid, intracellular calcium, excitatory amino acids, free fatty acids, nitric oxide, and oxygen free radicals. Second, it is important to distinguish between global and focal cerebral ischemia. In global ischemia, there is complete cessation of cerebral blood flow (CBF) for a period of time. Alternatively, during focal ischemia there is a heterogenity of CBF reductions so that a borderzone region of incomplete energy failure exists adjacent to the evolving infarction. This borderzone is termed the "ischemic penumbra." Third, depending on the occurrence of reperfusion there can be either permanent or transient ischemia. Fourth, damage following energy depletion can be purely functional, transient and completely reversible or structural, resulting in functional loss and cell death. The different molecular events of ischemia are closely interconnected, but for simplicity are discussed separately (Table 1).

ION HOMEOSTASIS

Ion gradients are important for any type of cell. Excitable cells like neurons use these gradients to accomplish their function of signal transfer. The maintenance of ion gradients consumes ATP which must be continuously replenished. Sodium and potassium gradients are a prerequisite for the occurrence of sodium action potentials and of voltage-, transmitter- or second messenger-gated re-/hyperpolarization of the cell membrane. Many transport systems in the plasma membrane of all cells use the driving force stored in the sodium gradient, its importance exceeds its role in signal processing. Sodium and potassium gradients are maintained by means of the electrogenic Na^+/K^+-ATPase located in the cell membrane. Lack of ATP results in an efflux of K^+ and an influx of Na^+. During ischemia, the marked increase in extracellular K^+ accompanied by a decrease in intracellular K^+ is due to both impaired ATPase-function and opening of K^+-channels (8, 9). Both mechanisms eventually lead to membrane depolarization. In conjunction with Na^+-influx, chloride ions flow into neurons thereby contributing to cell swelling during the initial stages of ischemia (10).

Table 1   **Some postulated mechanisms of ischemic-reperfusion injury**

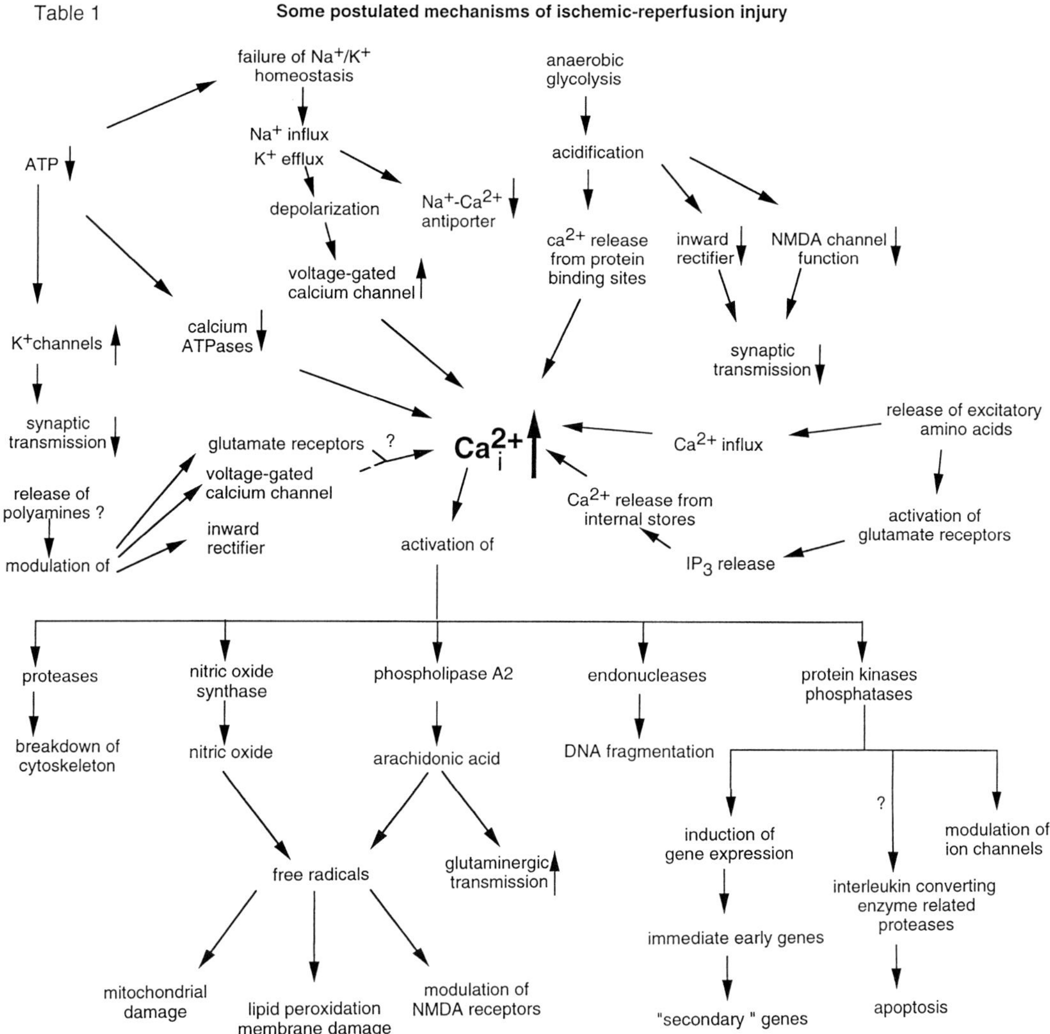

Calcium participates in signaling processes across the cytoplasmic membrane. In addition, Ca^{2+} serves as an intracellular second messenger. Calcium has many key functions in all cells and its intracellular concentration is tightly regulated. Calcium homeostasis is complex and not completely understood. Normally, the concentration gradient of 1/10,000 across the cell membrane provides an enormous driving force for the influx of calcium. The membrane permeability for this ion is controlled by voltage-, transmitter- or second messenger-gated ion channels. Under nonischemic conditions, cytosolic Ca^{2+}-concentration is maintained by means of a high affinity, low capacity Ca^{2+}-pumping ATPase (11–13) and during higher Ca^{2+}-loads by a low-affinity Na^+/Ca^{2+}-exchanger in the plasma membrane (14). Ischemia evokes an influx of Ca^{2+} across the cell membrane due to elevated extracellular concentrations of excitatory amino acids and through opening of voltage-gated Ca^{2+}-channels. Increased intracellular Na^+-concentration during ischemia may even reverse the direction of the Na^+/Ca^{2+}-exchanger, thus transporting Ca^{2+} into the cell (15, 16). Additional buffering capacity is provided by cytosolic Ca^{2+}-binding proteins, such as calmodulin, calbindin, and parvalbumin (11, 17). Their Ca^{2+}-buffering capacity may play a role in ischemia-resistance.

Calcium Homeostasis

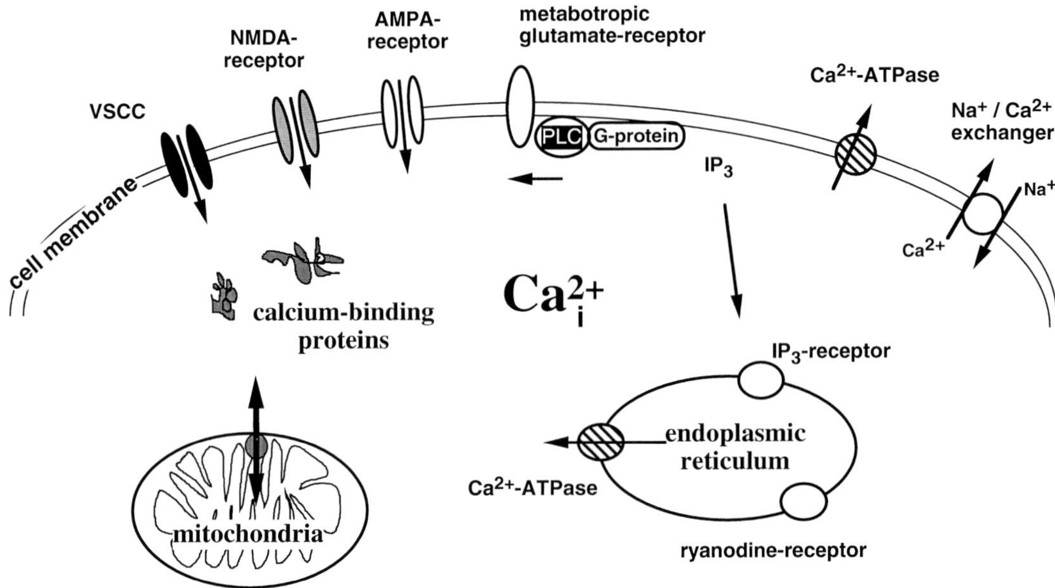

Figure 1. Cellular components involved in calcium homeostasis with impact on ischemia.

For example, in granule cells of the dentate gyrus the presence of calbindin is associated with survival after ischemia (18).

The endoplasmic reticulum (ER) and the mitochondria exhibit important Ca^{2+}-storing capacity. Release of Ca^{2+} from the ER is regulated by two receptors. One receptor-channel appears to be opened by inositol-triphosphate (IP_3). The opening of the IP_3-receptor (IP_3R) is modulated by cytosolic Ca^{2+} in a bell-shaped manner with the lowest channel activity during low and high Ca^{2+}-concentrations (19). The second type of receptor, the ryanodine receptor (RyR), seems to be regulated by the cytoplasmic Ca^{2+}-concentration (19). IP_3R and RyR are unequally distributed in the brain suggesting a possible contribution to ischemic cell damage: in the hippocampus IP_3R is predominantly found in the ischemia-sensitive CA1-neurons and RyR in the more resistant neurons of area CA3 and the dentate gyrus (20). In addition to the Ca^{2+}-releasing sites, the ER-membrane possesses a Ca^{2+}-pumping ATPase (11). Thus, the ER releases or takes up Ca^{2+} depending on the actual cytosolic concentration of Ca^{2+}, IP_3, and ATP. Mitochondria possess a low-affinity, high-capacity Ca^{2+}-importer in their inner membrane that uses the electrochemical gradient built up during oxidative phosphorylation (21, 22). Taken together, energy deprivation disables the ATP-dependent Ca^{2+} regulating mechanisms and, by creating an increased level of IP_3 (see below), results in an increase in cytosolic Ca^{2+}-concentration due to transmembrane influx and intracellular release (23) (Fig. 1).

Ischemia leads to a fall in intra- and extracellular pH. Partly responsible for this acidification is the production of lactate during anaerobic glycolysis; isolated hypoglycemia results in slight alkalinization (24). Regulation of neuronal pH is achieved by a Na^+/H^+ antiporter (25) and the Na^+-dependent Cl^-/HCO_3^--exchanger located in the cell membrane (26). As they utilize the Na^+-gradient, these regulators are indirectly ATP-dependent and thus reduced in their efficacy during ischemia. Acidosis leads to a decrease in synaptic transmission (27, 28).

POTASSIUM CHANNELS

In the early phase of energy depletion, opening of K^+-channels results in a membrane hyperpolarization in most neuronal populations

(29–31) and exerts a depressing effect on neuronal excitability (32). However some neurons, like those in the brainstem, depolarize during hypoxia and seem not to open a K^+-conductance (33). The opening of K^+-conductances might represent a kind of emergency measure to limit energy expenditure by decreasing electrical activity and K^+ efflux. The early K^+-channels are probably ATP-dependent (34, 35) and are closed with normal intracellular ATP-concentrations. At least in glucose depletion, these K^+-channels are not Ca^{2+}-dependent (36).

Since there is an increase in cytosolic Ca^{2+} during ischemia, other Ca^{2+}-dependent (37) or Na^+-dependent (38) classes of K^+-conductances are relevant, which likewise sense indirectly the energy status of the neuron. Certain inwardly rectifying K^+-channels show reduced current flow in a range of low extracellular pH which occurs during ischemia (39). These inward rectifiers normally stabilize the resting membrane potential, but also act as a filter promoting larger depolarizations. Their blockade impairs excitability and limits K^+-loss. The initial hyperpolarization due to ATP- and Ca^{2+}- or Na^+-regulated K^+-channels can delay release and impair postsynaptic efficacy of neurotransmitter. Together with blockade of inward rectifiers, these K^+-channels prevent opening of voltage-sensitive transmitter-gated channels like the NMDA-receptor and of voltage-gated Ca^{2+} or Na^+-channels thereby reducing neuronal activity and energy consumption. But this "emergency measure" is effective only for a short period. When a cell becomes depolarized, voltage-gated calcium channels open, further increasing the intracellular Ca^{2+}-concentration. Increased inactivation of voltage-gated Na^+-channels due to declining ATP-level may also limit the energy expenditure following Na^+-influx during action potentials (40). In summary, the changes in K^+-conductance are mainly responsible for the delay in membrane depolarization and the limitation of energy expenditure in the early phase of energy depletion.

NEUROTRANSMITTERS

Excitatory amino acids are regarded as important in neurodegenerative processes and acute brain injury (41). High increases in the concentration of glutamate have been measured during cerebral ischemia (42). This is due to an increased synaptic release caused by presynaptic Ca^{2+}-influx, but may also be secondary to an impairment of the Na^+-dependent, and thus ATP-dependent, uptake system in neurons and glial cells (43). Glutamate acts via a variety of receptors either containing an ion channel or coupling to membrane bound enzyme via G-proteins (44). Glutamate contributes by at least three mechanisms to the increase in intracellular Ca^{2+} (Fig. 1): 1) N-methyl-D-aspartate (NMDA)- and some α-amino-3-hydroxy-5-methyl-4-isoxazole propionic acid (AMPA)-receptors allow direct influx of Ca^{2+}. 2) AMPA/kainate receptors allow influx of small cations, resulting in membrane depolarization and opening of voltage-gated calcium channels. 3) glutamate activates phospholipase C via metabotropic receptors, which leads to the production of IP_3 and diacylglycerol (DAG) (45). IP_3 releases Ca^{2+} from internal stores (19).

The ischemia-related acidification can influence glutaminergic transmission by a direct effect on NMDA-receptors and indirectly by interacting with the glutamate-evoked arachidonic acid release: 1) the function of NMDA-receptors is attenuated by increasing concentration of protons (46, 47). Thus acidosis decreases synaptic glutamate responses (48). This corresponds to earlier results showing a depressing effect of acidification on synaptic transmission in vivo (27) and in vitro (28). 2) by inhibiting phospholipase A_2, acidification attenuates glutamate-evoked release of arachidonic acid (49). This diminishes the enhancing effect of arachidonic acid on glutaminergic synaptic transmission (50) and interrupts the positive feed back loop. In ischemia, these two mechanisms somewhat restrain the over-excitation caused by glutamate through negative feed back loops.

In addition to glutamate, the extracellular concentration of a variety of neurotransmitters, like adenosine and GABA, has been found to be elevated during ischemia (42, 51, 52) with possible depressing effects on synaptic transmission.

POLYAMINES

Three polyamines, putrescine, spermidine, and spermine, are present in all eukaryotic cells. A role in cell differentiation and growth is attributed to these polycationic molecules. Despite their modulation of important enzymatic pathways like the phosphoinositide cascade (53), their physiological significance is poorly understood.

Polyamines attracted attention since expression and activity (54, 55, 56) of ornithine decarboxylase (ODC), the key enzyme in polyamine synthesis, is markedly increased several hours after reperfusion, particularly in the hippocampal area CA1 (57). This results in high tissue levels of putrescine (56), accentuated in the ischemia-sensitive CA1 area (58). S-adenosylmethionine decarboxylase (SAMD) contributes to the conversion of putrescine to spermine and spermidine. In contrast to ODC, SAMD activity is depressed after reperfusion, hence tissue concentrations of spermine and spermidine are relatively unchanged or only slightly increased compared to normal (55, 58, 59, 60). These results suggest a contribution of polyamines to delayed cell death after ischemia.

Although blockade of polyamine synthesis did not prevent but rather enhanced glutamate neurotoxicity in cell cultures (61), ODC-inhibitors showed a protective effect against neuronal death in *in vivo* ischemia-reperfusion models (56, 62, 63). There is only one study reporting no beneficial effect (59), but the technique used to measure infarct size in this study may be less accurate than those used in other studies.

Studies to elucidate the effects of polyamines on ion channels yield no simple explanation for their effect on ischemia-induced neuronal damage. Patch clamp experiments with isolated neuroblastoma cells demonstrate an enhancing effect of putrescine on the activity of L-type Ca^{2+}-channels by an increase in open time (64). In isolated neurons, spermine potentiates glutamate/NMDA-responses by blocking the proton inhibitory site on the NMDA-receptor (65). Alternatively, polyamines exert a voltage-dependent, rectifying block of NMDA- and AMPA-channels (66) and a reduction of glutamate affinity to NMDA-receptors (67). These contradictory data may be explained by different NMDA- and AMPA-receptor subtypes with various regulatory sites for protons and polyamines and with different pore compositions (67). Spermine partly provides the rectifying property of inwardly rectifying potassium channels, thus increasing cellular excitability (68). However, spermine depresses synaptic transmission in brain slices (69) in contrast to the

excitation-promoting effects seen in isolated cells. To complicate matters further spermine and spermidine interact indirectly with Ca^{2+}-homeostasis by increasing the sensitivity of phosphoinositol production to stimuli (53). However, spermine activates mitochondrial Ca^{2+}-uptake (70). In summary, the effects of polyamines on certain neuronal populations might depend on the regionally different composition of ion channels. Further studies are necessary to define the role of polyamines during ischemia and reperfusion.

FREE RADICALS

Free radicals have been implicated in the pathophysiology of reperfusion injury. While reperfusion restores energy supply essential for neuronal survival, it produces oxygen radicals that exacerbate neuronal damage (71, 72). One source of free radicals in ischemic cells is arachidonic acid, released by membrane phospholipids under the action of Ca^{2+}-activated phospholipase A2. Arachidonic acid is the substrate for cyclo-oxygenase and lipoxygenase reactions, which produce prostaglandins, leukotrienes, and oxygen free radicals (73). Another source of free radicals during ischemia is xanthine oxidase. Normally, xanthines are oxidized by a dehydrogenase enzyme that transfers electrons to NAD^+. Tissue disruption and Ca^{2+} influx during ischemia, can convert xanthine dehydrogenase into the oxidase form, which uses O_2 as an electron acceptor, and releases superoxide radicals ($O_2^{\cdot-}$) (74). Hypoxanthine and xanthine, derived at high levels from the ATP pool during ischemia, are substrates for xanthine oxidase.

Several oxygen radical species besides superoxide radicals are produced following the initial reduction of oxygen, including perhydroxyl ($HO_2^{\cdot}$), hydrogen peroxide (H_2O_2) and hydroxyl ($\cdot OH$) (74). The damage occurring after ischemia may be caused in part by biochemical perturbations produced by elevated levels of $O_2^{\cdot-}$ and $\cdot OH$. Superoxide radicals have been shown to change phospholipid and protein structure (75). Hydroxyl radicals are the most reactive and are known to initiate lipid peroxidation (76), cause protein oxidation (77), and damage DNA in cells (78). Peroxidation of polyunsaturated fatty acids damages cell membranes and disrupts transmembrane ionic gradients. The products of lipid peroxidation are aldehydes, hydrocarbon gases, and other metabolites that can cause cytotoxic and vasogenic edema, alter vascular endothelial and blood-brain barrier permeability, and produce inflammation and chemotaxis (79). Furthermore, these products may also alter phospholipase activity, thereby increasing the release of arachidonic acid and the subsequent formation of prostaglandins.

The endogenous scavenging antioxidants include superoxide dismutase, glutathione peroxidase, and catalase. However, during reperfusion, it is likely that these antioxidative defense mechanisms are perturbed as a result of overproduction of oxygen radicals, inactivation of detoxification systems, and the failure to adequately replenish them in the ischemic brain tissue (80). There have been many studies which establish the role of endogenous antioxidants during ischemia-reperfusion. In hippocampal CA1 neurons of gerbils subjected to global ischemia, copper-zinc superoxide dismutase (CuZn-SOD) mRNA signals were induced at 3 and 24 hours of reperfusion. However, CuZn-SOD protein was not increased by the ischemic insult, suggesting a possible translation block (81).

Transgenic mice overexpressing SOD-1 genes have been used to elucidate the significance of oxidative stress following ischemia. After temporary focal ischemia, the volume of infarction was significantly reduced in transgenic mice which also showed elevated levels of antioxidants including glutathione and ascorbic acid in the penumbra region (82, 83). These data suggest that overexpression of SOD-1 activity increases resistance to reperfusion-induced oxidative stress. In permanent ischemia without reperfusion, overexpression of CuZn-SOD yields no neuroprotection (84). Because of the high probability of formation of free radicals and the difficulties in detection, free radical studies are focused on their effects and reactions rather than on direct demonstration of their presence, making the understanding of their role difficult.

NITRIC OXIDE

The role of nitric oxide (NO) in the pathophysiology of cerebral ischemia has generated much controversy. NO is involved in diverse physiological processes such as regulation of cerebrovascular tone (85, 86), neurotransmission (87, 88) and in various pathological processes including cerebral ischemia (89). In addition to neurons, astrocytes (90), perivascular nerves and cerebrovascular endothelium (91, 92) may form NO during cerebral ischemia.

NO can mediate neuronal death through production of the potent oxidant peroxynitrite ($ONOO^-$) (88) and other reactive oxygen species such as the hydroxyl free radical ($^{\cdot}OH$) and the radical nitrogen dioxide (NO_2) which can activate lipid peroxidation (93). NO and its degradation products can also cause neurotoxicity through formation of iron-NO complexes with several enzymes of the mitochondrial electron transport complex I and II, oxidation of protein sulfhydryls and DNA nitration (88, 94). NO-mediated ADP-ribosylation inhibits glyceraldehyde-3-phosphate dehydrogenase with detrimental effects as this enzyme is involved in both glycolysis and the hexose monophosphate shunt and is vital for $NADP^+$ synthesis (95).

After middle cerebral artery occlusion, NO increases more than 100-fold in the cortex within minutes (96). Administration of NO donors increases blood flow within the ischemic tissue and decreases infarct size (97–99), suggesting that endothelial and perivascular NO may have an indirect neuroprotective role. However, increasing CBF may promote free radical formation during reperfusion (100). On the other hand, inhibition of nitric oxide synthase (NOS), with low dose of NG-nitro-L-arginine methylester (L-NAME) attenuated brain acidosis independent of cerebral blood changes during intermittent focal cerebral ischemia in rabbits (101). It has been proposed that NO mediates NMDA toxicity. In cortical cultures, NOS inhibitors blocked NMDA-induced neuronal death (102). Depletion of L-arginine, the substrate of NO production, attenuated NMDA receptor-mediated toxicity (102).

Ischemia-induced NMDA receptor over-activation increases intracellular calcium and thereby promotes NO production via the $Ca^{2+}/$ calmodulin activated NOS. Alternatively, phosphorylation of NOS induced by glutamate activation of protein kinase C may inhibit its activity (103) providing a negative feed back mechanism. However, it has also been shown that NO inhibits NMDA currents depending on its redox state (104). In vivo studies yield conflicting data reporting either increases or reductions in infarct volume after NOS inhibition (105–107). Some of the discrepancies may be due to the different doses of NOS inhibitors used in different studies (108–110) and/or differences in administration schedule of NOS inhibitors (e.g. repetitive or continuous infusion) (107, 109, 111).

Whether increased NO production in the brain parenchyma is neurotoxic or neuroprotective depends on the redox state of NO and coexisting free radicals. For example, NO^- is suggested to account for the neurotoxic action of NO whereas NO^+ reacts with the thiol group of the NMDA receptor and blocks its function, and therefore may be neuroprotective (104). The controversy of the role of NO reflects its importance to the diversity of factors which impact on cerebral ischemia. Strategies which modify NO synthesis and/or metabolism may assume therapeutic importance in the future but not until there is a greater understanding of the tissue compartments generating NO, the activities of NOS that are inducibly and constitutively expressed, and the redox state of NO during different stages of ischemic injury.

PROTEIN KINASES AND PHOSPHATASES

For many cellular processes like receptor-regulation and gene expression, an exact interplay between protein phosphorylation and dephosphorylation is necessary. Recently the number of protein kinases was estimated as 2000 for the human genome, emphasizing the complexity of the phosphorylation system (112). An equally large number of phosphatases can be assumed. Some of the relevant kinases and phosphatases are activated by calcium. Therefore, it seems probable that energy depletion interferes with the phosphorylation balance via ATP depletion and calcium increase. Since this regulation network is still being deciphered, a unifying scheme cannot be described. Nevertheless there are already data highlighting some activation pathways.

Ca^{2+}/calmodulin-dependent protein kinase II (CaM PK II), a ubiquitous serine/threonine-protein kinase, is involved in longterm processes like memory. It undergoes autophosphorylation following stimulation with Ca^{2+} resulting in a prolonged Ca^{2+}-independent, activated state

(113). Activation of the NMDA subtype of glutamate receptors results in the intracellular translocation of the enzyme (114). Surprisingly in regard to the increase in Ca^{2+} following receptor activation, NMDA attenuates the activity of CaM PKII in all subcellular compartments (115). Equally after ischemia-reperfusion, the activity and expression of CaM PK II is decreased (116) and its neuronal sublocalization changed (116–118). Depressed enzyme activity is not related to altered autophosphorylation but seemingly to posttranslational changes decreasing affinity to ATP (119). In ischemia-resistant neuronal populations like the CA3 area and the dentate gyrus the CaM-PK II signal recovers several days postischemia (114, 118, 120), depending on the duration of ischemia (121), whereas in ischemia-sensitive CA1 neurons, the CaM PK II signal remains altered (114, 118). These ischemic changes in CaM-PKII distribution and activity can be prevented by NMDA antagonists (122). Evidence against an interpretation of these phenomena as epiphenomena and for an active role of CaM PKII in neuronal survival comes from experiments with genetically engineered mice. Knock-out mice lacking the alpha subunit of CaM-PKII develop greater infarction volumes after focal ischemia than normal animals or even heterozygotes (123). Since CaM PKII inhibits presynaptic transmitter release, e.g. glutamate (124), an explanation for the detrimental effect of CaM PKII-inactivity in these knock-out mice could be an increase in glutamate release. These results are complemented by seemingly conflicting data from *in vitro* experiments. Activation of NMDA receptors in neuronal cell cultures generates the Ca^{2+}-independent, activated CaM PKII (125). CaM PKII phosphorylates AMPA/kainate-receptors (126, 127) and enhances kainate- (128) and AMPA currents (129). A similar effect on AMPA receptors can be achieved by inhibition of phosphatases pointing to a certain phosphorylation level under normoxic conditions (130, 131). Postischemic CA1 neurons *ex vivo* show enhanced AMPA- but not kainate-currents (132). Keeping in mind the discussed data and the protective effects of AMPA antagonists given after ischemia (133, 134) and of NMDA antagonists given during ischemia (122) two hypothesis are suggested. First, the translocation of CaM PKII results in a locally enhanced enzyme activity responsible for the altered characteristics of AMPA receptors which together with the overall reduction of CaM PKII activity is detrimental for the survival of vulnerable neurons. Second, the AMPA phenomenon may be caused independently by decreased activity of phosphatases and may potentiate the injuring effect of reduced CaM PKII activity.

Tyrosine phosphorylation plays an important role in the signaling cascades of growth, differentiation, and survival after various cellular stress situations. After ischemia-reperfusion, tyrosine phosphorylation is augmented in ischemia-resistant brain areas and reduced in sensitive neuronal populations (135). Tyrosine phosphorylation can also influence NMDA receptors: nonischemic isolated spinal neurons *in vitro* exhibit enhanced NMDA responses upon treatment with protein-tyrosine kinase or after inhibition of protein tyrosine phosphatases (136). Postischemic CA1 neurons surviving 24 to 48 hours show reduced NMDA currents (132). Thus a postischemic increase in the activity of specific protein tyrosine phosphatases may account for the attenuated NMDA response. Data supporting such a hypothesis is still lacking.

Casein kinase II (CKII) is a protein kinase involved in growth factor signaling. After ischemia-reperfusion, its activity is decreased in vulnerable and increased in ischemia-resistant neuronal populations probably due to a phosphorylation of the enzyme (137). Although it has been suggested that CKII rescues neurons after ischemia, the data remain to be generated. Indirect support for this hypothesis comes from experiments with mice transgenic for basic fibroblast growth factor. These animals show a reduced susceptibility for cerebral ischemia (138).

Mitogen-activated protein kinase (MAP kinase), a member of the serine/threonine kinase family of MAP kinases, plays an important part in the signal cascade converting extracellular signals into altered gene expression. MAP kinase is activated by stimulation with glutamate via NMDA- and metabotropic receptors involving a protein kinase C- and a Ca^{2+}-dependent pathway (139). Tyrosine phosphorylation of the microtubulin-associated protein (MAP) kinase occurs after transient global ischemia and seems to involve the activation of glutamate receptors and a rise in intracellular calcium (140).

Calcineurin, Ca^{2+}/calmodulin-activated serine/threonine phosphoprotein phosphatase IIB, is abundant in the brain and colocalizes with CaM PKII in neuronal somata and dendrites (141). The expression of calcineurin is transiently depressed in the ischemia-resistant dentate gyrus and CA3 area after ischemia-reperfusion, followed by an increase lasting for days (142). Maintained calcineurin immunoreactivity is observed in the vulnerable CA1 area followed by a decrease parallel to cell death (114). It has been shown by Lieberman (143) that NMDA channels of neurons isolated from the dentate gyrus are inhibited by calcineurin. Additionally, calcineurin mediates dephosphorylation of tau, a component of the cytoskeleton, induced by NMDA receptor activation or failure of mitochondrial calcium buffering (144, 145). Dephosphorylated tau is more susceptible to degradation by the calcium-activated proteolysis (146). Since neurons from CA1 and the dentate gyrus exhibit a different susceptibility to ischemic damage and a different temporal profile of calcineurin expression, calcineurin may play a role in neuronal survival.

In summary, ischemia leads to disruption of phosphorylation balance. Only cells that can recover from this phase and can exert a compensating expression of certain enzymes, seem to have the potential for survival. The importance of protein kinases and phosphatases in the ischemia-induced cascade of events remains to be defined, but they seem to play an executing role for other cell programs.

CYTOSKELETON

The cytoskeleton supplies a cell with a membrane-free compartmentation. It determines the shape of the cells thereby influencing their volume and helps to anchor cells to their environment. Its active elements support cell movement. Furthermore, the cytoskeleton provides the scaffold and the kinetic elements for the transport of organelles and probably for the arrangement of receptors in the cell membrane (147). It is not static, but highly dynamic in its formation. Ischemia-reperfusion causes alterations of the cytoskeleton (148, 149).

MAP2 (microtubuline-associated protein 2), related to the microtubule-scaffold in dendrites and cell soma, shows a marked redistribution after hypoxia with a decrease in the dendrites and slight increase in the somata (149). These changes are accompanied by cell swelling (149) assuming loss of stabilization through the microtubular system. Certain neurofilaments (150, 151), MAP's (MAP1, MAP2, tau) (146, 152), and the actin-anchoring spectrin (152) are targets of calpain I, a calcium-activated cysteinprotease. Very early after ischemia, spectrin fragments were detected in the CA1 area pointing to an early activation of calpain (153). Sustained activation of calpain I is localized in selectively ischemia-sensitive neurons (154). Thus, calpain I may contribute to the structural cell damage seen in these neurons. This hypothesis is supported by experiments where inhibition of proteases leads to diminished spectrin proteolysis and less neuronal injury in CA1 (155). Despite the multiple changes in cytoskeletal structure during the course of ischemia, it remains to be shown whether any of these play an active role in neuronal cell damage.

GENE EXPRESSION

An essential part of regulation of gene expression is the induction or activation of specific transcription factors. Immediate early genes (IEGs) participate in the regulation of gene transcription by coding for transcription factors. These proteins bind to specific DNA sequences in the regulatory regions of target genes and increase or decrease their rate of transcription. For example, the IEG-proteins fos and jun dimerize to form a specific transcription factor, the activating protein 1 (AP-1). Hence, IEGs are termed "third messengers" that convert extracellular stimuli into alterations of cellular functions by regulating target gene expression.

Ischemia leads to activation of glutamate-receptors (NMDA- and non-NMDA subtypes) and to activation of Ca^{2+}-channels. Under non-ischemic conditions, influx of Ca^{2+} through these channels stimulates IEG induction e.g. by a Ca^{2+}-calmodulin-dependent protein kinase activating a cascade of phosphorylation events (156). In contrast, it is well established that cerebral ischemia results in a relatively lasting impairment of neuronal protein synthesis in general, (157, 158) despite elevated mRNA levels (159). Ischemia induces a variety of changes in gene expression and stress response of the brain. The range of altered gene expression that

occurs in response to cerebral ischemia remains to be fully characterized (Fig. 2).

IMMEDIATE-EARLY GENES

Many studies have demonstrated that ischemia, both focal and global, produces increases in the transcription of c-fos, c-jun, jun-B, zif 268, NGFI-A, and Krox-20 into mRNAs, as well as translation to their respective protein products (160–162). As an example, brief periods of ischemia induce transient expression of c-fos and c-jun several hours after ischemia (163). In the hippocampus, the distribution of expression of c-fos and c-jun is unequal with high levels in the dentate gyrus and CA3-area and low levels in the vulnerable CA1 region (164). The first transient peak of expression is followed by a second increase of c-fos- and c-jun expression 24 to 48 hours postischemia (160). Activation of NMDA receptors can potentiate the DNA binding activity of transcription factors like AP-1, thereby enhancing the effect of c-fos and c-jun (165). Hyperglycemia pretreatment has been shown to enhance neuronal injury following ischemia and abolish the increase in c-fos expression (166). Therefore, c-fos may be involved in repair and compensatory mechanisms after ischemia-reperfusion.

The proteins encoded by genes of the zinc finger family serve as transcription factors which utilize the so-called zinc-finger motif to bind nucleic acids (167). In a study by Abe and coworkers (168), mRNA of zinc finger genes (zfg) was transiently increased in the rat cerebral cortex after ischemia with a maximum expression at one hour of reperfusion. Correspondingly, the induction of zfg was detected in infarcted cortex. As zfg may be involved in differentiation and the regulation of cell growth, it is postulated that the transient increase in mRNA reflects some adaptive neuronal response during the recovery and repair process after ischemia (168). Krox-20, an IEG, encodes a transcription factor of the zinc finger family. It is present in both embryonic and adult CNS, suggesting that it may play a role in normal neuronal function (169, 170). After short ischemic periods, Krox-20 mRNA was induced in ischemic cortex whereas extended ischemia led to additional induction in non-ischemic, ipsilateral brain areas (171). The significance of the rapid and transient induction of the Krox-20

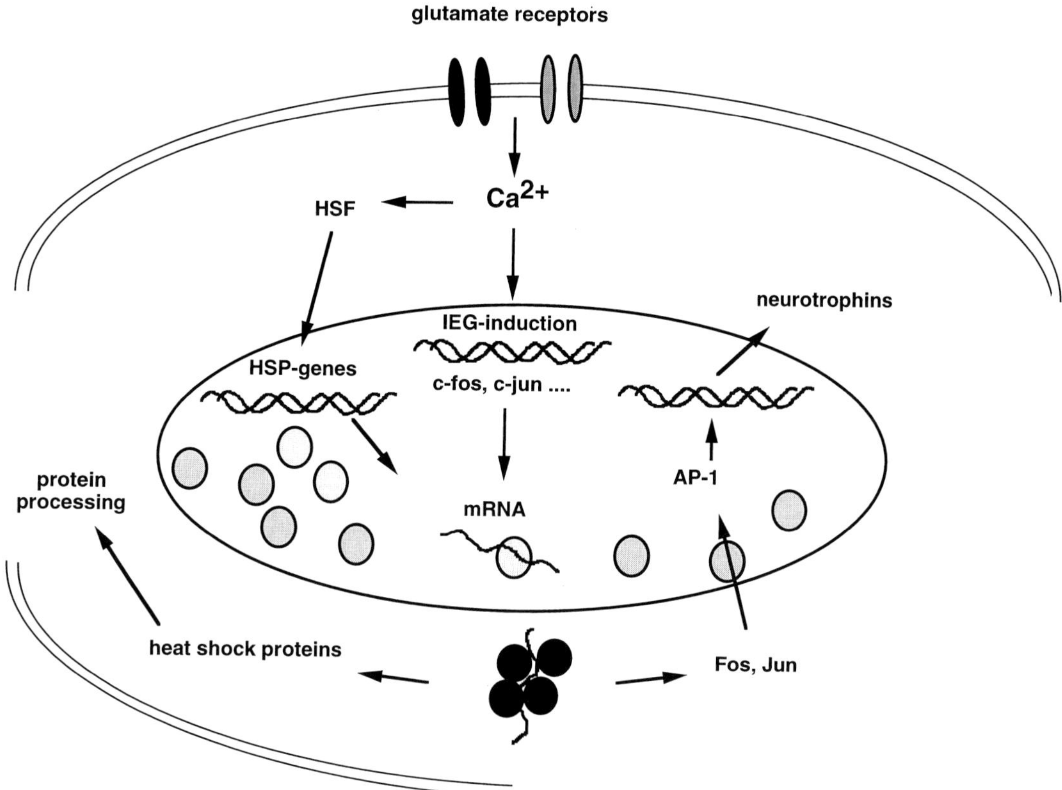

Figure 2. Genetic events resulting from ischemia-reperfusion. A calcium-activated protein kinase cascade induces immediate early gene (IEG) expression. The resulting proteins (e.g. Fos, Jun) form transcription factors (AP-1) and thereby increase the expression of other genes, e.g. neurotrophin genes.

Elevated intracellular calcium and activation of protein kinases probably evoke the formation of heat shock factors (HSF), which in turn regulate the transcription of heat shock genes (HSP-genes). The resulting heat shock proteins have multiple functions in posttranslational protein processing.

gene expression after ischemia remains unclear. Krox-20 is normally involved in the cell proliferation process (172) and may therefore be involved in functional recovery and remodeling after injury.

HEAT-SHOCK/STRESS RESPONSE

The induction of heat-shock proteins (HSPs) is a highly conserved cellular response to various harmful stresses, such as high temperature, inflammation and ischemia (173). HSPs are thought to be essential for posttranslational protein assembly and intracellular protein trafficking (174). Involvement of calcium and protein kinases in the induction cascade has been suggested (175). However, calcium does not appear to be an indispensable factor for the activation

of heat shock genes (176). Cellular stress evokes the formation of trimeric heat shock factors (HSF) which bind to heat shock elements on DNA regulating transcription of the corresponding heat shock genes (177).

Hsp72, a highly inducible member of the family of 70 kDa heat shock/stress proteins and a widely studied component of the generalized cellular response to injury, is detected in the brain after ischemia (178). Hsp72 mRNA is preferentially induced in neurons after global ischemia, and the duration of its expression is well correlated with the relative susceptibility of individual neuron populations to such insults (179). After ischemia as brief as two minutes, hsp72 immunoreactivity is selectively detected in the vulnerable CA1 pyramidal cells and the hilar interneurons (180). Electrical stimulation of the perforant path induces hsp72 only when the stimulus is strong enough to cause neuronal death (181). This suggests that hsp72 induction is associated with cell injury.

Hsp72 is also strongly expressed in regions of reduced but persistent blood flow (182). Thus, the immunoreactive protein is expressed strikingly in surviving neurons adjacent to the infarct, with a narrow zone of positive glia at the infarct rim (183). The cellular distribution of hsp72 protein expression is dependent on the duration of the insult. Brief ischemia results in pronounced neuronal hsp72 immunoreactivity whereas longer insults cause less induction when examined after 24 hours of reflow (184). These observations indicate that hsp72 induction identifies those discrete populations of surviving cells that are metabolically challenged, but not irreversibly damaged after ischemia (185).

Several studies have demonstrated that hsp72 expression may also contribute to mechanisms of induced tolerance to global ischemia, whereby brief ischemic insults that are capable of inducing a stress response result in an apparent protection of susceptible neurons against ischemic challenges (186, 187). However, there is no proven involvement of hsp72 or the stress response as a whole in the induction of tolerance. Taken together, the induction of IEGs which generally accompanies hsp72 expression provides an indication of the complex secondary cascades of altered gene expression that may be associated with the progression of injury or recovery following such insults.

TROPHIC FACTORS

There are several trophic factors which regulate survival and growth of neurons in the brain. There is a growing interest in the role of trophic factors in response to cerebral ischemic injury. These trophic factors include nerve growth factor (NGF), brain-derived neurotrophic factor (BDNF), and fibroblast growth factor (FGF).

NGF is essential for the survival, development, and maintenance of sensory and sympathetic neurons in the central and peripheral nervous system (188). The highest concentrations of NGF and NGF mRNA are found in the cerebral cortex and the hippocampus (189). In-

creased expression of BDNF and NGF mRNAs were observed subsequent to the expression of IEGs in the ischemic cortex and adjacent areas in a biphasic pattern (161), suggesting that increased IEG expression leads to increased AP-1 binding activity, which in turn has been linked to the enhanced expression of neurotrophin genes. NGF levels increase in the hippocampus and the cortex after hypoxic injury (190). Shozuhara and coworkers have shown that (191) NGF levels in the rat hippocampus decreased 2 days after ischemia but increased after 30 days coinciding with marked reactive astrocytosis. NGF injected into the lateral ventricle immediately before or after ischemia may have a protective effect on the delayed neuronal death of hippocampal neurons after transient forebrain ischemia in gerbils (192). Implantation of genetically engineered fibroblasts producing NGF protect the vulnerable CA1-CA2 hippocampal neurons in rat subjected to transient forebrain ischemia (193). There are also reports in which NGF did not ameliorate ischemic damage.

BDNF, a well characterized neurotrophic factor in the NGF family, may be especially important in the degenerative changes that occurs in hippocampal neuronal cells after ischemia. The hippocampus, relative to other brain regions, has the highest BDNF mRNA content (194). In a study by Lindvall and coworkers (195), BDNF mRNA was markedly increased in the dentate gyrus 2 h after transient forebrain ischemia and neurotrophin 3 (NT-3) mRNA was reduced in the dentate granule cell and in regions CA2 and medial CA1 of the hippocampus. However, Tsukahara and others (196) reported that BDNF mRNA was enhanced by transient ischemia both in the rat hippocampus and in the cerebral cortex as well. BDNF administered as a continuous intraventricular infusion prior to transient forebrain ischemia significantly increased the number of surviving pyramidal cells in the vulnerable CA1 sector of the hippocampus (196, 197).

The protein tyrosine kinases TrkA, TrkB and TrkC are signal-transducing receptors for neurotrophins. TrkB is a component of a high affinity receptor for BDNF. TrkB mRNA was transiently increased in the dentate gyrus following cerebral ischemia (198) and followed the same course and distribution as the rise in BDNF mRNA. The precise mechanism underlying these trophic effects has not yet been fully elucidated. It is thought that the changes of mRNA expression may lead to alterations in the availability of neurotrophic factors, and thus influence the functional outcome and neuronal necrosis following ischemic insults.

Fibroblast growth factor exists in acidic (aFGF) and basic (bFGF) forms (199, 200). FGF has been shown to promote the survival of cultured cortical and hippocampal neurons (201, 202). bFGF has also been shown to increase neuronal survival and neurite extension and to antagonize the excitotoxicity of glutamate in hippocampal neurons *in vitro* (203). After transient focal ischemia in the rat, the increase in bFGF-like immunoreactivity in cortical neurons (204) and appearance of bFGF binding sites on dorsolateral striatal neurons (205) may contribute to their repair after focal ischemia in rats. Continuous infusion of bFGF into the cerebral ventricle has been shown to rescue axotomized (fimbria-fornix transected) basal forebrain cholinergic neurons (206). Although a single dose of bFGF was not protective against neuronal injury in rats (207, 208), continuous intraventricular infusion of aFGF or bFGF has been reported to prevent CA1 neuronal damage following cerebral ischemia (209, 210). The mechanism by which growth factors protect against ischemic neuronal death is still unclear. However, Maiese and others (211) have shown that hippocampal neuronal death due to NO toxicity can be prevented by pretreatment with either bFGF or epidermal growth factor (EGF) or the combination of both. There is some evidence which suggests that bFGF may increase microcirculatory blood flow (212).

Insulin-like growth factors I and II (IGF-I and -II) are thought to play a role in neural growth and differentiation in the CNS (213). Bergstedt and Wieloch (214) demonstrated an upregulation of IGF-1 receptors in rat hippocampal CA1 and CA3 regions after brain ischemia but intracerebroventricular injections of IGF-1 (2 μg) showed no neuroprotection suggesting that the intracellular signal transduction chain activated by the IGF-1 receptor may be interrupted. Stephenson and coworkers (215) reported an increase in IGF-II receptor in neocortical neurons within the core of the ischemic infarct in rat at 4 days after permanent focal ischemia. A continuous intraventricular infusion of insulin and IGF-I in rats subjected to forebrain ischemia reduced neuronal damage (216). It is proposed that their neuroprotective effects may be mediated via a growth factor mechanism. Lateral ventricular administration of 1 μg rhIGF-1 2 hr after cerebral ischemia to fetal sheep delayed postischemic seizures and reduced neuronal loss (217). This suggests that growth factors may be involved with lesion-induced plasticity. It is important to note that although the above discussion emphasizes studies with positive effects of growth factors on ischemia-induced injury, there are a number of experiments which have failed to demonstrate an effect.

APOPTOSIS

Depending on the duration and severity of ischemic energy deprivation, neurons do not react with a transient breakdown of function, but undergo structural death. Cell death can occur very early after energy deprivation and is characterized by swelling of the neuron and lysis of its membranes. Based on swelling as a key feature, the name oncosis has been coined for that type of cell death (218). In cerebral ischemia, this apoplectic cell destruction in the core of infarction is accompanied by a delayed form of cell death of neurons (219) especially in the penumbra (220). From other tissues, the delayed cell death is also known as apoptosis, originally termed shrinkage necrosis (221). The end point for both types of cell death is necrosis and phagocytosis of the remnants. The pathway to this end stage is very different. Apoptosis is an active process involving expression of certain genes and synthesis of the corresponding proteins (131). As in the case of oncogenes and tumor suppressor genes, apoptosis-promoting and -suppressing genes have been identified. The exact mechanisms by which these genes cause or prevent cell death is the subject of many on-going studies.

Apoptosis means "cell death by schedule", a certain program of gene expression is started despite the fact that the concerned cells are not destined to die under normal circumstances. Apoptosis is therefore sometimes called cell suicide or programmed cell death. Programmed cell death is properly restricted to genetically determined cell death. This distinction is often not made and "apoptosis" and "programmed cell death" are used synonymously. Both share the feature of an active process with specific gene expression. Programmed cell death is a key event in development and adult tissue homeostasis. It might be regarded as the counterpart to mitosis. Programmed cell death and apoptosis are involved in a vast variety of cellular reactions reaching from embryogenesis to lymphocytic responses. During ontogenesis, the original high number of neural cell is reduced by apoptosis (222). In the nervous system, cells which are not connected to the appropriate target cell are eliminated by means of programmed cell death. Neural cells in culture die by apoptosis upon withdrawal of growth factors, which are provided normally by the target cells (223). In adrenalectomized rats, sudden withdrawal of glucocorticoids leads to apoptosis of granule cells in the dentate gyrus (224). In cancer, one mechanism for metastatic growth is an imbalance between mitotic activity and apoptosis (225). In other cell systems, apoptosis is induced not by deprivation, but by addition of a factor or a noxious agent like ionizing radiation (226). Thus apoptosis is not simply a withdrawal phenomenon, but more the common final pathway in various physiological and pathological settings.

Apoptosis is characterized morphologically by condensation and packing of chromatin along the nuclear membrane, a typical feature in electron microscopic studies. Ca^{2+}-dependent endonucleases cleave the DNA at specific points producing internucleosomal fragments. These segments can be detected in Southern blots yielding the typical "DNA laddering" pattern and by the so-called nick end labeling, marking the specific breaking point (227). Later

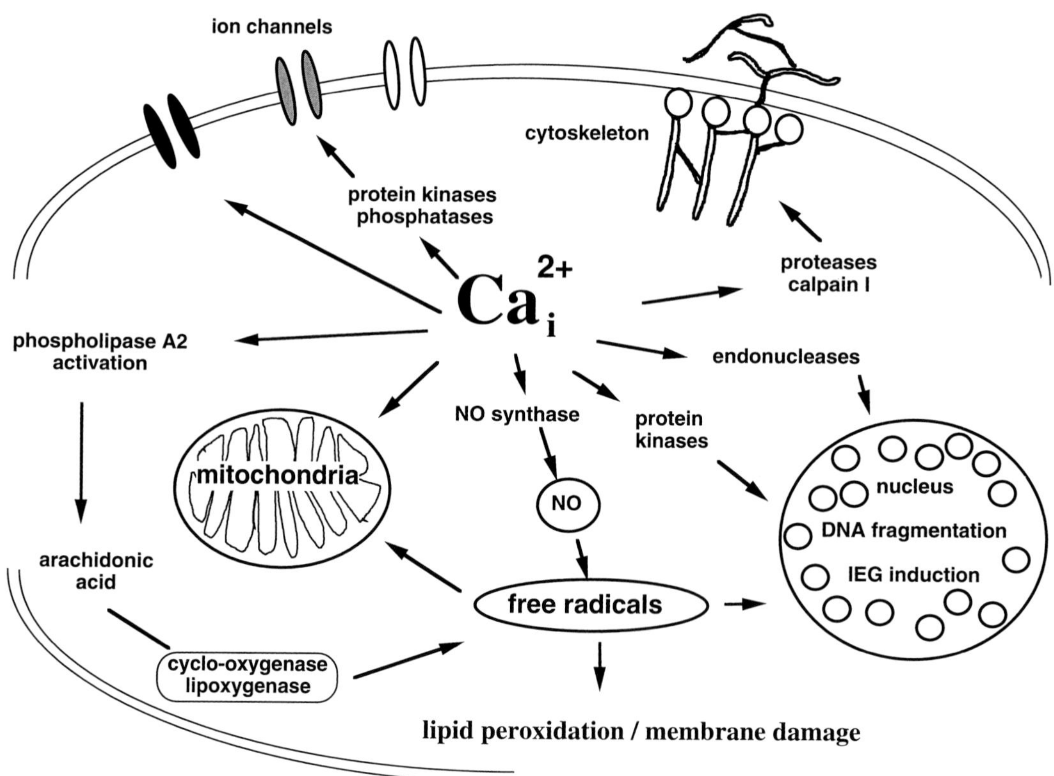

Figure 3. Downstream events following increase in cytosolic calcium caused by ischemia: Modification of ion channel characteristics directly by calcium or via activation of protein kinases or phosphatases, breakdown of cytoskeletal components by activated proteases, induction of gene expression mediated by protein kinases, DNA fragmentation by calcium activated endonucleases, formation of free radicals by increased availability of nitric oxide (NO) and arachidonic acid, impairment of mitochondrial function caused by calcium overload and free radicals, and lipid peroxidation and membrane damage exerted by free radicals.

the nucleus fragments, the cell shrinks, and budding of the cell occurs. These membrane-surrounded "buds" of the plasma membrane often contain organelles and nuclear fragments. Finally these buds separate (apoptotic bodies) and the cell breaks up. In contrast to oncosis, there is almost no swelling of organelles.

In cerebral ischemia, apoptosis affects primarily sensitive neuronal populations, like the CA1 pyramidal cells (228). With prolonged or more severe energy depletion the penumbra (220) and less sensitive cell groups are included (229). Apoptosis was detected using Southern blots (220, 228) and nick end labeling (230) and was confirmed by ultrastructural studies (231). Correspondingly, an increase in the activity of Ca^{2+}-dependent endonucleases was shown in ischemic brain areas (232).

As already mentioned, apoptosis is further characterized by an altered expression of certain genes. These genes are highly conserved during evolution. In mammals the genes *bcl-2* and *bcl-x*, and their corresponding proteins bcl-2 and bcl-x, are examples of genes associated with the blockade of apoptosis. Not surprisingly, these genes act as proto-oncogenes in other cellular contexts. Representative of apoptosis-promoting genes are bcl-xs and bax (233).

In cerebral ischemia, high levels of bax and correspondingly low levels of bcl-2 and bcl-x had been detected in ischemia-sensitive cell populations (234). The bcl-2 protein was seen in the penumbra or less injured cell, pointing to a possible role in cell survival (235). Association of bcl-2 expression with neuroprotection has also been confirmed in conditioning experiments. Here, a short ischemic period without infarction attenuated the damaging effect of a following prolonged ischemia. The conditioning ischemia showed an expression of bcl-2 in normally sensitive CA1-neurons, where unconditioned ischemia lead to a decreased expression (236). The significance of these data have been underlined by experiments with overexpression of the bcl-2 gene. Using herpes simplex virus vectors, an overexpression of bcl-2 was achieved in cell cultures (237) and *in vivo* (237). The bcl-2 overexpressing cells showed an increased resistance against ischemia (237) but also against other apoptosis-inducing stimuli like oxygen radicals and glutamate (237). Similarly, overexpression of bcl-2 in transgenic

mice resulted in a reduced infarct volume upon ischemia (238).

Recently, another class of genes, coding for interleukin converting enzyme related proteases (IRPs), have been identified as apoptosis-messengers in a broad spectrum of cell systems (239, 240). These enzymes are cysteine proteases and cleave the nuclear enzyme poly (ADP-ribose) polymerase. Their place in the cascade leading to apoptosis is not yet defined, but they seem to be involved in early steps of the process (241). In thymocytes, a classical apoptosis model, IRP genes respond to certain stimuli distinct from other apoptotic inductors (242, 243). The specific stimuli of IPRs during cerebral ischemia are not yet identified.

Since apoptosis can be elicited by a broad variety of stimuli in different cell systems, additional evidence is necessary to elucidate possible signal pathways from cerebral ischemia to delayed, apoptotic cell death. One trigger is the ischemia-induced rise in intracellular Ca^{2+} (244). The special pattern and amplitude of the Ca^{2+}-signal may induce the expression of IEGs, which in turn may act as third messengers inducing or blocking apoptosis-regulating genes.

Another candidate as link between ischemia and apoptotic cell death is oxidative stress. From other cell systems it is known that not only oxidative stress but also loss of intracellular reduction potential leads to apoptosis (245). As already discussed, cerebral ischemia and reperfusion result in the production of a variety of reactive oxygen species. It may be hypothesized that mild, sublethal oxidative stress induces the "death program" when compensating mechanisms fail, while a stronger insult kills the cells immediately (246).

CONCLUDING REMARKS

The complex molecular events which occur during cerebral ischemia are interconnected. There are two principal forms of cell death with implications for future therapeutic strategies:

1) severe energy depletion causing acute cell death. In this setting the breakdown of ion homeostasis and cell swelling are the key events. Shortening of the ischemic period (i.e. intravascular clot lysis) and eventually agents acting on ion channels and cell swelling may ameliorate injury.

2) the subacute, delayed cell death. A key role can be attributed to alterations in cellular Ca^{2+}-homeostasis (Fig. 3). However, many factors converge to the final common pathway of apoptosis-like cell death. This explains why so many different agents like glutamate receptors antagonists, free radical scavengers and NOS inhibitors, and manipulations of the expression of protein kinases may influence the outcome following ischemia. Future strategies for treatment could include a) a combination of different protectors to achieve a more potent synergistic effect, the "cocktail approach" or b) attempts to modulate the common final pathway(s), the "genetic approach."

Acknowledgment

This work was supported by NIH grant 25 374.

REFERENCES

1. Tymianski, M., and Tator, C. H.: Normal and abnormal calcium homeostasis in neurons: A basis for the pathophysiology of traumatic and ischemic central nervous system injury. Neurosurg. *38:*1176–95, 1996.
2. Siesjo, B. K., Katsura, K., Mellergard, P., *et al.*: Acidosis-related brain damage. Prog. Brain Res. *96:*23–48, 1993.
3. Wahl, M., Schilling, L., Unterberg, A., *et al.*: Mediators of vascular and parenchymal mechanisms in secondary brain damage. Acta Neurochir. Suppl. *57:*64–72, 1993.
4. Hossmann, K. A.: Glutamate-mediated injury in focal cerebral ischemia: The excitotoxin hypothesis revised. Brain Pathol. *4:*23–36, 1994.
5. Morley, P., Hogan, M. J., and Hakim, A. M.: Calcium-mediated mechanisms of ischemic injury and protection. Brain Pathol. *4:*37–47, 1994.
6. Lassen, N. A.: Cerebral blood flow and oxygen consumption in man. Physiol. Rev. *39:*183–197, 1959.
7. Lipton, P.: Regulation of glycogen in the dentate gyrus of the in vitro guinea pig hippocampus; effect of combined deprivation of glucose and oxygen. J. Neurosci. Methods *28:*147–154, 1988.
8. Jiang, C., and Haddad, G. G.: Effect of anoxia on intracellular and extracellular potassium activity in hypoglossal neurons in vitro. J. Neurophysiol. *66:*103–111, 1991.
9. Jiang, C., and Haddad, G. G.: Differential responses of neocortical neurons to glucose and/or O_2 deprivation in the human and rat. J. Neurophysiol. *68:*2165–2173, 1992.
10. Jiang, C., Agulian, S., and Haddad, G. G.: Cl^- and Na^+ homeostasis during anoxia in rat hypoglossal neurons: Intracellular and extracellular in vitro studies. J. Physiol. *448:*697–708, 1992.
11. Clapham, D. E.: Calcium signaling. Cell *80:*259–268, 1995.
12. Monteith, G. R., and Roufogalis, B. D.: The plasma membrane calcium pump—a physiological perspective on its regulation. Cell Calcium *18:*459–470, 1995.
13. Werth, J. L., Usachev, Y. M., and Thayer, S. A.: Modulation of calcium efflux from cultured rat dorsal root ganglion neurons. J. Neurosci. *16:*1008–1015, 1996.
14. Nachshen, D. A., Sanchez-Armass, S., and Weinstein, A. M.: The regulation of cytosolic calcium in rat brain synaptosomes by sodium-dependent calcium efflux. J. Physiol. *381:*17–28, 1986.
15. Waxman, S. G., Ransom, B. R., and Stys, P. K.: Nonsynaptic mechanisms of Ca(2+)-mediated injury in CNS white matter. TINS *14:*461–468, 1991.
16. Lobner, D., and Lipton, P.: Intracellular calcium levels and calcium fluxes in the CA1 region of the rat hippocampal slice during in vitro ischemia: Relationship to electrophysiological cell damage. J. Neurosci. *13:*4861–4871, 1993.
17. Baimbridge, K. G., Celio, M. R., and Rogers, J. H.: Calcium-binding proteins in the nervous system. TINS *15:*303–308, 1992.
18. Goodman, J. H., Wasterlain, C. G., Massarweh, W. F., *et al.*: Calbindin-D28k immunoreactivity and selective vulnerability to ischemia in the dentate gyrus of the developing rat. Brain Res. *606:*309–314, 1993.
19. Ehrlich, B. E.: Functional properties of intracellular calcium-release channels. Curr. Opin. Neurobiol. *5:*304–309, 1995.
20. Sharp, A., McPherson, P. S., Dawson, T. M., *et al.*: Differential immunohistochemical localization of inositol 1,4,5-triphosphate- and ryanodine-sensitive Ca^{2+} release channels in rat brain. J. Neurosci. *13:*3051–3063, 1993.
21. Pozzan, T., Rizzuto, R., Volpe, P., *et al.*: Molecular and cellular physiology of intracellular calcium stores. Physiol. Rev. *74:*595–636, 1994.
22. Werth, J. L., and Thayer, S. A.: Mitochondria buffer physiological calcium loads in cultured rat dorsal root ganglion neurons. J. Neurosci. *14:*348–356, 1994.
23. Mitani, A., Yanase, H., Sakai, K., *et al.*: Origin of intracellular Ca^{2+} elevation induced by in vitro ischemia-like conditions in hippocampal slices. Brain Res. *601:*103–110, 1993.
24. Spuler, A., Endres, W., and Grafe, P.: Metabolic origin of activity-related pH-changes in mammalian peripheral and central unmyelinated fibre tracts. Pflüger's Arch. *408:*R69, 1987.
25. Ou-yang, Y., Mellergard, P., and Siesjö, B. K.: Regulation of intracellular pH in single rat cortical neurons in vitro: A microspectrofluorometric study. J. Cereb. Blood Flow Metab. *13:*827–840, 1993.
26. Schwiening, C. J., and Boron, W. F.: Regulation of intracellular pH in pyramidal neurones from the rat hippocampus by Na(+)-dependent $Cl(-)$-HCO_3-exchange. J. Physiol. *475:*59–67, 1994.
27. Balestrino, M., and Somjen, G. G.: Concentration of carbon dioxide, interstitial pH and synaptic transmission in hippocampal formation of the rat. J. Physiol. *396:*247–266, 1988.
28. Walz, W., and Harold, D. E.: Brain lactic acidosis and

synaptic function. Can. J. Physiol. Pharmacol. *68:* 164–169, 1990.

29. Hansen, A. J., Hounsgaard, J., and Jahnsen, H.: Anoxia increases potassium conductance in hippocampal nerve cells. Acta Physiol. Scand. *115:*301–310, 1982.

30. Spuler, A., Endres, W., and Grafe, P.: Glucose depletion hyperpolarizes guinea pig hippocampal neurons by an increase in potassium conductance. Exp. Neurol. *100:*248–252, 1988.

31. Leblond, J., and Krnjevic, K.: Hypoxic changes in hippocampal neurons. J. Neurophysiol. *62:*1–14, 1989.

32. Glötzner, F.: Intrazelluläre Potentiale, EEG und corticale Gleichspannung an der sensomotorischen Rinde der Katze bei akuter Hypoxie. Arch. Psychiatr. Nervenkr. *210:*274–296, 1967.

33. Haddad, G. G., and Donnelly, D. F.: O_2 deprivation induces a major depolarization in brain stem neurons in the adult but not in the neonatal rat. J. Physiol. *429:*411–428, 1990.

34. Tromba, C., Salvaggio, A., Racagni, G., *et al.*: Hippocampal hypoglycaemia-activated K^+ channels: Single channel analysis of glucose and voltage dependence. Pflüger's Arch. *429:*58–63, 1994.

35. Mourre, C., Ben-Ari, Y., Bernardi, H., *et al.*: Antidiabetic sulfonylureas: Localization of binding sites in the brain and effects on the hyperpolarization induced by anoxia in hippocampal slices. Brain Res. *486:*159–164, 1989.

36. Knöpfel, T., Spuler, A., Grafe, P., *et al.*: Cytosolic calcium during glucose deprivation in rat hippocampal pyramidal cells of rats. Neurosci. Lett. *117:*295–299, 1990.

37. Hille, B.: Ionic channels of excitable membranes. Sunderland, Sinauer Associates, 1992.

38. Dryer, S. E.: Na^+-activated K^+ channels: A new family of large-conductance ion channels. TINS *17:* 155–160, 1994.

39. Coulter, K. L., Perier, F., Radeke, C. M., *et al.*: Identification and molecular localization of a pH-sensing domain for the inward rectifier potassium channel HIR. Neuron *15:*1157–1168, 1995.

40. Cummins, T. R., Jiang, C., and Haddad, G. G.: Human neocortical excitability is decreased during anoxia via sodium channel modulation. J. Clin. Invest. *91:*608–615, 1993.

41. Lipton, S. A., and Rosenberg, P. A.: Excitatory amino acids as a final common pathway for neurologic disorders. N. Engl. J. Med. *330:*613–622, 1994.

42. Hagberg, H., Lehmann, A., Sandberg, M., *et al.*: Ischemia-induced shift of inhibitory and excitatory amino acids from intra- to extracellular compartments. J. Cereb. Blood Flow Metab. *5:*413–419, 1985.

43. Kanai, Y., Smith, C. P., and Hediger, M. A.: The elusive transporters with a high affinity for glutamate. TINS *16:*359–356, 1993.

44. Nakanishi, S.: Molecular diversity of glutamate receptors and implications for brain function. Science *258:*597–603, 1992.

45. Pin, J.-P., and Bockaert, J.: Get receptive to metabotropic glutamate receptors. Curr. Opin. Neurobiol. *5:*342–349, 1995.

46. Tang, C.-M., Dichter, M., and Morad, M.: Modulation of the N-methyl-D-aspartate channel by extracellular H^+. Proc. Natl. Acad. Sci. U. S. A. *87:*6445–6449, 1990.

47. Traynelis, S. F., and Cull-Candy, S. G.: Proton inhibition of N-methyl-D-aspartate receptors in cerebellar neurons. Nature *345:*347–350, 1990.

48. Gottfried, J. A., and Chesler, M.: Endogenous H^+ modulation of NMDA receptor-mediated EPSCs revealed by carbonic anhydrase inhibition in rat hippocampus. J. Physiol. *478:*373–378, 1994.

49. Stella, N., Pellerin, L., and Magistretti, P. J.: Modulation of the glutamate-evoked release of arachidonic acid from mouse cortical neurons: Involvement of a pH-sensitive membrane phospholipase A_2. J. Neurosci. *15:*3307–3317, 1995.

50. Miller, B., Sarantis, M., Traynelis, S. F., *et al.*: Potentiation of NMDA receptor currents by arachidonic acid. Nature *355:*722–725, 1992.

51. Hagberg, H., Andersson, P., Lacarewicz, J., *et al.*: Extracellular adenosine, inosine, hypoxanthine, and xanthine in relation to tissue nucleotides and purines in rat striatum during transient ischemia. J. Neurochem. *49:*227–231, 1987.

52. Tan, W. K. M., Williams, C. E., During, M., *et al.*: Accumulation of cytotoxins during the development of seizures and edema after hypoxic-ischemic injury in late gestation fetal sheep. Pediatr. Res. 1996, in press.

53. Periyasamy, S., Kothapalli, M. R., and Hoss, W.: Regulation of the phosphoinositide cascade by polyamines in brain. J. Neurochem. *63:*1319–1327, 1994.

54. Dempsey, R. J., Carney, J. M., and Kindy, M. S.: Modulation of ornithine decarboxylase mRNA following transient ischemia in the gerbil brain. J. Cereb. Blood Flow Metab. *11:*979–985, 1991.

55. Paschen, W., Cleef, M., Röhn, G., *et al.*: Ischemia-induced disturbances of polyamine synthesis. Prog. Brain Res. *96:*147–160, 1993.

56. Kindy, M. S., Hu, Y., and Dempsey, R. J.: Blockade of ornithine decarboxylase enzyme protects against ischemic brain damage. J. Cereb. Blood Flow Metab. *14:*1040–1045, 1994.

57. Müller, M., Cleef, M., Röhn, G., *et al.*: Ornithine decarboxylase in reversible cerebral ischemia: An immunohistochemical study. Acta Neuropathol. *83:* 39–45, 1991.

58. Paschen, W., Hallmayer, J., and Mies, G.: Regional profile of polyamines in reversible cerebral ischemia of Mongolian gerbils. Neurochem. Pathol. *7:*143–156, 1987.

59. Sauer, D., Martin, P., Aallegrini, P. R., *et al.*: Differing effects of alpha-difluoromethylornithine and CGP40116 on polyamine levels and infarct volume in a rat model of focal cerebral ischemia. Neurosci. Lett. *141:*131–135, 1992.

60. Carter, C., Poignet, H., Carboni, S., *et al.*: Release of spermidine from the rat cortex following permanent middle cerebral artery occlusion. Fundam. Clin. Pharmacol. *9:*129–140, 1995.

61. Lombardi, G., Szekely, A. M., Bristol, L. A., *et al.*: Induction of ornithine decarboxylase by N-methyl-D-aspartate receptor activation is unrelated to po-

tentiation of glutamate excitotoxicity by polyamines in cerebellar granule neurons. J. Neurochem. *60:*1317–1324, 1993.

62. Gilad, G. M., and Gilad, V. H.: Polyamines can protect against ischemia-induced nerve cell death in gerbil forebrain. Exp. Neurol. *111:*349–355, 1991.

63. Zoli, M., Zini, I., Grimaldi, R., *et al.*: Effects of polyamine synthesis blockade on neuronal loss and astroglial reaction after transient forebrain ischemia. Int. J. Dev. Neurosci. *11:*175–187, 1993.

64. Herman, M. D., Reuveny, E., and Narahashi, T.: The effects of polyamines on voltage-activated calcium channels in mouse neuroblastoma cells. J. Physiol. *462:*645–660, 1993.

65. Traynelis, S. F., Hartley, M., and Heinemann, S. F.: Control of proton sensitivity of the NMDA receptor by RNA splicing and polyamines. Science *268:*873–876, 1995.

66. Koh, D.-S., Burnashev, N., and Jonas, P.: Block of native Ca^{2+}-permeable AMPA receptors in rat brain by intracellular polyamines generates double rectification. J. Physiol. *486:*305–312, 1995.

67. Johnson, T. D.: Modulation of channel function by polyamines. TIPS *17:*22–27, 1996.

68. Fakler, B., Brandle, U., Glowatzki, E., *et al.*: Strong voltage-dependent inward rectification of inward rectifier K^+ channels is caused by intracellular spermine. Cell *80:*149–154, 1995.

69. Ferchmin, P. A., Eterovic, V. A., Rivera, E. M., *et al.*: Spermine increases paired-pulse facilitation in area CA1 of hippocampus in a calcium-dependent manner. Brain Res. *689:*189–196, 1995.

70. Jensen, J. R., Lynch, G., and Baudry, M.: Allosteric activation of brain mitochondrial Ca^{2+} uptake by spermine and by Ca^{2+}: Developmental changes. J. Neurochem. *53:*1173–1181, 1989.

71. McCord, J. M.: Oxygen-derived free radicals in post-ischemic tissue injury. N. Engl. J. Med. *312:*159–163, 1985.

72. Ginsberg, M. D., Watson, B. D., Busto, R., *et al.*: Peroxidative damage to cell membranes following cerebral ischemia: A cause of ischemic brain injury. Neurochem. Pathol. *9:*171–193, 1988.

73. Keuhl, F. A., and Egan, R. N.: Prostaglandins, arachidonic acid, and inflammation. Science *210:*978–984, 1980.

74. Halliwell, B., and Gutteridge, J. M. C.: Oxygen toxicity, oxygen radicals, transition metals and disease. Biochem. J. *219:*1–14, 1984.

75. Brown, K., and Fridovich, I.: Superoxide radical and superoxide dismutase: Threat and defense. Acta Physiol. Scand. Suppl. *492:*9, 1980.

76. Watson, B. D., Busto, R., Goldberg, W. J., *et al.*: Lipid peroxidation in vivo induced by reversible glial ischemia in rat brain. J. Neurochem. *42:*268–274, 1984.

77. Carney, J. M., Starke-Reed, P. E., Oliver, C. N., *et al.*: Reversal of age-related increase in brain protein oxidation, decrease in enzyme activity, and loss in temporal and spatial memory by chronic administration of the spin-trapping compound N-tert-butyl-alpha-phenylnitrone. Proc. Natl. Acad. Sci. U. S. A. *88:*3633–3636, 1991.

78. Cathcart, R., Schwiers, E., Saul, R. L., *et al.*: Thymine glycol and thymidine glycol in human and rat urine: A possible assay for oxidative DNA damage. Proc. Natl. Acad. Sci. U. S. A. *81:*5633–5637, 1984.

79. Southorn, P. A., and Powis, G.: Free radicals in medicine. I. Chemical nature and biologic reactions. Mayo Clin. Proc. *63:*381–389, 1988.

80. Siesjo, B. K., Agardh, C. D., and Bengtsson, F.: Free radicals and brain damage. Cerebrovasc. Brain. Metab. Rev. *1:*165–171, 1989.

81. Matsuyama, T., Michishita, H., Nakamura, H., *et al.*: Induction of copper-zinc superoxide dismutase in gerbil hippocampus after ischemia. J. Cereb. Blood Flow Metab. *13:*135–144, 1993.

82. Kinouchi, H., Epstein, C. J., Mizui, T., *et al.*: Attenuation of focal cerebral ischemic injury in transgenic mice overexpressing CuZn superoxide dismutase. Proc. Natl. Acad. Sci. U. S. A. *88:*11 158–162, 1991.

83. Yang, G., Chan, P. H., Chen, J., *et al.*: Human copper-zinc superoxide dismutase transgenic mice are highly resistant to reperfusion injury after focal cerebral ischemia. Stroke *25:*165–170, 1994.

84. Chan, P. H., Kamii, H., Yang, G., *et al.*: Brain infarction is not reduced in SOD-1 transgenic mice after permanent focal cerebral ischemia. Neuroreport *5:*293–296, 1993.

85. Faraci, F. M.: Role of endothelium-derived relaxing factor in cerebral circulation: Large arteries vs. microcirculation. Am. J. Physiol. *261:* H1038–1042, 1991.

86. Tanaka, K., Gotoh, F., Gomi, S., *et al.*: Inhibition of nitric oxide synthesis induces a significant reduction in local cerebral blood flow in the rat. Neurosci. Lett. *127:*129–132, 1991.

87. Snyder, S. H., and Bredt, D. S.: Nitric oxide as a neuronal messenger. TIPS *12:*125–128, 1991.

88. Dawson, T. M., Dawson, V. L., and Snyder, S. H.: A novel messenger molecule in brain: The free radical, nitric oxide. Ann. Neurol. *32:*297–311, 1992.

89. Dawson, D. A.: Nitric oxide and focal cerebral ischemia: Multiplicity of actions and diverse outcome. Cerebrovasc. Brain. Metab. Rev. *6:*299–324, 1994.

90. Nakashima, M. N., Yamashita, K., Kataoka, Y., *et al.*: Time course of nitric oxide synthase activity in neuronal, glial, and endothelial cells of rat striatum following focal cerebral ischemia. Cell. Mol. Neurobiol. *15:*341–349, 1995.

91. Wahl, M., and Schilling, L.: Regulation of cerebral blood flow—a brief review. Acta Neurochir. Suppl. *59:*3–10, 1993.

92. Chen, F. Y., and Lee, T. J.: Arginine synthesis from citrulline in perivascular nerves of cerebral artery. J. Pharmacol. Exp. Ther. *273:*895–901, 1995.

93. Beckman, J. S.: The double-edged role of nitric oxide in brain function and superoxide-mediated injury. J. Dev. Physiol. *15:*53–59, 1991.

94. Stamler, J. S., Single, D. J., and Localzo, J.: Biochemistry of nitric oxide and its redox-activated forms. Science *258:*1898–1902, 1992.

95. MacDonald, L. J., and Moss, J.: Stimulation by nitric oxide of an NAD linkage to glyceraldehyde-3-phosphate dehydrogenase. Proc. Natl. Acad. Sci. U. S. A. *90:*6238–6241, 1993.

96. Malinski, T., Bailey, F., Zhang, Z. G., *et al.*: Nitric

oxide measures by porphyrininc microsensor in rat brain after transient middle cerebral artery occlusion. J. Cereb. Blood Flow Metab. *13:*355–358, 1993.

97. Morikawa, E., Huang, Z., and Moskowitz, M. A.: L-arginine decreases infarct size caused by middle cerebral arterial occlusion in SHR. Am. J. Physiol. *263:*H1632–1635, 1992.

98. Zhang, F., and Iadecola, C.: Nitroprusside improves blood flow and reduces brain damage after focal ischemia. Neuroreport *4:*559–562, 1993.

99. Morikawa, E., Moskowitz, M. A., Huang, Z., et al.: L-arginine infusion promotes nitric oxide-dependent vasodilatation, increases regional blood flow, and reduces infarction volume in the rat. Stroke *25:*429–435, 1994.

100. Traystman, R. J., Kirsch, J. R., and Koehler, R. C.: Oxygen radical mechanisms of brain injury following ischemia and reperfusion. J. Appl. Physiol. *71:*1185–1195, 1991.

101. Anderson, R. E., and Meyer, F. B.: Nitric oxide synthase inhibition by L-NAME during repetitive focal cerebral ischemia in rabbits. Am. J. Physiol. 1996, in press.

102. Dawson, V. L., Dawson, T. M., London, E. D., et al.: Nitric oxide mediate glutamate neurotoxicity in primary cortical culture. Proc. Natl. Acad. Sci. U. S. A. *88:*6368–6371, 1991.

103. Bredt, D. S., Ferris, C. D., and Snyder, S. H.: Nitric oxide synthase regulatory sites. Phosphorylation by cyclic AMP-dependent protein kinase, protein kinase C, and calcium/calmodulin protein kinase; identification of flavin and calmodulin binding sites. J. Biol. Chem. *267:*10 976–981, 1992.

104. Lipton, S. A., Choi, Y.-B., Pan, Z.-H., et al.: A redox-based mechanism for the neuroprotective effects of nitric oxide and related nitrosocompounds. Nature *364:*626–632, 1993.

105. Nowicki, J. P., Duval, D., Poignet, H., et al.: Nitric oxide mediates neuronal death after focal cerebral ischemia in the mouse. Eur. J. Pharmacol. *204:*339–340, 1991.

106. Yamamoto, S., Golanov, E. V., Berger, S. B., et al.: Inhibition of nitric oxide synthesis increases focal ischemic infarction in rat. J. Cereb. Blood Flow Metab. *12:*717–726, 1992.

107. Nishikawa, T., Kirsch, J. R., Koehler, R. C., et al.: Effect of nitric oxide synthase inhibition on cerebral blood flow and injury volume during focal ischemia in cats. Stroke *24:*1717–1724, 1993.

108. Dawson, D. A., Kusumoto, K., Graham, D. I., et al.: Inhibition of nitric oxide synthesis does not reduce infarct volume in a rat model of focal cerebral ischemia. Neurosci. Lett. *142:*151–154, 1992.

109. Nagafuji, T., Sugiyama, M., Matsui, T., et al.: A narrow therapeutical window of a nitric oxide synthase inhibitor against transient ischemic brain injury. Eur. J. Pharmacol. *248:*325–328, 1993.

110. Sancesario, G., Iannone, M., Morello, M., et al.: Nitric oxide inhibition aggravates ischemic damage of hippocampal but not of NADPH neurons in gerbils. Stroke *25:*436–443, 1994.

111. Moncada, C., Lekieffre, D., Arvin, B., et al.: Effect of NO synthase inhibition on NMDA- and ischemia-induced hippocampal lesions. Neuroreport *3:*530–532, 1992.

112. Hunter, T.: Protein kinases and phosphatases: The Yin and Yang of protein phosphorylation and signaling. Cell *80:*225–236, 1995.

113. Miller, S. G., and Kennedy, M. B.: Regulation of brain type II Ca^{2+}/calmodulin-dependent protein kinase by autophosphorylation: A Ca^{2+}-triggered molecular switch. Cell *44:861–870, 1986.*

114. Morioka, M., Fukunaga, K., Yasugawa, S., et al.: Regional and temporal alterations in Ca^{2+}/calmodulin-dependent protein kinase II and calcineurin in the hippocampus of rat brain after transient forebrain ischemia. J. Neurochem. *58:*1798–1809, 1992.

115. Churn, S. B., Limbrick, D., Sombati, S., et al.: Excitotoxic activation of the NMDA receptor results in inhibition of calcium/calmodulin kinase II activity in cultured hippocampal neurons. J. Neurosci. *15:*3200–3214, 1995.

116. Shackelford, D. A., Yeh, R. H., Hsu, M., et al.: Effect of cerebral ischemia on calcium/calmodulin-dependent protein kinase II activity and phosphorylation. J. Cereb. Blood Flow Metab. *15:*450–461, 1995.

117. Aronowski, J., Grotta, J. C., and Waxham, M. N.: Ischemia-induced translocation of Ca^{2+}/calmodulin-dependent protein kinase II: Potential role in neuronal damage. J. Neurochem. *58:*1743–1753, 1992.

118. Hu, B. R., Kamme, F., and Wieloch, T.: Alterations of Ca^{2+}/calmodulin-dependent protein kinase II and its messenger RNA in the rat hippocampus following normo- and hypothermic ischemia. Neurosci. *68:*1003–1016, 1995.

119. Churn, S. B., Taft, W. C., Billingsley, M. S., et al.: Global forebrain ischemia induces a posttranslational modification of multifunctional calcium- and calmodulin-dependent kinase II. J. Neurochem. *59:*1221–1232, 1992.

120. Hiestand, D. M., and Kindy, M. S.: Calcium/calmodulin dependent protein kinase II mRNA in the gerbil brain after cerebral ischemia. Neurosci. Lett. *144:*75–78, 1992.

121. Hanson, S. K., Grotta, J. C., Waxham, M. N., et al.: Calcium/calmodulin-dependent protein kinase II activity in focal ischemia with reperfusion in rats. Stroke *25:*466–473, 1994.

122. Aronowski, J., Waxham, M. N., and Grotta, J. C.: Neuronal protection and preservation of calcium/calmodulin-dependent protein kinase II and protein kinase C activity by dextrorphan treatment in global ischemia. J. Cereb. Blood Flow Metab. *13:*550–557, 1993.

123. Waxham, M. N., Grotta, J. C., Silva, A. J., et al.: Ischemia-induced neuronal damage: A role of calcium/calmodulin-dependent protein kinase II. J. Cereb. Blood Flow Metab. *16:*1–6, 1996.

124. Chapman, P., Frenguelli, B. G., Smith, A., et al.: The alpha-Ca^{2+}/calmodulin kinase II: A bidirectional modulator of presynaptic plasticity. Neuron *14:*591–597, 1995.

125. Kukunaga, K., Soderling, T. R., and Miyamoto, E.: Activation of Ca^{2+}/calmodulin-dependent protein kinase II and protein kinase C by glutamate in

cultures rat hippocampal neurons. J. Biol. Chem. *267*:22527–22533, 1992.

126. Tan, S. E., Wenthold, R. J., and Soderling, T. R.: Phosphorylation of AMPA-type glutamate receptors by calcium/camodulin-dependent protein kinase II and protein kinase C in cultured hippocampal neurons. J. Neurosci. *14*:1123–1129, 1994.

127. Yakel, J. L., Vissavajjhala, P., Derkach, V. A., *et al.*: Identification of a Ca^{2+}/calmoodulin-dependent protein kinase II regulatory phosphorylation site in non-N-methyl-D-aspartate glutamate receptors. Proc. Natl. Acad. Sci. U. S. A. *92*:1376–1380, 1995.

128. McGlade-McCulloh, E., Yamamoto, H., Tan, S. E., *et al.*: Phosphorylation and regulation of glutamate receptors by calcium/calmodulin-dependent protein kinase II. Nature *362*:640–642, 1993.

129. Wyllie, D. J. A., and Nicoll, R. A.: A role for protein kinases and phosphatases in the Ca^{2+}-induced enhancement of hippocampal AMPA receptor-mediated synaptic responses. Neuron *13*:635–643, 1994.

130. Figurov, A., Boddecke, H., and Müller, D.: Enhancement of AMPA-mediated synaptic transmission by the protein phosphatase inhibitor calyculin A in rat hippocampal slices. Eur. J. Neurosci. *5*:1035–1041, 1993.

131. Wyllie, A. H., Morris, R. G., Smith, A. L., *et al.*: Chromatin cleavage in apoptosis: Association with condensed chromatin morphology and dependence of macromolecules. J. Pathol. *142*:67–77, 1984.

132. Tsubokawa, H., Oguro, K., Robinson, H. P., *et al.*: Single glutamate channels in CA1 pyramidal neurones after transient ischaemia. Neuroreport *6*:527–531, 1995.

133. Sheardown, M. J., Nielsen, E. O., Hansen, A. J., *et al.*: 2,3-Dihydroxy-6-nitro-7-sulfamoyl-benzo(F)quinoxaline: A neuroprotectant for cerebral ischemia. Science *247*:571–574, 1990.

134. Sheardown, M. J., Suzdak, P. D., and Nordholm, L.: AMPA, but not NMDA receptor antagonism is neuroprotective in gerbil global ischemia, even delayed 24 h. Eur. J. Pharmacol. *236*:347–353, 1993.

135. Hu, B. R., and Wieloch, T.: Tyrosine phosphorylation and activation of mitogen-activated protein kinase in the rat brain following transient cerebral ischemia. J. Neurochem. *62*:1357–1367, 1994.

136. Wang, Y. T., and Salter, M. W.: Regulation of NMDA receptors by tyrosine kinases and phosphatases. Nature *369*: 233–235, 1994.

137. Hu, B. R., and Wieloch, T.: Casein kinase II activity in the postischemic rat brain increases in brain regions resistant to ischemia and decreases in vulnerable areas. J. Neurochem. *60*:1722–1728, 1993.

138. MacMillan, V., Judge, D., Wiseman, A., *et al.*: Mice expressing a bovine basic fibroblast growth factor transgene in the brain show increased resistance to hypoxemic-ischemic cerebral damage. Stroke *24*: 1735–1739, 1993.

139. Kurino, M., Fukunaga, K., Ushio, Y., *et al.*: Activation of mitogen-activated protein kinase in cultures rat hippocampal neurons by stimulation of glutamate receptors. J. Neurochem. *65*:1282–1289, 1995.

140. Campos-Gonzalez, R., and Kindy, M. S.: Tyrosine phosphorylation of microtubule-associated protein kinase after transient ischemia in the gerbil brain. J. Neurochem. *59*:1955*1958, 1992.*

141. Goto, S., Nagahiro, S., Korematsu, K., *et al.*: Cellular colocalization of calcium/calmodulin-dependent protein kinase II and calcineurin in the rat cerebral cortex and hippocampus. Neurosci. Lett. *149*:189–192, 1993.

142. Yamasaki, Y., Onodera, H., Adachi, K., *et al.*: Alteration in the immunoreactivity of the calcineurin subunits after ischemic hippocampal damage. Neurosci. *49*:545–556, 1992.

143. Lieberman, D. N., and Mody, I.: Regulation of NMDA channel function by endogenous Ca^{2+}-dependent phosphatase. Nature *369*:235–239, 1994.

144. Fleming, L. M., and Johnson, G. V.: Modulation of the phosphorylation state of tau in situ: The roles of calcium and cyclic AMP. Biochem. J. *309*:41–47, 1995.

145. Norman, S. G., and Johnson, G. V.: Compromised mitochondrial function results in dephophshorylation of tau through a calcium-dependent process in rat brain cerebral cortical slices. Neurochem. Res. *19*: 1151–1158, 1994.

146. Litersky, J. M., and Johnson, G. V.: Phosphorylation of tau in situ: Inhibition of calcium-dependent proteolysis. J. Neurochem. *65*:903–911, 1995.

147. Froehner, S. C.: Regulation of ion channel distribution at synapses. Ann. Rev. Neurosci. *16*:347–368, 1993.

148. Nakamura, M., Araki, M., Oguro, K., *et al.*: Differential distribution of 68 Kd and 200 Kd neurofilament proteins in the gerbil hippocampus and their early distributional changes following transient forebrain ischemia. Exp. Brain Res. *89*:31–39, 1992.

149. Kwei, S., Jiang, C., and Haddad, G. G.: Acute anoxia-induced alterations in MAP2 immunoreactivity and neuronal morphology in rat hippocampus. Brain Res. *620*:203–210, 1993.

150. Greenwood, J. A., Troncoso, J. C., Costello, A. C., *et al.*: Phosphorylation modulates calpain-mediated proteolysis and calmodulin binding of the 200-kDa and 160-kDa neurofilament proteins. J. Neurochem. *61*:191–199, 1993.

151. Kampfl, A., Zhao, X., Whitson, J. S., *et al.*: Calpain inhibitors protect against depolarization-induced neurofilament protein loss of septohippocampal neurons in culture. Eur. J. Neurosci. *8*:344–352, 1996.

152. Siman, R., and Noszek, J. C.: Excitatory amino acids activate calpain I and induce structural protein breakdown in vivo. Neuron *1*:279–287, 1988.

153. Seubert, P., Lee, K., and Lynch, G.: Ischemia triggers NMDA receptor-linked cytoskeletal proteolysis in hippocampus. Brain Res. *492*:366–370, 1989.

154. Roberts-Lewis, J. M., Savage, M. J., Marcy, V. R., *et al.*: Immunolocalization of calpain I-mediated spectrin degradation to vulnerable neurons in the gerbil grain. J. Neurosci. *14*:3934–3944, 1994.

155. Lee, K. S., Frank, S., Vanderklish, P., *et al.*: Inhibition of proteolysis protects hippocampal neurons from ischemia. Proc. Natl. Acad. Sci. U. S. A. *88*:7233–7237, 1991.

156. Bading, H., Ginty, D. D., and Greenberg, M. E.: Reg-

ulation of gene expression in hippocampal neurons by distinct calcium signaling pathways. Science *260:*181–186, 1993.

157. Araki, T., Kato, H., Inoue, T., *et al.*: Regional impairment of protein synthesis following brief cerebral ischemia in the gerbil. Acta Neuropathol. *79:*501–505, 1990.

158. Widmann, R., Kuroiwa, T., Bonnekoh, P., *et al.*: [14C]leucine incorporation into brain proteins in gerbils after transient ischemia: Relationship to selective vulnerability of hippocampus. J. Neurochem. *56:*789–796, 1991.

159. Kiessling, M., Stumm, G., Xie, Y., *et al.*: Differential transcription and translation of immediate early genes in the gerbil hippocampus after transient global ischemia. J. Cereb. Blood Flow Metab. *13:*914–924, 1993.

160. Wessel, T. C., Joh, T. H., and Volpe, B. T.: In situ hybridization analysis of c-fos and c-jun expression in the rat brain following transient forebrain ischemia. Brain Res. *567:*231–240, 1991.

161. Hsu, C. Y., An, G., Liu, J. S., *et al.*: Expression of immediate early gene and growth factor mRNAs in a focal ischemia model in the rat. Stroke *24:*178–78, 1993.

162. Collaco-Moraes, Y., Aspey, B. S., deBelleroche, J. S., *et al.*: Focal ischemia causes an extensive induction of immediate early genes that are sensitive to MK-801. Stroke *25:*1855–1860, 1994.

163. Uemura, Y., Kowall, N. W., and Moskowitz, M. A.: Focal ischemia in rats causes time-dependent expression of c-fos protein immunoreactivity in widespread regions of ipsilateral cortex. Brain Res. *552:*99–105, 1991.

164. Suga, S., and Nowak, T. S. J.: Localization of immunoreactive Fos and Jun proteins in gerbil brain: Effect of transient ischemia. J. Cereb. Blood Flow Metab. *11:*S352, 1991.

165. Ogita, K., and Yoneda, Y.: Selective potentiation of DNA binding activities of both activator protein 1 and cyclic AMP response element binding protein through in vivo activation of N-methyl-D-aspartate receptor complex in mouse brain. J. Neurochem. *63:*525–534, 1994.

166. Combs, D. J., Dempsey, R. J., Donaldson, D., *et al.*: Hyperglycemia suppresses c-fos mRNA expression following transient cerebral ischemia in gerbils. J. Cereb. Blood Flow Metab. *12:*169–172, 1992.

167. Struhl, K.: Helix-turn-helix, zinc-finger, and leucine-zipper motifs for eukaryotic transcriptional regulatory proteins. Trends Biochem. Sci. *14:*137–140, 1989.

168. Abe, K., Kawagoe, J., Sato, S., *et al.*: Induction of the 'zinc finger' gene after transient focal ischemia in rat cerebral cortex. Neurosci. Lett. *123:*248–250, 1991.

169. Wilkinson, D. G., Bhatt, S., Chavrier, P., *et al.*: Segment-specific expression of a zinc-finger gene in the developing nervous system of the mouse. Nature *337:*461–464, 1989.

170. Mack, K. J., Cortner, J., Mack, P., *et al.*: krox 20 messenger RNA and protein expression in the adult central nervous system. Brain Res. Mol. Brain Res. *14:*117–123, 1992.

171. An, G., Lin, T. N., Liu, J. S., *et al.*: Induction of Krox-20 expression after focal cerebral ischemia. Biochem. Biophys. Res. Commun. *188:*1104–1110, 1992.

172. Chavrier, P., Zerial, M., Lemaire, P., *et al.*: A gene encoding a protein with zinc fingers is activated during G0/G1 transition in cultured cells. EMBO J. *7:*29–35, 1988.

173. Welch, W. J., Kang, H. S., Beckmann, R. P., *et al.*: Response of mammalian cells to metabolic stress, changes in cell physiology and structure/function of stress proteins. Curr. Top. Microbiol. Immunol. *167:*31–55, 1991.

174. Beckmann, R. P., Mizzen, L. A., and Welch, W. J.: Interaction of Hsp 70 with newly synthesized proteins: Implications for protein folding and assembly. Science *248:*850–854, 1990.

175. Price, B. D., and Calderwood, S. K.: Ca^{2+} is essential for multistep activation of the heat shock factor in permeabilized cells. Mol. Cell. Biol. *11:*3365–3368, 1991.

176. Drummond, I. A., McClure, S. A., Poenie, M., *et al.*: Large changes in intracellular pH and calcium observed during heat shock are not responsible for the induction of heat shock proteins in Drosophila melanogaster. Mol. Cell. Biol. *6:*1767–1775, 1986.

177. Rabindran, S. K., Haroun, R. I., Cios, J., *et al.*: Regulation of heat shock factor trimer formation: Role of a conserved leucine zipper. Science *259:*230–234, 1993.

178. Nowak, T. J., and Jacewicz, M.: The heat shock/stress response in focal cerebral ischemia. Brain Pathol *4:*67–76, 1994.

179. Nowak, T. S. J.: Localization of 70 kDa stress protein mRNA induction in gerbil brain after ischemia. J. Cereb. Blood Flow Metab. *11:*432–439, 1991.

180. Simon, R. P., Cho, H., Gwinn, R., *et al.*: The temporal profile of 72-kDa heat-shock protein expression following global ischemia. J. Neurosci. *11:*881–889, 1991.

181. Sloviter, R. S., and Lowenstein, D. H.: Heat shock protein expression in vulnerable cells of the rat hippocampus as an indicator of excitation-induced neuronal stress. J. Neurosci. *12:*3004–3009, 1992.

182. Welsh, F. A., Moyer, D. J., and Harris, V. A.: Regional expression of heat shock protein-70 mRNA and c-fos mRNA following focal ischemia in rat brain. J. Cereb. Blood Flow Metab. *12:*204–212, 1992.

183. Gonzalez, M. F., Shiraishi, K., Hisanaga, K., *et al.*: Heat shock proteins as markers of neural injury. Brain Res. Mol. Brain Res. *6:*93–100, 1989.

184. Kinouchi, H., Sharp, F. R., Hill, M. P., *et al.*: Induction of 70-kDa heat shock protein and hsp79 mRNA following transient focal cerebral ischemia in the rat. J. Cereb. Blood Flow Metab. *13:*105–115, 1993.

185. Li. Y., Chopp, M., Garcia, J. H., *et al.*: Distribution of the 72-kd heat-shock protein as a function of transient focal cerebral ischemia in rats. Stroke *23:*1292–1298, 1992.

186. Liu, Y., Kato, H., Nakata, N., *et al.*: Protection of rat hippocampus against ischemic neuronal damage by

pretreatment with sublethal ischemia. Brain Res. *586:*121–124, 1992.

187. Glazier, S. S., O'Rourke, D. M., Graham, D. I., *et al.*: Focal induction of heat-shock protein-70 is associated with focal neuroprotection following forebrain ischemia in thei rat. J. Cereb. Blood Flow Metab. *13:*S452, 1993.

188. Levi-Montalcini, R.: The nerve growth factor 35 years later. Science *237:*1154–1162, 1987.

189. Shelton, D. L., and Reichardt, L. F.: Studies on the expression of the beta nerve growth factor (NGF) gene in the central nervous system: Level and regional distribution of NGF mRNA suggest that NGF functions as a trophic factor for several distinct populations of neurons. Proc. Natl. Acad. Sci. U. S. A. *83:*2714–2718, 1986.

190. Lorez, H., Keller, F., Ruess, G., *et al.*: Nerve growth factor increases in adult rat brain after hypoxic injury. Neurosci. Lett. *98:*339–344, 1989.

191. Shozuhara, H., Onodera, H., Katoh-Semba, R., *et al.*: Temporal profiles of nerve growth factor beta-subunit level in rat brain regions after transient ischemia. J. Neurochem. *59:*175–180, 1992.

192. Shigeno, T., Mima, T., Takakura, K., *et al.*: Amelioriation of delayed neuronal death in the hippocampus by nerve growth factor. J. Neurosci. *11:*2914–2919, 1991.

193. Pechan, P. A., Yoshida, T., Panahian, N., *et al.*: Genetically modified fibroblasts producing NGF protect hippocampal neurons after ischemia in the rat. Neuroreport *6:*669–672, 1995.

194. Hofer, M., Pagliusi, S. R., Hohn, A., *et al.*: Regional distribution of brain-derived neurotrophic factor mRNA in the adult mouse brain. EMBO J. *9:*2459–2464, 1990.

195. Lindvall, O., Ernfors, P., Bengzon, J., *et al.*: Differential regulation of mRNAs for nerve growth factor, brain-derived neurotrophic factor, and neurotrophin 3 in the adult rat brain following cerebral ischemia and hypoglycemic coma. Proc. Natl. Acad. Sci. U. S. A. *89:*648–652, 1992.

196. Tsukahara, T., Yonekawa, Y., Tanaka, K., *et al.*: The role of brain-derived neurotrophic factor in transient forebrain ischemia in the rat brain. Neurosurg. *34:*323–331, 1994.

197. Beck, T., Lindholm, D., Castren, E., *et al.*: Brain-derived neurotrophic factor protects against ischemic cell damage in rat hippocampus. J. Cereb. Blood Flow Metab. *14:*689–692, 1994.

198. Merlio, J. P., Ernfors, P., Kokaia, Z., *et al.*: Increased production of the TrkB protein tyrosine kinase receptor after brain insults. Neuron *10:*151–164, 1993.

199. Abraham, J. A., Mergia, A., Whang, J. L., *et al.*: Nucleotide sequence of a bovine clone encoding the angiogenic protein, basic fibroblast growth factor. Science *233:*545–548, 1986.

200. Thomas, K. A., Rios-Candelore, M., Gimenez-Gallego, G., *et al.*: Pure brain-derived acidic fibroblast growth factor is a potent angiogenic vascular endothelial cell mitogen with sequence homology to interleukin 1. Proc. Natl. Acad. Sci. U. S. A. *82:*6409–6413, 1985.

201. Morrison, R. S., Sharma, A., de Vellis, J., *et al.*: Basic fibroblast growth factor supports the survival of cerebral cortical neurons in primary culture. Proc. Natl. Acad. Sci. U. S. A. *83:*7537–7541, 1986.

202. Walicke, P., Cowan, W. N., Ueno, N., *et al.*: Fibroblast growth factor promotes survival of dissociated hippocampal neurons and enhances neurite extension. Proc. Natl. Acad. Sci. U. S. A. *83:*3012–3016, 1986.

203. Mattson, M. P., Murrain, M., Guthrie, P. B., *et al.*: Fibroblast growth factor and glutamate: Opposing roles in the generation and degeneration of hippocampal neuroarchitecture. J. Neurosci. *9:*3728–3740, 1989.

204. Kumon, Y., Sakaki, S., Kadota, O., *et al.*: Transient increase in endogenous basic fibroblast growth factor in neurons of ischemic rat brains. Brain Res. *605:*169–174, 1993.

205. Kato, T., Nakano, S., Kogure, K., *et al.*: The binding of basic fibroblast growth factor to ischemic neurons in the rat. Neuropathol. Appl. Neurobiol. *18:*282–290, 1992.

206. Anderson, K. J., Dam, D., Lee, S., *et al.*: Basic fibroblast growth factor prevents death of lesioned cholinergic neurons in vivo. Nature *332:*360–361, 1988.

207. Hara, H., Onodera, H., Kawagoe, J., *et al.*: Failure of basic fibroblast growth factor to prevent postischemic neuronal damate in the rat. Eur. J. Pharmacol. *209:*195–198, 1991.

208. Tenjin, N., Anderson, R. E., and Meyer, F. B.: Treatment with basic fibroblast growth factor following focal cerebral ischemia does not prevent neuronal injury. J. Neurol. Sci. *128:*66–70, 1995.

209. Sasaki, K., Oomura, Y., Suzuki, K., *et al.*: Acidic fibroblast growth factor prevents death of hippocampal CA1 pyramidal cells following ischemia. Neurochem. Int. *21:*397–402, 1992.

210. Nakata, N., Kato, H., and Kogure, K.: Protective effects of basic fibroblast growth factor against hippocampal neuronal damage following cerebral ischemia in the gerbil. Brain Res. *605:*354–356, 1993.

211. Maiese, K., Boniece, I., DeMeo, D., *et al.*: Peptide growth factors protect against ischemia in culture by preventing nitric oxide toxicity. J. Neurosci. *13:*3034–3040, 1993.

212. Regli, L., Anderson, R. E., and Meyer, F. B.: Basic fibroblast growth factor increases cortical blood flow in vivo. Brain Res. *665:*155–157, 1994.

213. Havrankova, J., Roth, J., and Brownstein, M.: Insulin receptors are widely distributed in the central nervous system of the rat. Nature *272:*827–829, 1978.

214. Bergstedt, K., and Wieloch, T.: Changes in insulin-like growth factor 1 receptor density after transient cerebral ischemia in the rat. Lack of protection against ischemic brain damage following injection of insulin-like growth factor 1. J. Cereb. Blood Flow Metab. *13:*895–898, 1993.

215. Stephenson, D. T., Rash, K., and Clemens, J. A.: Increase in insulin-like growth factor II receptor within ischemic neurons following focal cerebral infarction. J. Cereb. Blood Flow Metab. *15:*1022–1031, 1995.

216. Zhu, C. Z., and Auer, R. N.: Intraventricular administration of insulin and IGF-1 in transient forebrain

ischemia. J. Cereb. Blood Flow Metab. *14:*237–242, 1994.

217. Johnston, B. M., Mallard, E. C., Williams, C. E., *et al.*: Insulin-like growth factor-1 is a potent neuronal rescue agent after hypoxic-ischemic injury in fetal lambs. J. Clin. Invest. *97:*300–308, 1996.

218. Majno, G., and Joris, I.: Apoptosis, oncosis, and necrosis. An overview of cell death. Am. J. Pathol. *146*(w):3–15, 1995.

219. Kirino, T.: Delayed neuronal death in the gerbil hippocampus following ischaemia. Brain Res. *239:*57–69, 1982.

220. Li, Y., Chopp, M., Jiang, N., *et al.*: In situ detection of DNA fragmentation after focal cerebral ischemia in mice. Brain Res. Mol. Brain Res. *28:*164–168, 1995.

221. Kerr, J. F. R.: Shrinkage necrosis: A distinct mode of cellular death. J. Pathol. *105:*13–20, 1971.

222. Sanders, E. J., and Wride, M. A.: Programmed cell death in development. Int. Rev. Cytol. *163:*105–173, 1995.

223. Deckwerth, T. L., and Johnson, E. M.: Neurotrophic factor deprivation-induced death. Ann. NY Acad. Sci. *679:*121–131, 1993.

224. Sloviter, R. S., Dean, E., and Neubort, S.: Electron microscopic analysis of adrenalectomy-induced hippocampal granule cell degeneration in the rat apoptosis in the adult central nervous system. J. Comp. Neurol. *330:*337–351, 1993.

225. Holmgren, L., O'Reilly, M. S., and Folkman, J.: Dormancy of micrometastases; balanced proliferation and apoptosis in the presence of angiogenesis suppression. Nature Med. *1*(2):149–153, 1995.

226. Haimovitz, F. A., Kan, C. C., Ehleiter, D., *et al.*: Ionizing radiation acts on cellular membranes to generate ceramide and initiate apoptosis. J. Exp. Med. *180*(2):525–535, 1994.

227. Gavrieli, Y., Sherman, Y., and Ben-Sasson, S. A.: Identification of programmed cell death in situ via specific labeling of nuclear DNA fragmentation. J. Cell. Biol. *119*(3):493–501, 1992.

228. MacManus, J. P., Buchan, A. M., Hill, I. E., *et al.*: Global ischemia can cause DNA fragmentation indicative of apoptosis in rat brain. Neurosci. Lett. *164:*89–92, 1993.

229. Li, Y., Chopp, M., Jiang, N., *et al.*: Induction of DNA fragmentation after 10 to 120 minutes of focal cerebral ischemia in rats. Stroke *26:*1252–1258, 1995.

230. Linnik, M. D., Miller, J. A., Sprinkle-Cavallo, J., *et al.*: Apoptotic DNA fragmentation in the rat cerebral cortex induced by permanent middle cerebral artery occlusion. Brain Res. Mol. Brain Res. *32:*116–124, 1995.

231. Li, Y., Sharov, V. G., Jiang, N., *et al.*: Ultrastructural and light microscopic evidence of apoptosis after middle cerebral artery occlusion in the rat. Am. J. Pathol., *146:*1045–1051, 1995.

232. Tominaga, T., Kure, S., Narisawa, K., *et al.*: Endonuclease activation following focal ischemic injury in the rat brain. Brain Res. *608:*21–26, 1993.

233. Boise, L. H., Gottschalk, A. R., Quintans, J., *et al.*: Bcl-2 and Bcl-2-related proteins in apoptosis regulation. Curr. Top. Microbiol. Immunol. *200:*107–121, 1995.

234. Krajewski, S., Mai, J. K., Krajewska, M., *et al.*: Upregulation of bax protein levels in neurons following cerebral ischemia. J. Neurosci. *15:*6364–6376, 1995.

235. Chen, J., Graham, S. H., Chan, P. H., *et al.*: bcl-2 is expressed in neurons that survive focal ischemia in the rat. Neuroreport *6:*394–398, 1995.

236. Shimazaki, K., Ishida, A., and Kawai, N.: Increase in bcl-2 oncoprotein and the tolerance to ischemia-induced neuronal death in the gerbil hippocampus. Neurosci. Res. *20:*95–99, 1994.

237. Lawrence, M. S., Ho, D. Y., Sun, G. H., *et al.*: Overexpression of bcl-2 with herpes simplex virus vectors protects CNS neurons against neurological insults in vitro and in vivo. J. Neurosci. *16:*486–496, 1996.

238. Martinou, J. C., Dubois-Dauphin, M., Staple, J. K., *et al.*: Overexpression of bcl-2 in transgenic mice protects neurons from naturally occurring cell death and experimental ischemia. Neuron *13:*1017–1030, 1994.

239. Nicholson, D. W., Ali, A., Thornberry, N. A., *et al.*: Identification and inhibition of the ICE/CED-3 protease necessary for mammalian apoptosis. Nature *376:*37–43, 1995.

240. Kumar, S.: ICE-like proteases in apoptosis. TIBS *20:*198–202, 1995.

241. Lund, L. R., Romer, J., Thomasset, N., *et al.*: Two distinct phases of apoptosis in mammary gland involution: Proteinase-independent and -dependent pathways. Development *122:*181–193, 1996.

242. Kuida, K., Lippke, J. A., Ku, G., *et al.*: Altered cytokine export and apoptosis in mice deficient in interleukin-1 beta converting enzyme. Science *267:*2000–2003, 1995.

243. Li, W. W., Fishman, M. C., and Yuan, J. Y.: Prevention of apoptosis in CNTF-dependent neurons by a mutant ICE and by viral protein CRMA but not by proto-oncogen-product bcl-2. Cell Death Diff. *3:*105–112, 1996.

244. Choi, D. W.: Glutamate neurotoxicity and diseases of the nervous system. Neuron *1:*623–634, 1988.

245. Slater, A. F. G., Stefan, C., Nobel, I., *et al.*: Intracellular redox changes during apoptosis. Cell Death Diff. *3:*57–62, 1996.

246. Dawson, V. L., and Dawson, T. M.: Free radicals and neuronal cell death. Cell Death Diff. *3:*71–78, 1996.

CHAPTER 16

The Genetics of Intracranial Vascular Malformations

JOHN GOLFINOS, M.D., JOSEPH M. ZABRAMSKI, M.D.

INTRODUCTION

The genetic defects underlying the major human cerebrovascular diseases remain unknown. The recent discovery of large families with inherited cerebrovascular malformations has prompted the application of genetic mapping techniques to the search for the genetic defects involved (16, 85). Introduction of the polymerase chain reaction (PCR) and the discovery of new classes of highly polymorphic DNA markers such as restriction fragment length, microsatellite, and short tandem repeat polymorphisms have greatly improved the technology for mapping genetic diseases (10). Progress in sequencing the genome promises that the underlying pathogenetic mechanisms cerebrovascular disease will eventually be revealed.

This chapter reviews current understanding of the inheritance and molecular pathogenesis of the three major cerebral vascular malformations: cavernous malformations (sometimes referred to as cavernous angiomas), arteriovenous malformations, and aneurysms. A candidate gene for familial cavernous malformations has been identified (16). The possible involvement of these genes in related diseases, arteriovenous malformations and aneurysms is discussed. Finally, current knowledge of the genetic mechanisms of intracerebral lobar hemorrhage is reviewed.

CAVERNOUS MALFORMATIONS

Cerebral cavernous malformations are circumscribed conglomerations of dilated, thin-walled capillaries that form "cavernous" spaces (31, 52, 75). They occur throughout the central nervous system in rough proportion to the vol-

ume of the various compartments, 80% above the tentorium, 10 to 15% in the posterior fossa, and 5% in the spine. They usually present with seizures (50 to 60%), headache (20 to 30%) or focal neurological deficits (15 to 20%). In the familial form of the disease, 40% of patients are asymptomatic despite radiographic evidence of one or more cerebral cavernous malformations (90). Magnetic resonance imaging (MRI) is the study of choice for diagnosis. The signal characteristics of these lesions are sufficiently unique to allow accurate diagnosis in most patients without the need for pathologic confirmation (69). Although the details of their natural history are still being elucidated, cavernous malformations pose a life-long risk of hemorrhage, progressive neurological deficit, and debilitating epilepsy (12, 72, 90).

The possibility that cerebral cavernous malformations may be inherited was originally voiced in 1928 (39), but it was not confirmed until discovery in 1982 (26) of a single Mexican-American family that provided 122 individuals for study. Although genetic linkage studies in this family failed to identify an affected gene—few linkage markers were available at that time—the pedigree clearly demonstrated autosomal dominant inheritance with variable penetrance. Six unrelated Mexican-American families were subsequently studied (40, 90). Studies using MRI to detect clinically silent cases, demonstrated that the familial form of the disease is more common and the expression of the genetic defect is more complete than previously suspected. These findings further support an autosomal dominant mode of transmission. A higher incidence of multiple lesions was found in these familial cases; 80% of affected family members have three or more lesions (90). Subsequent reports have confirmed that the familial form of the disease is more prevalent than previously appreciated and that it occurs in many ethnic groups (13, 35, 83, 85).

The congenital nature of the disease has been established by discovery of (20, 76) cavernous malformations in neonates. Cavernous malformations present infrequently in infancy but with an incidence consistent with longitudinal studies that demonstrate an increase in the number and size of lesions in familial cases over time (90). Cases establish that the genetic defect can be expressed early in development (20, 76).

This evidence suggesting hereditary transmission of cavernous malformations prompted searches for the responsible gene using modern linkage markers and techniques. Linkage analysis in a large Hispanic kindred using short tandem repeat polymorphisms (STRPs) localized the gene responsible for the familial form of cerebral cavernous malformations (CCM1) to the long arm of chromosome 7 in the region from q11 to q22 (16). Linkage of the CCM1 to this same region of 7q has recently been confirmed (21, 24).

A large cooperative effort by 9 institutions and 16 laboratories has further narrowed the range of possible location of CCM1 gene on 7q from 33 centimorgans (cM) or 33 million base pairs to 4 cM. This eliminated a number of earlier candidate genes for CCM1, including those encoding elastin, the multiple drug resistant proteins 1 and 3, and the Type I procollagen α-chain (COL2A1) (9, 16, 30).

Other studies have sought clues to the genetic defect of CCM1 in rare familial syndromes that feature cavernous malformations. The association of cavernous malformations with genetic syndromes of limb malformation implicates a possible developmental defect in cartilage formation. One family had two members with both cerebral cavernous malformations and terminal transverse limb defects, several others with only cerebral cavernous malformations, two with retinal cavernous malformations, and still others with cutaneous or visceral cavernous malformations (17). One patient with Robert's syndrome, an autosomal recessive syndrome associated with limb malformations, has been found to have a cavernous malformation of the oculomotor nerve (58). Two alternative hypotheses are suggested by these reports. First, a molecu-

lar defect may be present in one of the 30 or more genes coding for the procollagen α-chains. Second, there may be an error in the post-transcriptional modification and assembly of the procollagen subunits that results in limb malformations and cavernous malformations. Two other familial syndromes with cerebral cavernous malformations have been described. One syndrome includes cerebral cavernous malformations, retinal cavernous malformations, and cutaneous vascular malformations (14). The other includes hepatic angiomas in addition to cerebral and retinal cavernous malformations (15). The molecular pathogenesis of these syndromes is unknown, and it remains unclear if they are separate diseases or just variants of the more common CCM1.

ARTERIOVENOUS MALFORMATIONS (AVMs)

In contrast to cavernous malformations, arteriovenous malformations (AVMs) contain neural parenchyma within their tangled vessels; however, this brain matter is gliotic, disorganized and nonfunctional (48). The vessels are both arterial and venous; the venous walls are markedly thickened. Familial AVMs are exceedingly rare. They are most frequently found in association with uncommon inherited systemic disorders such as Osler-Weber-Rendu disease (hereditary hemorrhagic telangiectasia) (89). Substantial confusion exists in the literature about familial AVMs; some reports likely include familial cavernous malformations (5, 7).

Several recent views, however, have documented familial AVMs (1, 6, 56, 89, 91). In a comprehensive review of 18 patients with multiple cerebral AVMs, 7 (39%) had a familial history of vascular disease while the remainder appeared to be spontaneous in origin (88). In those with a family history, 5 had Osler-Weber-Rendu disease, 1 had Wyburn-Mason syndrome, and 1 case could not be further categorized. Other reports of afflicted families also include cases of hereditary AVMs that cannot be associated with known angiodysplastic syndromes; however, pigmented cutaneous lesions are noted in some of these patients, suggesting that all familial AVM syndromes are related genetically and may even be allelic disorders (88, 91). Indeed, 2 members of a family with cerebral AVMs had pulmonary AVMs without known central nervous system malformations, strongly suggesting Osler-Weber-Rendu disease (91). In another family, the proband had hyperpigmented spots on his lip, raising the possibility of Osler-Weber-Rendu disease (6). The proportion of familial AVM cases related to an underlying angiodysplasia syndrome remains unknown but, based on the above review, may be as high as 50%

Congenital AVMs are a hallmark of the Wyburn-Mason syndrome (49, 61). Named for the authors of the first report in the English literature, this syndrome is characterized by retinal and mesencephalic AVMs and, in some cases, extensive facial nevi (58). The genetic defect is unknown. One case has been reported from the Netherlands Antilles where there is a high incidence of Osler-Weber-Rendu disease, again suggesting that these disorders may reflect different mutations of the same gene (28).

Members of families with Osler-Weber-Rendu disease (2, 28, 33, 36) have high incidences of cerebral AVMs as well as the more common angiodysplastic lesions of the disease, AVMs of the lung, the gastrointestinal system and the nasal mucosa (51). Moreover, multiple cerebral AVMs are not uncommon in this group, in contrast to their low incidence among cases of sporadic AVM (28, 33, 36, 38). Although most neurologic morbidity in this disorder is due to embolization from pulmonary AVMs, hemorrhage from cerebral lesions also contributes significantly (2).

Osler-Weber-Rendu disease is transmitted in autosomal dominant fashion with age-dependent penetrance. One of the genes responsible for this disorder has been identified (51). Linkage studies of a large kindred mapped the gene to chromosome 9 in the region q33-34 (81). Linkage analysis in other kindreds suggested the existence of a second disease locus. The locus on chromosome 9q has been identified as the endoglin gene (51). Endoglin is a receptor for transforming growth factor β (TGF-β) and is the most abundant TGF-β binding protein in endothelial cells (51). TGF-β is a potent angiogenesis factor and plays an important role in tissue repair, growth, and differentiation, especially vascular ingrowth. Endothelial cells lacking competent TGF-β receptors (endoglin) may form abnormal vessels because of a poor response to TGF-β (51). The existence of families affected by Osler-Weber-Rendu disease in which the genetic locus is not linked to 9q33-q34 suggests mutations in genes for other TGF-β receptors or in other unknown vascular genes. Whether defects in the TGF-β receptor genes are responsible for cases of sporadic AVMs remains unknown as does the etiology of AVMs in familial cases unassociated with underlying systemic disorders.

INTRACRANIAL ANEURYSMS

The pathogenesis of cerebral aneurysms remains controversial. As yet, a single molecular defect has not been identified. Controversy centers on the relative importance of acquired factors, such as atherosclerosis and hypertension, and genetically determined alterations in the structure of the arterial wall (84, 87). A combined pathogenesis is also feasible. A genetic lesion might lead to weakness of the vessel wall and increased susceptibility to aneurysm formation. Such a mechanism would explain the increased prevalence of aneurysms with age and the rarity of neonatal aneurysms, even in families with an indisputable inherited predilection (38, 84). Aneurysms also may be the common phenotypic endpoint of genetically heterogeneous diseases.

Evidence for a genetic lesion comes from numerous reports of familial cases of cerebral aneurysms, reports of monozygotic twins with aneurysms, and the existence of connective tissue disorders in which aneurysms play a prominent role (4, 44, 60, 73, 77, 78, 80). There are well-documented reports of families and twins afflicted by intracerebral aneurysms and subarachnoid hemorrhage without an underlying connective tissue disorder (80, 84, 86). Approximately 7% of all intracranial aneurysms are familial (56). Familial cases of aneurysms are characterized by aneurysm rupture at a younger age than in nonfamilial cases (84). Whether the incidence of multiple aneurysms in familial cases is higher than in nonfamilial cases is unclear. The reported pedigrees point to an autosomal dominant genetic defect (84), but the responsible gene has thus far eluded detection.

Efforts to identify the genetic defect have been aided by the recent characterization of the molecular disorders in inherited connective tissue diseases. Ehlers-Danlos syndrome is a heterogeneous group of inherited disorders characterized by hypermobile joints and skin abnormalities (77, 86). Molecular defects in collagen synthesis have been demonstrated for some forms of the disease. Type IV Ehlers-Danlos syndrome is characterized by vessel fragility and easy bruisability. Minor trauma can lead to extensive ecchymoses. Spontaneous dissection and rupture of large extracranial arteries and rupture of the intestines are prominent. These patients also have a high incidence of ruptured cerebral aneurysms and spontaneous carotid-cavernous fistulae (77). The molecular mutation in this form of the disease is in the Type III collagen gene, which encodes an important component of gastrointestinal and vascular connective tissue (77). Type III collagen is composed of three identical α-chains wound in a triple helix. The gene coding for Type III procollagen, COL3A1, has been localized to the distal end of the long arm of chromosome 2. At least eight different point mutations have been characterized in families with this syndrome (29, 37, 40, 57, 66–68). Mosaics that carry the gene but are asymptomatic have also been identified (37, 68).

The attractiveness of the possibility that a molecular defect might contribute to the pathogenesis of aneurysm formation has resulted in a search for Type III collagen defects in both familial and spontaneous cases of cerebral aneurysms. Indeed, several early studies suggested that there were abnormalities in Type III collagen in patients with aneurysms (55, 62); however, subsequent work has failed to confirm these findings (41, 43).

Marfan's syndrome is characterized by a combination of skeletal, ocular, and cardiovascular abnormalities (22, 63, 77). Aortic and mitral valve insufficiency, aneurysmal dilatation of the aortic root, and spontaneous dissection of the aorta are the typical cardiovascular manifestations of this disease. Dissection and aneurysm formation in medium-sized vessels are relatively infrequent. The cardiovascular complications are the cause of death in the vast majority of patients (47, 54, 71). When intracranial aneurysms are present in patients with Marfan's syndrome, they most often involve the cavernous segment of the carotid artery and become symptomatic with mass effect (11, 18, 25, 27, 50, 65, 74, 82). There are, however, reports of patients with Marfan's syndrome who presented with subarachnoid hemorrhage from rupture of an aneurysm (32, 59).

The basic molecular defect in patients with Marfan's syndrome is a mutation in the gene coding for the microfibrillary protein fibrillin (22, 77). Fibrillin is one of the major components of elastin-associated microfibrils. Elastin microfibrils are found in high concentrations in the heart valves and the walls of the large conducting vessels and, to a lesser extent, in smaller arteries. This pattern explains the distribution of the common vascular manifestations of this disease. The gene coding for fibrillin (FBN1) has been localized to chromosome 15 (34), and multiple mutations have been characterized in patients with this disease (19, 22, 53, 64). The prevalence of Marfan's syndrome is about 1 in 10,000 population (22). Marfan's syndrome is inherited as an autosomal dominant trait; however, about 30% of patients have no family history of the disease, and these cases are thought to be caused by new mutations. Fibrillin gene defects have not been reported in cases of familial aneurysms not associated with Marfan's syndrome or in sporadic aneurysms.

Patients with autosomal dominant polycystic kidney disease (ADPKD) suffer from an increased incidence of intracranial aneurysms and intracranial arterial dissections (8, 42, 77). Although the responsible gene in most cases of this disorder has been localized to chromosome 16p (the PKD1 locus), the molecular pathology has not yet been elucidated. The disease is known to be genetically heterogeneous, with 5 to 10% of cases not demonstrating linkage to the PKD1 locus (77). Moreover, intracranial aneurysms tend to occur in some families with ADPKD and not in others. In one report, two of three families with intracranial aneurysms showed linkage to the PKD1 locus (8). Demonstrating the molecular defect resulting from mutations at this locus may provide another clue to the etiology of intracranial aneurysms not related to ADPKD.

Repeated efforts to identify a genetic defect in sporadic cases of intracranial aneurysms have failed. This difficulty may reflect the multiple mutations in structural genes of arterial wall components that might result in aneurysm formation. A review of all cases of α1-antitrypsin deficiency seen at the Mayo Clinic over a 15-year period identified a possible association with ruptured intracranial aneurysms and cervical carotid artery dissection (29). α1-antitrypsin deficiency is implicated in abdominal aortic arterial dissections. Studies of α1-antitrypsin in sporadic cases of aneurysms have not been performed, but α1-antitrypsin deficiency might explain the possible role of smoking as a risk factor for subarachnoid hemorrhage (29). Smoking decreases the efficacy of α1-antitrypsin in its role as an antiproteolytic enzyme.

The ultimate pathogenesis of intracranial aneurysms may rely on contributions from several genes in combination with environmental influences such as smoking and hypertension. No doubt additional gene mutations will be found in familial cases and in other inherited connective tissue disorders. Sporadic cases may result from sporadic mutations or, more likely, from the effects of multiple alleles resulting in a genetically weaker arterial wall that becomes more predisposed to aneurysm formation with the passage of time and under the influence of other environmental factors.

OTHER FAMILIAL SYNDROMES OF VASCULAR MALFORMATIONS

There remains a group of rare, inherited diseases that feature cutaneous vascular malformations in conjunction with spinal or intracerebral vascular abnormalities. Osler-Weber-Rendu disease was discussed above because it is associated with intracranial AVMs. In Sturge-Weber syndrome (encephalotrigeminal angiomatosis), a cutaneous facial nevus is associated with a meningeal nevus composed of venous and capillary channels (49). Klippel-Trenaunay-Weber syndrome combines a cutaneous angioma in proximity to an underlying spinal AVM with occasional hypertrophy of the affected cutaneous region.

SPONTANEOUS INTRACEREBRAL HEMORRHAGE

The genetic defects in two familial forms of lobar intracerebral hemorrhage have been identified (4, 23). A mutation in the amyloid precursor gene causes the Dutch variant of hereditary cerebral hemorrhage with amyloidosis; a mutation in the cystatin C gene is responsible for the Icelandic variant (4, 23). Screening for these mutations in nonfamilial cases revealed no association with sporadic lobar hemorrhage.

CONCLUSION

The rapid evolution of genetic techniques in the past decade has led to an increased appreciation of the molecular pathogenesis of vascular disease. Genetic linkage has been established for the familial form of cavernous malformations as well as for some forms of familial AVMs and aneurysms. That these genetic defects do not account for all cases of these disorders stresses that genetic influences act in the context of environmental influences. Genotype in some diseases such as aneurysms and hemorrhagic stroke may only provide a predisposition and not an ineluctable genetic sentence. Further studies of familial forms of these diseases will uncover additional genetic mechanisms of cerebrovascular diseases.

Acknowledgment

The authors thank the staff of the Neuroscience Publications office for their help in preparing this manuscript.

REFERENCES

1. Aberfeld, D. C., and Rao, K. R. Familial arteriovenous malformations of the brain. Neurology *31:*184–186, 1981.
2. Aesch, B., Lioret, E., de Toffol, B., and Jan, M. Multiple cerebral angiomas and Rendu-Osler-Weber disease: case report. Neurosurgery *29:*599–602, 1991.
3. Aiba, T., Tanaka, R., Koike, T., *et al.* Natural history of intracranial cavernous malformations. J. Neurosurg. *83:*56–59, 1995.
4. Alberts, M. J. Genetic aspects of cerebrovascular disease. Stroke *22:*276–279, 1991.
5. Allard, J. C., Hochberg, F. H., Franklin, P. D., and Carter, A. P. Magnetic resonance imaging in a family with hereditary cerebral arteriovenous malformations. Arch. Neurol. *46:*184–187, 1989.
6. Boyd, M. C., Steinbok, P., and Paty, D. W. Familial arteriovenous malformation. J. Neurosurg. *62:*597–599, 1985.
7. Bucci, M. N., Chandler, W. F., Gebarski, S. S., and McKeever, P. E. Multiple progressive familial thrombosed arteriovenous malformations. Neurosurgery *19:*401–404, 1986.
8. Chauveau, D., Pirson, Y., Verellen-Dumoulin, C., *et al.* Intracranial aneurysms in autosomal dominant polycystic kidney disease. Kidney Int. *45:*1140–1146, 1994.
9. The Chromosome Coordinating Meeting. Human gene mapping: a compendium. 1994 (abstract).
10. Cooper, N. G. *The Human Genome Project: Deciphering the Blueprint of Heredity.* University Science Books, Mill Valley, CA, 1994.
11. Croisille, B., Deruty, R., Pialat, J., *et al.* Anévrysme de la carotide supra-clinoïdienne et méga-dolicho-

artères cervicales dans un syndrome de Marfan. Neurochirurgie *34:*342–347, 1988.

12. Del Curling, O., Jr., Kelly, D. L., Jr., Elster, A. D., and Craven, T. E. An analysis of the natural history of cavernous angiomas. J Neurosurg. *75:*702–708, 1991.

13. Dellemijn, P. L. I., and Vanneste, J. A. L. Cavernous angiomatosis of the central nervous system: usefulness of screening the family. Acta Neurol. Scand. *88:*259–263, 1993.

14. Dobyns, W. B., Michels, V. V., Groover, R. V., *et al.* Familial cavernous malformations of the central nervous system and retina. Ann. Neurol. *21:*578–583, 1987.

15. Drigo, P., Mammi, I., Battistella, P. A., *et al.* Familial cerebral, hepatic, and retinal cavernous angiomas: A new syndrome. Childs Nerv. Syst. *10:*205–209, 1994.

16. Dubovsky, J., Zabramski, J. M., Kurth, J., *et al.* A gene responsible for cavernous malformations of the brain maps to chromosome 7q. Hum. Mol. Genet. *4:*453–458, 1995.

17. Filling-Katz, M. R., Levin, S. W., Patronas, N. J., and Katz, N. N. K. Terminal transverse limb defects associated with familial cavernous angiomatosis. Am. J. Med. Genet. *42:*346–351, 1992.

18. Finney, H. L., Roberts, T. S., and Anderson, R. E. Giant intracranial aneurysm associated with Marfan's syndrome: case report. J. Neurosurg. *45:*342–347, 1976.

19. Francke, U., and Furthmayr, H. Genes and gene products involved in Marfan syndrome. Semin. Thorac. Cardiovasc. Surg. *5:*3–10, 1999.

20. Gangemi, M., Longatti, P., Maiuri, F., *et al.* Cerebral cavernous angiomas in the first year of life. Neurosurgery *25:*465–469, 1989.

21. Gil-Nagel, A., Dubovsky, J., Wilcox, K. J., *et al.* Familial cerebral angioma: an autosomal dominant gene localized to 15 cM interval on human chromosome 7q. Arch. Neurol. 1995, in press.

22. Godfrey, M. The Marfan Syndrome. In: *McKusick's Heritable Disorders of Connective Tissue*, edited by P. Beighton, p. 51. CV Mosby Co., St. Louis, 1993.

23. Graffagnino, C., Herbstreith, M. H., Roses, A. D., and Alberts, M. I. A molecular genetic study of intracerebral hemorrhage. Arch. Neurol. *51:*981–984, 1994.

24. Gunel, M., Awad, I. A., Anson, J., and Lifton, R. P. Mapping of a gene causing cerebral cavernous malformation to 7q11.2–q21. Proc. Natl. Acad. Sci. USA *92:*6620–6624, 1995.

25. Hainsworth, P. J., and Mendelow, A. D. Giant intracranial aneurysm associated with Marfan's syndrome: a case report. J. Neurol. Neurosurg. Psychiatry *54:* 471–472, 1991.

26. Hayman, L. A., Evans, R. A., Ferrell, R. E., *et al.* Familial cavernous angiomas: Natural history and genetic study over a 5-year period. Am. J. Med. Genet. *11:*147–160, 1982.

27. Higashida, R. T., Halbach, V. V., Hieshima, G. B., and Cahan, L. Cavernous carotid artery aneurysm associated with Marfan's syndrome: treatment by balloon embolization therapy. Neurosurgery *22:*297–300, 1988.

28. Jessurun, G. A. J., Kamphuis, D. J., van der Zande, F. H. R., and Nossent, J. C. Cerebral arteriovenous malformations in the Netherlands Antilles: high prevalence of hereditary hemorrhagic telangiectasia-related single and multiple cerebral arteriovenous malformation. Clin. Neurol. Neurosurg. *95:*193–198, 1993.

29. Johnson, P. H., Richards, A. J., Pope, F. M., and Hopkinson, D. A. A COL3A1 glycine 1006 to glutamic acid substitution in a patient with Ehlers-Danlos syndrome type IV detected by denaturing gradient gel electrophoresis. J. Inhert. Metab. Dis. *15:*426–430, 1992.

30. Johnson, E. W., Smith, L. M., Rich, S. S., *et al.* Refined localization of the cerebral cavernous malformation gene (CCM1) to a 4 cM interval of chromosome 7q contained in a well defined YAC contig. Genome Res. 1995, in press.

31. Johnson, P. C., Wascher, T. M., Golfinos, J. G., and Spetzler, R. F. Cavernous malformations: definition and pathologic features. In: *Cavernous Malformations*, edited by I. Awad and D. L. Barrow, p. 1. Park Ridge, IL, American Association of Neurological Surgeons, 1993.

32. Jourdan, C., Artru, F., Convert, J., *et al.* Anévrysme intracranien et dysplasie du tissue élastique: problemes pré et post-opératoires. Agressologie *31:*405–408, 1990.

33. Kadoya, C., Momota, Y., Ikegami, Y., *et al.* Central nervous system arteriovenous malformations with hereditary hemorrhagic telangiectasia: report of a family with three cases. Surg. Neurol. *42:*234–239, 1994.

34. Kainulainen, K., Pulkkinen, L., Savolainen, A., *et al.* Location on chromosome 15 of the gene defect causing Marfan syndrome. N. Engl. J. Med. *323:*935–939, 1990.

35. Kattapong, V. J., Hart, B. L., and Davis, L. E. Familial cerebral cavernous angiomas: clinical and radiologic studies. Neurology *45:*492–497, 1995.

36. Kikuchi, K., Kowada, M., and Sasajima, H. Vascular malformations of the brain in hereditary hemorrhagic telangiectasia (Rendu-Osler-Weber-Disease). Surg. Neurol. *41:*374–380, 1994.

37. Kontusaari, S., Tromp, G., Kuivaniemi, H., *et al.* Substitution of aspartate for glycine 1018 in the type III procollagen (COL3A1) gene causes type IV Ehlers-Danlos syndrome: the mutated allele is present in most blood leukocytes of the asymptomatic and mosaic mother. Am. J. Genet. *51:*497–507, 1992.

38. Kuchelmeister, K., Schulz, R., Bergmann, M., *et al.* A probably familiar saccular aneurysm of the anterior communicating artery in a neonate. Childs Nerv. Syst. *9:*302–305, 1993.

39. Kufs, H., Über heredofamiliäre Angiomatose des Gehirns und der Retina, ihre Beziehungen zueinander und zur Angiomatose der Haut. Z. Neurol. Psychiatra *113:*651–686, 1928.

40. Kuivaniemi, H. Single base mutation that substitutes glutamic acid for glycine 1021 in the COL3A1 gene and causes Ehlers-Danlos type IV. Am. J. Med. Genet. *46:*278–283, 1993.

41. Kuivaniemi, H., Prockop, D. J., Wu, Y., *et al.* Exclusion of mutations in the gene for type III collagen (COL3A1) as a common cause of intracranial aneurysms or cervical artery dissections: results from

sequence analysis of the coding sequences of type III collagen from 55 unrelated patients. Neurology *43:*2652–2658, 1993.

42. Larranaga, J., Rutecki, G. W., Whittier, F. C. Spontaneous vertebral artery dissection as a complication of autosomal dominant polycystic kidney disease. Am. J. Kidney Dis. *25:*70–74, 1995.

43. Leblanc, R., Lozano, A. M., van der Rest, M., and Guttman, R. D. Absence of collagen deficiency in familial cerebral aneurysms. J. Neurosurg. *70:*837–840, 1989.

44. Leblanc, R., Worsley, K. J., Melanson, D., and Tampieri, D. Angiographic screening and elective surgery of familial cerebral aneurysms: a decision analysis. Neurosurgery *35:*9–19, 1994.

45. Madhatheri, S. L., Tromp, G., Gustavason, K. H., and Kuivaniemi, H. Substitution of glutamic acid for glycine 589 in the triple-helical domain of type III procollagen (COL3A1) in a family with variable phenotype of the Ehlers-Danlos syndrome type IV. Hum. Mol. Genet. *3:*511–512, 1994.

46. Marchuk, D. A., Gallione, C. J., Morrison, L. A., *et al.* A locus for cerebral cavernous malformations maps to chromosome 7q in two families. Genomics *28:*311–314, 1995.

47. Marsalese, D. L., Moodie, D. S., Vacante, M., *et al.* Marafan's syndrome: natural history and long-term follow-up of cardiovascular involvement. J. Am. Coll. Cardiol. *14:*422–428, 1989.

48. Martin, N., and Vinters, H. Pathology and grading of intracranial vascular malformations. In: *Intracranial Vascular Malformations,* edited by D. L. Barrow, p. 1. American Association of Neurological Surgeons, Park Ridge, Il, 1990.

49. Martin, N. A., and Vinters, H. V. Arteriovenous malformations. In: *Neurovascular Surgery,* p. 875, edited by L. P. Carter, R. F. Spetzler, and M. G. Hamilton. McGraw-Hill, New York, 1995.

50. Matsuda, M., Matsuda, I., Handa, H., and Okamoto, K. Intracavernous giant aneurysm associated with Marfan's syndrome. Surg. Neurol. *12:*119–121, 1979.

51. McAllister, K. A., Grogg, K. M., Johnson, D. W., *et al.* Endoglin, a TGF-β binding protein of endothelial cells is the gene for hereditary harmorrhagic telangiectasia type 1. Nature Genet. *8:*345–351, 1994.

52. McCormick, W. F. Pathology of vascular malformations of the brain. In: *Intracranial Arteriovenous Malformation,* edited by C. B. Wilson, and B. M. Stein, p. 44. Baltimore, Williams & Wilkins, 1984.

53. Milewicz, D. M., Pyeritz, R. E., Crawford, E. S., and Byers, P. H. Marfan syndrome: Defective synthesis, secretion, and extracellular matrix formation of fibrillin by cultured dermal fibroblasts. J. Clin. Invest. *89:*79–86, 1992.

54. Murdock, J. L., Walker, B. A., Halpern, B. L., *et al.* Life expectancy and causes of death in the Marfan syndrome. N. Engl. J. Med. *286:*804–808, 1972.

55. Neil-Dwyer, G., Bartlett, J. R., Nicholls, A. C., *et al.* Collagen deficiency and ruptured cerebral aneurysms. a clinical and biochemical study. J. Neurosurg. *59:*16–20, 1983.

56. Norrgard, O., Angquist, K. A., Fodstad, H. Intracranial aneurysms and heredity. Neurosurgery *20:*236–239, 1987.

57. Nuytinck, L., DePaepe, A., Renard, J. P., *et al.* Single-strand conformation polymorphism (SSCP) analysis of the COL3A1 gene detects a mutation that results in the substitution of glycine 1009 to valine and causes severe Ehlers-Danlos syndrome type IV. Hum. Mutat. *3:*268–274, 1994.

58. Ogilvy, C. S., Pakzaban, P., and Lee, J. M. Oculomotor nerve cavernous angioma in a patient with Roberts syndrome. Surg. Neurol. *40:*39–42, 1993.

59. Ohtsuki, H., Sugiura, M., Iwaki, K., *et al.* A case of Marfan's syndrome with a ruptured distal middle cerebral aneurysm [Japanese]. No Shinkei Geka *12:*983–985, 1984.

60. Parekh, H. C., Gurusinghe, N. T., and Sharma, R. R. Cerebral berry aneurysms in identical twins: a case report. Surg. Neurol. *38:*277–299, 1992.

61. Patel, U., and Gupta, S. C. Wyburn-Mason syndrome: a case report and review of the literature. Neuroradiology *31:*544–546, 1990.

62. Pope, F. M., Narcisi, P., Neil-Dwyer, G., *et al.* Some patients with cerebral aneurysms are deficient in type III collagen. Lancet *1:*973–975, 1981.

63. Pyeritz, R. E. The Marfan Syndrome. In: *Connective Tissue and Its Heritable Disorders: Molecular, Genetic, and Medical Aspects,* edited by P. M. Royce and B. Steinmann, p. 437. New York, Wiley-Liss, 1993.

64. Pyeritz, R. E., and Francke, U. Conference report: the second international symposium on the Marfan syndrome. Am. J. Med. Genet. *47:*127–135, 1993.

65. Resende, L. A., Asseis, E. A., Costa, L. S., and Gallina, R. A. Sindroma de Marfan e aneurismas intracranionos gigantes: relato de um caso. Arq. Neuropsiquiatr. *42:*294–297, 1984.

66. Richards, A. J., Lloyd, J. C., Narcisi, P., *et al.* A 27-bp deletion from one allele of the type III collagen gene (COL3A1) in a large family with Ehlers-Danlos syndrome type IV. Hum. Genet. *88:*325–330, 1992.

67. Richards, A., Narcisi, P., Lloyd, J., *et al.* The substitution of glycine 661 by arginine in type III collagen produces mutant molecules with thermal stabilities and causes Ehlers-Danlos syndrome type IV. J. Med. Genet. *30:*690–693, 1993.

68. Richards, A. J., Ward, P. N., Narcisi, P., *et al.* A single base mutation in the gene for type III collagen (COL3A1) converts glycine 847 to glutamic acid in a family with Ehlers-Danlos syndrome type IV. An unaffected family members is mosaic for the mutation. Hum. Genet. *89:*414–418, 1992.

69. Rigamonti, D., Drayer, B. P., Johnson, P. C., *et al.* The MRI appearance of cavernous malformations (angiomas). J. Neurosurg. *67:*518–524, 1987.

70. Rigamonti, D., Hadley, M. N., Drayer, B. P., *et al.* Cerebral cavernous malformations: incidence and familial occurrence. N. Engl. J. Med. *319:*343–347, 1988.

71. Roberts, W. C., and Honig, H. S. The spectrum of cardiovascular disease in the Marfan syndrome: a clinico-morphologic study of 18 necropsy patients and comparison to 151 previously reported necropsy patients. Am. Heart J. *104:*115–135, 1982.

72. Robinson, J. R., Jr., Awad, I. A., and Little, J. R.

Natural history of the cavernous angioma. J. Neurosurg. *75:*709–714, 1991.

73. Ronkainen, A., Hernesniemi, J., Ryynanen, M., *et al.* A ten percent prevalence of asymptomatic familial intracranial aneurysms: preliminary report on 110 magnetic resonance angiography studies in members of 21 Finnish familial intracranial aneurysm families. Neurosurgery *35:*208–213, 1994.

74. Rose, B. S., and Pretorius, D. I. Dissecting basilar artery aneurysm in Marfan syndrome: case report. AJNR *12:*503–504, 1991.

75. Russel, D. S., and Rubinstein, L. J. *Pathology of Tumors of the Nervous System*, 4th Ed., p. 116. Williams & Wilkins, Baltimore, 1977.

76. Sakai, N., Yamada, H., Nishimura, Y., *et al.* Intracranial cavernous angioma in the first year of life and a review of the literature. Childs Nerv. Syst. *8:*49–52, 1992.

77. Schievink, W. I., Michels, V. V., and Piepgras, D. G. Neurovascular manifestations of heritable connective tissue disorders: a review. Stroke *25:*889–903, 1994.

78. Schievink, W. I., Mokri, B., Michels, V. V., and Piepgras, D. G. Familial association of intracranial aneurysms and cervical artery dissections. Stroke *22:*1426–1430, 1991.

79. Schievink, W. I., Prakash, U. B. S., Piepgras, D. G., and Mokri, B. a1-antitrypsin deficiency in intracranial aneurysms and cervical artery dissection. Lancet *343:*452–453, 1994.

80. Schievink, W. I., Schaid, D. J., Rogers, H. M., *et al.* On the inheritance of intracranial aneurysms. Stroke *25:*2028–2037, 1994.

81. Shovlin, C. L., Hughes, J. M. B., and Tuddenham, E. G. D., *et al.* A gene for hereditary hemorrhagic telangiectasia maps to chromosome 9q3. Nature Genet. *6:*205–209, 1994.

82. Speciali, J. G. Lison, M. P., and Junqueira, G. L. Aneurysma intracranio no syndrome de Marfan. Arq. Neuropsiquiatr *29:*453–457, 1971.

83. Steichen-Gersdorf, E., Felber, S., Fuchs, W., *et al.* Familial cavernous angiomas of the brain: Observations in a four generation family. Eur. J. Pediatr. *151:*861–863, 1992.

84. ter Berg, H. W. M., Diederik, W. J. D., Limburg, M., *et al.* Familial intracranial aneurysms: a review. Stroke *23:*1024–1030, 1992.

85. Traverso, F., Passeri, F., Pedrinazzi, E., and Reduzzi, L. A family with hereditary intracerebral cavernous angiomas. Nuova Rivista di Neurologia *61:*71–73, 1991.

86. Weir, B. Medical, neurologic, and ophthalmologic aspects of aneurysms. In: *Aneurysms Affecting the Nervous System*, p. 54. Williams & Wilkins, Baltimore, 1987.

87. Weir, B. Pathology. In: *Aneurysms Affecting the Nervous System*. Williams & Wilkins, Baltimore, 1987.

88. Willinsky, R., Lasjaunia, P., Terbrugge, K., and Burrows, P. Multiple cerebral arteriovenous malformations (AVMs). Neuroradiology *32:*207–210, 1990.

89. Yokoyama, K., Asano, Y., Murakawa, T., *et al.* Familial occurrence of arteriovenous malformation of the brain. J. Neurosurg. *74:*585–589, 1991.

90. Zabramski, J. M., Wascher, T. M., Spetzler, R. F., *et al.* The natural history of cavernous malformations: Results of an ongoing study. J. Neurosurg. *80:*422–432, 1994.

91. Zellem, R. T., and Bucheit, W. A. Multiple intracranial arteriovenous malformations: case report. Neurosurgery *17:*88–93, 1985.

CHAPTER 17

Molecular Changes with Subarachnoid Hemorrhage and Vasospasm

R. LOCH MACDONALD, M.D., Ph.D., F.R.C.S.(C), XIAOYU WANG, Ph.D., JOHN ZHANG, M.D., Ph.D., LINDA S. MARTON, Ph.D.

INTRODUCTION

Of the 3521 patients with aneurysmal subarachnoid hemorrhage (SAH) in the most recent cooperative study on the timing of aneurysm surgery, 75% were in good condition on admission (59). After 6 months, 26% were dead, and 58% had recovered fully. Seventy-five percent of the morbidity and mortality was attributable to 3 causes: direct effect of the SAH (25%), vasospasm (32%), and rebleeding (18%). Improvements in outcome for patients with SAH may come through earlier detection and treatment of aneurysms before they rupture, early surgery to prevent rebleeding, and better treatments for the brain damage that results from SAH and vasospasm. The last will require understanding of the molecular basis of the pathophysiology of SAH and vasospasm. This chapter reviews our current knowledge of these events.

ACUTE EFFECTS OF SUBARACHNOID HEMORRHAGE

Nornes measured intracranial pressure during rebleeding from aneurysms in 10 patients and concluded that cessation of bleeding resulted from tamponade of the aneurysm by an increase in intracranial pressure to equal the diastolic blood pressure (108). Blood coagulation also is important. Small hemorrhages not associated with loss of consciousness probably do not cause great increases in intracranial pressure, but severe SAH associated with altered consciousness and a rapid, marked increase in intracranial pressure produces some degree of immediate global cerebral ischemia (32). This has largely been ignored experimentally.

Fein reported that SAH caused impaired brain glucose and oxygen metabolism, an increase in cerebrospinal fluid (CSF) lactate, a depletion of brain high-energy phosphates, an increase in cerebrovascular resistance, and a decrease in cerebral blood flow independent of changes in intracranial pressure, suggesting that subarachnoid blood exerts deleterious effects on the brain (21). Subarachnoid hemorrhage in cats and rats is associated with brain cellular depolarization, inhibition of the Na^+,K^+-ATPase, increased extracellular potassium, and decreased extracellular Ca^{++} (47, 170). This results in cell membrane destabilization, osmotic imbalance, and altered brain electrical conductance (47, 85). Alterations in brain arachidonic acid metabolism may be responsible for some of the alterations in cerebral blood flow and metabolism that occur after SAH (27). The basis for these changes is otherwise unknown. There is induction of c-fos-like immunoreactivity in the brainstem of rats hours after SAH (110). Changes in gene expression following SAH have not otherwise been investigated.

VASOSPASM

Mechanism of Vasospasm

Vasospasm is reversible arterial narrowing that occurs 4 to 12 days after SAH (157). Smooth muscle contraction or vasoconstriction is the primary process that causes this narrowing, although contraction by other cells, alterations in the passive-elastic characteristics of the artery, endothelial proliferation, and mural thrombosis may contribute in some cases (22, 60, 67, 80, 157, 158). While there is no question that endothelial proliferation occurs after SAH, the number and volume of proliferating cells in the arterial wall are not sufficient to cause vasospasm (76, 92, 113). Many of the possible stimuli that might lead to endothelial proliferation also cause smooth muscle contraction, supporting the theory that proliferation is an epiphenomenon or marker of how much vasospasm occurred (34, 62, 143). Smooth muscle cell and endothelial cell damage is associated with endothelial proliferation, and the causes of damage to these cells during spasm include increased shear stress and, possibly, arterial wall hypoxia or some response to prolonged contraction. Oxidative stress from free radicals produced during the oxidation of oxyhemoglobin may be important, as may other unidentified factors (79). The endothelins (ET) and growth factors such as platelet-derived growth factor and insulin-like growth factor-1 are smooth muscle mitogens that also may be involved (34, 62). The factors in hemorrhagic CSF that cause the proliferative responses remain unidentified (143).

Changes in Cerebrospinal Fluid and Release of Potential Spasmogens

Because smooth muscle contraction is the primary process in vasospasm, many studies have attempted to identify vasoactive substances in hemorrhagic CSF (15, 26–28, 53, 56, 78, 86, 87, 111, 125, 132, 136, 157, 158). Limitations of this approach are that concentration of substances in CSF may not reflect their abundance in the arterial wall, that the experiments usually involve short-term responses, and that the interactions that occur *in vivo* between CSF, blood clot, and the artery are neglected. Incubation *in vitro* of blood mixed with CSF results in hemolysis and release of oxyhemoglobin from the erythrocytes (78). Spontaneous oxidation of oxyhemoglobin to methemoglobin occurs with release of heme from globin. *In vivo*, cells in the arachnoid provide heme oxygenase and biliverdin reductase to form biliverdin and bilirubin from heme (73, 78, 102). Other processes associated with the breakdown of sub-

arachnoid blood *in vivo* that do not occur *in vitro* are inflammation, cell death and cell proliferation, and fibrosis.

Numerous experiments show that the component of blood necessary for vasospasm to develop is the erythrocyte, that hemolysis releases a vasoactive substance from the erythrocyte, that this substance is oxyhemoglobin or hemoglobin, and that hemoglobin and its breakdown products are present in CSF during vasospasm (78, 157, 158). Other compounds that bind to hemoglobin or that are present in trace amounts in hemoglobin solutions may account for some of the vasoactivity. For example, Smith *et al.*, found that the factor in CSF that contracted fibroblast-populated collagen lattices was heat stable and had a molecular weight less than 6000 (132). The molecular weight of the hemoglobin tetramer is 64,000, and that of heme is 617. Endotoxin, erythrocyte membrane components, and other stromal proteins may contaminate hemoglobin solutions and be responsible for some of the vasoactivity that has been observed in previous studies (10, 82). Hemoglobin breakdown products are also vasoactive and, furthermore, effects of the intact hemoglobin molecule may differ from those of its metabolites (73, 102). For example, hemoglobin augmented, but ferric and ferrous iron diminished, interleukin-1β-induced nitric oxide synthesis in cultured rat aortic smooth muscle cells (138).

ATP binds avidly to hemoglobin and is present in millimolar quantities in erythrocyte hemolysate (171). ATP caused significant elevations in intracellular Ca^{++} in smooth muscle cells and significant contractions of dog basilar artery *in vitro*. Investigations by Aoki *et al.* also showed that while oxyhemoglobin was vasoactive, its activity was increased to equal that of erythrocyte hemolysate by combining it with a hemolysate fraction of molecular weight 0.5 to 2.0 kD (4). The molecular weight of ATP is 550. Further studies using refined biochemical and purification techniques will be required to determine the exact contributions of ATP and of different components of erythrocyte hemolysate to vasospasm *in vivo*.

Numerous other substances are elevated in CSF after SAH. Interest has focused on vasoactive eicosanoids, endothelins, free radicals, interleukins and other compounds that mediate inflammation, the lipid autocoid platelet activating factor, and mediators of coagulation and fibrinolysis (14, 15, 17, 25–28, 36, 43, 53, 70, 78, 79, 86, 87, 105, 111, 125, 136, 137). Many are elevated in relation to vasospasm, although their direct role in causing spasm is uncertain. Some may be elevated in response to the inflammation or the brain damage associated with SAH (17, 105) and, therefore, may be epiphenomena only secondarily related to vasospasm.

A more fruitful method of investigation may be to measure compounds in subarachnoid clot. Duff's group reported that hemin and bilirubin, breakdown products of hemoglobin, accumulate in subarachnoid clots and cause contraction and increased uptake of Ca^{++} into smooth muscle cells (72, 102, 148).

ROLE OF SMOOTH MUSCLE IN VASOSPASM

Intracellular Ca^{++} and Physiological Smooth Muscle Contraction

A change in intracellular Ca^{++} ($[Ca^{++}]_i$) is the principle regulator of vascular smooth muscle tone (99, 134). This may occur in response to a variety of electrical, mechanical, or chemical stimuli. Elevation of $[Ca^{++}]_i$ results in the binding of Ca^{++} with its receptor protein calmodulin and activation of calmodulin-dependent myosin light-chain kinase, producing a phosphorylated form of myosin that can interact with actin to cause smooth muscle contraction. Four sources of Ca^{++} are available to increase $[Ca^{++}]_i$ in vascular smooth muscle: 1) sarcoplasmic reticulum; 2) extracellular space; 3) Ca^{++} bound to the plasmalemma; and 4) mitochondria. The first two are the most important in smooth muscle. Membrane-bound Ca^{++} probably contributes only minimally to excitation-contraction coupling since only small amounts of Ca^{++} are bound compared with the total requirement for contraction. The Ca^{++} in the mitochondrial matrix of vascular smooth muscle can be mobilized, but its relevance to contraction is still in question, and its efflux pathway is poorly understood (134).

Ca^{++} Release

The sarcoplasmic reticulum is an intracellular system of tubules that functions in Ca^{++} uptake, release, and storage and plays a role in both contraction and relaxation of smooth muscle. Ca^{++} can be released from it by inositol 1,4,5-triphosphate (IP_3) acting on IP_3 receptor or by Ca^{++}-induced Ca^{++} release via the ryanodine receptor. Binding of cell surface receptors by agonists leads to activation of phospholipase C via a G protein-mediated interaction. Phospholipase C forms IP_3 and diacyl glycerol from phosphatidylinositol 4,5-bisphosphate. Diacyl glycerol participates in activation of protein kinase C.

The smooth muscle IP_3 receptor has been isolated from bovine aorta and rat vas deferens (99). The purified receptor is a single polypeptide with a molecular weight of 224–260 kD that probably functions as a tetramer to form the channel. A ryanodine binding protein that functions as a Ca^{++}-induced Ca^{++}-release channel in artificial lipid bilayers has been isolated from skeletal and cardiac muscle. The cDNAs encoding ryanodine receptors in skeletal and cardiac muscle and brain have been cloned, and they share sequence homology with the IP_3 receptor and probably also function as tetramers to form the channel.

Zhang and colleagues studied Ca^{++} release from both IP_3- and ryanodine-sensitive stores in freshly isolated smooth muscle cells from rat basilar artery using fura-2 microfluorimetry (171). Caffeine produces a large transient Ca^{++} release in the presence or absence of external Ca^{++}. This transient release is inhibited by ryanodine, suggesting that caffeine releases Ca^{++} from ryanodine-sensitive stores. KCl causes contraction by membrane depolarization, opening of voltage-gated Ca^{++} channels, and Ca^{++} entry. It may also indirectly activate the ryanodine receptor since KCl-induced Ca^{++} entry triggers Ca^{++} release from Ca^{++} stores, and co-application of KCl with ryanodine enhances the $[Ca^{++}]_i$ level induced by KCl alone (Fig. 1). Receptor agonists such as serotonin and ET-1 generate IP_3 and release Ca^{++} from IP_3-sensitive stores in cerebral smooth muscle cells (Fig. 2) (142). Caffeine increases $[Ca^{++}]_i$ by acting on the ryanodine receptor and releasing Ca^{++}. ATP acts on cell surface purinoceptors and produces a biphasic Ca^{++} elevation: a transient spike followed by a prolonged plateau phase, which is abolished in the absence of extracellular Ca^{++} (171). Pre-incubation of cells with caffeine attenuates the $[Ca^{++}]_i$ response to ATP, and pre-treatment with thapsigargin, a Ca^{++} pump inhibitor that depletes internal Ca^{++} stores, also attenuates the $[Ca^{++}]_i$ peak response to ATP and caffeine.

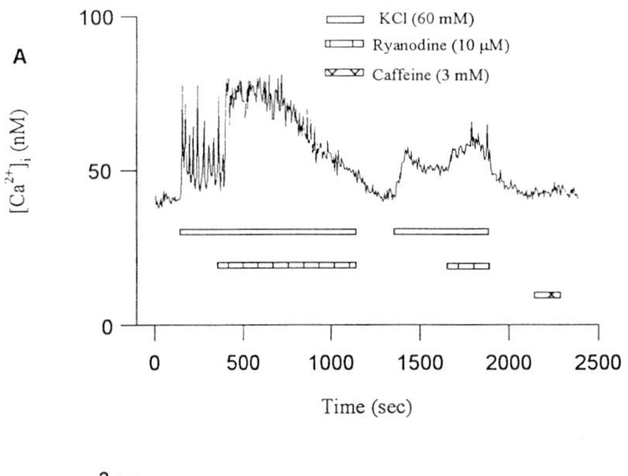

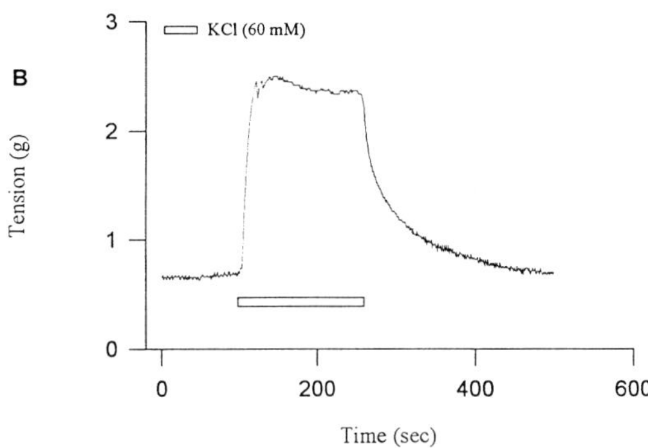

Figure 1. (*A*) Graph of fura-2 microfluorimetric imaging of intracellular Ca^{++} in isolated cerebrovascular smooth muscle cells (171). KCl (60 m*M*) elevates basal $[Ca^{++}]_i$ and induces oscillation. The addition of ryanodine (10 μ*M*) maintains $[Ca^{++}]_i$ to the level of the peak of the oscillation. This increase in $[Ca^{++}]_i$ slowly reverses in the presence of KCl and ryanodine. Subsequent application of KCl elevates $[Ca^{++}]_i$ without inducing oscillation, showing that the oscillation reflects Ca^{++}-induced Ca^{++} release from a ryanodine-sensitive store. Additional ryanodine causes a smaller elevation of $[Ca^{++}]_i$ because of partial depletion of the Ca^{++} stores. Subsequent application of caffeine also fails to increase $[Ca^{++}]_i$ because the stores are depleted. This shows that KCl depolarizes the membrane and causes Ca^{++} influx. The increased $[Ca^{++}]_i$ triggers Ca^{++}-induced Ca^{++} release from ryanodine-sensitive stores. (*B*) KCl produces a sustained contraction when applied to a ring of dog basilar artery suspended under isometric tension.

This suggests that the IP_3-sensitive and ryanodine-sensitive stores in rat basilar smooth muscle cells overlap.

Ca^{++} Influx

Ca^{++} influx from the extracellular space through Ca^{++} channels is important in the maintenance of the tonic phase of smooth muscle contraction. Cell membrane Ca^{++} channels may be activated by depolarization, by an in-

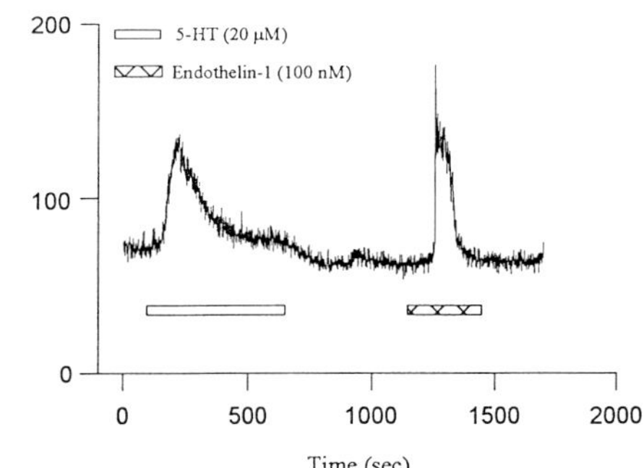

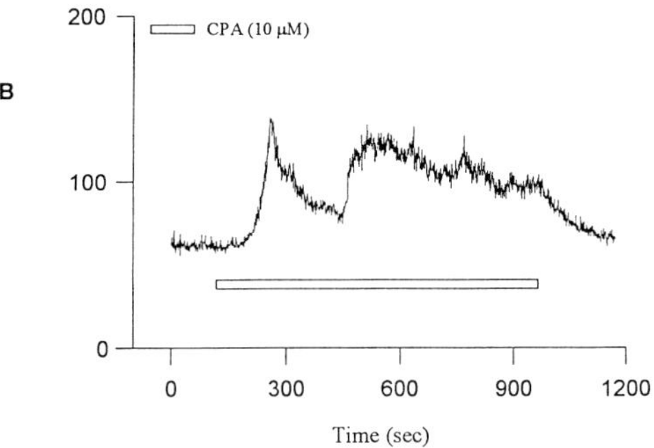

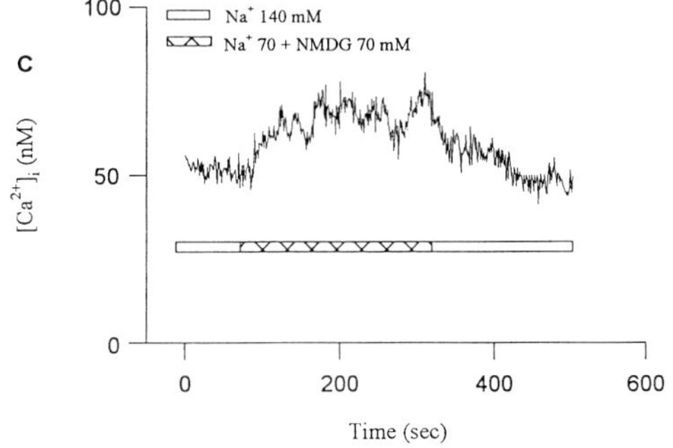

Figure 2. (*A*) Graph of fura-2 microfluorimetric imaging of intracellular Ca^{++} in isolated cerebrovascular smooth muscle cells (171). Serotonin (20 μ*M*) slowly elevates $[Ca^{++}]_i$ that decays within 3 minutes to a level slightly above resting $[Ca^{++}]_i$. ET-1 (100 n*M*) causes a sharp $[Ca^{++}]_i$ spike after a 1-minute delay, which declines to resting $[Ca^{++}]_i$ after 2 to 3 minutes. Both serotonin and ET-1 generate IP_3 after binding to S_2 and ET_A receptors, respectively. (*B*) Cyclopiazonic acid (CPA, 10 μ*M*) in the presence of extracellular Ca^{++} causes a slow increase in $[Ca^{++}]_i$ to a peak followed by a plateau. CPA depletes the Ca^{++} stores by inhibiting the Ca^{++}-ATPase on the sarcoplasmic reticulum. The second increase in $[Ca^{++}]_i$ reflects Ca^{++} influx to refill the stores; the mechanism of this is unknown. (*C*) Replacement of 50% of the Na^+ in the bath solution with N-methyl-D-glucamine produces a 20 to 30 n*M* elevation in $[Ca^{++}]_i$ by reducing the Na^+ available for Na^+-Ca^{++} exchange.

crease in $[Ca^{++}]_i$ produced by release of Ca^{++} from intracellular stores, or by direct opening upon binding of an agonist to its surface-membrane receptor (99).

Multiple Ca^{++} channels have been described in smooth muscle cells, but the L-type Ca^{++} channel plays the dominant role in the upstroke of the action potential and the influx of Ca^{++} during membrane depolarization. The L-type Ca^{++} channels, which are sensitive to dihydropyridines and other organic and inorganic blockers, show a threshold for activation around -40 mV and are fully activated around 0 mV (130). The Ca^{++} flux through these channels is regulated by receptor agonists such as noradrenaline, angiotensin II, ET, serotonin, and ATP, as well as by the membrane potential (99, 160).

Ca^{++} influx also can be triggered by depletion of intracellular Ca^{++} stores (Fig. 2). The exact mechanism of this store-operated Ca^{++} entry is unknown, but it is theorized that an intracellular second messenger tells the plasma membrane channels the state of filling of the stores (99, 134). One theory is that the luminal Ca^{++} in the sacroplasmic reticulum activates a tyrosine phosphatase that shifts a 130-kD protein toward a dephosphorylated state. Depletion of the Ca^{++} stores favors phosphorylation of the 130-kD protein, which then gates a Ca^{++}-permeable membrane channel. Other possibilities are that the luminal Ca^{++} content is signalled to the plasma membrane by a cytochrome P450-dependent mechanism or by a cyclic GMP-mediated signalling system (99).

Contraction and $[Ca^{++}]_i$

There is not a direct relationship between $[Ca^{++}]_i$ and smooth muscle contraction (Fig. 3). Contraction may persist in the absence of high $[Ca^{++}]_i$ or increased myosin light chain phosphorylation (35, 158). Contractions to some agonists develop with minimal or no elevation of intracellular Ca^{++} (39). At least two processes have been postulated to explain prolonged tension development in the absence of increased intracellular Ca^{++} and myosin light chain phosphorylation: a latch state or another regulatory mechanism such as one attributable to phosphorylation of other cytoplasmic proteins by, for example, protein kinase C (35, 39, 114, 158).

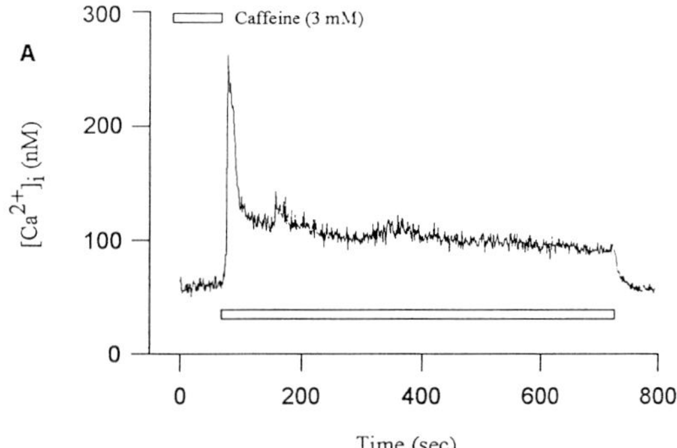

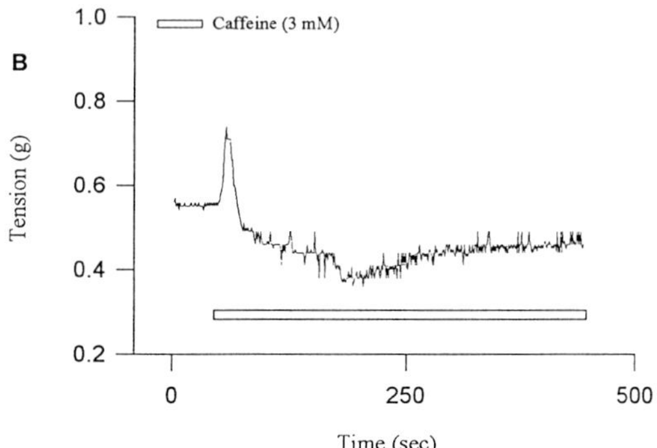

Figure 3. The indirect relationship between $[Ca^{++}]_i$ and contraction is demonstrated. (*A*) Application of caffeine (3 m*M*) to isolated smooth muscle cells (see Fig. 1) causes a rapid increase in $[Ca^{++}]_i$, followed by a prolonged plateau. (*B*) Application of caffeine (3 m*M*) to a ring of dog basilar artery causes a transient contraction, followed by a prolonged relaxation. The relaxation could also manifest the effects of caffeine on endothelial cells.

Molecular Changes in Smooth Muscle during Vasospasm

Studies of isolated cerebrovascular smooth muscle cells show that hemoglobin or erythrocyte hemolysate causes prolonged elevations in $[Ca^{++}]_i$ that are associated with cell contraction, membrane bleb formation, and cell death (79, 135, 139–142). Different experiments on single cells have found these changes are caused by free radicals and by activation of phospholipase C and myosin light chain kinase. During vasospasm in dogs, $[Ca^{++}]_i$ in the basilar artery has been reported to be unchanged or decreased (119, 161). Given the indirect relation between $[Ca^{++}]_i$ and contraction, the significance of these changes remains uncertain.

The ability of smooth muscle cells to regulate $[Ca^{++}]_i$ may be disrupted during vasospasm

(69), or the contractile apparatus may be more sensitive to a given $[Ca^{++}]_i$ (99, 161), leading to unregulated contraction. Further support for this theory is that the plasma membrane Ca^{++}-ATPase that pumps Ca^{++} out of cells and lowers $[Ca^{++}]_i$, is significantly decreased in basilar artery smooth muscle following SAH in dogs (155).

Zhang *et al.* studied the effects of erythrocyte hemolysate on $[Ca^{++}]_i$ in smooth muscle cells (171). Hemolysate released Ca^{++} from cyclopiazonic acid- and thapsigargin-sensitive intracellular stores and promoted Ca^{++} entry via the store-operated Ca^{++} influx pathway. The effect of hemolysate on $[Ca^{++}]_i$ was mediated mainly by small molecules released from erythrocytes, but not by hemoglobin since purified oxyhemoglobin failed to raise $[Ca^{++}]_i$. ATP created effects on $[Ca^{++}]_i$ that were similar to the effects of hemolysate, suggesting that it was the vasoactive component released by hemolysis.

As discussed above, tonic smooth muscle contraction is not usually associated with persistent, high levels of myosin light chain phosphorylation (35, 39, 158). In vasospastic arteries, contractile proteins are decreased and levels of myosin light chain phosphorylation are not markedly elevated (37, 80, 89, 98, 144, 147).

Calponin inhibits the actin-myosin interaction that is the basis of contraction (18, 158). Its action is accentuated when it is phosphorylated by protein kinase C or Ca^{++}-calmodulin-dependent protein kinase II. A decrease in calponin in vasospastic rat femoral arteries could promote vasoconstriction (18). Contractions to a calmodulin inhibitor, trifluoperazine, were increased in spastic dog basilar artery *in vitro*, although trifluoperazine had minimal effect on vasospasm *in vivo* in dogs (112).

Protein kinase C, which is activated by diacyl glycerol in conjunction with IP_3-induced Ca^{++} release, may be involved in tonic smooth muscle contraction and in vasospasm (88, 90). Topical application of the relatively nonspecific protein kinase C inhibitors H-7 and staurosporine reversed vasospasm in dogs (88, 90). The diacyl glycerol content of the basilar artery was elevated and correlated with vasospasm in one study, although this finding was not replicated by other investigators (168). Several investigations support a role for protein kinase C activity in contraction of spastic arteries as evidenced by the increase in the ratio of membrane-bound to soluble activity after SAH in dogs (107, 146, 168). Again, although this ratio was increased, it did not correlate with the time of vasospasm in one study in dogs (120). Numerous forms of protein kinase C have been identified. Only one study of analysis of the isoforms of protein kinase C found a decrease in α and ϵ, but not ζ, isoforms (147). Involvement of IP_3 and protein kinase C in vasospasm was also suggested by observations that oxyhemoglobin elevates intracellular Ca^{++} and IP_3 in cultured smooth muscle cells and that these responses are blocked by neomycin, an inhibitor of phospholipase C (152).

Calpains are neutral proteases that, when activated by increased $[Ca^{++}]_i$, will break down cytoskeletal and contractile proteins and protein kinases, leading in part to activation of these kinases, including protein kinase C (72, 97, 156, 164). Some of the pathways that are activated lead to smooth muscle contraction. The decrease in contractile proteins and in caldesmon, the demonstrated activation of calpain proteolysis, and the efficacy of inhibitors of calpeptin against vasospasm in rats, dogs, and rabbits supports a role for Ca^{++}-activated proteolysis in vasospasm (72, 97, 144, 156, 164).

Smooth muscle cells rely on high energy phosphate compounds such as ATP and GTP in normal contractions and relaxations. Deficiencies, particularly of ATP, can result in rigor in smooth muscle, a state that has some similarities to vasospasm (67, 80, 151). Vasospasm has been associated with a progressive reduction in high-energy phosphates, and there is evidence that hemoglobin and bilirubin can decrease ATP levels, at least in cultured smooth muscle cells (102, 109, 148, 149, 169).

It is clear from the above that our knowledge of physiological smooth muscle contraction is still incomplete, and this probably precludes a complete understanding of the mechanisms of vasospasm at present.

ROLE OF ENDOTHELIUM IN VASOSPASM

Physiological Roles

In addition to being a physical barrier that contains blood in blood vessels, the endothelium plays a critical role in regulation of blood vessel tone and responses to various physiological and pathological stimuli (19, 75). Endothelium produces endothelium-derived relaxing and contracting factors under basal conditions and in response to neurotransmitters, hormones, and physical stimuli. Major alterations in endothelial function are associated with SAH and probably contribute to the pathogenesis of vasospasm.

Endothelium-Derived Relaxing Factors

Vasodilatory substances released from endothelial cells include endothelium-derived relaxing factor (EDRF), prostacyclin, and endothelium-derived hyperpolarizing factor (EDHF) (19, 150). EDRF is nitric oxide (NO) or a NO-containing compound, although its exact identity in the cerebral circulation remains open to question (3, 117). The identity of EDHF remains unclear (29).

Nitric oxide synthase (NOS) catalyzes the conversion of L-arginine into NO and citrulline (19). Three distinct NOSs have been identified and exist predominately in endothelial cells, macrophages, and brain (9, 16, 24, 30, 84, 127). Brain tissue NOS is located predominately in the cytosol (soluble) and endothelial NOS is associated mostly with the plasma membrane (particulate) (24). Brain and endothelial forms are constitutively expressed, resulting in NO release under basal conditions, and are dependent on Ca^{++} and calmodulin for activity, whereas the macrophage enzyme is inducible and has no identified dependence on Ca^{++} and calmodulin for activity (24, 100, 124). Induction of NOS may occur in cells that normally do not express NOS, such as vascular smooth muscle cells, as well as in cells such as endothelia that constitutively express NOS. Stimuli for induction include lipopolysaccharide and cytokines (19).

Basal release of EDRF is augmented by shear stress and a variety of receptor agonists (24, 44). EDRF causes vascular smooth muscle relaxation by activating soluble guanylate cyclase in smooth muscle, resulting in a rise in $3',5'$-guanosine monophosphate (cGMP) (100). Nitrovasodilators such as nitroglycerin and sodium nitroprusside also dilate vessels by this mechanism. Nitric oxide also inhibits platelet aggregation, leucocyte adhesion to endothelial cells, and vascular smooth muscle proliferation and may have an important role in neurotransmission in the peripheral nervous system (24).

Endothelins and Endothelium-Derived Contracting Factors

In 1985, Hickey and colleagues noted release of an endothelium-derived contracting factor from endothelial cells (40). The factor was purified, identified as a 21 amino acid peptide, and named endothelin (ET) in 1988 (165). Three isoforms exist (ET-1, ET-2 and ET-3) that are synthesized from three different genes (50, 133). The ETs are synthesized as large (203 amino acids) preprotein precursors (ppET) that are processed by dibasic pair-specific endopeptidases and carboxypeptidases to yield 30 amino acid intermediates (big ETs). Big ETs, which generally have lower vasoconstrictive activity than their daughter peptides, are converted to ETs by endothelin converting enzyme(s) (133, 165). The ETs are not stored in cells but are secreted constitutively with regulation at the levels of transcription and possibly metabolism (167). They act locally in an autocrine or paracrine fashion and probably do not exert significant endocrine effects (2, 14, 33). Phosphoramidon, a metalloprotease inhibitor, reduces conversion of big ET-1 to ET-1 *in vitro* (49, 95) and *in vivo* (123). The ETs show substantial sequence homology to vasoactive intestinal contractor and 4 sarafotoxins found in snakes (133).

The ETs act via specific receptors (7, 133). ET_A, ET_B, and ET_C receptor subtypes have been identified by molecular genetic analysis (7, 74, 133). The ET_A receptor is selective for ET-1 and ET-2 and is located predominantly on smooth muscle where it mediates contraction (5). The ET_B receptor does not discriminate among the three ET isoforms and is expressed by endothelial cells where the binding of ET causes the release of NO and vasodilation (20, 116, 121). There is substantial variability in the numbers and distribution of ET receptors between different vascular beds and different species. In some cases, ET_B receptors are located on smooth muscle cells where they mediate contraction (83, 126). Pharmacological studies suggest that the situation may be even more complex and not fully explained by the present classification of receptors (7). Despite these differences, infusion of ETs *in vivo* generally causes hypertension although transient hypotension may occur. ET-1 and, at least in primates, ET-3, are potent constrictors of cerebral arteries. The ET_C receptor has high affinity for ET-3 and at present has been identified in mammals in anterior pituitary cells only (122). The ET_A and ET_B receptor polypeptides are seven-looped G-protein coupled receptors (5, 121). The complete intracellular signal transduction pathways for ET-induced vasoconstriction are currently unknown but may involve both opening of cell membrane voltage-gated Ca^{++} channels and activation of phospholipase C (31, 64, 115, 145, 166).

ETs and ET receptors are expressed in many different tissues, and their role extends beyond modulation of vascular tone. They induce smooth muscle proliferation (34). Mice that are deficient in ET-1 are hypertensive and develop with deformities of the first pharyngeal arch (71). Mice lacking ET-3 or the ET_B receptor have defects in neural crest-derived structures manifest by skin depigmentation (piebald appearance) and megacolon resembling Hirschsprung's disease in man (6, 46).

A reduction in NO production or release of cyclooxygenase metabolites or superoxide anion may also be involved in endothelium-dependent contractions, although whether these contractions result from actual release of diffusable substances from endothelial cells is less well documented (150).

EDRF and Changes after SAH

Endothelium-dependent relaxation is impaired in large cerebral arteries after SAH in animals and humans (38, 44, 57, 65, 66, 103, 104). There is evidence that hemoglobin and bloody CSF mediate this impairment, although the exact mechanisms are subject to debate (56, 78). SAH causes endothelial cell denudation and desquamation in cerebral arteries that could reduce NO production although, paradoxically, evidence reviewed below suggests that the same damage is associated with an increase in another endothelium-derived substance, ET-1 (22, 80, 103, 104). Hemoglobin binding of NO may complement the reduced production of NO by endothelial cells, in causing inhibition of endothelium-dependent relaxation after SAH (38, 44, 45, 57, 65, 78, 103). Oxyhemoglobin also undergoes spontaneous oxidation with formation of superoxide anion, a compound that breaks down NO (19, 54). Finally, SAH may decrease GTP in smooth muscle or impair the function of guanylate cyclase in smooth muscle, rendering the muscle unable to relax in response

to NO (63, 66, 68). Evidence from a variety of experimental models indicates that each of these mechanisms may be acting alone, or in concert with others, to reduce endothelium-dependent relaxations, but the exact mechanism involved in man is unclear.

Changes in ETs and ET Receptors after SAH

Cisternal injection of ET-1 into cats and dogs or incubation of canine basilar arteries with ET-1 is associated with potent and long-lasting constriction, indicating that the peptide might be involved in vasospasm (48, 96). This theory is supported by reports that ET-1 and, in some cases, ET-3, are elevated in CSF of patients with SAH, and that higher levels of ET are associated with vasospasm (70, 125, 136, 137). Other studies, however, found no increase or only transient increases (14, 26, 27, 36, 91). Since ETs act by an autocrine or paracrine mechanism, levels in CSF may not reflect those at their site of action in the arterial wall (33). An immunoassay to measure ET-1 in the basilar artery of dogs after SAH found an increase after 2 days that had returned to control levels by 7 days after SAH, although significant vasospasm persisted at day 7 (163). Since ET synthesis is transcriptionally regulated, changes in ppET mRNA levels should directly reflect ET levels in the absence of changes in mechanisms that breakdown ETs. In monkeys, no significant increase in ppET-1 mRNA or protein was observed in vasospastic cerebral arteries 7 days after SAH despite a marked ability of an antagonist of ET_A receptors, BQ-123, to prevent the vasospasm (41, 42). Changes at earlier times were not assessed. Finally, although most studies show that vasospastic arteries have reduced contractile ability (55, 57, 67), arteries may be more sensitive to ETs after SAH, resulting in more vasoconstriction in the presence of low levels of ETs (1). These results are consistent with the unproven hypothesis that vasospasm is caused by prolonged constriction induced by early, transient changes in the ET system.

Further evidence of a role for ETs in vasospasm is the effect of ET receptor antagonists in SAH models (Table 1) (11, 13, 23, 41, 51, 52, 91, 106, 118, 129, 159). Caution is necessary when drawing conclusions about the pathophysiology of a disease based solely on the effect of high doses of a drug that may have multiple or

TABLE 1
Studies of the Effects of ET Antagonists on Experimental Vasospasm

Author, Year	Model	Treatment	Effect on Vasospasm
Matsumura et al., 1991[91]	2-hemorrhage dog	Phosphoramidon, bolus intracisternal, therapeutic	Decreased
Clozel et al., 1993[11]	1-hemorrhage rat	BQ-123 intravenous bolus, therapeutic	No effect
		BQ-123 intracisternal bolus, therapeutic	Decreased
Cosentino et al., 1993[13]	2-hemorrhage dog	Phosphoramidon, bolus intracisternal, prophylactic	No effect
		BQ-123 bolus intracisternal, prophylactic	No effect
Nirei et al., 1993[106]	2-hemorrhage dog	FR139317, bolus intracisternal, prophylactic	Decreased
Itoh et al., 1993[51]	2-hemorrhage dog	BQ-485, continuous intravenous infusion, prophylactic	Decreased
Itoh et al., 1994[52]	2-hemorrhage dog	BQ-123, continuous intracisternal, prophylactic	Decreased
Willette et al., 1994[159]	2-hemorrhage dog	($\pm$)-SB209670, intravenous prophylactic	No effect
		($\pm$)-SB209670, continuous intracisternal, prophylactic	Decreased
Foley et al., 1994[23]	1-hemorrhage rabbit	Topical ET antagonist, therapeutic	Decreased
Roux et al., 1995[118]	2-hemorrhage dog	Bosentan, intravenous bolus, therapeutic	Decreased
Shigeno et al., 1995[129]	2-hemorrhage dog	Bosentan, intravenous bolus, prophylactic	Decreased
Hino et al., 1995[41]	Primate	BQ-123, continuous intracisternal, prophylactic	Decreased
		Bosentan, bolus intracisternal, prophylactic	No effect

nonspecific effects. Few studies have included biochemical measurement of endothelin in models of vasospasm. Studies of ET antagonists against vasospasm show that synthetic peptide (BQ-123, BQ-485) and nonpeptide antagonists (($\pm$)-SB 209670, bosentan) are effective only when administered intracisternally to rats, dogs, rabbits, and monkeys. Failure of bosentan, phosphoramidon, and BQ-123 to prevent vasospasm in some models may reflect experimental design, mode of drug administration, or other factors.

Several investigators have found changes in ET receptors following SAH (42, 52, 118). Cerebral ischemia and other disorders are associated with an increase in ET_B receptor expression (52). In monkey cerebral arteries there is a predominance of ET_A receptor. Vasospastic monkey cerebral arteries show a significant increase in ET_B receptor mRNA at 7 days after SAH that is associated with an increase of ET_B receptor protein (52). A similar shift in expression from ET_A to ET_B receptors occurs after SAH in dogs (118). Itoh et al., however, found an increase in ET_A receptor mRNA 3 days after SAH but not at 7 days in dogs (42).

Inhibition of ET synthesis could prevent the development of vasospasm (128). Actinomycin D, which inhibits RNA and DNA synthesis, was used before the period of vasospasm at a subtherapeutic dose for tumors in dogs. Vasospasm after SAH was prevented completely. Yanagisawa et al. observed specific inhibition of mRNA expression of human ET gene by actinomycin D (166).

CHANGES IN THE EXTRACELLULAR MATRIX DURING VASOSPASM

Role of Changes in the Extracellular Matrix

In addition to those described above, vasospastic-affected arteries undergo other major pathological and pharmacological changes (22, 80, 92, 157, 158). Within 7 days of SAH in dogs, about 75% of angiographic vasospasm can be reversed with papaverine, indicating that most of the spasm is caused by reversible smooth muscle contraction (81). The component of vasospasm attributable to contraction decreased with increasing time from SAH and with increasingly severe vasospasm. Pharmacologically, these changes correlated with progressive decreases in arterial contractility and compliance. Others, notably Vorkapic and coworkers using a rabbit model, have reported similar findings (8, 67, 153, 154). These changes have generally been attributed to arterial wall fibrosis, edema, inflammation, and infiltration with myofibroblasts, although this hypothesis has not been rigorously tested (22, 80, 131, 132, 153, 154, 162). It is equally possible that the pharmacological changes result not from changes in the extracellular matrix but from changes in smooth muscle cells, such as development of rigor, a state associated with similar pharmacological findings (67, 151). The molecular basis of the pharmacological and pathological changes is unknown.

Normal Extracellular Matrix

Extracellular matrix consists of collagens, elastins, glycoproteins, glycosaminoglycans, and proteoglycans. Collagen is the primary component (12, 93, 94). The major structural collagens of the arterial wall are types I and III. These form the fibrils of collagen in the adventitia, media, and intima of cerebral arteries (93). Type IV collagen is found in basement membranes that are formed by and support the endothelial and smooth muscle cells. Basement membranes also contain laminin, heparan sulfate proteoglycan, and entactin. Types V, VI, and VIII collagen are also found in the arterial wall. There are molecular connections between actin in smooth muscle cells, cell membrane structures (that contain vinculin, talin, α-actinin, and integrin receptors), extracellular fibronectin, and the rest of the extracellular matrix so that when the smooth muscle cell contracts, it pulls on the extracellular matrix of the arterial wall to accomplish constriction. Arterial smooth muscle and endothelial cells make up the extracellular matrix, and the matrix, in turn, influences smooth muscle differentiation, migration, and proliferation. Changes in the amount or molecular composition of the extracellular matrix reflect a modification of ongoing synthesis and/or degradation and should alter the mechanical properties of a tissue.

Involvement of Other Cells in the Arterial Wall

Microscopy and immunohistochemistry have been used to characterize cells grown by explant culture from vasospastic human cerebral arteries (131, 132, 162). The cells have characteristics of myofibroblasts such as few thick myofilaments, low positivity for α-actin, and the ability to contract collagen lattices. Myofibroblasts contract healing wounds; they are probably derived from perivascular fibroblasts in vasospastic arteries and cause abnormal contractions and vasospasm (162). They also synthesize type V collagen and extracellular matrix

material that could cause the decreased arterial compliance and fibrosis of vasospasm.

Changes in Extracellular Matrix with Vasospasm

Most reports of matrix changes associated with cerebral vasospasm are only descriptions of light and electron microscopic observations (22, 77, 157, 158). Qualitative accounts of changes in extracellular collagen or other matrix components in vasospastic arteries are unreliable. Several semiquantitative and quantitative studies, however, suggest that arterial fibrosis does occur and that there is an increase in fibronectin in the extracellular matrix. However these changes appear only after angiographic vasospasm has run its course (77, 101, 131). These findings are consistent with a report that mRNA levels for types I and III collagen are increased threefold at 7 and 14 days after blood clot placement around the femoral arteries of rats. The expression of transforming growth factor-beta, a regulator of matrix synthesis, precedes this, suggesting that it is a proximate cause of increased expression of the collagen gene expression (61).

The gross and histopathologic changes in the arterial wall that accompany vasospasm resemble those found in atherosclerosis, hypertension, and after balloon angioplasty (22, 58). Smooth muscle cell proliferation and increased extracellular matrix synthesis are found (34). The hypertrophy of smooth muscle in hypertension is associated with a reduction in elastin and an increase in interstitial collagen that reduce arterial compliance (34). The similarities, however, do not establish that the inciting stimuli (either molecular or other) are the same or that proliferative responses in the arterial wall contribute to vasospasm (76, 92, 113). The factor or factors engendering the active component of vasospasm may also promote smooth muscle hypertrophy or proliferation. For example, angiotensin II, thromboxane A2, and ET-1 are potent vasoconstrictors that also promote growth and some mitogenic growth factors, such as EGF and PDGF, are also vasoactive (34). Stimulation of smooth muscle by external factors can modulate levels of endogenous growth promoters and inhibitors that function in autocrine loops (58).

SUMMARY

Understanding of SAH and vasospasm is quite rudimentary. This reflects the complexity of these phenomena and inadequate knowledge of the normal physiology, molecular biology and genetics, and biochemistry of the arterial wall. Genetic factors predisposing to aneurysm formation, cerebral ischemia, and altered cerebrovascular physiology are incompletely deciphered. Advancement in the field will continue to depend on cooperative efforts of basic scientists and clinicians.

REFERENCES

1. Alafaci, C., Jansen, I., Arbab, M. A. R., *et al.* Enhanced vasoconstrictor effect of endothelin in cerebral arteries from rats with subarachnoid haemorrhage. Acta Physiol Scand *138:*317–319, 1990.
2. Alberts, G. F., Peifley, K. A., Johns, A., *et al.* Constitutive endothelin-1 overexpression promotes smooth muscle cell proliferation via an external autocrine loop. J. Biol. Chem. *269:*10112–10118, 1994.
3. Angus, J. A., and Cocks, T. M. Endothelium-derived relaxing factor. Pharmacol. Ther. *41:*303–352, 1989.
4. Aoki, T., Takenaka, K., Suzuki, S., *et al.* The role of hemolysate in the facilitation of oxyhemoglobin-induced contraction of rabbit basilar arteries. J. Neurosurg. *81:*261–266, 1994.
5. Arai, H., Hori, S., Aramori, I., *et al.* Cloning and expression of a cDNA encoding an endothelin receptor. Nature *348:*730–732, 1990.
6. Baynash, A. G., Hosoda, K., Giaid, A., *et al.* Interaction of endothelin-3 with endothelin-B receptor is essential for development of epidermal melanocytes and enteric neurons. Cell *79:*1277–1285, 1994.
7. Bax, W. A., and Saxena, P. R. The current endothelin receptor classification: time for reconsideration? Trends Pharmacol. Sci. *15:*379–386, 1994.
8. Bevan, J. A., Bevan, R. D., and Frazee, J. G. Functional arterial changes in chronic cerebrovasospasm in monkeys: an in vitro assessment of the contribution to arterial narrowing. Stroke *18:*472–481, 1987.
9. Bredt, D. S., and Snyder, S. H. Nitric oxide, a novel neuronal messenger. Neuron *8:*3–11, 1992.
10. Chang, T. M. S. Blood substitutes based on modified hemoglobin prepared by encapsulation or crosslinking: an overview. Biomat. Art Cells Immob. Biotech. *20:*159–179, 1992.
11. Clozel, M., and Watanabe, H. BQ-123, a peptidic endothelin ET$_A$ receptor antagonist, prevents the early cerebral vasospasm following subarachnoid hemorrhage after intracisternal but not intravenous injection. Life Sci. *52:*825–834, 1993.
12. Clyman, R. I., McDonald, K. A., and Kramer, H. Integrin receptors on aortic smooth muscle cells mediate adhesion to fibronectin, laminin, and collagen. Circ. Res. *67:*175–186, 1990.
13. Cosentino, F., McMahon, E. G., Carter, J. S., and Katusic, Z. S. Effect of endothelin$_A$ antagonist BQ-123 and phosphoramidon on cerebral vasospasm. J. Cardiovasc. Pharmacol. *22*(Suppl 8):S332–S335, 1993.
14. Cosentino, F., and Katusic, Z. S. Does endothelin-1 play a role in the pathogenesis of vasospasm? Stroke *25:*904–908, 1994.
15. D'Avella, D., Germano, A., Santoro, G., *et al.* Effect of experimental subarachnoid hemorrhage on CSF eicosanoids in the rat. J. Neurotrauma *7:*121–129, 1990.
16. Dinerman, J. L., Lowenstein, C. J., and Snyder, S. H. Molecular mechanisms of nitric oxide regulation: potential relevance to cardiovascular disease. Circ. Res. *73:*217–222, 1993.
17. Diringer, M. N., Kirsch, J. R., Ladenson, P. W., *et al.* Cerebrospinal fluid atrial natriuretic factor in intracranial disease. Stroke *21:*1550–1554, 1990.
18. Doi, M., Allen, B. G., Walsh, M. P., *et al.* Involvement of calcium proteins in the development of arterial spasm. In: *Cerebral Vasospasm*, edited by J. M. Findlay. Elsevier, Amsterdam, 1993, pp. 109–112.
19. Faraci, F. M., and Brian, J. E., Jr. Nitric oxide and the cerebral circulation. Stroke *25:*692–703, 1994.
20. Feger, G. I., Schilling, L., Ehrenreich, H., and Wahl, M. Endothelin-induced contraction and relaxation of rat isolated basilar artery: effect of BQ-123. J. Cereb. Blood Flow Metab. *14:*845–852, 1994.
21. Fein, J. M. Cerebral energy metabolism after subarachnoid hemorrhage. Stroke *6:*1–8, 1975.
22. Findlay, J. M., Weir, B. K. A., Kanamaru, K., and Espinosa, F. Arterial wall changes in cerebral vasospasm. Neurosurgery *25:*736–746, 1989.
23. Foley, P. L., Caner, H. H., Kassell, N. F., and Lee, K. S. Reversal of subarachnoid hemorrhage-induced vasoconstriction with an endothelin receptor antagonist. Neurosurgery *34:*108–113, 1994.
24. Forstermann, U., Pollack, J. S., and Nakane, M. Nitric oxide synthases in the cardiovascular system. Trends Cardiovasc. Med. *3:*104–108, 1993.
25. Foy, P. M., and Shaw, M. D. Does thrombin prevent cerebral vasospasm following aneurysmal subarachnoid haemorrhage. Br. J. Neurosurg. *6:*313–319, 1992.
26. Fujimori, A., Yanagisawa, M., Saito, A., *et al.* Endothelin in plasma and cerebrospinal fluid of patients with subarachnoid hemorrhage. Lancet *336:*633, 1990.
27. Gaetani, P., Marzatico, F., and Rodriguez, Y., Baena, R., *et al.* Arachidonic acid metabolism and pathophysiologic aspects of subarachnoid hemorrhage in rats. Stroke *21:*328–332, 1990.
28. Gaetani, P., Rodriguez, Y., Baena, R., Grignani, G., *et al.* Endothelin and aneurysmal subarachnoid haemorrhage: a study of subarachnoid cisternal cerebrospinal fluid. J. Neurol. Neurosurg. Psychiatry *57:*66–72, 1994.
29. Garland, C. J., Plane, F., Kemp, B. K., and Cocks, T. M. Endothelium-dependent hyperpolarization: a role in the control of vascular tone. Trends Pharmacol. Sci. *16:*23–30, 1995.
30. Geller, D. A., Lowenstein, C. J., Shapiro, R. A., *et al.* Molecular cloning and expression of inducible ni-

tric oxide synthase from human hepatocytes. Proc. Natl. Acad. Sci. USA *90:*3491–3495, 1993.

31. Goto, K., Kasuya, Y., Matsuki, N., *et al.* Endothelin activates the dihydropyridine-sensitive, voltage-dependent Ca^{2+} channel in vascular smooth muscle. Proc. Natl. Acad. Sci. USA *86:*3915–3918, 1989.

32. Grote, E., and Hassler, W. The critical first minutes after subarachnoid hemorrhage. Neurosurgery *22:*654–661, 1988.

33. Hahn, A. W. A., Resink, T. J., Scott-Burden, T., *et al.* Stimulation of endothelin mRNA and secretion in rat vascular smooth muscle cells: a novel autocrine function. Cell Regulation *1:*649–659, 1990.

34. Hahn, A. W. A., Resink, T. J., Kern, F., and Buhler, F. R. Peptide vasoconstrictors, vessel structure, and vascular smooth-muscle proliferation. J. Cardiovasc. Pharmacol. *22*(Suppl 5):S37–S43, 1993.

35. Hai, C. M., and Murphy, R. A. Ca^{2+}, crossbridge phosphorylation, and contraction. Annu. Rev. Physiol. *51:*285–298, 1989.

36. Hamann, G., Isenberg, E., Strittmatter, M., and Schimrigk, K. Absence of elevation of big endothelin in subarachnoid hemorrhage. Stroke *24:*383–386, 1993.

37. Harada, T., Seto, M., Sasaki, Y., *et al.* The time course of myosin light-chain phosphorylation in blood-induced vasospasm. Neurosurgery *36:*1178–1183, 1995.

38. Hatake, K., Wakabayashi, I., Kakishita, E., and Hishida, S. Impairment of endothelium-derived relaxing factor after subarachnoid hemorrhage. Stroke *23:*1111–1117, 1992.

39. Heaslip, R. J., and Sickels, B. D. Evidence that prostaglandins can contract the rat aorta via a novel protein kinase C-dependent mechanism. J. Pharmacol. Exp. Ther. *250:*44–51, 1989.

40. Hickey, K. A., Rubanyi, G. M., Paul, R. J., and Highsmith, R. F. Characterization of a coronary vasoconstrictor produced by endothelial cells in culture. Am. J. Physiol. *248:*C550–C556, 1985.

41. Hino, A., Weir, B., Macdonald, R. L., *et al.* Prospective, randomized, double-blind trial of BQ-123 and bosentan for prevention of vasospasm following subarachnoid hemorrhage in monkeys. J. Neurosurg., 1995 (in press).

42. Hino, A., Tokuyama, Y., Kobayashi, M., *et al.* Increased expression of endothelin B receptor mRNA following subarachnoid hemorrhage in monkeys, 1995 (submitted).

43. Hirashima, Y., Edno, S., Ohmori, T., *et al.* Platelet-activating factor (PAF) concentration and PAF acetylhydrolase activity in cerebrospinal fluid of patients with subarachnoid hemorrhage. J. Neurosurg. *80:*31–36, 1994.

44. Hongo, K., Kassell, N. F., Nakagomi, T., *et al.* Subarachnoid hemorrhage inhibition of endothelium-derived relaxing factor in rabbit basilar artery. J. Neurosurg. *69:*247–253, 1988.

45. Hongo, K., Ogawa, H., Kassell, N. F., *et al.* Comparison of intraluminal and extraluminal inhibitory effects of hemoglobin on endothelium-dependent relaxation of rabbit basilar artery. Stroke *19:*1550–1555, 1988.

46. Hosoda, K., Hammer, R. E., Richardson, J. A., *et al.* Targeted and natural (piebald-lethal) mutations of endothelin-B receptor gene produce megacolon associated with spotted coat color in mice. Cell *79:*1267–1276, 1994.

47. Hubschmann, O. R., and Nathanson, D. C. The role of calcium and cellular membrane dysfunction in experimental trauma and subarachnoid hemorrhage. J. Neurosurg. *62:*698–703, 1985.

48. Ide, K., Yamakawa, K., Nakagomi, T., *et al.* The role of endothelin in the pathogenesis of vasospasm following subarachnoid haemorrhage. Neurol. Res. *11:*101–104, 1989.

49. Ikegawa, R., Matsumura, Y., Tsukahara, Y., *et al.* Phosphoramidon, a metalloproteinase inhibitor, suppresses the secretion of endothelin-1 from cultured endothelial cells by inhibiting big endothelin-1 converting enzyme. Biochem. Biophys. Res. Commun. *171:*669–675, 1990.

50. Inoue, A., Yanagisawa, M., Kimura, S., *et al.* The human endothelin family: three structurally and pharmacologically distinct isopeptides predicted by three separate genes. Proc. Natl. Acad. Sci. USA *86:*2863–2867, 1989.

51. Itoh, S., Sasaki, T., Ide, K., *et al.* A novel endothelin ET_A receptor antagonist, BQ-485, and its preventive effect on experimental cerebral vasospasm in dogs. Biochem. Biophys. Res. Commun. *195:*969–975, 1993.

52. Itoh, S., Sasaki, T., Asai, A., and Kuchino, Y. Prevention of delayed vasospasm by an endothelin ET_A receptor antagonist, BQ-123: change of ET_A receptor mRNA expression in a canine subarachnoid hemorrhage model. J. Neurosurg. *81:*759–764, 1994.

53. Itoyama, Y., Fujioka, S., Takaki, S., *et al.* Significance of elevated thrombin-antithrombin III complex and plasmin-α_2-plasmin inhibitor complex in the acute stage of nontraumatic subarachnoid hemorrhage. Neurosurgery *35:*1055–1060, 1994.

54. Kajita, Y., Suzuki, Y., Oyama, H., *et al.* Combined effect of L-arginine and superoxide dismutase on the spastic basilar artery after subarachnoid hemorrhage in dogs. J. Neurosurg. *80:*476–483, 1994.

55. Kamata, K., Nishiyama, H., Miyata, N., and Kasuya, Y. Changes in responsiveness of the canine basilar artery to endothelin-1 after subarachnoid hemorrhage. Life Sci. *49:*217–224, 1991.

56. Kanamaru, K., Waga, S., Kojima, T., *et al.* Endothelium dependent relaxation of canine basilar arteries. Part 2: Inhibition by hemoglobin and cerebrospinal fluid from patients with aneurysmal subarachnoid hemorrhage. Stroke *18:*938–943, 1987.

57. Kanamaru, K., Weir, B. K. A., Findlay, J. M., *et al.* Pharmacological studies on relaxation of spastic primate cerebral arteries in subarachnoid hemorrhage. J. Neurosurg. *71:*909–915, 1989.

58. Karim, M. A., Miller, D. D., Farrar, M. A., *et al.* Histomorphometric and biochemical correlates of arterial procollagen gene expression during vascular repair after experimental angioplasty. Circulation *91:*2049–2057, 1995.

59. Kassell, N. F., Torner, J. C., Haley, E. C., Jr., *et al.* The international cooperative study on the timing of

aneurysm surgery. Part 1: Overall management results. J. Neurosurg. *73:*18–36, 1990.

60. Kassell, N. F., Shaffrey, M. E., Shaffrey, C. I. Cerebral vasospasm following aneurysmal subarachnoid hemorrhage. In: *Brain Surgery. Complication Avoidance and Management*, edited by M. L. J. Apuzzo. Churchill-Livingstone, New York, 1993, pp. 847–856.

61. Kasuya, H., Weir, B. K. A., Shen, Y., *et al.* Procollagen types I and III and transforming growth factor-beta gene expression in the arterial wall after exposure to periarterial blood. Neurosurgery *33:*716–722, 1993.

62. Kasuya, H., Weir, B. K. A., Shen, Y., *et al.* Insulin-like growth factor-1 in the arterial wall after exposure to periarterial blood. Neurosurgery *35:*99–105, 1994.

63. Kasuya, H., Weir, B. K., Nakane, M., *et al.* Nitric oxide synthase and guanylate cyclase levels in canine basilar artery after subarachnoid hemorrhage. J. Neurosurg. *82:*250–255, 1995.

64. Kasuya, Y., Takuwa, Y., Yanagisawa, M., *et al.* Endothelin-1 induces vasoconstriction through two functionally-distinct pathways in porcine coronary artery: contribution of phosphoinositide turnover. Biochem. Biophys. Res. Commun. *161:*1049–1055, 1989.

65. Kim, P., Sundt, T. M., and Vanhoutte, P. M. Alterations in endothelium-dependent responsiveness of the canine basilar artery after subarachnoid hemorrhage. J. Neurosurg. *69:*239–246, 1988.

66. Kim, P., Lorenz, R. R., Sundt, T. M., Jr., and Vanhoutte, P. M. Release of endothelium-dependent relaxing factor after subarachnoid hemorrhage. J. Neurosurg. *70:*108–114, 1989.

67. Kim, P., Sundt, T. M., Jr., and Vanhoutte, P. M. Alterations in mechanical properties in canine basilar arteries after subarachnoid hemorrhage. J. Neurosurg. *71:*430–436, 1989.

68. Kim, P., Schini, V. B., Sundt, T. M., Jr., and Vanhoutte, P. M. Reduced production of cGMP underlies the loss of endothelium-dependent relaxations in the canine basilar artery after subarachnoid hemorrhage. Circ. Res. *70:*248–256, 1992.

69. Kim, P., Yoshimoto, Y., Iino, M., *et al.* Alteration of calcium permeability of the smooth muscle cell membrane in the spastic cerebral arteries. In: *Cerebral Vasospasm*, edited by J. M. Findlay. Elsevier, Amsterdam, 1993, pp. 101–104.

70. Kraus, G. E., Bucholz, R. D., Yoon, K. W., *et al.* Cerebrospinal fluid endothelin-1 and endothelin-3 levels in normal and neurosurgical patients: a clinical study and literature review. Surg. Neurol. *35:*20–29, 1991.

71. Kurihara, Y., Kurihara, H., Suzuki, H., *et al.* Elevated blood pressure and craniofacial abnormalities in mice deficient in endothelin-1. Nature *368:*703–710, 1994.

72. Lee, K. S., Foley, P. L., Vanderklish, P., *et al.* The role of calcium-activated proteolysis in vasospasm after subarachnoid hemorrhage. In: *Cerebral Vasospasm*, edited by J. M. Findlay. Elsevier, Amsterdam, 1993, pp. 85–88.

73. Letarte, P. B., Lieberman, K., Nagatani, K., *et al.* Hemin: levels in experimental subarachnoid hematoma and effects on dissociated vascular smooth muscle cells. J. Neurosurg. *79:*252–255, 1993.

74. Lin, H. Y., Kaji, E. H., Winkel, G. K., *et al.* Cloning and functional expression of a vascular smooth muscle endothelin-1 receptor. Proc. Natl. Acad. Sci. USA *88:*3185–3189, 1991.

75. Luscher, T. F., Yang, Z., Diederich, D., and Buhler, F. R. Endothelium-derived vasoactive substances: potential role in hypertension, atherosclerosis, and vascular occlusion. J. Cardiovasc. Pharmacol. *14*(Suppl. 6):S63–S69, 1989.

76. Macdonald, R. L., Weir, B. K. A., Grace, M. G. A., *et al.* Morphometric analysis of monkey cerebral arteries exposed in vivo to whole blood, oxyhemoglobin, methemoglobin, and bilirubin. Blood Vessels *28:*498–510, 1991.

77. Macdonald, R. L., Weir, B. K. A., Young, J. D., and Grace, M. G. A. Cytoskeletal and extracellular matrix proteins in cerebral arteries following subarachnoid hemorrhage in monkeys. J. Neurosurg. *76:*81–90, 1992.

78. Macdonald, R. L., and Weir, B. K. A. A review of hemoglobin and the pathogenesis of cerebral vasospasm. Stroke *22:*971–982, 1991.

79. Macdonald, R. L., and Weir, B. K. A. Free radicals and vasospasm. Free Radical Biol. Med. *16:*633–644, 1994.

80. Macdonald, R. L. Cerebral Vasospasm. Neurosurg. Q. *5:*73–97, 1995.

81. Macdonald, R. L., Zhang, J., Sima, B., and Johns, L. Papaverine-sensitive vasospasm and arterial contractility and compliance following subarachnoid hemorrhage in dogs. Neurosurgery, 1995 (in press).

82. Macdonald, V. W., and Winslow, R. M. Oxygen delivery and myocardial function in rabbit hearts perfused with cell-free hemoglobin. J. Appl. Physiol. *72:*476–483, 1992.

83. MacLean, M. M. R., McCulloch, K. M., and Baird, M. Endothelin ET_A- and ET_B-receptor-mediated vasoconstriction in rat pulmonary arteries and arterioles. J. Cardiovasc. Pharmacol. *23:*838–845, 1994.

84. Marletta, M. A. Nitric oxide synthase structure and mechanism. J. Biol. Chem. *268:*12231–12234, 1993.

85. Marzatico, F., Gaetani, P., Rodriguez, Y., Baena, R., *et al.* Experimental subarachnoid hemorrhage. Lipid peroxidation and Na^+,K^+-ATPase in different rat brain areas. Mol. Chem. Neuropathol. *11:*99–107, 1989.

86. Mathiesen, T., Andersson, B., Loftenius, A., and von Holst, H. Increased interleukin-6 levels in cerebrospinal fluid following subarachnoid hemorrhage. J. Neurosurg. *78:*562–567, 1993.

87. Mathiesen, T., Fuchs, D., Wachter, H., and von Holst, H. Increased CSF neopterin levels in subarachnoid hemorrhage. J. Neurosurg. *73:*69–71, 1990.

88. Matsui, T., Takuwa, Y., Johshita, H., and Asano, T. Possible role of protein kinase C-dependent smooth muscle contraction in the pathogenesis of chronic cerebral vasospasm. J. Cereb. Blood Flow Metab. *11:*143–149, 1991.

89. Matsui, T., Sugawa, M., Johshita, H., *et al.* Activation of the protein kinase C-mediated contractile system

in canine basilar artery undergoing chronic vasospasm. Stroke *22*:1183–1187, 1991.

90. Matsui, T., Takuwa, Y., Nagafuji, T., *et al.* PKC and chronic cerebral vasospasm. In: *Cerebral Vasospasm*, edited by J. M. Findlay. Elsevier, Amsterdam, 1993, pp. 113–116.

91. Matsumura, Y., Ikegawa, R., Suzuki, Y., *et al.* Phosphoramidon prevents cerebral vasospasm following subarachnoid hemorrhage in dogs: the relationship to endothelin-1 levels in the cerebrospinal fluid. Life Sci. *49*:841–848, 1991.

92. Mayberg, M. R., Okada, T., and Bark, D. H. The significance of morphological changes in cerebral arteries after subarachnoid hemorrhage. J. Neurosurg. *72*:626–633, 1990.

93. Mayne, R. Collagenous proteins of blood vessels. Arteriosclerosis *6*:585–593, 1986.

94. McDonald, J. A. Extracellular matrix assembly. Ann. Rev. Cell. Biol. *4*:183–207, 1988.

95. McMahon, E. G., Palomo, M. A., Moore, W. M., *et al.* Phosphoramidon blocks the pressor activity of porcine big endothelin-1 (1–39) in vivo and conversion of big endothelin-1 (1–39) to endothelin-1 (1–21) in vitro. Proc. Natl. Acad. Sci. USA *88*:703–707, 1991.

96. Mima, T., Yanagisawa, M., Shigeno, T., *et al.* Endothelin acts in feline and canine cerebral arteries from the adventitial side. Stroke *20*:1553–1556, 1989.

97. Minami, N., Tani, E., Maeda, Y., *et al.* Effects of inhibitors of protein kinase C and calpain in experimental delayed cerebral vasospasm. J. Neurosurg. *76*:111–118, 1992.

98. Minami, N., Tani, E., Maeda, Y., *et al.* Immunoblotting of contractile and cytoskeletal protein of canine basilar artery in vasospasm. In: *Cerebral Vasospasm*, edited by J. M. Findlay. Elsevier, Amsterdam, 1993, pp. 141–144.

99. Missiaen, L., De Smedt, H., Droogmans, G., *et al.* Calcium ion homeostasis in smooth muscle. Pharmacol. Ther. *56*:191–231, 1992.

100. Moncada, S., Palmer, R. M. J., and Higgs, E. A. Nitric oxide: physiology, pathophysiology, and pharmacology. Pharmacol. Rev. *43*:109–142, 1991.

101. Nagasawa, S., Handa, H., Naruo, Y., *et al.* Experimental cerebral vasospasm arterial wall mechanics and connective tissue composition. Stroke *13*:595–600, 1982.

102. Nagatani, K., Masciopinto, J. E., Letarte, P. B., *et al.* The effect of hemoglobin and its metabolites on energy metabolism in cultured cerebrovascular smooth muscle cells. J. Neurosurg. *82*:244–249, 1995.

103. Nakagomi, T., Kassell, N. F., Sasaki, T., *et al.* Impairment of endothelium-dependent vasodilation induced by acetylcholine and adenosine triphosphate following experimental subarachnoid hemorrhage. Stroke *18*:482–489, 1987.

104. Nakagomi, T., Kassell, N. F., Sasaki, T., *et al.* Effect of subarachnoid hemorrhage on endothelium-dependent vasodilation. J. Neurosurg. *66*:915–923, 1987.

105. Nakashima, T., Takenaka, K., Nishimura, Y., *et al.* Phospholipase C activity in cerebrospinal fluid following subarachnoid hemorrhage related to brain damage. J. Cereb. Blood Flow Metab. *13*:255–259, 1993.

106. Nirei, H., Hamada, K., Shoubo, M., *et al.* An endothelin ET_A receptor antagonist, FR139317, ameliorates cerebral vasospasm in dogs. Life Sci. *52*: 1869–1874, 1993.

107. Nishizawa, S., Nezu, N., and Uemura, K. Direct evidence for a key role of protein kinase C in the development of vasospasm after subarachnoid hemorrhage. J. Neurosurg. *76*:635–639, 1992.

108. Nornes, H. The role of intracranial pressure in the arrest of hemorrhage in patients with ruptured intracranial aneurysm. J. Neurosurg. *39*:226–234, 1973.

109. Nozaki, K., Okamoto, S., Uemura, Y., *et al.* Changes of glycogen and ATP contents of the major cerebral arteries after experimentally produced subarachnoid hemorrhage in the dog. Acta Neurochir. (Wien) *104*:38–41, 1990.

110. Nozaki, K., Boccalini, P., and Moskowitz, M. A. Expression of c-fos-like immunoreactivity in brainstem after meningeal irritation by blood in the subarachnoid space. Neuroscience *49*:669–680, 1992.

111. O'Neill, P., Walton, S., Foy, P. M., and Shaw, M. D. Role of prostaglandins in delayed cerebral ischemia after subarachnoid hemorrhage. Neurosurgery *30*: 17–22, 1992.

112. Peterson, J. W., Candia, G., Spanos, A. J., and Zervas, N. T. The calmodulin antagonist trifluoperazine provides mild prophylactic protection against cerebral vasospasm after subarachnoid hemorrhage, but no therapeutic value. Neurosurgery *25*:917–922, 1989.

113. Pluta, R. M., Zauner, A., Morgan, J. K., *et al.* Is vasospasm related to proliferative vasculopathy? J. Neurosurg. *77*:740–748, 1992.

114. Rasmussen, H., Takuwa, Y., and Park, S. Protein kinase C in the regulation of smooth muscle contraction. FASEB J. *1*:177–185, 1987.

115. Resink, T. J., Scott-Burden, T., and Buhler, F. R. Endothelin stimulates phospholipase C in cultured vascular smooth muscle cells. Biochem. Biophys. Res. Commun. *157*:1360–1368, 1988.

116. Riezebos, J., Watts, I. S., and Vallance, P. J. T. Endothelin receptors mediating functional responses in human small arteries and veins. Br. J. Pharmacol. *111*:609–615, 1994.

117. Rosenblum, W. I. Endothelium-derived relaxing factor in brain blood vessels is not nitric oxide. Stroke *23*:1527–1532, 1992.

118. Roux, S., Loffler, B. M., Gray, G. A., *et al.* The role of endothelin in experimental cerebral vasospasm. Neurosurgery *37*:78–86, 1995.

119. Sakaki, S., Ohue, S., Kokno, K., Takeda, S. Impairment of vascular reactivity and changes in intracellular calcium and calmodulin levels of smooth muscle cells in canine basilar arteries after subarachnoid hemorrhage. Neurosurgery *25*:753–761, 1989.

120. Sako, M., Nishihara, J., Ohta, S., *et al.* Role of protein kinase C in the pathogenesis of cerebral vasospasm after subarachnoid hemorrhage. J. Cereb. Blood Flow Metab. *13*:247–254, 1993.

121. Sakurai, T., Yanagisawa, M., Takuwa, Y., *et al.* Clon-

ing of a cDNA encoding a non-isopeptide-selective subtype of endothelin receptor. Nature *348:*732–735, 1990.

122. Samson, W. K., Skala, K. D., Alexander, B. D., and Huang, F. S. Pituitary site of action of endothelin: selective inhibition of prolactin release in vitro. Biochem. Biophys. Res. Commun. *169:*737–743, 1990.

123. Sawamura, T., Kimura, S., Shinmi, O., *et al.* Characterization of endothelin converting enzyme activities in soluble fraction of bovine endothelial cells. Biochem. Biophys. Res. Commun. *169:*1138–1144, 1990.

124. Schmidt, H. H. H. W., Lohmann, S. M., and Walter, U. The nitric oxide and cGMP signal transduction system: regulation and mechanism of action. Biochem. Biophys. Acta *1178:*153–178, 1993.

125. Seifert, V., Loffler, B. M., Zimmermann, M., *et al.* Endothelin concentrations in patients with aneurysmal subarachnoid hemorrhage. Correlation with cerebral vasospasm, delayed ischemic neurological deficits, and volume of hematoma. J. Neurosurg. *82:*55–62, 1995.

126. Seo, B., Oemar, B. S., Siebenmann, R., *et al.* Both ET_A and ET_B receptors mediate contraction to endothelin-1 in human blood vessels. Circulation *89:*1203–1308, 1994.

127. Sessa, W. C., Harrison, J. K., Luthin, D. R., *et al.* Genomic analysis and expression patterns reveal distinct genes for endothelial and brain nitric oxide synthase. Hypertension *21:*934–938, 1993.

128. Shigeno, Y., Mima, T., Yanagisawa, M., *et al.* Possible role of endothelin in the pathogenesis of cerebral vasospasm. J. Cardiovasc. Pharmacol. *17*(Suppl. 7):S480–S483, 1991.

129. Shigeno, T., Clozel, M., Sakai, S., *et al.* The effect of bosentan, a new potent endothelin receptor antagonist, on the pathogenesis of cerebral vasospasm. Neurosurgery *37:*87–91, 1995.

130. Simard, J. M. Calcium channel currents in isolated smooth muscle cells from the basilar artery of the guinea pig. Pflügers Arch. *417:*528–536, 1991.

131. Smith, R. R., Clower, B. R., Grotendorst, G. M., *et al.* Arterial wall changes in early human vasospasm. Neurosurgery *16:*171–176, 1985.

132. Smith, R. R., Yamamoto, Y., Clower, B. R., and Bernanke, D. H. Cerebrospinal fluid factors following subarachnoid haemorrhage accelerate collagen lattice contraction by fibroblasts. Neurol. Res. *12:*41–44, 1990.

133. Sokolovsky, M. Endothelins and sarafotoxins: physiological regulation, receptor subtypes and transmembrane signaling. Pharmacol. Ther. *54:*129–149, 1992.

134. Somlyo, A. P., and Somlyo, A. V. Smooth muscle: excitation-contraction coupling, contractile regulation, and the cross-bridge cycle. Alcohol Clin. Exp. Res. *18:*138–143, 1994.

135. Steele, J. A., Stockbridge, N., Maljkovic, G., and Weir, B. K. Free radicals mediate actions of oxyhemoglobin on cerebrovascular smooth muscle cells. Circ. Res. *68:*416–423, 1991.

136. Suzuki, H., Sato, S., Suzuki, Y., Oka, M., *et al.* Endothelin immunoreactivity in cerebrospinal fluid of patients with subarachnoid haemorrhage. Ann. Med. *22:*233–236, 1990.

137. Suzuki, R., Masaoka, H., Hirata, Y., *et al.* The role of endothelin-1 in the origin of cerebral vasospasm in patients with aneurysmal subarachnoid hemorrhage. J. Neurosurg. *77:*96–100, 1992.

138. Suzuki, S., Takenaka, K., Kassell, N. F., and Lee, K. S. Hemoglobin augmentation of interleukin-1β-induced production of nitric oxide in smooth-muscle cells. J. Neurosurg. *81:*895–901, 1994.

139. Takanashi, Y., Fujitsu, K., Fujii, S., and Kuwabara, T. Altered reactivity of hemolysate-treated cultured smooth-muscle cells from rabbit basilar artery determined by digital imaging microscopy. J. Neurosurg. *75:*82–90, 1991.

140. Takanashi, Y., Weir, B. K. A., Vollrath, B., *et al.* Time course of changes in concentration of intracellular free calcium in cultured cerebrovascular smooth muscle cells exposed to oxyhemoglobin. Neurosurgery *30:*346–350, 1992.

141. Takenaka, K., Yamada, H., Sakai, N., *et al.* Cytosolic calcium changes in cultured rat aortic smooth-muscle cells induced by oxyhemoglobin. J. Neurosurg. *74:*620–624, 1991.

142. Takenaka, K., Yamanda, H., Sakai, N., *et al.* Intracellular Ca^{++} changes in cultured vascular smooth muscle cells by treatment with various spasmogens. Neurol. Res. *13:*168–172, 1991.

143. Takenaka, K., Kishino, J., Yamada, J., *et al.* DNA synthesis and intracellular calcium elevation in porcine cerebral arterial smooth muscle cells by cerebrospinal fluid from patients with subarachnoid hemorrhage. Neurol. Res. *14:*330–334, 1992.

144. Takenaka, K., Goto, Y., Kassell, N. F., and Lee, K. S. Modification of vascular smooth muscle proteins in rabbit basilar artery after subarachnoid hemorrhage. In: *Cerebral Vasospasm*, edited by J. M. Findlay. Elsevier, Amsterdam, 1993, pp. 93–96.

145. Takuwa, Y., Kasuya, Y., Takuwa, N., *et al.* Endothelin receptor is coupled to phospholipase C via a pertussis toxin-insensitive guanine nucleotide-binding regulatory protein in vascular smooth muscle cells. J. Clin. Invest. *85:*653–658, 1990.

146. Takuwa, Nishizawa, S., Nezu, N., and Uemura, K. Direct evidence for a key role of protein kinase C in the development of vasospasm after subarachnoid hemorrhage. J. Neurosurg. *76:*635–639, 1992.

147. Takuwa, Y., Matsui, T., Abe, Y., *et al.* Alterations in protein kinase C activity and membrane lipid metabolism in cerebral vasospasm after subarachnoid hemorrhage. J. Cereb. Blood Flow Metab. *13:*409–415, 1993.

148. Trost, G. R., Nagatani, K., Goknur, A. B., *et al.* Bilirubin levels in subarachnoid clot and effects on canine arterial smooth muscle cells. Stroke *24:*1241–1245, 1993.

149. Tsukahara, T., Kassell, N. F., Hongo, K., *et al.* Metabolic alterations in rabbit cerebral arteries caused by subarachnoid hemorrhage. Stroke *19:*883–887, 1988.

150. Vanhoutte, P. M. Other endothelium-derived vasoactive factors. Circulation *87*(Suppl. V):V-9–V-17, 1993.

151. Vinall, P. E., and Simeone, F. A. Effects of oxygen

and glucose deprivation on vasoactivity in isolated bovine middle cerebral arteries. Stroke *17:*970–975, 1986.

152. Vollrath, B. A. M., Weir, B. K. A., Macdonald, R. L., and Cook, D. A. Intracellular mechanisms involved in the responses of cerebrovascular smooth muscle cells to haemoglobin. J. Neurosurg. *80:*261–268, 1994.

153. Vorkapic, P., Bevan, R. D., and Bevan, J. A. Pharmacologic irreversible narrowing in chronic cerebrovasospasm in rabbits is associated with functional damage. Stroke *21:*1478–1484, 1990.

154. Vorkapic, P., Bevan, R. D., and Bevan, J. A. Longitudinal time course of reversible and irreversible components of chronic cerebrovasospasm in the rabbit basilar artery. J. Neurosurg. *74:*951–955, 1991.

155. Wang, J., Ohta, S., Sakaki, S., *et al.* Changes in Ca^{++}-ATPase activity in smooth-muscle cell membranes of the canine basilar artery with experimental subarachnoid hemorrhage. J. Neurosurg. *80:*269–274, 1994.

156. Wang, K. K. W., Yuen, P. W. Calpain inhibition: an overview of its therapeutic potential. Trends Pharmacol. Sci. *15:*412–419, 1994.

157. Weir, B. *Aneurysms affecting the nervous system.* Williams & Wilkins, Baltimore, 1987.

158. Weir, B. The pathophysiology of cerebral vasospasm. Br. J. Neurosurg. *9:*375–390, 1995.

159. Willette, R. N., Zhang, H., Mitchell, M. P., *et al.* Nonpeptide endothelin antagonist. Cerebrovascular characterization and effects on delayed cerebral vasospasm. Stroke *25:*2450–2456, 1994.

160. Xiong, Z., and Sperelakis, N. Regulation of L-type calcium channels of vascular smooth muscle cells. J. Mol. Cell Cardiol. *27:*75–91, 1995.

161. Yamada, T., Tanaka, Y., Fujimoto, K., *et al.* Relationship between cytosolic Ca^{++} level and contractile tension in canine basilar artery of chronic vasospasm. Neurosurgery *34:*496–504, 1994.

162. Yamamoto, Y., Smith, R. R., and Bernanke, D. H. Accelerated nonmuscle contraction after subarachnoid hemorrhage: culture and characterization of myofibroblasts from human cerebral arteries in vasospasm. Neurosurgery *30:*337–345, 1992.

163. Yamaura, I., Tani, E., Maeda, Y., *et al.* Endothelin-1 of canine basilar artery in vasospasm. J. Neurosurg. *76:*99–105, 1992.

164. Yamaura, I., Tani, E., Maeda, Y., *et al.* Calpain-calpastatin system of canine basilar artery in vasospasm. In: *Cerebral Vasospasm,* edited by J. M. Findlay. Elsevier, Amsterdam, 1993, pp. 137–140.

165. Yanagisawa, M., Kurihara, H., Kumura, S., *et al.* A novel potent vasoconstrictor peptide produced by vascular endothelial cells. Nature *332:*411–415, 1988.

166. Yanagisawa, M., Inoue, A., Takuwa, Y., *et al.* The human preproendothelin-1 gene: possible regulation by endothelial phosphoinositide turnover signaling. J. Cardiovasc. Pharmacol. *13*(Suppl. 5): S13–S17, 1989.

167. Yanagisawa, M. The endothelin system: a new target for therapeutic intervention. Circulation *89:*1320–1322, 1994.

168. Yokota, M., Peterson, J. W., Kaoutzanis, M. C., *et al.* Protein kinase C and diacyl glycerol content in basilar arteries during experimental cerebral vasospasm in the dog. J. Neurosurg. *82:*834–840, 1995.

169. Yoshimoto, Y., Kim, P., Sasaki, T., and Takakura, K. Temporal profile and significance of metabolic failure and trophic changes in the canine cerebral arteries during chronic vasospasm after subarachnoid hemorrhage. J. Neurosurg. *78:*807–812, 1993.

170. Yufu, K., Itoh, T., Edamatsu, R., *et al.* Effect of hyperbaric oxygenation on the Na^+,K^+-ATPase and membrane fluidity of cerebrocortical membranes after experimental subarachnoid hemorrhage. Neurochem. Res. *18:*1033–1039, 1993.

171. Zhang, H., Weir, B., Marton, L. S., *et al.* Mechanisms of hemolysate-induced calcium elevation in smooth muscle cells—significance for cerebral vasospasm. Am. J. Physiol. 1995 (in press).

PART V

Mechanisms and Treatment of Nervous System Trauma

CHAPTER 18

Molecular Basis of Head Injury

JACK WILBERGER M.D., F.A.C.S.

INTRODUCTION

The past decade has witnessed a rapid accumulation of information about the pathophysiology of head injury. Over 500 articles have been published exploring diverse cellular and molecular mechanisms such as calcium homoestasis, free radical production excitatoxic neurotransmitters, and inflammation, and their potential contributions to the brain damage secondary to head injury. Recently, the involvement of apoptosis and cellular repair mechanisms have been studied. This research effort is motivated by the conviction that understanding the molecular events leading to traumatic brain injury will lead to interventions capable of limiting the damage or enhancing repair of the damage. Attention to the clinical fundamentals of head injury, i.e. early surgical intervention when indicated, avoidance of hypoxia and hypotension, and maintenance of cerebral perfusion, has led to a significant decline in the mortality of closed head injury in the past 20 years (Fig 1). Manipulation, pharmacological or otherwise, of the molecular events leading to secondary injury may lead to a further improvement in the outcome of closed head injury. The amelioration of secondary injury is one of the major goals of current head injury research.

MECHANISMS OF SECONDARY BRAIN INJURY AFTER TRAUMA

Data from both laboratory and clinical studies of head injury have strongly supported the concept that damage from trauma can be divided into primary, that occurring at the time of impact, and secondary, that occurring after the impact. Impact causes primary anatomic and cellular disruption that initiates a cascade of physiologic, biochemical and genetic events leading to secondary brain injury. The events causing secondary injury evolve over hours and days. The molecular events leading to secondary injury are multifactorial and interrelated. Separating the various components, while somewhat artificial, is necessary for discussion below (Fig 2).

GENERATION OF FREE RADICALS

The contribution of free radicals to secondary brain injury has been well established (5,13,22,28,29). Potential sources for the generation of trauma induced free radicals include components of the arachidonic acid cascade, oxidation of extravasated blood, and neutrophilic infiltration of an area of tissue damage. The vascular endothelium can generate large amounts of free radicals, especially superoxide, in the presence of trauma induced loss of autoregulation and blood brain barrier disruption. Especially important are oxygen containing free radicals generated after head injury, including the superoxide free radical, the hyydroxyl free radical, hydrogen peroxide, singlet oxygen, and nitrous oxide. These free radicals can disrupt cellular function by oxidizing proteins or lipids of the cell membrane, mitochondrial membranes and lysosomal membranes. Sufficient lipid peroxidation, the combination of a free radical with unsaturated fatty acid phospholipid side chains, can lead to disruption of the oxidized membrane.

Under normal circumstances, the small amount of free radicals produced by cellular metabolic process are "quenched" by endoge-

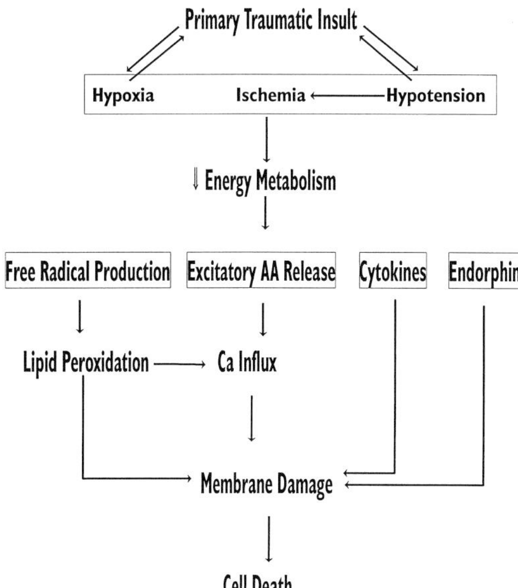

Figure 1. Mortality statistics, closed head injury, 1970–1990.

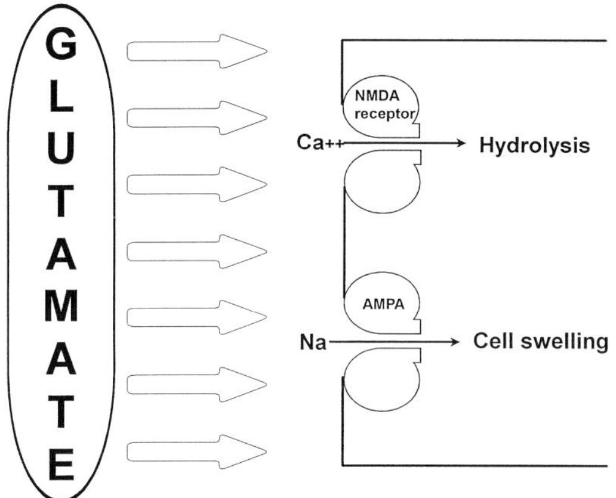

Figure 2. Molecular mechanisms of secondary brain injury.

nous anti-oxidants such as vitamins C and E and intracellular enzymes such as superoxide dismutase. In the presence of head injury, the production of free radicals can overwhelm these "quenching" mechanisms, leaving free radicals available to cause oxidative damage to the cell.

Free radical production by the arachidonic acid cascade has been extensively studied (29,30). Closed head injury produces a transient increase in the level of free arachidonic acid. Superoxide is a by-product of the normal metabolism of arachidonic acid via the cyclo-oxygenase and lipooxygenase pathways. The increased levels of arachidonic acid present after head injury leads to increased superoxide production as the acid is metabolized via these pathways.

Mitochondrial oxidative phosphorylation is another normal source of free radical production in the cell. Production of ATP by mitochondria involves the generation of superoxide when an electron is removed from the oxygen molecule. After trauma, oxygen consumption by the mitochondria is increased, while ATP production is decreased. This uncoupling of oxidation and ATP synthesis leads to overproduction of superoxide (33,53), which can then oxidize lipids of the mitochondrial membrane.

Iron can serve as a catalyst for free radical mediated oxidation. The presence of iron in hemorrhagic tissue may lead to enhanced secondary tissue damage, as tissue oxidation by free radicals in this tissue is increased by the catalytic activity of iron released from hemoglobin.

Once lipid peroxidation by free radicals has occurred, a chain reaction is begun that eventually causes the loss of membrane integrity with resultant ion fluxes leading to cell death.

DISRUPTION OF CALCIUM HOMEOSTASIS

Brain trauma causes extensive neuronal membrane depolarization. Voltage sensitive calcium channels are opened in a nonspecific fashion in the face of this depolarization, leading to influx and abnormal accumulation of intracellular calcium in neurons and glia (48,52). The abnormal increase in intracellular calcium initiates a cascade of events resulting in activation of lipolytic enzymes, proteolytic enzymes, protein kinases, and protein phosphatases, dissolution of microtubules, initiation of the arachidonic acid cascade, and altered gene expression (56). These events disrupt the cytoskeleton, arrest axoplasmic transport, and disrupt cellular membranes.

Abnormal calcium influx can also be initiated by overstimulation of excitatory neurotransmitter receptors (3,8). Traumatic insults to the brain have been shown to lead to excessive release of excitatory amino acid neurotransmitters, such as glutamate, glycine, and aspartate (16,27,37,46).

PEG - SOD in Head Injury
Outcome at 3 Months

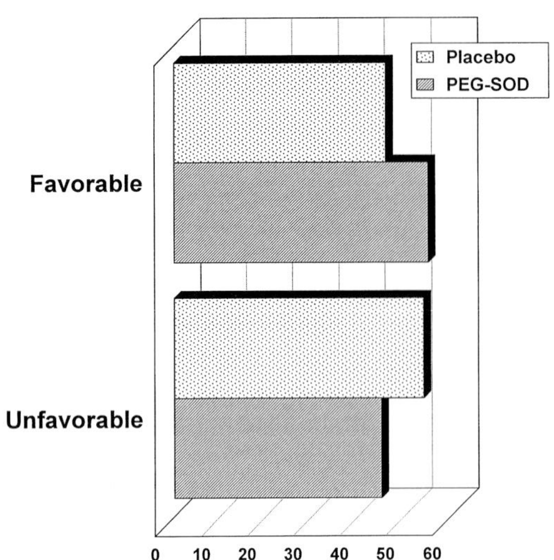

Figure 3. Mechanisms of neurotransmitter excitatotoxicity.

Glutamate, the most extensively studied, activates three distinct post-postsynaptic receptors named for neurotransmitter analogs that bind to them. The a-amino-3-hydroxyl-5-methyl-isoxazole proprionic acid (AMPA) receptor mediates monovalent cation (sodium, potassium, and hydrogen) influx. Activation of the N-methyl-D-aspartate (NMDA) receptor results in sodium, potassium, calcium influx. The third receptor is the 1-aminocyclopentane 15,3R-dicarboxylic acid (ATCD) receptor. Normally, changes in membrane polarization induced by ion fluxes initiated by activation of these receptors are quickly reversed by rapid changes in potassium and chloride permeability. The excess intracellular cations are then pumped out of the cell, using ATP-linked transport pumps. In the face of continuing glutamate release, which occurs after trauma, these normal homeostatic mechanisms can be overwhelmed, leading to chronic membrane depolarization. The resulting high levels of intracellular calcium can lead to cell destruction by the mechanisms listed above.

EXCITATORY NEUROTRANSMITTER MEDIATED TOXICITY

The excitatory amino acids, glutamate, aspartate, and glycine, alter membrane potentials by

Head Injury Mortality Trends
1980 - 1993

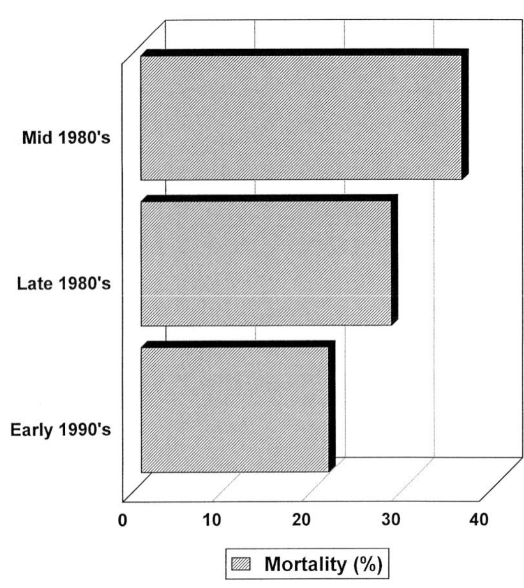

Figure 4. Glasgow outcome scales in dismutec head injury study 1995.

binding to post-synaptic receptors, which in turn control membrane ion channels (37). Excessive excitatory neurotransmitter leads to over stimulation of the receptors and eventually to cell swelling, vacuolization, and cell death. As mentioned above, at least some of these effects involve abnormally high intracellular calcium concentrations. Abnormal release of excitatory amino acids has been documented in experimental head injury models and recently, using microdialysis techniques, in human brain after significant head trauma (8,34,39,46).

For several days following head injury, levels of glutamate and aspartate in areas of the brain near the injured site are elevated (43). This elevation has been suggested to play an important role in secondary brain injury via an NMDA receptor mediated mechanism. Excessive activation of this receptor is hypothesized to lead to neuronal injury through one of a number of mechanisms, one of which may be calcium influx, as described above (11,12). Associated with the influx of cations caused by the activated receptor, an influx of water follows, resulting in cell volume expansion and possibly membrane rupture. If the cell is not irreversibly damaged by water influx, the cytotoxic effects of calcium influx, occurring over the next few hours, may also lead to cell death (3,27).

EFFECTS OF CYTOKINES

A portion of the acute response to traumatic brain damage involves the accumulation of polymorphonuclear leukocytes (PMNs) and macrophages in the area of damage. Early PMN accumulation has been correlated with the extent of post-traumatic edema formation (10). Cytokines, proteins synthesized and released by white blood cells in response to a number of stimuli, including trauma, are widely held to be the effectors of many of the responses seen after traumatic injury (41). Cytokines are active both as growth factors and as mediators of the inflammatory response to injury. More than 15 different cytokines have been identified. Three of these, interleukin-1 (IL-1), interleukin-6 (IL-6), and tumor necrosis factor (TNF), have been extensively studied in CNS trauma (1,18,20).

IL-1 was originally described as "endogenous pyrogen" because of its ability to cause fever when given intravenously. High dose infusion causes systemic shock-like effects. IL-6, also known as hepatocyte stimulating factor, appears responsible for the increased liver metabolism seen in the acute phase response. TNF, named because of its ability to lyse tumor cells, results in cachexia when given intravenously. This effect has been associated with an increase in metabolic rate. TNF may be responsible for the increased catabolism seen after trauma.

Elevated levels of all three of these cytokines have been documented in both the blood and brain tissue following experimental head injury. In vitro studies demonstrating cytokine mediated CNS tissue injury have been confirmed in animal studies. Recent clinical studies of patients with severe head injury have documented increased levels of all three cytokines in the CSF and brain of injured patients. The degree and time course of cytokine elevation correlates with outcome in head injury studies (36,38).

OTHER MECHANISMS OF SECONDARY DAMAGE

A number of other mechanisms have been implicated in delayed traumatic brain injury. Some other areas currently being studied include:

1. Opiate receptor activation. Increased levels of various endogenous opioids have been described after experimental head injury. The elevations detected correlate well with the amount of injury and with alterations in regional blood flow. Opiate receptor antagonists have been shown to decrease brain damage and attenuate physiologic changes in a fluid percussion model of traumatic brain injury (21,24,32).
2. Alterations in magnesium concentration. Magnesium is an NMDA receptor antagonist. Decreased intracellular magnesium concentrations have been demonstrated in the brain following trauma. This decrease may potentiate the cascade of events initiated by NMDA receptor over-stimulation. Administration of intravenous magnesium as much as 1 hour after injury reduces edema formation and improves outcome in a rat head injury model.

CLINICAL APPLICATIONS

Research into the events occurring in the brain after head injury has led to a number of potential therapies aimed at preventing secondary brain damage. Many of these proposed therapies have shown efficacy in animal models. Transfer of these results to the clinical settings has been slow; many results have been equivocal. The schemes used and studies performed are described below.

FREE RADICAL SCAVENGERS

Glucocorticoids in high doses inhibit free radical mediated lipid peroxidation. Despite promising studies in experimental head injury, as yet no clinical study has convincingly demonstrated a beneficial effect of steroids in patients with severe head injury. In one controlled trial using a 30 mg/kg bolus of methylprednisolone in patients with severe head injury (Glasgow coma score of 3 to 8), increased survival and lessened disability was reported in the experimental group (17). However, this improvement in outcome was only seen after significant post-hoc manipulation of the data and was detected only in patients less than 40 years of age.

A new steroid group, 21 amino steroids, of which tirilazad is the current clinical prototype, has also been investigated in head injury. After demonstration of efficacy in animals, a large clinical trial was begun in the U.S. and Europe. The U.S. trial enrolled a total of 1155 patients before being halted by the observation that the subgroup of patients with pretreatment hypotension had increased mortality when given tirilazad. The data from this study are being carefully reviewed. One interpretation suggests that the placebo patients were doing better than predicted, accounting for the apparent deleterious effect of the steroid. The results of the European trial are being awaited.

Another free radical scavenger used in clinical trials is the naturally occurring enzyme superoxide dismutase. To increase serum half life and to decrease immunogenicity, the enzyme has been conjugated to ethylene glycol for clinical use. A large multicenter randomized trial of the conjugate (commercial name dismutec) has accrued over 1000 patients. Analysis of the first 463 patients demonstrated that those patients receiving dismutec (10,000 U/kg) less than 8 hours after injury had an improved outcome. The effect did not reach statistical significance (55). Analysis of the data from all patients will not be forthcoming until late 1996.

CALCIUM CHANNEL BLOCKERS

Based on the rationale that much of the secondary damage seen after head injury is caused by abnormal influx of calcium into cells, the effect of calcium channel antagonists on outcome from head injury has been studied. Nimodipine has been used in two European trials that accrued more than 1000 patients with severe head trauma. In these placebo controlled trials, nimodipine was given at a dose of 1 to 2 mg/hour for up to seven days after injury. Neither deleterious effects on blood pressure nor positive benefits on intracranial pressure was seen in the treated group. No statistically significant difference in outcome was detected (2). Interestingly, in the group of patients with traumatic subarachnoid hemorrhage detected on their initial CT scan, a reduction in unfavorable outcome from 61% to 41% (p < 0.025) was observed in the patients receiving nimodipine compared to the placebo group (26).

NMDA RECEPTOR ANTAGONISTS

Several groups have demonstrated that outcome after experimental brain trauma is improved by the use of NMDA receptor antagonists. In one study using a fluid percussion model of head injury, the NMDA receptor antagonist MK801 produced a dose dependent decrease in mortality with an associated improvement in post-recovery memory and motor function. In an experimental subdural hematoma model, the seven fold increase in glutamate levels in the cortex directly below the hematoma and the increased glucose metabolism in the surrounding area seen in the placebo group was completely abolished by pretreatment with D-CPP-ene, an NMDA receptor antagonist (9). In addition, the zone of infarction under the clot was reduced by 54% in the treated animals.

A number of Phase II clinical studies using different NMDA receptor antagonists have been reported. While no major safety issues have been identified, prominent CNS effects including psychiatric symptoms, agitation, hallucinations, and respiratory depression have been noted. Because these side effects should not be an issue in the comatose, mechanically ventilated posthead injured patient, phase III trials of two inhibitors have begun.

DEPLETION OF IRON

Because iron potentiates the lipid peroxidation by free radicals, iron chelating drugs have been used to treat experimental head injury. Deferoxamine has been shown to decrease lipid peroxidation and stabilize transmembrane ion flux.

ADRENOCORTICTROPIC HORMONE ANALOGS

The vasoactive analog of adrenocorticotropic hormone, GMM2, has been effective in reversing the early hypoperfusion, blood brain barrier disruption, and elevation in intracranial pressure seen after experimental head injury (19).

GANGLIOSIDES

Gangliosides are important components of normal neuronal membranes. They have a number of beneficial effects when administered in experimental models of brain injury. Acutely, gangliosides may protect against toxicity induced by excess excitatory neurotransmitter. Subacutely, they may stimulate the production of neurotrophic factors related to neuronal differentiation and repair (50).

ENDOGENOUS NEUROPROTECTIVE FACTORS

One approach to improve from head injury is to induce repair of damage that occurs either primarily or secondarily. The lack of regenerative capacity of mature neurons may be caused by a genetically determined shut down of membrane biosynthesis in these cells. Activation of early response genes and heat shock genes may turn on the genes controlling membrane biosynthesis. Induction of these repair genes may be important in potential repair of neuronal membranes following ischemia and reperfusion (15,31,45,48).

In addition to membrane repair, regeneration of synaptic connections is a crucial event in repair of traumatic brain damage. Recently, the gene encoding the protein agrin, a major mediator of synaptogenesis, has been cloned. In regions of the brain known for significant postnatal plasticity, such as the hippocampus and olfactory bulb, agrin levels are elevated throughout life. In other regions of the brain with little or no plasticity, agrin expression is only present until completion of postnatal synaptogenesis (14). Further work on potential repair mechanisms is needed before they can be manipulated to treat head injury.

Neurotrophic factors such as basic fibroblast growth factor, ciliary neurotrophic factor, and the insulin-like growth factors are important during brain growth and development. They are actively expressed during brain development, but are down-regulated in the adult brain. These factors can be produced by neurons and glial cells after injury. They may play a role in repair of cellular damage (35,54).

CONCLUSIONS

The rapid acquisition of information about the molecular events occurring during and after head trauma has significantly advanced the understanding of the interrelationships and cascades responsible for the damage produced. The understanding of these events has led to proposed schemes for preventing or treating the damage using compounds that control, block, modulate, or reverse the events leading to permanent brain damage. A number of clinical trials are underway to test these schemes. Additional trials are sure to open in the near future. Because of the multifactorial, complex, time dependent interaction involved in head injury, it may be that one drug or treatment is not enough to improve outcome by preventing or reversing secondary brain damage. A combination of treatments, interfering with the development of secondary injury at multiple places, may be the only way to achieve success.

REFERENCES

1. Akira, S., Hirano, T., Tasa, T., Kishimoto, T. Biology of multifunctional cytokines IL-6 and related molecules. FASEB J *4:*2860–2867, 1992.
2. Bailey, I., Bell, A., Gray, J., et al. A trial of the effect of nimodipine on outcome after head injury. Acta Neurochir *110:*97–105, 1991.
3. Becker, D.P., Katayama, Y., Tamura, T., et al. Excitotoxic ion fluxes and neuronal dysfunction following traumatic brain injury. J CBF Metabol 9 (suppl 1): 302, 1989.
4. Bielenberg, G.W., Beck, T., Sauer, D., et al. Effects of cerebroprotective agents on cerebral blood flow and on postischemic energy metabolism in the rat's brain. J Cereb Blood Flow Metabol. *7:*480–488, 1987.
5. Braughler, J.M., Hall, E.D. CNS trauma and stroke. Biochemical considerations for oxygen radical formation and lipid peroxidation. Free Rad Biol Med. *6:*289–301, 1989.
6. Buchan, A., Li, H., Cho, S., et al. Blockade of the AMPA receptor prevents CA1 hippocampal injury following severe but transient forebrain ischemia in adult rat. Neurosci Lett *132:*255–258, 1991.
7. Busto, R., Globus, M.Y.T., Dietrich, W.D., et al. Effect of mild hypothermia on ischemia induced release of neurotransmitters and free fatty acids in rat brain. Stroke *20:*904–910, 1989.
8. Bullock, R., Fujisawa H. The role of glutamate antagonists for the treatment of CNS injury. J Neurotrauma *19*(suppl 20:S443–S462, 1992.
9. Chen, M.H., Bullock, R., Graham, D.I., et al. Ischemic neuronal damage after acute subdural hematoma in the rat. Effects of pretreatment with a glutamate antagonist. J Neurosurg *74:*944–950, 1991.
10. Chiolero, R., Schultz, Y., Lemaerchand, T. Hormonal and metabolic changes following severe head injury or noncranial injury. J Parent Ent Nutr. *13:*5–12, 1989.
11. Choi, D.W. Ionic dependence of glutamate neurotoxicity. J Neurosci *7:*369–379, 1987.
12. Choi, D.W. Calcium-mediated neurotoxicity. Relationship to specific channel types and role in ischemic damage. Trends Neurosci. *11:*465–469, 1988.
13. Demopoulos, H.B., Flamm, E.S., Pietrongrio, D.D., et al. The free radical pathology and the microcirculation in the major central nervous system disorders. Acta Physiol Scand. (suppl 1) *492:*91–119, 1980.

14. Deyst, K.A., Ma, J., Fallon, J.R. Agrin: toward a molecular understanding of synapse regeneration. Neurosurg. *37:*71–77, 1995.

15. Deshaies, R.J., Coch, B.D., Schekman, R. The role of stress proteins in membrane bigenesis. TIBS. *13:* 384–388, 1988.

16. Faden A.I., Demediuk, P., Panter, S.S., Vink, R. The role of excitatory amino acids and NMDA receptors in traumatic brain injury. Science. *244:*289–800, 1989.

17. Gianotta, S.L., Weiss, M.H., Apuzzo, M.L.J., Martin, E. High-dose glucocorticoids in the management of severe head injury. Neurosurg. *1597*–105, 1991.

18. Gluckman, P., Klempt, N., Guan, J., et al. A role for IGF1 in the rescue of central nervous system neurons following hypoxic-ischemic injury. Biochem Biophys Res Comm. *182:*593–599.

19. Goldman, H., Morehead, M., Murphy, S. Use of adrenocroticotrophic hormone analog to minimize brain injury. Ann ER Med. *22:*1035–1040, 1993.

20. Goodman, J.C., Robertson, C.S., Grossman, R.G., Narayan, R.K. Elevation of tumor necrosis factor in head injury. J Neuroimmunol. *30:*213–217, 1990.

21. Hall, E.D., Wolf, D.L., Althaus, J.S., et al. Beneficial effects of the K-Opoid receptor antagonist U-50488H in experimental acute brain and spinal cord injury. Brain Res. *435:*174–180, 1987.

22. Hall, E.D., Yonkers, P.A., Andrus, J.K., et al. Biochemistry and pharmacology of lipid antioxidants in acute brain and spinal cord injury. J Neurotrauma. *9*(suppl 2):S425–S442, 1992.

23. Hall, E.D. Lipid antioxidants in acute CNS injury. Ann ER Med. *22:*1022–1027, 1993.

24. Hayes R.L., Galinat, B.J., Kulkarne, P., et al. Effects of naloxone on systemic and cerebral responses to experimental concussive brain injury in cats. J Neurosurg. *58:*720–728, 1983.

25. Hayes, R.L., Jenkins, L.W., Lyeth, B.G. Neurotransmitter mediated mechanisms of traumatic brain injury: Acetylcholine and excitatory amino acids. J Neurotrauma. *9*(suppl 1)S173–S188, 1992.

26. Karieka, A., Braakman, R., Shakel, E.H. Traumatic subarachnoid hemorrhage. Importance in treatment perspective with nimodipine. J Neurotrauma. *10*(suppl 1):193, 1993.

27. Katayama, Y., Becker, D.P., Tamura, T., Hovda, D.A. Massive increases in extracellular potassium and the indiscriminate release of glutamate following a concussive brain injury. J Neurosurg. *73:*889–900, 1990.

28. Knotos, H.A., Povlishok, J.T. Oxygen radicals in brain injury. CNS Trauma. 257–263, 1986.

29. Kontos, H.A., Wei, E.P. Superoxide production in experimental brain injury. J Neurosurg. *64:*803–807, 1986.

30. Kukreja, R.C., Kontos, H.A., Hess, M.L., et al. PGH synthetase and lipooxygenase generate superoxide in the presence of NADH or NADPH. Circ Res. *59:* 612–619, 1986.

31. Linquist, S. The heat shock response. Annl Rev Biochem. *55:*1151–1191, 1986.

32. Lyeth, B.J., Hayes, R.L. Cholinergic and opoid mediation of traumatic brain injury. J Neurotrauma. *9*(suppl 2):S463–S474, 1992.

33. Mahler, L.M., Phillips, J.W., Peterson, P.L. Effects of compression concussion on brain mitochondrial bioenergetics in the rat. Soc Neurosci. *13:*1634, 1987 Abstract.

34. Marion D.W., Obrist, W.D., Carlier, P.M. The use of moderate therapeutic hypothermia for patients with severe head injury: a preliminary report. J Neurosurg. *79:*354–362, 1993.

35. Mattson, M.P., Scheff, S.W. Endogenous neuroprotection factors and traumatic brain injury. Mechanisms of action and implications for therapy. J Neurotrauma. *11:*3–33, 1994.

36. McClain, C.J., Cohen, D., Phillips, R., et. al. Increased plasma and ventricular fluid interleukin 6 levels in patients with head injury. J Lab Clin Med *118:*225–231, 1991.

37. McIntosh, T.K., Ving, R., Smith D.H., et al. Excitatory amino acids and traumatic nervous system injury in Meldrum, B.S., Morrini, F., Simon, R.P. (editors). *Excitatory Amino Acids.* Raven Press. 1991:695–701.

38. Medary, M., Ku, K., Hariri, R.J., et al. Outcome from severe traumatic brain injury: correlation with CSF interleukin-6 levels. AANS Annual Meeting Abstract Book, 1995:358.

39. Myseros, J., Bullock, M.R., Marmarou, T., et al. Monitoring intracerebral excitatory amino acids following severe human head injury. AANS Anual Meeting Abstract Book, 1994, pp219–220.

40. Olney, J.W. Inciting excitotoxic cytocide among central neurons. Adv Exp Med Biol *203:*631–645, 1986.

41. Ott, L., McClain, C.J., Gillespie, M., Young, B. Cytokines and metabolic dysfunction after severe head injury. J Neurotrauma. *11:*447–472, 1994.

42. Ozyurt, E., Graham, D.I., Woodruff, G., McCulloch, J. Protective effect of the glutamate antagonist MK-801 in focal cerebral ischemia in the cat. J Cereb Blood Flow Metab. *8:*138–143, 1988.

43. Palmer, A.M., Marion, D.W., Botscheller, M.L., et al. Traumatic brain injury-induced excitotoxicity assessed in a controlled cortical impact model. J Neurochem. *61:*2015–2014, 1993.

44. Panter S.S., Braughler, J.M., Hall, E.D. Dextran-coupled deferoxamine improves outcome in a murine model of head injury. J Neurotrauma. *9:*47–53, 1992.

45. Pelham, H.R.B. Speculations of the functions of the major heat shock proteins and glucose regulated proteins. Cell *46:*959–969, 1986.

46. Robertson, D.P., Gopinath, S.P., Robertson, C.S., et al. Neurochemical monitoring in the neurosurgical intensive care unit using microdialysis. AANS Annual Meeting Abstract Book, 1994:216–217.

47. Rothman, S.M., Olney, J.W. Glutamate and the pathophysiology of hypoxic ischemic brain damage. Ann Neurol. *19:*105–110, 1986.

48. Sheng, M., Greenberg, M.E. The regulation and function of C-fos and other immediate early genes in the nervous system. Neuron. *4:*477–485, 1990.

49. Siesjo, B. The role of calcium in cell death. In Price, D., Aguayo, A., Thoenen, H. (Editors). *Neurodegenerative Disorders. Mechanisms and Prospects for Therapy.* John Wiley and Sons LTD, United Kingdom, 1994, pp35–59.

50. Skaper, S.D., Leon, A. Monosialogangliosides, neuro-

protection and neuronal repair processes. J Neurotrauma. *9*(suppl 1):S507–S516, 1992.

51. Steinberg, G.K., Kunis, D., Saleh, J., DeLaPaz, R. Protection after focal cerebral ischemia by the NMDA antagonist dextrophan is dependent on brain and plasma levels. J Cereb Blood Flow Metabol. *8:*790–798, 1988.

52. Shapira, Y., Yadid, G., Cotev, S., et al. Accumulation of calcium in the brain following head trauma. Neurol Res. *11:*169–172, 1989.

53. Vink, R., Head, V.A., Rogers, P.J., et al. Mitochondrial metabolism following traumatic brain injury in rats. J Neurotrauma. *21:*73, 1990.

54. Wanaka, A., Johnson, E.M., Millbrandt, J. Localization of FGF receptor in RNA in the adult rat CNS by in situ hybridization. Neuron. *5:*267–281, 1990.

55. Waxman, K., Wilberger, J.E., et al. Report of the six-month outcome of a clinical trial of PEG-SOD in severely head injured patients. J Neurotrauma. *12:*418–419, 1995.

56. Young, W. Calcium paradox in neural injury: a hypothesis. J Neurotrauma. *3:*235–251, 1986.

CHAPTER 19

The Molecular Biology of Regeneration in the CNS

D. H. BHATT, M.D., B. A. GREEN, M.D.

INTRODUCTION

One of the greatest challenges of modern medical science is the successful treatment of neurodegenerative diseases and neuronal trauma. Regeneration of a damaged central neuron with functional recovery is limited. As Cajal pointed out in 1911, "...aborted restorative processes are incapable of bringing about a complete or definitive repair of interrupted paths." (37). Cajal's student, F. Tello, showed that segments of peripheral nerve stimulate new growth of nerve fibers (174), providing an early insight into the significance of neuronal-glial interactions in development and regeneration. Recently, the molecular characteristics and pathological implications of neuronal interactions have raised some interesting questions concerning neuronal development, plasticity and regeneration. Central nervous system (CNS) and peripheral nervous system (PNS) components such as extra-cellular matrix proteins (174), integrins, cytoskeletal elements (206), cytokines (20, 40, 129, 142, 159, 191, 217), growth factors (20, 58, 122, 158, 200, 217), trophins (26, 86, 110, 126, 200), neurotransmitters (12, 12, 14, 15, 38, 47), astrocytes (40, 62, 63, 121, 137, 165, 167, 175, 178, 217), and oligodendrocytes (169–174), and Schwann cells (and their derivatives) (2, 4, 33, 34, 35, 65, 79, 108, 111, 140, 214) have all been attributed roles in development and regeneration. Factors that are conducive to neurite outgrowth during development may become restrictive upon maturation (4, 24, 29, 73, 173, 174, 175). While peripheral regeneration has been shown to occur in mammalian, avian, marsupial, fish, and amphibian systems, the adult central nervous system of higher vertebrates possesses limited capacity to regenerate interrupted fiber tracts (4, 24, 173, 174, 175).

Grafting CNS neurons into a PNS environment enables the neurons to extend processes (173, 174, 175). On the other hand, PNS neurons are unable to exhibit outgrowth in a CNS milieu (173, 174, 175). In experiments designed to explore the possible differences in levels of neurotrophic factors within and outside the blood-brain-barrier, a three compartment culture chamber with bridges of peripheral and central tissue was used. Neurons were grown in the central chambers and given trophic support. Several thousand axons were found to grow through the sciatic bridge and non through the optic bridge, demonstrating the nonpermissive substrate effect of CNS tissue.

The long standing notion of the inherent inability of neurons from the CNS to regenerate, cast in stone by Cajal, has been disproven for most neuronal types. As a consequence, ideas on the mechanisms underlying the process of regeneration involving neurons, glia, and their environment before and after injury, are leading to fascinating discoveries. Recent literature cites four distinct phases during the regenerative response observed in a lesioned CNS axon (173, 174, 175). These are: sprouting of the proximal stump, elongation, target recognition and formation of appropriate synapses (174, 175).

The process of axonal regeneration can be observed within the CNS in some lower vertebrates and during early development in higher vertebrates. In the lower vertebrates, the optic system has been the subject of extensive study. Mechanisms necessary for both axonal guidance and appropriate synapse formation have been shown to be present throughout life (4, 6, 13, 14, 46, 132, 139). Guidance is achieved using both positive and negative substrate molecules and chemotropic signals (29, 144, 169, 173, 174, 175, 205). Mechanisms responsible for target recognition are broad although some of these processes undergo fine tuning, even in the adult. The processes that mark regeneration in the adult are the same as those that occur during development, thus providing further evidence of the possibilities for repair and renewal in the lesioned adult (24, 50, 122, 131, 158, 174). Recent studies on the dedifferentiating capabilities of adult mammalian neurons and the presence of unrecruited 'dormant' neurons in the adult human brain, have led neuroscientists to reconsider old, outmoded ideas; (6, 7; figure 1).

The significance of neuronal-glial interactions during development has been documented from the time of Cajal (37). In recent years, the molecular characteristics and pathological implications of such interactions have been investigated with respect to neuronal development, plasticity and regeneration. Astrocytes, oligodendrocytes (OL), Schwann cells, and their derivatives have all been assigned roles in development and regeneration. Neuronal development and regeneration involve target

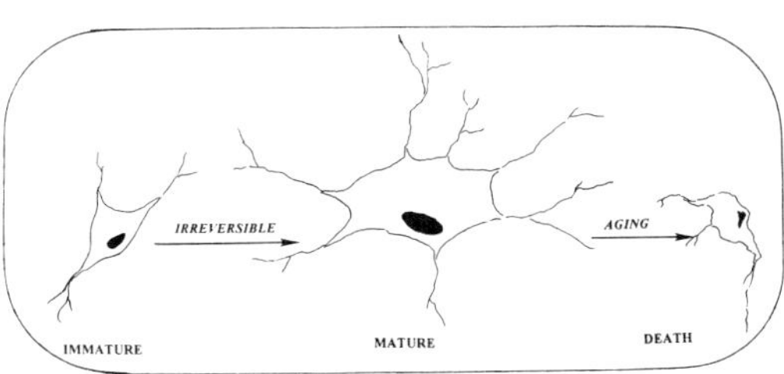

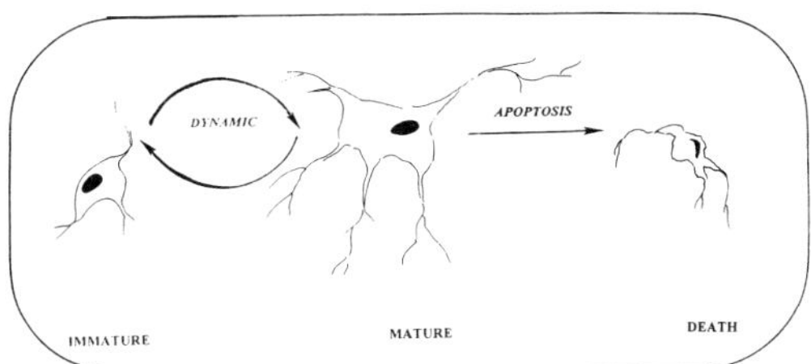

Figure 1. This figure illustrates how the traditional linear model of a neuronal plasticity and function requires reformulation in light of recent developmental and regenerative research findings. The more dynamic model is suggested by Whitaker-Azmitia and Azmitia (209).

specificity. Factors that inhibit growth are equally important in guidance and organization as factors that promote growth. The history of neuroscience is replete with descriptions of growth promoting elements (Harrison, 1910; Ramon y Cajal, 1928, 1929). The discovery of nerve growth factor (NGF) (Cohen, 1960; Levi-Montalcini & Hamburger, 1951) has led to the neurotrophic factors hypothesis (84). This hypothesis is being amended and refined as new information on families of soluble factors with neurite growth promoting, survival, mitogenic, and differentiation effects increases. As a result of the growth in significance of cell-cell and cell-matrix interactions, membrane bound and extracellular matrix (ECM) proteins were sought and analyzed for their role in neurite outgrowth, cell adhesion, and axon guidance, but the focus has been on the growth promoting aspects of these signals.

The evidence of inhibitors of nerve fiber growth in the CNS of higher vertebrates has been provided by experiments involving the grafting of neurons into PNS and CNS environments. CNS neurons were able to extend processes in a PNS system, but PNS neurons were unable to exhibit outgrowth in a CNS milieu (5). To access the possible difference in levels of neurotrophic factors within and outside the BBB (as suggested by Tello in 1911, Schwab & Thoenen), experiments were performed in which three compartment chambers with bridges of peripheral and central tissue were plated with neurons (in the central chamber) and given trophic support (170). Several thousand axons were found to grow through the sciatic implant and non through the optic bridge, indicating the nonpermissive substrate effect of CNS tissue. Experiments similar to those done by Schwab and Thoenen, but utilizing frozen sections of adult rat peripheral nerves or various CNS regions as substrates and performed on rat sensory and sympathetic neurons or neuroblastoma cells, gave similar results (53).

NI 35/250 is a protein isolated from CNS tissue (specifically oligodendroglial myelin) that strongly inhibits neurite outgrowth (171). The presence of inhibiting substances in myelin has led to the investigation of inhibitory neuronglial interactions (17, 53, 199). Distinct differences in the inhibitory characteristics of different glial sub-populations were observed in coculture experiments involving dissociated glial cells and neurons (5, 16, 53, 171). Astrocytes and OL precursor cells provided a favorable environment for neurite outgrowth (62, 63). This was in contrast to the marked inhibition in the presence of mature OL (5, 16, 171). Mature OL inhibit neurite outgrowth from a variety of neuronal populations, as well as neuroblastomas and PC 12 cells, even in the presence of neurotrophic factors (84).

To further characterize the OL inhibition, video time-lapse studies were performed (16, 17). Dorsal root ganglia (DRG) were grown on a laminin substrate in the presence of NGF. Contact of the tips of filopodia with OL processes was sufficient to completely arrest growth cone elongation, implicating second messenger involvement. The effect was rapid, localized (fibers on the same neuron that did not come into contact with an OL or any of its processes continued to grow), and long lasting (hours). These studies showed that inhibition of growth is dependent on physical contact with OL (16, 17). Furthermore, no neuritic growth activity could be recovered using OL conditioned media (see Fig. 2). Immediately preced-

ing growth cone collapse, there was a significant and rapid increase in intracellular calcium. Dantrolene, an inhibitor of calcium release from caffeine-sensitive intracellular stores, also prevented growth cone collapse.

When CNS myelin and OL membrane fraction enriched cultures were used as substrates for neurons, inhibition was marked (199). SDS-PAGE analysis of the proteins from these membrane fractions, followed by liposomal reconstitution, revealed two active fractions of 35 kD and 250 kD (termed Neurite Inhibitors (NI) 35 and 250); the smaller one is now thought to be part of the heavier one (174). Protein purification by SDS-PAGE and HPLC and subsequent partial amino acid sequencing revealed no homology to known proteins. NI 35/250 activity has been found in all white matter regions of the CNS, except in the goldfish, trout (19), and certain regions of the Xenopus (115), which could explain the regenerative capabilities of the CNS of these and other lower vertebrates (16, 174). A neutralizing antibody to NI 35/250, IN-1, was used in *in vivo* experiments of axonal growth (164, 172). Either irradiated OL precur-

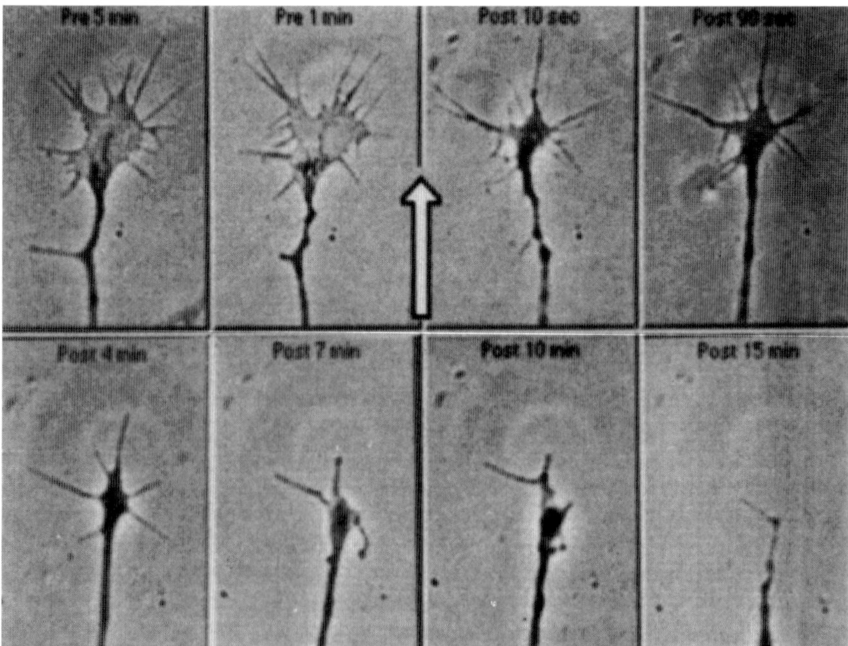

Figure 2.   Studies done by Bandtlow, et al., on the role of intracellular calcium in NI-35-evoked collapse of neuronal growth cones (17). Phase-contrast photomicrographs demonstrate the response of a DRG growth cone responds to NI-35-containing liposomes. The application of the liposomes is indicated by the open arrow. The subsequent retraction and collapse over time is evident.

sor cells of newborn rats or IN-1 producing hybridoma cells were placed in newborn rat brains (169, 172). The spinal cords of these rats were then completely transected, and regeneration of corticospinal tract (CST) fibers was compared with that in untreated, lesioned rats. In control animals, fiber growth extended a maximum of 1 mm from the lesion site. Experimentally treated rats showed a maximal CST fiber elongation of 10 to 20 mm, with an average growth of 4–7 mm (172). Developmental studies revealed that CST fibers grew aberrantly into adjacent areas in the rostral cord with frequent, dense infiltration into the gray matter (173). Similar paradigms have been used to study axonal regeneration after a fetal OL cell graft (29, 30). Axonal growth around and through the graft was greatly enhanced in experimentally treated rats. Grafted animals without IN-1 treatments showed greater elongation than control animals (non-grafted), but not to the extent seen in Ab treated rats. The fetal graft enhancement is thought to be primarily due to its rich source of trophic factors. The most prolific and longest sprouting and elongation occur when both IN-1 and NT3 are used; see figure 3.

Several studies have correlated failure of regrowth with onset of myelination (174). In the rat optic nerve, inhibitory activity and appearance of GalC positive OL is coincident, but predates by 5 to 7 days, the onset of myelination (49). This and other studies (16, 17) have led to the suggestion that NI 35/250 mediated inhibition provides boundary guides for late growing CNS tracts and, in target areas, can restrict collateral access of fibers to certain regions and layers. The presence of the protein in the adult also suggests that stabilization of organization is required. The role played by NI 35/250, and other as yet unknown inhibitory molecules, may be crucial in understanding how neurons "know" when and where to grow. Understanding these inhibitory influences may also lead to advancement in the therapeutics of traumatic and degenerative neurological disorders.

Besides OL and their derivatives, subpopulations of astrocytes and their derivatives can provide inhibitory influences on axonal growth. Silver and colleagues have examined the role of proteoglycans, a component of the extra cellular matrix (ECM), which is secreted by some neurons, astrocytes, and neuroepithelial cells (180).

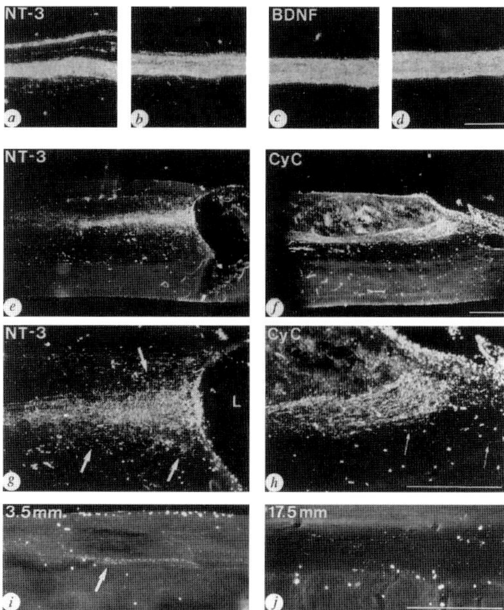

Figure 3. Shown are darkfield photomicrographs of the CST, at the thoracic level, of a 5-day old rat. a–d show NT-3 and BDNF-induced premature sprouting. e–h show transected CST's. f and h show cytochrome c labeling. i shows the presence of a bundle of regenerating fibers growing in the dorsal funiculus in an IN-1/NT-3 treated animal, 3.5 mm rostral to the lesion. j shows fibers in the same animal, 17.5 mm. rostral to the lesion. The bars represent 100 μm in a–d, and 500 μm in e–j. (169).

Proteoglycans add to the nonpermissive character of the adult CNS and are associated with boundary regions such as the dorsal root entry zone. They are made of a protein core attached to various glycosaminoglycan side chains. Substrate assays have shown that one type of proteoglycan, heparin sulfate, interacts with laminin and/or other growth factor to promote neurite outgrowth (180). In contrast, keratin and chondroitan sulfate proteoglycans are potent inhibitors of neurite outgrowth. Utilizing rat retinal development as a model, chondroitan sulfate has been shown to play an important role in directing and limiting neuronal differentiation and axon growth in the retina (31). Once in place, ECM forms a barrier for regeneration.

Glial cells associated with proteoglycans are found in areas of the developing CNS that are non-permissive for axonal elongation (63, 121, 130, 178, 180). Astrocytes serve many functions including providing a radial tract for neuronal migrations, secreting trophic support, storing glycogen, buffering extracellular ion levels, taking up and releasing of neuroactive substances, and participating in the immune response, as well as forming scar tissue after injury (63, 178). Their functional diversity is achieved through subpopulations and in the receptor-signaling plasticity of astrocytes (63, 121, 130). For example reactive astrocytes are believed to arise from either hypertrophied 'normal' astrocytes, or from astrocytic precursor cells which proliferate before growing in size (63, 178). Given the diversity in neuronal type, and the diversity in glial populations, the difficulty in characterizing the nature of the scar becomes apparent. However, since the lesion and subsequent glial scar have been shown to confer a huge obstacle to regenerating fibers, it has become a major focus in the study of CNS regeneration. As with astrocytes, scar tissue presents the dichotomy of being both restrictive and permissive (initially) to axon growth (130).

Using electrolytic lesioning of the CST in the upper cervical region, Li and Raisman (121) have investigated the relationship of the astrocytic scar to axonal sprouting. Labeling of glial fibrillary acid protein (GFAP) showed substantial hypertrophy of astrocytic processes in and beyond the lesion site. Axonal tracing showed that the cut ends of fibers, and adjacent uncut axons, exhibited large end varicosities. Furthermore, these varicosities gave off sprouts that entered the macrophage and Schwann cell infested lesion area. Sprouting persisted during the height of the scarring (9.5–13 weeks). The arborizations entering the scar site were also found to be either myelinated or ensheathed by invading peripheral Schwann cells (121).

Risling et al. have studied the axonal growth permissible characteristics of scars in the dorsal and ventral funiculi of feline spinal cords (160, 161). Scar tissue compromises the BBB as evidenced by the loss of transferrin and connexin 43 immunoreactivity (160, 161). This results in two broad implications: (1) the entry of blood borne macrophages and related cytokines and, (2) greater accessibility to trophic support. Astrocytes in the lesioned area show a transient upregulation of trkB mRNA. Upregulation of many other growth factors that stimulate the product of ECM molecules such as collagen types I, III, IV, the alpha-subunit of laminin and a species of tenascin has also been shown (160, 161, 180).

There is also a great deal of evidence pointing to the scar-cord interface as the source of inhibitory influences (40, 62, 63, 121, 137, 160, 161, 165, 166, 175, 178, 217). In rat lesion models in which IN-1 antibody is used, many regenerating axons terminate at the cavern wall or at the interface with solid scar tissue. These models contained regenerating axons which were morphologically and functionally different from the sprouting fibers described by Li and Raisman (121). The inhibitory effects of scar tissue was also demonstrated by creating lesions perinatally in the rat in the future area of the CST at P2. The gliotic scar resulted in complete blockage of CST growth past this point (175).

Inhibition of regeneration in the CNS may occur only in those cases in which scars are involved. Kawaguchi's group has been able to experimentally produce conditions under which no dense scar tissue forms subsequent to lesioning (101). Transection of the spinal cord of Wistar rats ranging in ages from birth to three months at the level of T10–T11, either sharply, with a razor, or bluntly, by cauterization, resulted in clear regeneration in some animals up to 25 days old, but regeneration was absent or abortive in all cases showing glial scar formation. In an accompanying experiment, neonatal rats were subjected to transection and removal of one and a half to two segments at the T10–T11 level. The gap was then filled with embryonic homologous segments, in the proper orientation. Controls had their embryonic grafts placed either in inverted dorsoventral or rostrocaudal orientations, had PNS graft, or had no grafts at all. Neural connectivity was examined morphologically, electrophysiologically and behaviorally. The results showed almost normal, functional connectivity (in all of the parameters examined), but only in cases where the embryonic graft was inserted in the proper orientation relative to the host cord (96, 101). These results clearly reiterate the capacity of CNS neurons not only to regenerate, but also to self organize.

Silver et al. utilized an implant paradigm to study the expression of both adhesive and inhibitory factors found in the postinjury milieu (180). The implant, made of nitrocellulose fibers, was placed into a previously made stab lesion site within the cerebral cortex of neonatal rats. The implants were removed after one month and their contents were determined immunohistochemically. Along with GFAP-positive astrocytes, the filters contained associated growth permissive substrates such as fibonectin, collagen IV, and laminin. The same experiments performed in adult rats revealed the presence of two additional molecules, chondroitan sulfate and tenascin. Upregulation of these two factors has been demonstrated a variety of adult CNS lesion models. To determine the effect of the gliotic environment on neurite outgrowth, the implants were used as substrate for axon outgrowth from embryonic CNS and PNS tissue. In all cases, outgrowth was minimal when the substrate used was from an adult. Neurites were longer and more plentiful when the substrate was from neonatal scar tissue. Furthermore, treatment of adult implants with lyase resulted in increased neurite outgrowth, often to levels seen with the neonate scar samples. Thus, both growth permissive and inhibitory (chondroitin sulfate proteoglycan) molecules exist in adult gliosis. The authors suggest that there may be an imbalance in adults favoring inhibitory molecules that leads to regenerative failure (180).

Silver's group has isolated various isoforms of chondroitin sulfate proteoglycan. They found that beta-amyloid peptide can induce glial cells, in vitro and in vivo, to deposit chondroitin sulfate proteoglycan in the local matrix. These reactive astrocytes may then begin to deposit growth inhibitory substances near the neuron, impairing its survival and ability to regenerate (180).

TROPHICS

The concept of neurotrophic factors arose from the observation that, during development, target tissues provide limited support for their innervating neurons. This ensures that the size of the neuronal population approximates the size of the target cell population, (149). NGF represents the classical target-derived and retrogradely transported molecule that regulates survival, neurite outgrowth, and differentiation (26). Other members of the NGF neurotrophin family are brain-derived neurotrophic factor (BDNF), NT-3, NT-4/5, and NT-6. Each neurotrophin has its own specific receptors: trk A, B, and C (18, 26, 44, 56, 87, 99, 126). Other trophins worthy of report in the context of CNS regeneration are ciliary neurotrophic factor (CNTF), leukemia inhibitory factor (LIF), the family of fibroblast growth factors (FGF), insulin-like growth factors (IGF), and neurotransmitters. Attempts to find strict correlations between neurotrophins and the neuron subtypes they affect have not been very successful (110). Any discussion of the current state of research in CNS regeneration would require an exploration of the role trophins play in repair.

The magnitude of influence that neurotrophins exert on cell survival and 'pruning' during development, as well as on synaptic plasticity and neurotransmitter release, make them attractive molecules for treatment of neurodegenerative disease and trauma. IGF-1 and 2, and CNTF have already entered the clinical arena in trials for the treatment of neuropathies such as ALS (although CNTF has been shown to have intolerable side effects). The fact that growth factor levels and effects have been linked to neurons involved in spinal cord and brain injuries, Parkinson's disease, Alzheimer's disease, and Huntington disease, emphasizes the need for further study into the mechanisms involved. These studies should lead to strategies that best utilize the regenerative/restorative properties of such molecules and their receptors.

Frans Hefti outlined the steps involved in the clinical use of a neurotrophic factor (86). It is important to note that these steps can only be undertaken after demonstrating that the neurotrophin in question is associated with the affected neuron in the disease being considered and that the target population of neurons express the receptor(s) for the trophin being used.

Cell culture studies have lead to the purification and isolation of growth factors. Cells used in these cultures were of fetal or transformed origin, and thus are more reflective of developmental states rather than those found in the adult. In a second step, these factors could be tested for their efficacy in an appropriate disease model (86). Models for progressive neurodegenerative diseases are usually produced *in vivo* through transgenic techniques and acute injury models have also been used. It is important to note that these models only approach, in varying degrees, the pathology involved in the human situation.

Neurotrophic factor therapy has been used to enhance the survival and maintain the expression of deficient neurotransmitter levels. In vitro, these effects are displayed by a variety of neurotrophins, growth factors and cytokines-

BDNF, NT4/5, glial derived neurotrophic factor (GDNF), IGF1, IGF2, epidermal growth factor (EGF), transforming growth factor (TGF) and interleukin (IL). In vitro results are encouraging, not only because of possible in vivo links, but also because they may be useful in the pretreatment of cells used in a transplantation therapy. The stimulatory and supportive effects of NGF administration have already been shown to improve adrenal medullary grafts (148). BDNF and NT4/5 treatments, after nigrastriatal transection in rats, have not provided any remarkable results, probably because the trk-B receptor is not highly expressed in this region (86).

FGF's play an interesting role in Parkinson's disease. Evidence shows that receptors for FGF1 (FGFR1) and FGF2 (FGFR2) exist in the substantial nigra and striatum (10). Pathological analysis of Parkinsonian brains shows a dramatic loss of FGF2 levels in the substantia nigra (193). Additionally, intracerebral injection of FGF2 into adult mice pretreated with MPTP leads to recovery of dopaminergic function (150).

ALZHEIMER'S

Much of the current research in Alzheimer's disease centers around the characterization and manipulation of plaque and neurofibrillary tangle formation. It is also clear that the selective loss of forebrain cholinergic input to the hippocampus has serious behavioral consequences. The neurons that are lost include those that are selectively responsive to NGF during development (86). NGF does prevent the atrophy of cholinergic neurons, as seen in Alzheimer's, and induces hypertrophy in those cholinergic neurons that survive any experimental or age related insult (86). In initial clinical trials utilizing NGF administration for Alzheimers, one of the patients exhibited encouraging results (48). Two obstacles must be overcome in the use of NGF, however; the high degree of selectivity which limits the scope of trophism, and the often detrimental collateral sprouting that occurs. In regards to the latter, the site of administration (usually intraventricular) poses great problems in the directionality and extent of efficient neurite outgrowth (as will be discussed later). Because of NGF's selectivity, other growth factors will be needed to provide the

broad spectrum of protection needed to combat the neuronal degeneration associated with Alzheimer's.

The traditional concept of neurotrophins has been challenged by the existence of alternative paths or sources of trophic support, e.g., bFGF anterograde signaling in retinal ganglion cells; paracrine mechanisms; and autocrine pathways, as have been shown for some BDNF and FGF neurons; Figure 4. "As neurotrophins and their receptors are coincidentally expressed in the same neuronal cell type and also reveal broad tissue distribution in nonneuronal cells and tissues (e.g., testis, ovaries, platelets), pleiotropism and overlapping biological activities of neurotrophic factors have been recognized" (26).

Although neurotrophins are being used in clinical trials for the treatment of neurodegenerative disorders such as Alzheimer's, Parkinson's, and ALS (26, 86, 109, 125, 127, 148, 155, 182), much less attention has been given to their regenerative capabilities (24, 128). The best studied neurotrophin in regenerative models is NGF. An *in vivo* assay for the regenerative effect of NGF involves lesioning of the medial septal-hippocampal projection by means of fimbria-fornix tract transections in adult rats (73, 195). Upon complete transection of this tract, the hippocampus is totally deafferented of its cholinergic input. Exogeneous administration of NGF leads to little or no improved regeneration (73, 195, 200), but degeneration of medial septal cholinergic neurons is prevented (Fig. 5) (58, 73, 82, 151, 195, 200).

Studies involving the use of a sciatic nerve explant bridge have been used to quantify the effect of NGF on axonal growth by determining the number of fibers crossing imaginary lines (46, 151, 200). The cholinergic fiber growth into the bridge reached a maximum at one month after the lesion. The rate of entry showed a marked decrease beyond the first mm of the bridge (Figure 6) (200). In this model, the distance from PNS support tissue occurs as a spatial temporal gradient away from the lesion, as opposed to a spatially defined area. Hagg et al. have suggested that cholinergic regeneration requires NGF along the regrowth pathway and eventual target, as well as in the cell body (82). To test this hypothesis, NGF was infused into the medial septum. This led to a great reduction in the number of fibers invading the fresh nerve

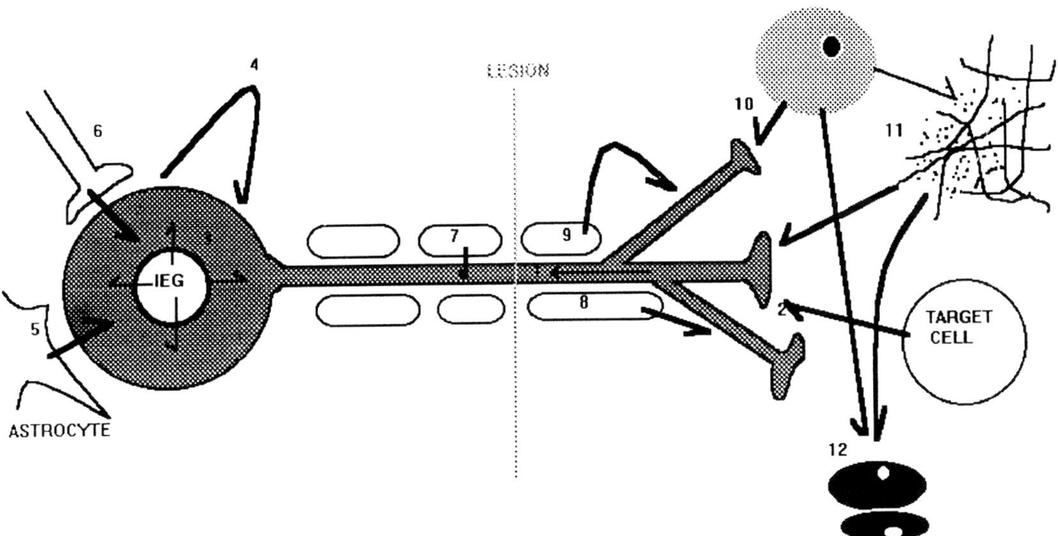

Figure 4. Diagrammatic representation of possible post-lesion neurotrophic strategies in peripheral, and perhaps central, neural regeneration. A lesioned neuron with trophic deficiency due to impaired retrograde axonal support (1) and/or loss of target derived neurotrophic factors (2) might obtain trophic support at its perikaryon by immediate early gene (IEG)-induced synthesis of trophic molecules involved in either intracrine (3) and/or autocrine pathways (4), by specific uptake of trophic factors from activated perineural glial cells (5) or from afferents via anterograde transport (6). Retrograde trophic support may be received from axon-ensheathing and intact Schwann cells via axo-glial trophic interactions (7). At the site of the lesion, multiple sources for neurotrophic factors or cytokines exist, e.g., injured Schwann cells (8) and/or activated Schwann cells induced by macrophage derived cytokines (9), recruited macrohpages and their secretory products (10) or in the ECM by macrophage-induced proteolytic release of sequestered cytokines (11) which may act as maintenance and/or axonal sprouting factors. Lesion-induced cytokines, for example, from recruited macrophages or ECM, may also stimulate proliferation of non-neuronal elements involved in tissue repair and vascularization (12). Trophic support or impairment is indicated by bold or broken arrows. Plain arrows indicate inductive signals. Shading indicates lesion-induced activation. Adapted from (26).

bridge and prolific sprouting within the septum towards the infusion (82, 200). Similar results have been obtained using retinal ganglion cells (6). Findings included sprouting and tremendously long outgrowth away from the junction of the bridge. The procedure used for measuring activity caused a puncture in the vitreous (at a position opposed to the area of the bridge), which proved to be a rich source of trophin (6).

An NGF sensitive model in sensory DRG neuron axotomy has recently been established (151). Certain parameters in this model were addressed; i.e., "the definition of (1) the lesion and bridge implantation modalities, (2) the identification of the axons under study (by either natural or experimental labels) and their quantification, (3) baseline and time course studies of spontaneous regeneration events, and eventually (4) modalities and effects of exogenous NGF administrations" (200). This DRG/NGF model involves the removal of a small

segment of the dorsal funiculus, which is then replaced by a peripheral nerve bridge (either fresh or predegenerated). Three days before the end of the experiment, central sensory fibers were labeled through retrograde choleratoxin B (CTB) staining of the ipsalateral sciatic nerve. CTB immunostaining elucidated axonal regrowth caudal and rostral to the graft. The results indicated that the use of predegenerated peripheral explants is much more attractive to axons due to various factors including debris phagocytosis and Schwann cell proliferation (151, 200). Rostral infusion of NGF increased both distance into and number of DRG fibers in the cord. However, not all of the sensory fibers at the end of the graft were attracted into the spinal cord by the NGF infusion (151, 200). This may be due to the fact that only about half of the DRG neurons in the adult rat are believed to be responsive to NGF (151). Although this model has extended the regenerative scope of

LNGFR   ChAT

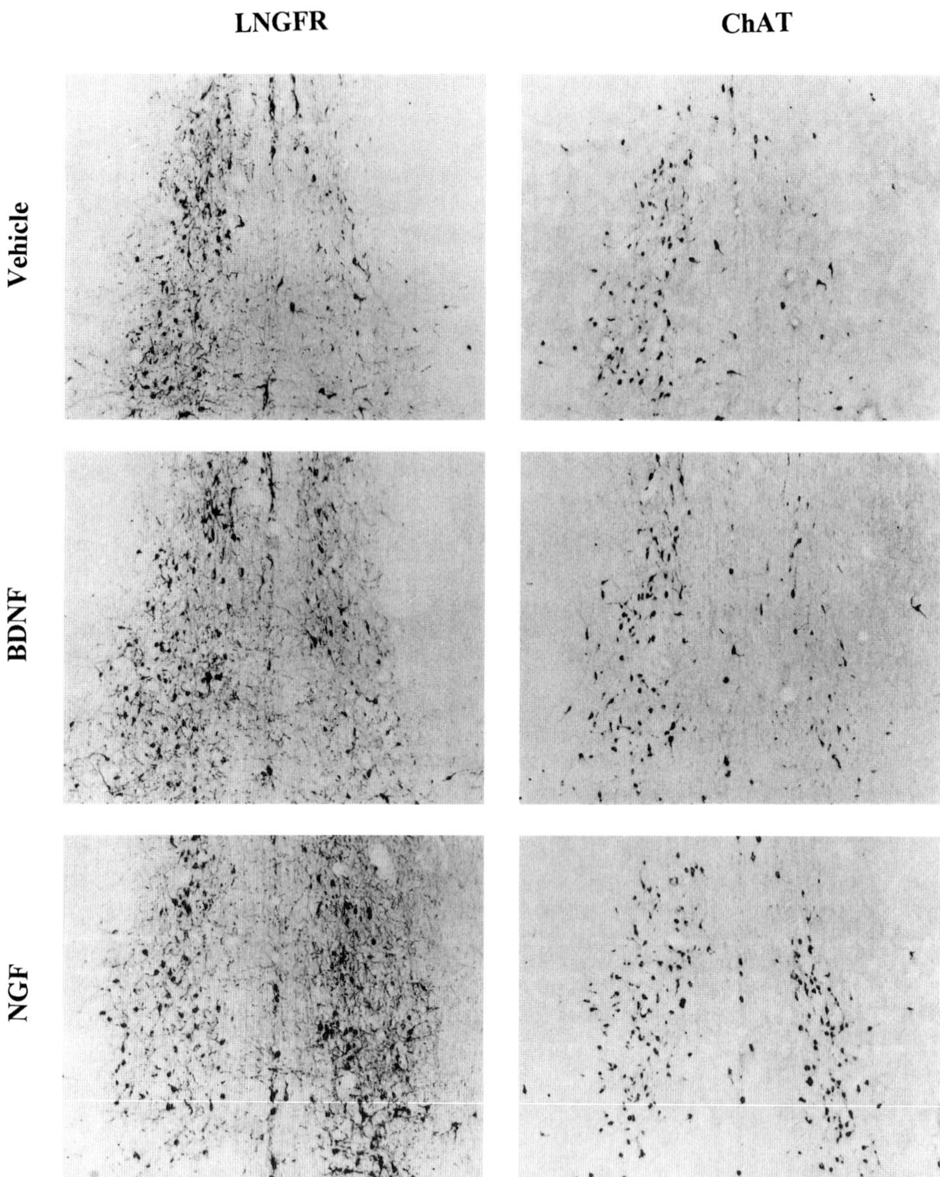

Figure 5. Photomicrographs showing the effects of fimbria-fornix transection on the number of septal neurons immunopositive for either LNGFR or ChAT, in animals intracerebroventricularly treated with NGF, BDNF or vehicle. The intact side of the septum is towards the left. Scale bar, 150 μm. Adapted from (141).

NGF to areas outside of the septo-hippocampal system, it reinforces the role of other neurotrophins and the differential responsiveness of subpopulations of neurons to various growth factors.

The aforementioned models quantify the ability of regrowth, but none addresses the question of whether proper synaptic reorganization is established after regeneration. In the fimbria-fornix transection model, a remarkable similarity in the cholinergic staining pattern (Figure 7) in the unlesioned adult rat hippocampus and the re-establishment of cholinergic axons has been demonstrated (50, 200). Using a

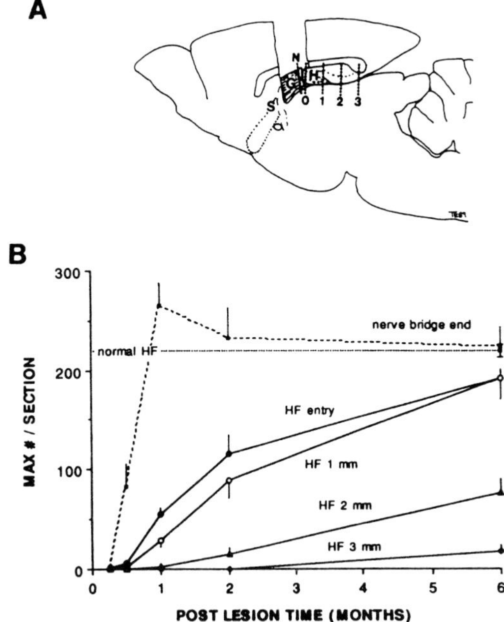

Figure 6. The septohippocampal cholinergic regeneration model presented by Varon and Conner. A. Sagittal diagram indicates the oriented nerve bridge (G) grafted between septum (S) and hippocampal formation (H) and the imaginary lines at the bridge end (N), the HF entrance (O), at different depths within the HF (1 mm, 2 mm, 3 mm), and the intersections of which by AChE-stained fibers permit quantitation of the regeneration. B. Time course of the axonal advances to the bridge end and into the hippocampal tissue. Adapted from (200).

potent anti-NGF polyclonal antibody and immunostaining, Varon and Conner examined how the distribution of endogenous NGF affected hippocampal formation (50, 200). Their results showed NGF-immunoreactivity (IR) within the cell body only in the basal forebrain cholinergic neurons. They also unexpectedly found extrasomal NGF-IR in the hilus of the dentate gyrus and in the CA2 and CA3 (but not in CA1) regions of the hippocampus (50). The extrasomal area of NGF-IR had clearly defined boundaries, suggesting a relationship with local structures that differed from the hippocampal pattern of cholinergic innervation in that the CA regions and laminar patterns closely resembled mossy fiber pattern formation (Figure 8) (50). "Selective localization and extrasomal anchorage are two attributes that would be required if endogenous NGF were to serve as a marker for axonal routes and axonal endfields" (50). Cur-

rent research centers on ways to enhance the number of sensory fibers entering the spinal cord and the distances they can reach once inside (200).

Features under study include the spatial distribution of the infused NGF, as well as dosage and timing. Modification to this model should provide a corresponding paradigm for the descending motor axons of the CST and their regenerative capabilities given the appropriate trophic, neuritogenic, and tropic factors. Identification of such factors is currently being sought using *in vitro* (CST neurons) and *in vivo* (adult axotomized CST neurons) models (5, 24, 26, 200).

Recent information obtained from NGF gene knockout in mice has confirmed earlier immunodepletion studies in which the extent of NGF influence during development was investigated. The mice were shown to have virtually no sympathetic neurons and a greater than seventy percent depletion of DRG neurons (52). Notably, there was a relatively normal population of basal forebrain cholinergic neurons. As a possible explanation for these results, and in light of the aforementioned septal cholinergic studies, the activity of an alternative trophic factor was considered, as will be discussed later.

Studies of NGF receptor expression have also given insight into the trophin's role during regeneration. The p75 molecule is the low affinity receptor for NGF, which is also slow to bind the whole family of NGF-related trophins (44, 45). The p75 receptor has been fully characterized but its role and implication in axonal regeneration remains a point of speculation. p75 is upregulated following transection (especially in Schwann cells) (44, 45). Whether the p75 receptor has a physiological role in increasing the ligand binding to the trk class of high affinity receptors remains an area of debate (21, 44, 45, 93, 161, 201). However, degrees of interaction between different receptor types may be responsible for the varied influence of neurotrophins on different populations of neurons. The signal transduction capabilities of p75 have only recently been described through structural analysis and studies on the cytoplasmic domain of the receptor which implicate a tumor necrosis factor (TNF)-like G-protein linkage (44, 189, 202). It is generally accepted that the trk high affinity receptors trkA, trkB, and trkC, a family of tyrosine kinase receptors, carry the signal trans-

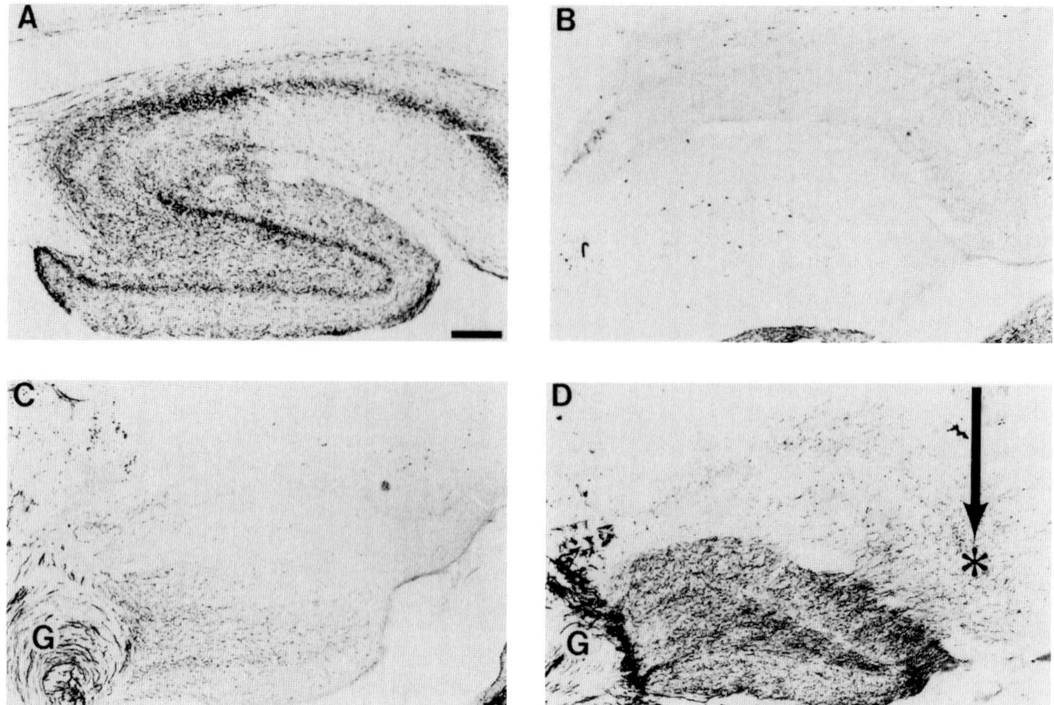

Figure 7.   Intrahippocampal NGF promotes cholinergic axonal regeneration into the hippocampus. A, Sagittal section of a normal AChE-stained hippocampus, scale bar, 250 μm. B, One month post ff transection, the hippocampus of gelfoam-implanted animals show no AChE fiber labeling. C, With sciatic nerve graft (G), many fibers show regrowth into the hippocampus. D, NGF infusion for 1 month into the dorsal hippocampus, along with the peripheral nerve graft (G), showing significant increase in hippocampal innervation by AChE-labeling fibers. Asterix, marks site of infusion. Adapted from (82).

duction load for the regenerative or outgrowth actions of the neurotrophins.

Each of the neurotrophins has a preferred receptor as depicted in Figure 9, with NT-3 showing the most 'cross-talk' capability (18, 94). The binding of neurotrophins elicits a biphasic response. Initially there is dimerization or oligomerization of the ligand-receptor complex which initiates autophosphorylation of their intracellular tyrosine residues (Figure 10) (18, 97, 168). These phosphorylated sites then serve as anchors for other molecules (enzymes and adaptors), activating them (18, 60, 168), and leading to the various downstream effects. Activation of trk kinases is also implicated in malignant transformation, but such changes are NT-independent, suggesting the presence of elements that discriminate between proliferation and growth/differentiation pathways (18). As far as regenerative responses are concerned, no specific trk substrates have been identified. TrkB expression has been shown to increase the

number of glial cells the hippocampus and dorsal funiculus of the spinal cord after transection, but no change has been seen in neurons (71). There is also an observed transient increase in expression of trkB transcripts in cerebral ischemia, kindling induced hippocampal seizures and hypoglycemic coma (18, 70, 71). Much of what is known about trk levels and expression has been examined in the context of development and survival, and much work remains to be done to elucidate the role these receptors may play in facilitating trophin-mediated regeneration.

Ibanez et al. have done extensive work in the structural analysis of the NGF-family of neurotrophins (90). Chimeric proteins were produced from NGF molecular replacements or homologous recombination with the BDNF molecule and were assessed with respect to their NGF-like trophism and/or their BDNF-like trophism. Findings included the ability of the NGF molecule to retain its trophism despite large re-

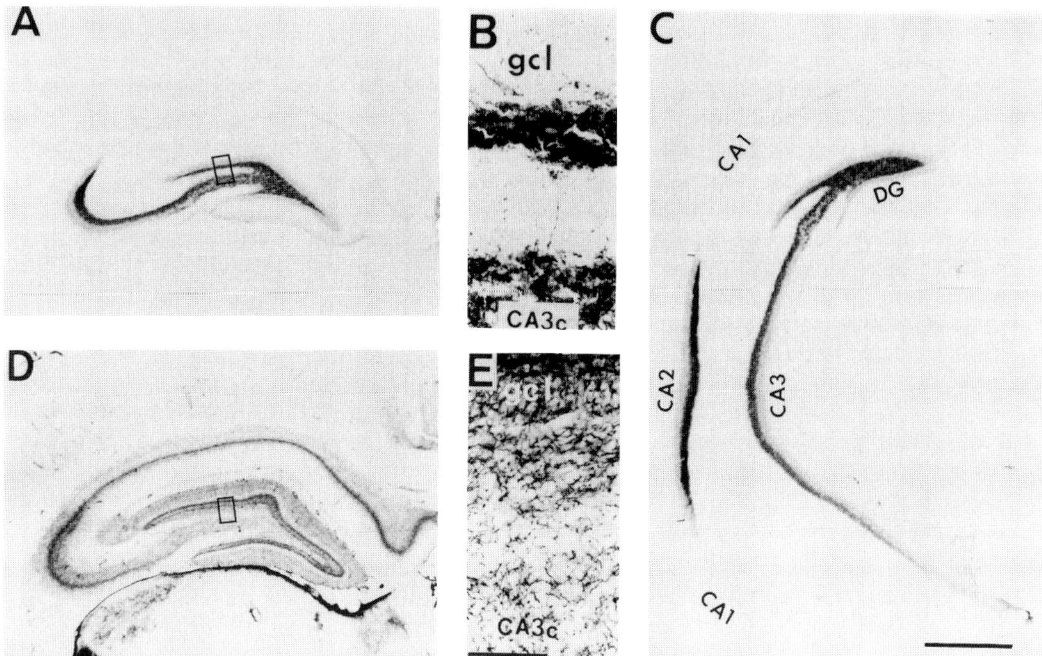

Figure 8.   NGF-like and LNGFR IR in the adult rat hippocampus. A, NGF-like IR localized to the dorsal hippocampus. B, 10× of inset from A, illustrating NGF IR in the dentate gyrus. C, NGF-like IR in the posterior hippocampus. Labeling was intensified adjacent to CA2 and was missing throughout CA1. D and E, Section adjacent to the one shown in A, illustrating LNGFR immunoreactivity in the dorsal hippocampus. Scale bar as shown in panel C, represents 1 mm. and is given for A, C, and D. Scale bar in E represents 100 μm and is given for B and E (gel-granule cell layer, DG-dentate gyrus). Adapted from (50).

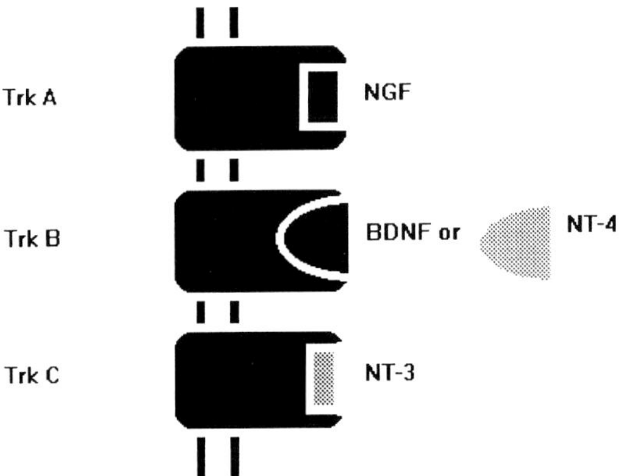

Figure 9.   Cartoon representing the ligand/trophin interaction with the NGF-family of NT's and the corresponding Trk family of receptors. These represent primary interactions and do not include the secondary interactions seen between NT-3 and all three Trk subtypes.

placements in its variable region. Additionally, these experiments revealed that homologous replacement of certain areas of the variable region

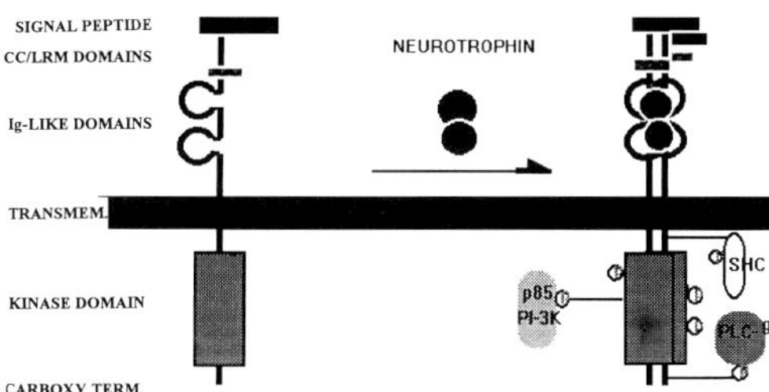

Figure 10.   This schematic represents the overall mechanism involved in the activation of the Trk family of tyrosine kinase receptors. The different domains of the receptor are indicated on the left side. After binding, dimerization is shown as are some of the proteins known to be directly phosphorylated from NT mediated activation of the Trk receptor. Adapted from (18, 97).

can endow a molecule both NGF and BDNF-like trophism (Fig. 11).

An interesting issue is the question of how the same neurotrophin can affect different responses such as differentiation and cell growth. Constitutive expression of certain proteins that are in the Ras pathway (a second messenger

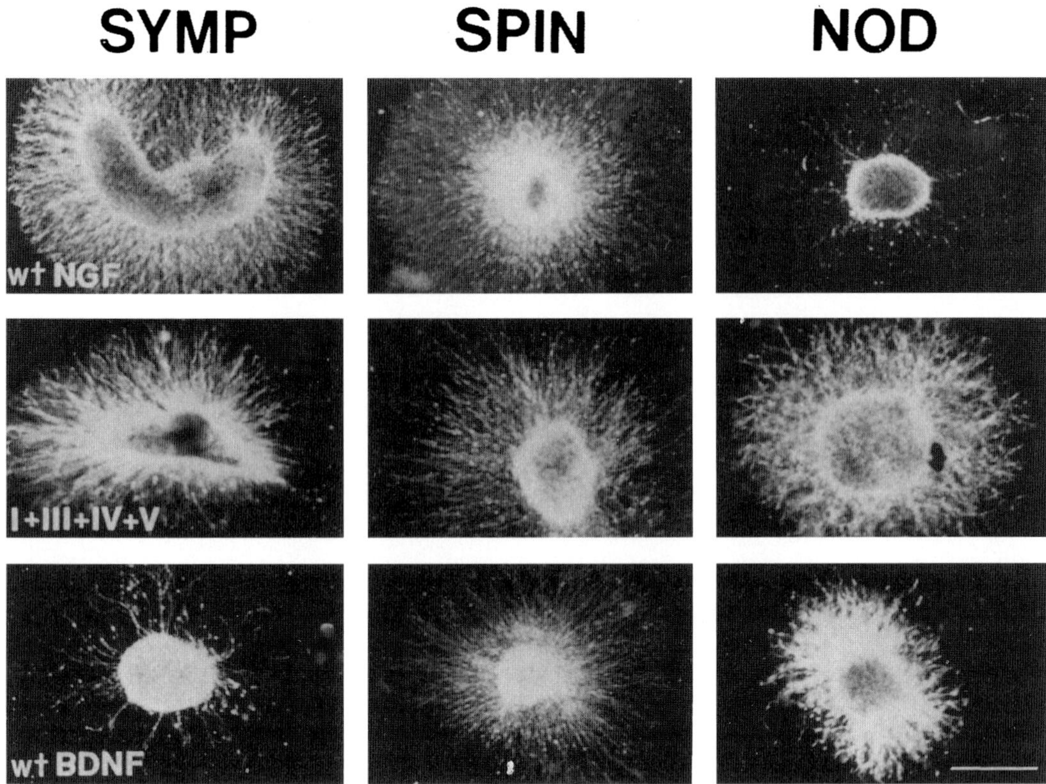

Figure 11. Shown are the neurite outgrowth activities of wild type NGF, BDNF and the chimeric molecule, I, III, IV, V, in embryonic explants of sympathetic (SYMP), spinal dorsal root (SPIN) and nodose (NOD) ganglion. The chimeric is able to evoke neurite outgrowth from both typically NGF-responsive ganglia (SYMP) and typically BDNF-responsive ganglia (NOD). Adapted from (90).

pathway activated by NT-trk binding), has been suggested to lead to neurite outgrowth (146, 192). Kaplan et al. have compiled a comprehensive review of signaling proteins that respond rapidly to NGF binding (as seen in PC12 cells) (100).

High and low affinity receptors are present at significant levels during embryonic development, but are extremely rare in the adult (80, 90, 126, 160, 161). It is noteworthy to mention that adult motor neurons that retain trkA-IR appear to be the ones spared in degenerative diseases such as amylotrophic lateral sclerosis (148, 160, 161). The role and expression of NGF-family trophic factors and receptors have been well studied in the PNS (especially spinal motor nerves) (24, 126, 149, 208). TrkA expression has been shown to become more pronounced after nerve transection, and subside upon completion of physiological regenerative events (26,

160, 161). This receptor expression is not always accompanied by an increased sensitivity to NGF, which implicates the role of NGFr protein in a family of neurotrophins (160, 161). Experiments done by Risling et al. reveal re-expression of trkA-IR in adult spinal cat motor-neurons after intermedullary axotomy (160). The re-expression of trkA in motorneurons after peripheral lesions may be the result of target derived signal, or be associated with periods of axonal regrowth and maturation (26, 110).

In scar tissue, the lesioned area may provide trophic factors, which in turn may lead to increased receptor synthesis (for a permitted time course) (160, 161). A lesion in the CNS could result in deficient BBB leading to an influx of serum NGF, in addition to the mesodermal intra-scar production of the trophin (20, 40, 129, 159, 160, 161, 217). Additionally, there may be infiltration of glial factors and cytokines that may affect both NGF and trkA production (20, 159). IL-1 may be involved in the central regenerative process in a variety of ways. IL-1 is produced by activated macrophages and glia and has a role in astrocytic proliferation (which is initially helpful to axonal regeneration); IL-1 is also known to direct NGF production in non-neuronal cell types (20, 40, 73, 159, 195).

Gage and Tuszynski have reviewed the role NGF may have in central trauma and regeneration (73, 195). Initial lesioning would lead to both direct neuronal damage and perforation of the BBB. Terminal degeneration and debris could activate the glia (microglia and astrocytes) which would then secrete IL-1 into the surrounding environment and induce the proliferation of astrocytes. Activated astrocytes release NGF which is an attractant to those fibers (cholinergic, for example) that express NGF receptor.

Bregman and Kunkel-Badgen have performed extensive studies on the role of NT's in graft related survival and regeneration in models of spinal cord lesion (27, 28, 29, 30, 112). The requirements for anatomical and functional repair in the cord may be considerably more complicated than recovery from other neurodegenerative disorders, which may only involve restoration of neurotransmitter levels (27, 29, 30). As mentioned previously, experiments have shown that PNS and embryonic explants are capable of promoting survival and regeneration of CNS neurons, including those of the spinal cord. Bregman's group performed a comprehensive study of the role played by the family of NGF-related NT's I axonal regrowth (as opposed to survival studies).

The immature spinal cord responds to trauma with greater anatomical reorganization than that observed following the same injury in the adult (30). Rerouting the late developing pathways and more enthusiastic axonal sprouting are two possible reasons for this difference (27, 29, 32, 39). Axonal sprouting in the neonate involves not only a greater density of innervation, but also a greater area (27, 29, 30). The increased anatomical plasticity that is found in the mature spinal cord varies with different tracts (27, 29, 30, 112). For example, injury to the immature rubrospinal tract results in massive death of axotomized neurons, whereas injury to the mature pathway results in neuronal atrophy and increase gliosis within the nucleus, but little cell loss (27, 29). In the immature circumstance, axons are closer to the cell body than in the adult and this may result in the increase appearance of cell death (46, 139). Coincidental with anatomical maturation is functional maturation, i.e., locomotion, which complicates measurement of functional regeneration after injury, relative to age (132).

Following spinal cord lesions at birth, fetal cord transplants rescue immature axotomized brainstem-spinal neurons from injury-induced retrograde cell death in a target specific fashion (27, 29, 96, 132). Neurons from the immature host regenerate through the fetal transplant and reach normal targets caudal to the graft. Additionally, neurons from the graft send axons into the host spinal cord. Thus, the transplanted graft serves both as a bridge for host axons and as a *de novo* source of axons for the injured cord (27, 29, 96, 132).

In the adult, axons from the fetal graft are able to send out axons into the host (corticospinal, raphe-spinal, coeruleospinal, intraspinal, and dorsal root). Adult axons have been shown to synapse in graft tissue. However, there is no growth of host fibers through the graft, caudal to the lesion (27, 29, 30, 96, 101). The fetal graft can therefore be seen to serve as a relay for supraspinal control for areas caudal to the transplant. Thus, just as the sprouting capabilities of axons after a lesion are greater at birth than in adulthood, so is transplant mediated regeneration (30, 96, 101).

Double fluorescent tracers were used to determine whether axons growing through the transplant originated from axotomized neurons and were, therefore, regenerating, or whether they arose from the fetal tissue (27, 29, 30). This paradigm involved a mid-thoracic spinal cord hemisection in a rat and temporally spaced retrograde tracing with fluorescent fast tracers: fast blue (FB) and diamindino yellow (DY). FB was introduced at the site of the lesion and given time to be taken up and transported. A transplant of embryonic day 14 spinal cord tissue was placed into the lesion site and after, 3–6 weeks, DY was injected caudal to the lesion. Late developing axons would not be exposed to FB, but could be exposed to DY, so neurons labeled only with DY were considered to be late growing. Neurons axotomized at the mid-thoracic level would be exposed to FB, so if they grew after the lesion, through the transplant and further caudals, they could also be DY labeled. These double-labeled axons would be considered to be regenerating neurons. Axotomized neurons that did not grow through the graft would only be labeled by FB. Bregman's group also used a pump to deliver BDNF, NT-3, or NT-4/5 to the site of the lesion. A schematic diagram of the progressive restriction of corticospinal plasticity with increasing age at the time of lesion is shown in Fig. 16 (29).

When fetal spinal cord tissue is transplanted into the adult after spinal cord injury, host axons grow into the transplants but their growth is limited to 2 mm adjacent to the transplant border. The exogenous administration of NT-3, BDNF, or NT-4/5 after fetal transplants into adult rats resulted in dramatic increase of brainstem spinal axonal growth into the graft. Infusion of NT-3 and BDNF was also shown to greatly enhance the growth of collaterals into the fetal graft (30). The authors suggest that exogenous administration of BDNF, NT-3, or NT-4/5 may rescue mature neurons from degeneration and death as well as enhance the growth environment of the fetal graft (30). In further unpublished results by Bregman's group, utilizing the same paradigm, the use of NT-3 and NT-4/5 revealed a marked increase in serotonin labeling. Administration of BDNF resulted in an increase in both 5-HT and DBH noradrenergic immunoreactivity (30). This is clinically significant since serotonergic and norandrenergic fibers in the spinal cord have been shown to carry all of the locomotive capabilities of the organism.

NGF has also been used to support adrenal medullary grafts in Parkinson's disease. NGF infusion helps both chromaffin cell survival and neuronal transformation and significantly improves adrenal medullary graft transplant efficacy (148). NGF treatment may also be shown to be helpful in Alzheimer's disease although the disease has no direct effect on any NGF mediated mechanism (148). Olson et al have suggested that NGF treatment may be used to retard or inhibit cholinergic denervation (involved in cognitive and memory function loss) and induce sprouting of these fibers (148). The wide range of animal evidence supporting the use of NGF has led to its recent introduction into clinical trials (125).

To substantiate a potential role for BDNF in the maintenance of forebrain cholinergic neu-

rons in the adult brain, Morse et al. studied the trophin's ability to sustain the medial septal cholinergic neuronal phenotype after a unilateral transection of the fimbria (141). Their studies showed that infusion of BDNF into the brains of adult rats from an implanted osmotic pump rescued basal forebrain cholinergic neurons from axotomy-induced degeneration and death. When BDNF was delivered into the parenchyma at the level of the septum, its effects were comparable to those reported for NGF infusion via an intracerebroventricular route. However, as opposed to NGF, which diffuses well from the CSF space into the brain parenchyma, BDNF displays an extremely limited penetration through the ependymal cells and glial end feet which make up the ventricular lining (56, 141). The reason for this may be the high level expression on astrocytes and ependymal cells of a truncated form of trkB, the high affinity BDNF receptor (126).

BDNF has also been suggested for the treatment of Alzheimer's disease. As mentioned earlier, NGF studies have been promising, but the high specificity of the trophin may limit its positive effects. For this reason, the broader spectrum of influence of BDNF lends itself to investigation. Due to the lack of any relevant animal model for Alzheimer's, BDNF has been studied by its application to various brain regions, and the assessment of its influence on morphology, neurochemistry, and behavior (87, 88, 109, 126, 141, 155). Infusion of BDNF into the hippocampus, cortex or striatum leads to dramatic changes in levels of several neuroactive peptides including substance P, dynorphin, and CCK (20). Changes in the peptide levels induced by BDNF were generally opposite to those seen in the Alzheimer's disease state (51, 143, 155). The effects of BDNF on cognitively impaired aged rats and chemically lesioned animals are current areas of research (56).

BDNF was the first fully characterized NT that was found to promote the survival of embryonic rat nigral dopaminergic neurons (87). BDNF has also been shown to provide protection against the neurotoxic effects of 6-hydroxydopanine (6-OHDA) and MPTP (183) suggesting a role for BDNF in the treatment of Parkinson's disease (125). The finding that BDNF protects dopaminergic neurons from 6-OHDA toxicity by a mechanism which decreases oxidative stress may have great importance, if indeed oxidative stress is an important component of neurodegenerative diseases such as Parkinson's (183).

Hyman's group has recently shown that BDNF also promotes survival of nigral GABAergic neurons (87, 88). The *in vitro* survival promoting effects of BDNF on striatal GABAergic neurons indicates its possible usefulness in Huntington's disease studies (88, 126).

Localization of the expression of BDNF mRNA using *in situ* hybridization methods has both supported and extended previous findings of the presence of BDNF in various brain regions (57, 126, 143, 155). The presence of BDNF mRNA is a subpopulation of dorsal root ganglion cells (having no afferent input) is consistent with the possibility that BDNF may serve an autocrine function (155). Treatment with BDNF antisense oligonucleotides leads to selective neuronal death of DRG neurons (with no effect using sense strands) (126). In the adult CNS, autocrine NT loops may be a common mechanism which ensures neuronal survival once the appropriate period of 'pruning' has plateaued (126). If this is true, any decrease in autocrine NT levels as a result of aging, disease or trauma may lead to neuronal loss (or loss of function) and possibly be a component of the etiology of one or more neurodegenerative diseases. For example, significant loss of BDNF mRNA levels in post mortem tissue samples from the hippocampal formation of Alzheimer's patients has been noted (155).

Mey and Thanos looked at how retinal ganglion cells (RGC) were affected after optic nerve transection and BDNF treatment (190). NT's were injected into the vitreous body of adult rats that were sacrificed at different times; the survival and size of RGC's were then determined. It is important to emphasize that a variety of trophic factors may be involved in the maintenance of injured neurons. Their experiments suggested the importance of a time window of effectiveness, successful treatment based on the site of delivery, and the inherent resistance to degradation exhibited by larger RGC's (190).

A third member of the NGF-related gene family is neurotrophin-3 (NT-3). In tissue culture studies, there is a marked overlap in effects between BDNF and NT-3 (87, 88, 92, 165, 166, 182). This may be due to the colocalization of the high affinity receptors for both BDNF and NT-3 (trkB and trkC, respectively) and the fact that NT-3 can act at the BDNF receptor, albeit at a higher concentration (8, 94, 114, 182). This finding is evident in the effect of NT-3 on basal cholinergic neurons (9); in vitro, NT-3 is much less potent that BDNF in promoting the survival and differentiation of these cells and, in vivo, is less vigorously retrogradely transported than BDNF to septal cholinergic neurons following hippocampal injection of either ligand (56, 126).

In 1991, Hallbook et. al. cloned a fourth member of the NGF-related family from Xenopus: neurotrophin-4/5 (NT-4/5) (83). Berkemeier et al., in 1992 (91), subsequently cloned the human gene. Most of the studies done with NT-3, -4/5, as with BDNF, are survival studies, and the literature is replete with findings on this subject (9, 22, 46, 87, 92, 109, 123, 139, 141, 158, 165, 169). With regard to regeneration in the CNS, these latter NT's have only been preliminarily assayed in some of the same models presented for NGF.

Nicholl's group has studied the developing CNS of the opposum (Monodelphis domestics), as it can be isolated and maintained in vitro for periods of a week or longer (194). Lesioning studies have shown that the developing opposum CNS has a great ability to regenerate which decreases dramatically with the onset of glial development. The authors are currently investigating how treatment with NGF, BDNF, NT-3, and NT-4/5 and inhibitors of oligodendroglial associated molecules (IN-1 and IN-2) affect regeneration (194).

Aguayo et. al. have investigated the molecular events surrounding optic nerve injury and regeneration in the retino-tectal system of adult rats (5, 6, 46, 132). They grafted segments of peripheral nerve (PN) to the ocular stump of severed ON's and used them to provide the axotomized retinal ganglion cells with PNS substrates rich in peripheral ECM and Schwann cells (35). Additionally, they administered various NT's intravitreally before and after ON transection (6). In mature rats, the majority of RGC's express the high affinity trkB receptor that can mediate BDNF and NT-4/5 trophism (106, 107, 182); a smaller population of RGCs exhibit the trkC receptor (6). Truncated forms of trkB that predominate in glial cells (166) decrease abruptly in the ON after axotomy (6,

132). Furthermore, while glia in transected ON's do not significantly up-regulate mRNA's for several NT's, PN segments show a marked and sustained increase. This data may help to explain why ON transections result in the apoptopic death of nearly 90% of all RGC's within two weeks, while PN grafts enhance RGC survival and axonal elongation. The delivery of either BDNF or NT-4 by intravitreal injection transiently rescues most injured RGC's and stimulates intra-retinal axonal growth (Fig. 12) (5, 6, 46, 132).

NT-4/5 cause a dose dependent increase in intravitreal neurite outgrowth with one half maximal effects at approximately 0.5 ng/ml and maximal effects at 5 ng/ml (46). In explants treated for seven days, the influence of NT-4/5 was similar to that of BDNF (46, 132). NT-3 has been shown to stimulate RGC sprouting and its administration is associated with a distinct pattern of GAP-43 expression in RGC's (132). Growth factors expressed within the lesioned eye can also protect RGC's from dying soon after axotomy.

On the other hand, neither the intravitreal administration of NT's nor their availability from endogenous sources has resulted in increased innervation of the PN grafts by RGC's, which suggests that an appropriate substrate may be needed for axons to extend from the retina to the grafts (Fig. 12) (5, 6, 46, 132).

Schnell et al. have investigated the effects of NGF, NT-3, and BDNF in concert with IN-1 in the corticospinal tract of lesioned adult rat spi-

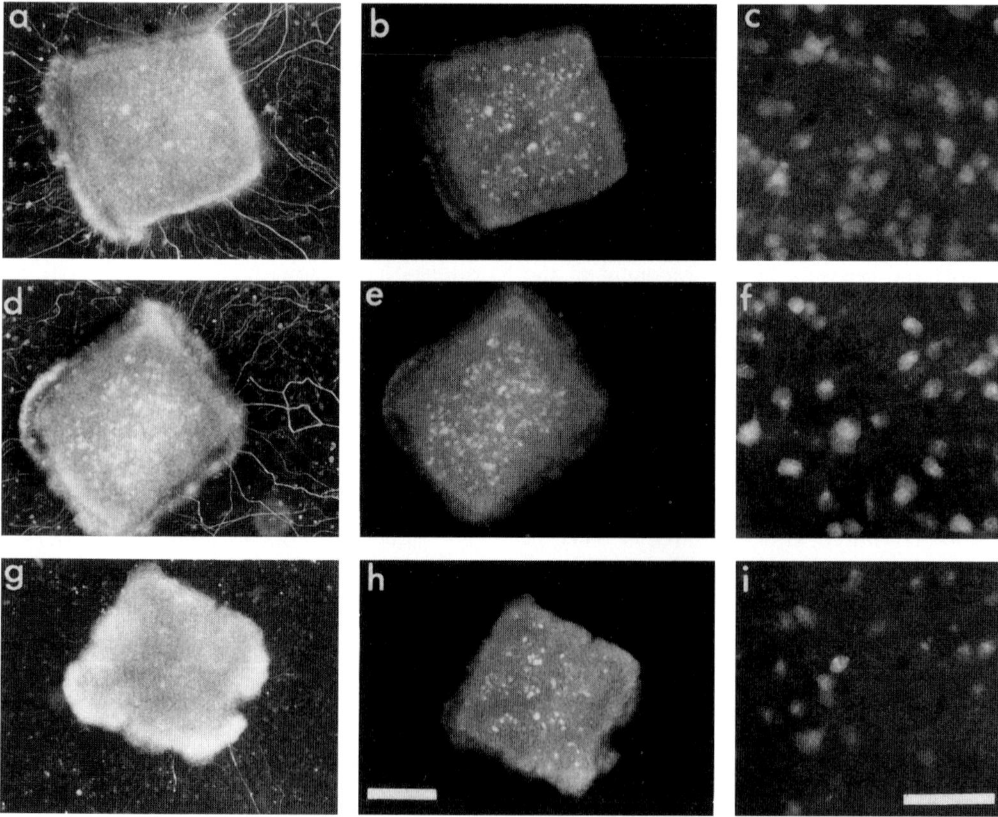

Figure 12. Increased survival and promotion of neurite outgrowth of RGC's in retinal explants treated with NT-4/5 or BDNF. FG prelabelled RGC's cultured for 7 days in the presence of controlled media or media + NT-4/5 (50 ng/ml). Immunolabelled with RT97 (a,d,g), BDNF (d,e,f), or no added trophic factor (g,h,i). The morphology and degree of fasciculation were comparable for neurites exposed to NT-4/5 and BDNF. Neurite outgrowth from the explants was observed on the surface of migrating glia (GFAP-positive cells), as well as on laminin. The degree of glial migration was similar in both control and treated specimens. Adapted from (46).

nal cord (169). In these experiments, the dorsal half of spinal cords of rats aged 4–7 weeks were bilaterally transected at the lower thoracic level. The NT's were injected immediately rostral to the lesion. In half of the experimental animals, hybridoma cells, secreting monoclonal IN-1 (or a control substance) were injected into the left parietal cortex and lateral ventricle. This led to the formation of tumors that would supply the cord with IN-1 via the CSF. Parasagittal sections were used to quantify regenerating axons and, as seen in figure 3, there were marked difference in the length of elongating axons as a function of the antibody and the NT used. In the controls, elongation was rarely past sprouting length, whereas growth over the greatest distances was observed in the animals receiving IN-1 with NT-3. In this group, axons reached the lower lumbar and sacral portions of the cord. These and developmental data suggest that NT-3 is the NT of choice for developing CST fibers (169).

CNTF and FGF are neurotrophic factors that are unrelated to the NGF-family of molecules. The two major FGF's and CNTF are relatively abundant as compared to the other NT's, as they are not readily secreted and tend to accumulate. In addition to crucial roles in tissue development and differentiation, these factors also have characteristics relevant to the traumatic-regenerative response. A large supply of trophic support in the cytoplasm may serve as an immediate local source for delivery after injury. In fact, CNTF and its receptors have functional and structural homology to IL's and other cytokines intimately associated with defense and inflammatory responses (119, 177).

CNTF was identified and named through its association with the survival of chick ciliary neurons (1, 145, 177). Human CNTF has been structurally characterized and cloned (113, 177). In the adult rat CNS, highest levels of CNTF are found in the optic nerve, olfactory bulb, and spinal cord. Other areas of the brain contain varying levels of CNTF, but none has been demonstrated in frontal cortex or the retina (177). CNTF mRNA has been shown to increase rapidly in the adult CNS after lesions involving the hippocampus or cortex (95, 177). The increase is seen in both mRNA and protein levels and found to be sustained for a minimum of three weeks (95). Immuno-precipitation (Ip) has revealed that a large source of this CNTF is

the reactive astrocyte. Interestingly, IFN-gamma can cause an increase in CNTF transcription (42, 177). IFN-gamma is a cytokine not normally found in the CNS, and its affect on astrocytes may be a general response of these glial cells when exposed, through trauma, to cells of the immune system. CNTF expression can be repressed upon activation of adenylate cyclase and treatment with beta-adrenergic agonists (42). Thus, neurotransmitters may keep astrocytic production of CNTF in check in the uninjured CNS. At a lesion, where neuronal input is comprised and there is loss of neurotransmitter mediated suppression, a possible breach of the BBB and hypertrophy of astrocytes (i.e., formation of the gliotic scar), may lead to unhindered production of CNTF. CNTF has been shown to promote the survival and differentiation of a variety of neuronal populations in the prenatal rat. In the adult, CNTF exerts neuroprotection over certain cells in ways other than merely preventing degeneration. Evidence shows that CNTF may protect hippocampal cells from glutamate toxicity (181) as well as protecting retinal photoreceptor cells against deleterious effects of constant fluorescent light (116). The capability of CNTF to promote survival has also been examined in various transection models. CNTF infusion can rescue various populations of septal neurons (including NGF sensitive cholinergic neurons) in fornix-fimbria transections (80). Administration of CNTF has been shown to save dopaminergic cells of the substantia nigra after nigrostriatal transection, and neurons of the dorsal and anteroventral thalamic nuclei after cingulum bundle transection (81). The precise *in vivo* role of CNTF is still very unclear, but there are clues that may be more important in the adult than in the developing nervous system. CNTF levels are extremely low in the embryo, and knockout experiments in mice have revealed that these animals develop and thrive normally but show a great deal of muscle atrophy and motor neuron loss in adulthood (134). Because of this, CNTF was used in clinical trials for ALS patients. Furthermore, CNTF levels are known to rise dramatically after injury, via Schwann cell and astrocyte production (95, 177). These expression patterns point to the fact that CNTF may play a key role in the response to injury and in long term maintenance in the adult nervous system.

Elucidation of the mechanisms involved in CNTF binding occurred in parallel with related cytokine studies. CNTF binds to a three component receptor complex, CNTF-alfa, LIF-beta, and gp130 (185). Although binding requires the presence of all three, only the last two are involved in phosphorylation events eliciting intracellular signal transduction (185). It is of interest to note that LIF binds to two receptors LIF-beta and gp130, forming a heterodimer (184), while IL-6 also binds to two receptors, both gp130, forming a homodimer (103). The gp130 subunit is found in many cells, as is LIF-beta. Tissue specificity is conferred by the presence (or absence) of the CNTF-alpha subunit, found rather exclusively in neurons (185). These findings may explain the cross-talk of LIF and CNTF.

Characterization of the CNTF-receptor complex may also provide much information regarding other members of the cytokine family. As mentioned earlier, the beta subunits are responsible for tyrosine kinase activity (55). The tyrosine kinase activity is from the family of Jak/Tyk kinases prelinked to the beta subunits and activated by ligand driven dimerization (186). Jak/Tyk activity results in phosphorylation of many proteins, including a novel signaling protein that is a DNA-binding transcriptional activator-STAT 88/90 (185). Although STAT 88/90 is exclusively activated by CNTF, there are many other tyrosine inducible phosphorylations that overlap with other neurotrophic factors such as NGF and FGF. This type of collaboration between cytokines and growth factors, both acting through receptor tyrosine kinases, has been well documented in the hematopoeitic system (Figure 13) (185).

The family of FGF's consists of nine members (59). The first two discovered, acidic FGF (aFGF or FGF1) and basic FGF (bFGF or FGF2), are also the best characterized and are considered representative of the family. Both FGF1 and FGF2 are present in high amounts in the CNS (59). The cellular localization of FGF's in still a matter of debate but it is known that these two factors are the primary mitogens in the adult CNS. In optic nerve lesion models, an appreciable rise in FGF2 levels is observed. Furthermore, the source of this factor has been shown to be astrocytes (59).

Four high affinity receptors for FGF's have been isolated and sequenced, and subsequent cloning has revealed that the two most common receptor types (FGFR-1 and FGFR-2) are splice variants (59, 98). Over the last few years, a large number of FGF receptor splice variants have been characterized. Each splicing is not the sole mechanism involved in conferring selectivity. Receptors from the four different genes that do not exhibit variance in the splicing of the third Ig domain (where variance has the greatest affect on selectivity and ligand affinity) may still exhibit differing binding affinities (98). Moreover, the high affinity FGF receptors belong to a family of transmembrane tyrosine kinases. Phosphorylation of phospholipase C-gamma appears to play a role in signal trans-

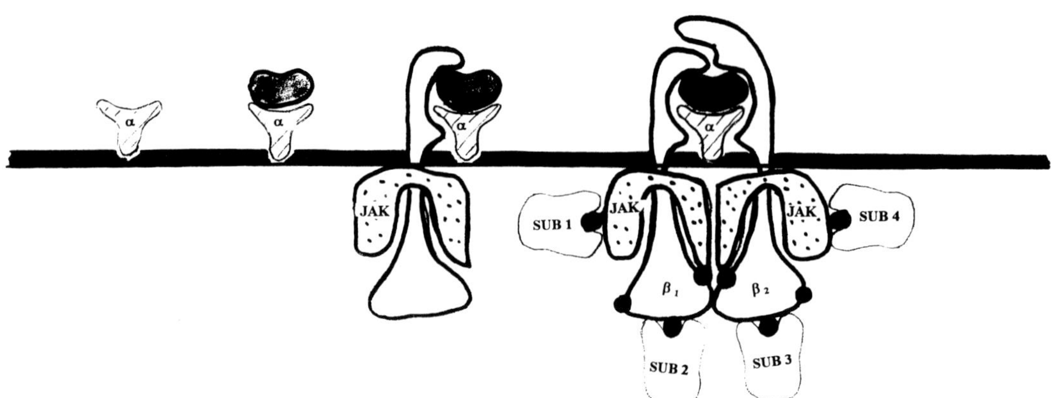

Figure 13.   From left to right is depicted a schematic for the stepwise events of CNTF binding leading to an activated receptor form (generically shown). More detail of the sequence of events and the specific molecules involved in this process is given in the text. Adapted from (183).

duction (36). Localization of the different high affinity FGFR's reveals that FGFR-1 is associated with neurons (204) and FGFR2 and 3, with glial cells (11); all three of these receptors are found predominately in their IIIc splice forms (with variation at the third Ig domain). These isoforms, by themselves, would make it difficult for the cell to distinguish between FGF-1 and FGF-2.

The fact that the growth factor and its receptors all interact with heparan sulfate proteoglycans (HSPG) implicates a role for these molecules in FGF binding specificity and selectivity (59). Although FGF's do not bind to HSPG with affinity greater than to FGFR's, HSPG's are preferred over other sulfated proteoglycans (59). This fact and the fact that FGF's are found bound to the surface suggests that HSPG could be the low affinity FGF receptor. Characterization of these and other relevant low affinity proteoglycans is underway, but two molecules have been shown to be significant. Syndecan and glypican are surface bound heparan proteoglycans (41, 59, 102). Glypican, which is much more abundant in the mature CNS than syndecan, has been shown to bind FGF-2 with intermediate affinity (102). Depletion of heparan sulfate from the cell surface greatly reduces the ability of FGF to activate FGFR phosphorylation (156). Findings such as this have resulted in the following proposal for FGF-HSPG-FGFR interactions (59, 104). Free FGF requires heparan sulfate binding to conformationally activate it, thus making it presentable to the FGFR. This hypothesis is advanced by observations that FGF does indeed undergo conformational changes upon HSPG binding, and that HSPC binding alone can activate the FGF receptor (104).

FGF's display a wide range of effects which detract from their specificity. The mitogenic response to FGF is the most common effect observed in cells from the ectoderm and mesoderm. Oligodendrocytes, Schwann cells and astrocytes have been implicated as the primary target for FGF mediated mitogenesis (59). FGF-1 and FGF-2 have also been shown to promote survival of cerebral cortical and hippocampal neurons (176). Post-lesion protective effects of FGF-2 on MPTP treated substantia nigra and axotomized septal cholinergic neurons have also been observed (59). FGF-1 has

been reported to promote regeneration in some of these lesioned systems.

The mechanisms involved in FGF's trophism include the upregulation of neurotransmitter receptors (136) and ion channel expression (54), in addition to an increase in the production of cell adhesion molecules (137) and other neurotrophins (217). These observations are largely derived from *in vitro* studies. Cells may have access to FGF's in the extracellular space in vivo. Thus, elucidation of the processes involved in the release and delivery of FGF's is integral to the understanding of this molecule's function.

The family of FGF's contradict with the traditional view of target derived neurotrophins in two ways (59); FGF's possess remarkably broad mitogenic capabilities and their neurotrophism displays relatively little specificity. One hypothetical model for FGF action has been suggested by Eckenstein, using the motor neuron, which express both FGF-1 and FGFR-1 (59). In this model, secreted FGF's may promote division of developing motor neurons in the neuroepithelium and provide target derived trophism during apoptotic signaling. Sufficient evidence to support this part of the hypothesis is not available, since the expression of extracellular FGF does not reach significant levels until well after the period of programmed cell death, i.e. apoptosis. It has been shown that, after axotomy, immature motor neurons are more likely to degenerate while mature cells will more likely regenerate. This propensity for regeneration coincides with an increase in FGF-1 expression levels and a concomitant increase in intracellular stores. Eckenstein suggests that, upon injury, the plasma membrane is compromised, leading to spillage of the stores that contain almost 10^3 times more FGF than other traditionally secreted factors. This mechanism would provide a sufficient source of extracellular FGF, leading to receptor binding and activation. Therefore, FGF-1 can act as a messenger of motor neuron damage and an initiator of the repair response. This response would not only promote motor neuron survival and aid regeneration by directly acting on the neuron, but would also recruit support through astrocytic, oligodendrocytic, and Schwann cell proliferation (59). This hypothetical model is far from proven, but many of its ideas are consistent with the data.

In the context of regeneration, IGF's have been studied primarily in the PNS. However, in situ hybridization experiments have localized IGF-1 and IGF-2 regions of the brain (117). Both IGF's bind to specific surface bound receptors. The structure of the IGF-1 receptor closely resembles that of the insulin receptor in that it exists as a heterotetrameric integral membrane glycoprotein, with two extracellular, ligand interactive alpha subunits and two transmembrane/cytoplasmic beta subunits (117, 147, 163, 196). The cytoplasmic domains contain an ATP binding and a typical tyrosine kinase domain. IGF binding at the alpha subunit leads to a conformational change in the associated beta subunit, leading to autophosphorylation and activation of tyrosine kinase (163). Downstream phosphorylation of various substrates leads to the relevant biological consequences of the growth factor. The IGF-2 receptor is completely different, being composed of a single polypeptide chain with large extracellular and short cytoplasmic domains. There is no tyrosine kinase region but this receptor is thought to have a G-protein binding domain (147). The fact that both the receptors and growth factors have been found in the brain suggests that they have a role in the CNS. For example, *in vitro*, the presence of the IGF's and their receptors is associated with synaptogeneiss, neurite outgrowth, myelination, and cell proliferation (117).

As important as the recruitment of dendritic and axonal cytoskeleton proteins are to regeneration, cellular metabolism must also be maintained to facilitate the demands of growth. The BBB chiefly regulates the degree of glucose uptake in the CNS. IGF-1 has been reported to effect transcription of Glut-1, a glucose transporter protein (117, 203, 207). In the neonate, it is thought that Glut-1 is the primary internal transporter for glucose metabolism (203, 207). However, increased glucose metabolism is seen only in glial cells and not in neurons (117, 207). IGF-1 stimulates the proliferation of glial progenitro cells and the differentiation of oligodendrocytes. Increased Glut-1 synthesis leads to the proliferation of astroglial cells. LeRoith and others hypothesize that IGF-1 and IGF binding proteins (IGF-B's) provide a set of signals controlling the protein's neurotrophic effects (117). IGF-1 is synthesized and released and used in an autocrine or paracrine fashion (Figure 14) which is regulated by receptor and IGF-BP lev-

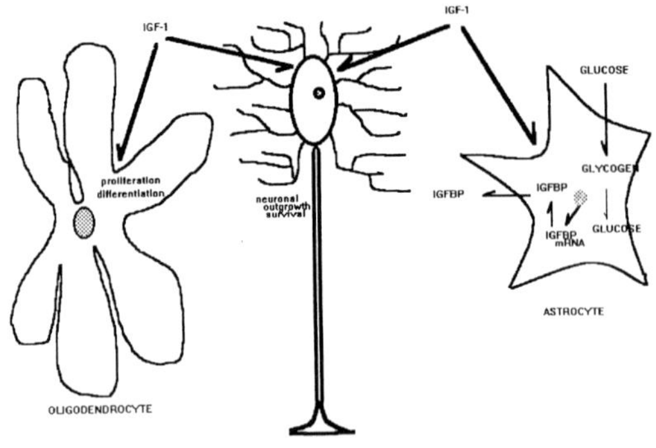

Figure 14.   This cartoon shows the hypothetical effects if IGF-1 on neurons and glia. In astrocytes, IGF-1 receptor activation leads to Glut1 gene expression and increased glucose transport. This results in the build up of glycogen. Additionally, the expression of the IGF-BP gene and release of binding proteins (BP's), may serve to regulate the astrocyte-directed actions of IGF-1. In neurons, IGF-1 stimulates survival and outgrowth and in oligodendrocytes, IGF-1 leads to proliferation and differentiation. Adapted from (117).

els. The involvement of glial cells in addition to the neurons provides great sensitivity to changes in the environment. Thus, a mechanism exists in which a neuron may react to a gliotic or a hypoglycemic situation (117).

Another avenue of study involves the differential gene expression in lesioned and regenerating neurons. Immediate early genes have been shown to be preferentially upregulated in PNS axotomy models. It has been suggested that initial patterns of gene expression are similar following axotomy in the CNS. Immediate early genes are activated by growth factors and can rapidly and transiently effect a multitude of changes in the cell. These changes differ based on the diversity of growth factor responses and differences in neuronal/glial phenotypes. The most commonly studied immediate early genes in the neuron are c-jun, c-fos, egr1, krox20, nur77, and scip (most closely linked to the Schwann cell proliferation). These genes have also been implicated in many of the long-term developmental changes associated with neuronal plasticity.

A suitable environment for regeneration could also be provided by introduction of cells to the injured area. Much of the work involving the transplantation of supportive Schwann cells (SC) has been undertaken by Bunge's group at the Miami Project. SC display many vital qual-

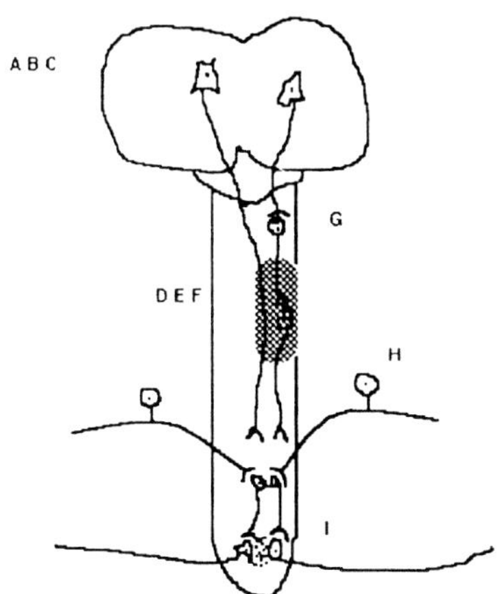

Figure 15. Possible mechanisms for repair. This schematic diagram illustrates several potentail mechanisms by which transplants of fetal CNS tissue may repair the injured spinal cord and mediate recovery of function. ABC show how the graft may provide target specific support for either late developing or regenerating axons to grow into or through the graft. The DEF area shows how the graft may provide a more favorable environment at the site of injury (perhaps through trophic factors). G and H illustrate how the graft may act as a bridge and relay for supraspinal control; H figure based on figure in (29).

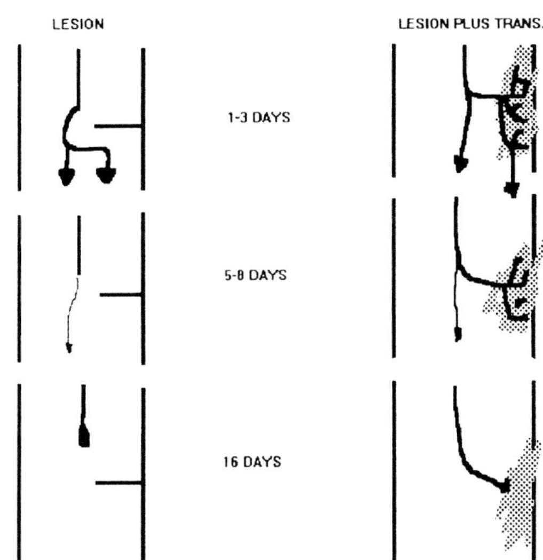

Figure 16. Diagram of the progressive restriction of corticospinal tract regenerative capability with increasing age at the time of lesion. Adapted from (29).

ities that make them key elements in peripheral regeneration. SC's are important regulators of ensheathment and myelination. When injured axons degenerate, SC's clear the debris and maintain their original position in the basal lamina so as to form faciliatory conduits, termed bands of Bungner, through which regenerating axons grow (35). Studies in which cellular composites were removed from peripheral nerve grafts revealed that only grafts with viable cells were able to allow regeneration of damaged axons from the CNS. The classic fornix-fimbria transection model has also served to demonstrate the ability of SC's to allow for CNS axonal regeneration (35, 111). Septal cholinergic axons that traverse this region show extremely limited regenerative capabilities. However, in the presence of a collagen-supported SC graft, regenerating axons reaching the hippocampus within two weeks (collagen only grafts had no effect). Axons of retinal ganglion cells have also been shown to be responsive, in a regenerative fashion, to SC's (4). A paradigm similar to the fornix-fimbria model has been undertaken to study spinal cord regeneration (152). Purified populations of SC's were grown

and expanded *in vitro* and seeded within tubular guidance channels, which were then inserted at the site of the lesion (connecting the distal and proximal stumps of the cord). The initial studies were performed using a dense collagen support (213, 214, 215). To avoid the possible barrier to elongation this may have presented, semipermeable polyacrylonitrile/polvinylchloride (PAN/ PVC) guidance channels were used (which have previously been shown to be effective in peripheral nerve regeneration) (2, 3, 33). Stumps, created by photochemical lesioning at T8, were placed 1 mm into openings of the graft/channel (33). One month post-grafting, a highly vascularized cable was used to connect the stumps of the cord, creating a bridge. Some channels were closed at the distal end and others were open at both ends, in order to discriminate between ascending and descending input into the graft (Fig. 17) (215).

The vast majority of axons that regenerated into the graft were from the spinal gray matter, and the mean number of myelinated axons was almost double when both ends of the channel were open (153). The key technical advantages of this channel are the versatility in length, width, and content. These guidance channels also serve to limit the invasion of scar tissue, or other inhibitory substances. SC's were purified and expanded from peripheral nerve segments

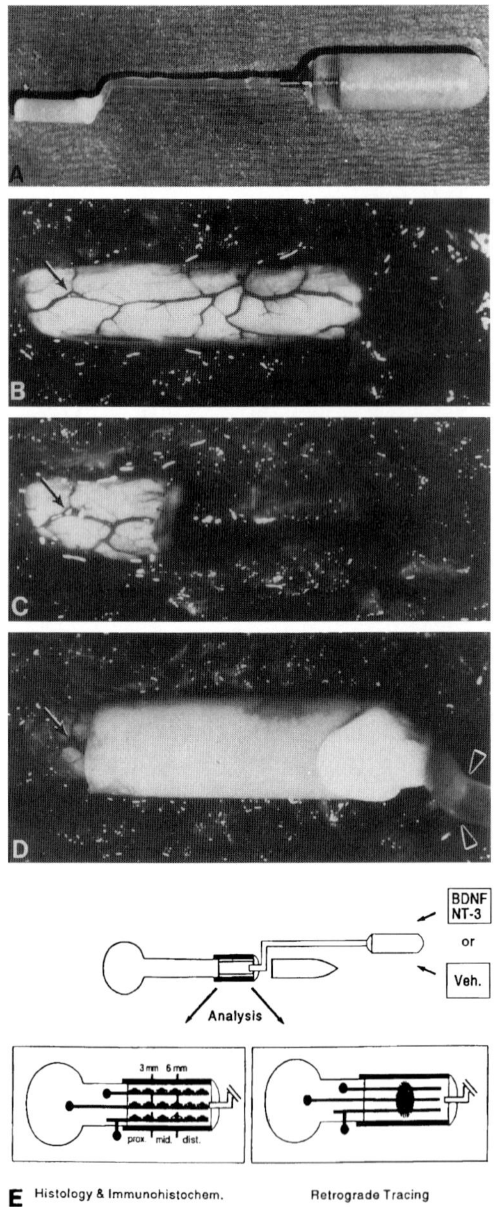

Figure 17. A, Schwann cell filled guidance channel connected to an Alzet pump, immediately prior to implantation (A); (B) is the dorsal exposure of four segments of the spinal cord (T8–T11); (C) shows the transection of T8–9, and removal of the portion of the cord rostral to this, to allow for, (D) grafting of the channel into the gap, with insertion of the rostral stump 1–1.5 mm into the channel. The arrowheads show where the tubing is attached to the capped distal end of the channel. Gross damage to blood vessels during the procedure was kept to a minimum. (E) demonstrates the orientation of the implanted apparatus in this paradigm, utilized by Bunge et al. (215).

of adult rats, a procedure that has only recently become technically feasible. Thus, the use of fetal tissue, which brings a great deal of ethical and political concerns to many can be avoided. Additionally, the development of methods which utilize adult cells has potential use in autografting (as in autologously derived human epidermal cells used for burn victims).

Morrisey's laboratory has developed protocols to efficiently purify and expand large populations of SC's from adult peripheral nerve explants of rats (140). The cells are exposed to appropriate mitogens and the resulting populations are fully functional, conferring both regenerative and myelinating support to damaged neurons. Similar methods have been applied to human adult peripheral nerve SC's, but the identification of the appropriate mitogenic factors has been difficult and is ongoing. Glial growth factors (GGF), a recently characterized, potent rat SC mitogen, has led to the discovery of a family of proteins which includes heregulins (HRG), neu-differentiation factor and acetylcholin (Ach) receptor inducing activity, all of which are alternative splice products of the same gene (61, 75, 120). Levi et al. have shown the effectiveness of one of the members of this family, HRG, as a human, adult SC mitogen (120). Furthermore, they have shown that HRG treatment, in the presence of cAMP elevating factors, induces a relatively pure expansion of cells. HRG receptor binding, causes a receptor tyrosine kinase (a putative $p185^{erbB2}$) to be phosphorylated (120). Presence of $p185^{erbB2}$ has been demonstrated in human adult SC's, suggesting that participation of this protein in mediating the mitogenic response of human SC's (120).

As the next logical extension, Bunge et al. examined the regenerative/myelinating effects of HRG expanded and purified human SC's *in vivo* (33, 79). They utilized the same paradigm as discussed earlier, SC seeded in Matrigel and PAN/PVC guidance channels. Following a T8 spinal cord transection, the rostral stump was placed 1 mm into the channel. After 30 days, the animals were sacrificed and sections were analyzed by EM, thin section microscopy and immunohistochemical techniques. Initial studies in rat-rat syngeneic transplants showed growth of propriospinal axons but retrograde fast blue labeling showed no supraspinal regenerative input. To achieve brainstem input, neurotrophins were administered into the PAN/PVC bridge via an Alzet minipump at a rate of 12 micrograms per day. Both BDNF and NT-3 were infused, separately, and both showed an increase in propriospinal innervation, from cell bodies as far rostral as C3 and a far caudal as S3, and dorsal root ganglion axons. Most significant was the entry of supraspinal neurons, evidenced through 5-HT and DBH staining fibers. The mean number of myelinated regenerating axons also increased upon the addition of NTs. A similar result, i.e., raphe nuclei and locus coeruleus contribution to the graft, was seen with the administration of methylprednisilone (MP) at the time of graft transplantation. MP treated animals showed three times as many myelinated axons and four times as many neurons contributing to the graft.

Most recently, human SC's in the PAN/PVC guidance channel paradigm have shown the most promising results (33, 35, 79, 215). There was a significant increase in the mean number of myelinated axons up to 3 mm from the rostral stump-graft interface. Suprisingly, the human SC seeded bridges showed the presence of serotonergic and dopaminergic supraspinal neurons within the cable in the absence of NT or MP treatment. These studies highlight the effectiveness and feasibility of using human SC grafts to provide a suitable "bridge" that could facilitate, or even "induce," axonal regeneration to re-establish functional connectivity of the spinal cord. Questions regarding the mechanistic molecular biology underlying the efficacy of the above experiments is based on the role SC's play in the PNS. SCs possess a remarkable ability to produce a wide variety of trophic factors (NGF, BDNF, CNTF, S100) (35). Due to their intimate contact with developing and injured axons, SC's also exhibit varied cell surface adhesion and recognition molecules in addition to growth permissive ECM components, such as laminin (108). SC's have also recently been shown to re-establish conduction by affecting central remyelination (in concert with oligodendrocytes) (65). SC's enter the CNS through the dorsal roots to restore relatively normal functional. It is the combined regenerative and remyelinating potential of SC's that make them such an attractive tool in CNS repair. The guidance channel approach allows for modification in the controlled cellular content and volume, to select for the optimal SC medi-

ated response (33, 35). The fact that axons find the bridge environment conducive to regrowth and that these axons may use the bridge to reach targets caudal to the graft is encouraging.

Injury through trauma, especially in the spinal cord, is further complicated by the formation of gliotic scars and cysts. These factors become even more important when considering the trauma involved during insertion of the grafts. There has been a great deal of effort invested in studying how these mircocysts can be modified or subdued. The current research seeks not only to identify different types of cysts, but also their inhibitory (and stimulatory) characteristics.

The past decade has seen neurotransmitters adopt the role of NT's in addition to their classic role as molecules of impulse transmission (Figure 18). As with the NT's, neurotransmitters intimately affect changes that occur during development and synapse formation. Transient changes in transmitter and receptor levels during 'critical' periods of development have been well documented. It is important to note that modulation of structural and physiological con-

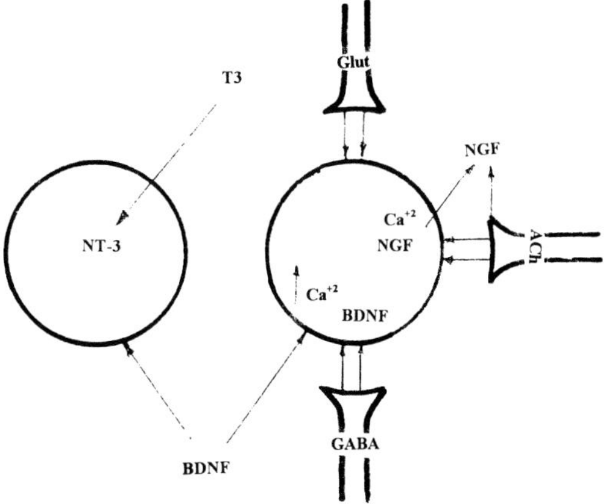

Figure 18. This diagram represents roles for three neurotransmitters in the regulation of neurotrophin synthesis and release. Release of ACh or glutamate has been shown to produce an increase in NGF and BDNF mRNA. In turn, NGF and BDNF have been shown to increase ACh production in septal cholinergic neurons. GABA, on the other hand, has been shown to reduce NT mRNA levels. Glucocorticoids shown to stimulate NGF synthesis and triiodothyronine (T3) can lead to increase NT-3 mRNA synthesis. BDNF can also stimulate NT-3 production as well as increase intracellular calcium levels in hippocampal neurons. Adapted from (124).

nectivity via neurotransmitters and their receptors has been observed in the adult as well as the developing system. In fact, the extent of influence that neurotransmitters exert on plasticity and the period of time over which this potential exists demands a review of how we define neurotransmitters and age related plasticity.

Serotonin (5-HT) lends itself to in-depth analysis as a NT. Serotonin is an ancient molecule and can be seen early in ontogeny; in other species, its presence has been shown to precede the development of any neuronal tissue. Seminal work by Azmitia et al. illustrates how serotonin may work in an autoregluatory loop with S100 (118, 209, 210). Receptor agonist studies reveal how low concentrations of 5-HT may activate 5-HT1B receptors, leading to inhibition of neuronal differentiation. As concentrations of serotonin (or certain analogs) increase, the 5-HT1A receptor is activated, leading to stimulation of outgrowth. The 1A

receptor has been shown to be present on glial cells, and it is believed that the high concentrations of 5-HT results in release of S100, itself a promoter of neuronal outgrowth (118, 209, 210).

Protein assembly and stability would be integral parts of any regenerative process, and this is especially true when considering how inseparable a neuron's cytoarchitecture and functionality are. Studies have shown that serotonin can dramatically affect immunoreactivity of microtubule associated proteins (MAP's). Bhatt's group is currently studying the mechanism related to serotonin mediated protein stability (69). Experiments involve the pharmacological manipulation of the serotonin receptor, either through receptor antagonists or agonists. Preliminary, unpublished data indicates that inactivation of the 5-HT 1A receptor leads to increased phosphorylation of MAP. The manner in which this affects the stability of MAP and

SEROTONIN - A TROPHIC LIKE FACTOR

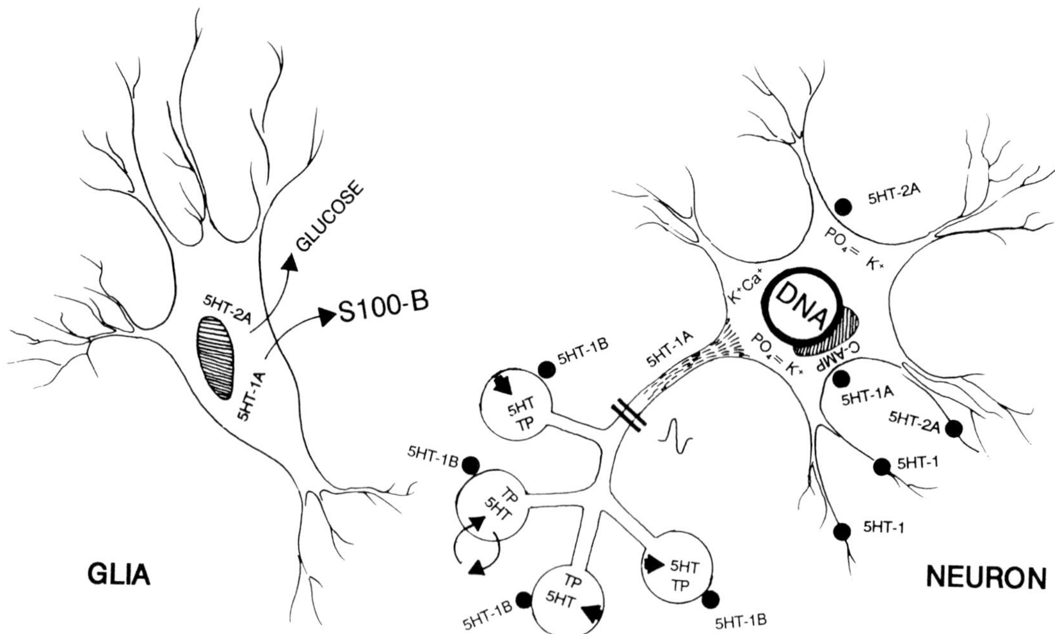

Figure 19.   This schematic represents the role that serotonin (5-HT) may play as a neurotrophin. The figure shows the homologous regulation of neuron growth, via different serotonin receptors (5-HT1a, 1b and 2a). Serotonin released from the neuron may autoregulate its growth (i.e., be inhibitory) via the 1b receptor. Higher concentrations could lead to glial production of the S100-B neurotrophin. S100-B, acting via the 1a and 2a receptors, could stimulate dendritic outgrowth. Serotonin receptor activation (and inactivation) by 5-HT may play a role in the stability of cytoskeletal proteins via the cAMP cascade. Adapted from (209).

the structural integrity of the cell is currently under investigation.

L-Glutamate is regarded as the chief excitatory neurotransmitter in the CNS. The trophic effect of this excitatory amino acid varies greatly with age, with immature neurons being insensitive to the glutamate toxicity felt by mature neurons (118). In vitro studies utilizing embryonic cells from the hippocampus, cerebellum, and spinal cord show dendritic outgrowth and increased survival upon exposure to receptor agonist (47). This trophism is calcium dependent, as evidenced by inhibition and reversal of trophic effects upon calcium channel blocking (15). As with the situation *in vivo*, trophism changes to toxicity with aging of these cultures. The reason for this change has been speculated to involve changes in receptor density, receptor stability and activity and/or diminishing sensitivity to intracellular calcium concentrations (38).

Glutamate has been shown to act as an inhibitor of neurite outgrowth in developing hippocampal neurons (135). Interestingly, this inhibition is neutralized by FGF-2. It is thought that the balance between the two is an important homeostatic component of hippocampal physiology (135). The degenerative state may be due to a disruption of this balance in favor of glutamate. However, not all glutamate-NT relationships are contradictory. For example, in Purkinje cells of the cerebellum (upon which excitatory amino acids have been shown to exert trophic effects), glutamates and NGF have been shown to act synergistically in motivating dendritic outgrowth (118).

Gamma-aminobutryic acid (GABA) uptake and release mechanisms have been demonstrated in growth cones of neonatal rat neurons (190). It is well known that GABA stimulates protein synthesis in the adult rat brain (118). The catecholamines have had limited scrutiny in their roles as NT's, however. Dopamine has been shown to greatly inhibit neurite outgrowth, as has norepinephrine (in rat cerebellar development). Van Hoof et. al. have suggested a role for Ach in neurite outgrowth. Specifically, activation of the muscarinic receptor leads to inauguration of the phosphatidyl inotisol pathway resulting in growth associated protein 43 (GAP43) phosphorylation (198). Although the physiological significance of this is not completely understood, GAP43 phosphorylation has been linked to signal transduction at the growth cone. Although GAP43 immunoreactivity has been shown to increase as a neuronal process is extending, exogenous stimulation of GAP43 expression does not lead to regeneration or outgrowth.

The obvious significance of elucidating developmental cues in axon outgrowth has led to a barrage of recent studies suggesting some specific target derived chemorepellents, as well as attractants. Netrin-1 has been shown to be a diffusable protein that is secreted by target cells into the surrounding tissue (48, 133). Studies have shown that netrin-1 is manufactured on the ventral surface of the floor plate of the developing spinal cord. The protein has been shown to help guide axons of commissural neurons that relay pain and temperature sensation to the brain. These neurons originate on the dorsal surface of the spinal cord and must move ventrally to the floor plate before they travel to the brain. Netrin-1 may provide the signal to attract these axons ventrally (133). Researchers believe that many such proteins may exist and that repellent molecules would exert an interactive role. To date, three such diffusable repellent proteins have been found. Semaphorin II, semaphorin III, and netrin-1 (in a dual role) have been shown to be secreted in the developmental CNS environment where they affect the axon guidance/growth of several different neuronal populations (133). Experiments involving the use of embryonic trochlear motor neurons, which function to control eye movement, revealed the chemorepellent behavior of netrin-1 (48). In contrast to commissural axons, trochlear axons grow away from the floor plate, which led to the hypothesis that nectrin-1 may exert a repellent effect on these fibers. Colamarino and Tessier-Lavigne used an assay system which entails culturing two samples of neuronal tissue, separated by some distance, on a collagen gel matrix. When floor plate tissue and trochlear neurons were assayed together it was found that the latter grew away from the floor plate. To prove the role of netrin-1, nonneuronal cells were transfected with the netrin-1 gene. The repellent effect of this protein on trochlear neurons is demonstrated in Figure 20. Murakami et al. have shown floor plate repellence of brain neurons which is suggestive of the fact that many different types of neurons

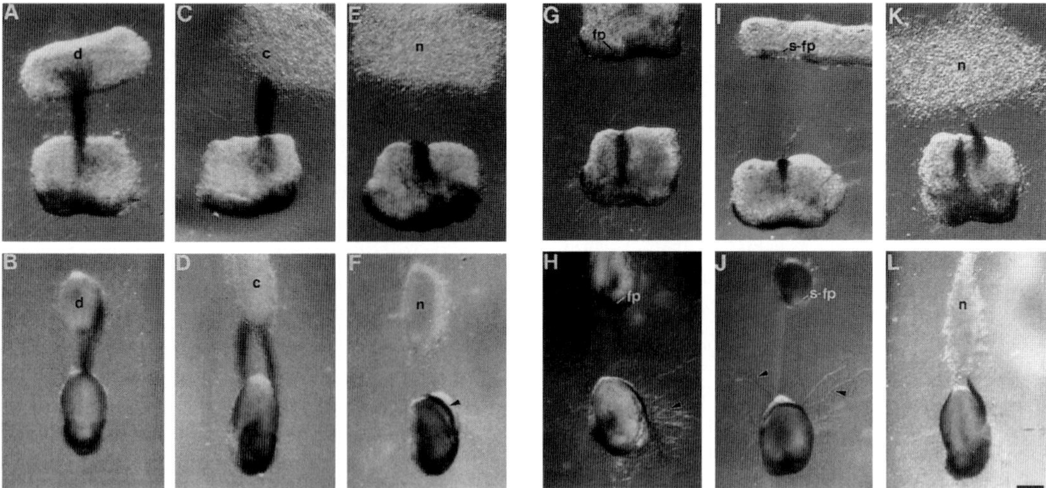

Figure 20.   Side views (A,C,E,G,I,K) and transverse views (B,D,F,H,J,L) of HMJ explants stained for F84.1 expression after 40 hrs. of culture in collagen gels opposite various tissues (explants on top); A and B, dorsal spinal explants; C and D, COS control cells; G and H, other ventral HMJ explants; I and J spinal cord floor plate; E,F,K,L, netrin-1 secreting COS cells. (c-control COS cells, d-dorsal spinal explants, fp-floor plate in ventral HMJ explants, n-netrin-1 secreting COS cells, s-fp, spinal cord floor plate. Scale bars, 160 μm. Adapted from (48).

may utilize the same guidance and growth mechanisms (133).

Semaphorin III/collapsin was discovered through the growth inhibition it rendered when encountered by a nearby growth cone. In the adult, both sets of sensory neurons enter the dorsal horn: whereas temperature and pain fibers synapse in the dorsal horns, mechanoreceptors travel across the cord to synapse in the ventral horn. Assays with embryonic rat derived cells show that semaporin III repels pain and temperature sensory neurons but has no effect on muscle stretch and propioceptive sensory neurons. It is also interesting to note that semaphorin III is produced in the ventral horn, putting it in the right place to serve as a molecular 'gate-keeper'. Many members of the semaphorin family have been identified in many species, including humans. Although the roles for each of these molecules is not yet known, the differing expression patterns of the individual members of the semaphorin family in different tissues endows the protein with great potential for specificity in guiding axons. It also remains to be seen whether semaphorins can also act as chemoattractants (133). It seems clear that these mechanisms could help to explain both the precision and accuracy of axon guidance and growth in both the CNS and PNS.

Furthermore, a clearer understanding of these and similar proteins would be advantageous in efforts to assist in the reconstruction of an injured nervous system.

PROBLEMS/LIMITATIONS

The single greatest limitation to the use of neurotrophic therapy disease and trauma is the same that faces all pharmacology: side effects. The ubiquity of trk receptors ensures cross-reactivity with other neuronal and non-neuronal cell types as well as other NT and growth factor receptors. A large concern is the mitogenic features of the many NT's in different cell populations. In conjunction with formulating effective delivery mechanisms, it will be important to understand the immunological (especially if administration is peripheral) and dose-related repercussions of chronic infusions of NT's (86). A variety of routes that may be pursued in the delivery of NT's to the CNS include:
- Intracerebral infusion via a mechanical pump (has been performed experimentally on animals and humans)
- Slow release implants within viable polymers These could be position during a single surgical procedure. Aebischer's (3) group has been involved in the development of these

'biodegradable transporters' and in protein modifications to allow for efficient shuttling.

- The implantation of cells that are genetically engineered to produce the necessary NT(s). Such experiments have already been performed using cells that produce recombinant NGF and CNTF. Whittemore's group has also been able to immortalize cell lines that may be used in similar transplantation schemes (211). The addition of temperature sensitive promoters to the modified cell's genome could allow for control of proliferation. NT's are being used to select for the differentiation of neuronal subpopulations. Bhatt and Eaton are examining these cells using cytoskeletal protein stability and phosphorylation events to ascertain how serotonin receptor expression can affect the cells' ability to regenerate (69).

- Gene therapy would allow for the manipulation of endogenous cells to produce NT's. The peptide production could be enhanced either pharmacologically or by introduction of the gene (and promoter elements) directly. There exists a variety of ways, theoretically, in which the gene can be delivered to the tissue of choice. Most of these methods would necessitate a recombination event or the expression of the gene to be dependent upon a genetic element (a specific promoter, for example) that is only active in the cell or tissue type that is the target of therapy.

- Use of NT fragments or analogs. This would bypass many of the difficulties associated with the use of natural, protein growth factors. Currently, the compounds K-252a and b exist as drugs that selectively inhibit the trk receptor and allow for the interrupted function of IGF, EGF, and platelet derived growth factor (PDGF) mediated effects. K-252b has also been shown to exclusively enhance NT-3 mediate effects.

- Use of endogenous effectors of NT expression. NGF levels in the brain have been shown to be sensitive to testosterone, and p75 receptor expression seems to be influenced by estrogen receptor activation by cholinergic neurons in the basal forebrain.

- Recent reports by Fernandez-Sanchez and Novelli, and Koh' group suggest that glutamate neurotoxicity is thought to be NMDA receptor mediated, and tropin interaction with this process may lead to potentiated neurotoxicity (66).

The neurotrophic situation following injury becomes even more complex with the introduction of several multifunctional polypeptide growth factors (cytokines) in hematopoeisis, inflammation, and the immune response. A variety of transgenic and knockout experiments are beginning to elucidate the roles of various growth factors (bFGF, FGF2, IGF, LIF), interleukins and glial factors.

Transplantation provides a two pronged remedy to the injured system: it replaces lost neurons and replenishes the microenvironment with a more favorable 'regenerative stage' (Fig. 15) (29, 132). When fetal substantia nigra (or adrenal medulla) is grafted into the striatum of 6-OHDS and MPTP lesioned animals, depleted neurotransmitter levels can be restored (23, 132, 183). Currently, the greatest problem facing transplant efficacy, besides the political and ethical questions surrounding the use of fetal donor tissue, is the survivability of grafted tissue.

CONCLUSION

Investigations into a multitude of factors, positive and negative, that influence the regenerative characteristics of the CNS have been undertaken. The family of NGF-related NT's plays a somewhat obvious and yet subtle role in this process. Although much work has been done on the survival enhancing effects of NT's in the PNS, the field of research into subpopulations of CNS neurons is in its infancy. The various redundancies in trophism reveal the potential breadth and complexity of interactions between different classes of NT's. It is evident that neurons differ in their responsiveness to NT's depending upon their age, sub-population, and environment. Knockout studies involving either the gene for a NT (or its receptor), or a protein relevant for a regenerative response (such as a cytoskeletal protein) will continue to provide insight into the role that these molecules play in development, and thus provide strategies for formulating a regenerative/reparative campaign. The signal transduction actions of the trophic factors, and the congeniality of the surface to extracellular environment interaction, will help us to understand the molecular characteristics underlying the diversity (and overlap) of action, and help provide a broader base for intervention strategies.

This chapter has merely given a glance on how basic science is endeavoring to affect CNS recovery. The overall list of strategies includes all of the trophic factors found in the CNS and peripheral PNS, growth factors, tropic factors, cytokines, glial associated molecules, extracellular matrix components, inhibitory molecules, and neurotransmitters (many of which overlap, in terms of their influences). Furthermore, in our quest to deliver answers, we come across even more questions; What is the distinction between tropism and trophism? How does the architecture of the CNS change from a growth permissive one during development to a growth restrictive one later? Hopefully, it will not take a resolution of the deep issues before further progress, of clinical significance, is attained in regeneration.

Acknowledgments

The authors thank all of the contributors listed as well as the contributions of Dr. H.C. Bhatt and Prof. M.H. Bhatt. We also thank the Miami Project to Cure Paralysis, the Narayan Foundation, Dr. E.C. Azmitia, and Dr. Narayan Swarupdasji for their support and guidance.

REFERENCES

1. Adler, R., Landa, K. B., Manthorpe, M., and Varon, S. Cholinergic neurotrophic factors: intraocular distribution of trophic activity for ciliary neurons. Science 204: 1434–1436, 1979.
2. Aebischer, P., Guenard, V., and Brace, S. Peripheral nerve regeneration through semi-permeable guidance channels: effect of the molecular weight cutoff. J. Neurosci. 9: 3590–3595, 1989.
3. Aebischer, P., Guenard, V., and Valentini, R. F. The morphology of regenerating peripheral nerves is modulated by the surface microgeometry of polymelic guidance channels. Brain Res. 351: 211–218, 1990.
4. Agauyo, A. J. Axonal regeneration from injured neurons in the adult mammalian CNS. In: Synaptic Plasticity, edited by C. W. Cotman, pp. 457–484. Guilford Press, New York, 1985.
5. Aguayo, A. J., Bray, G. M., Rasminsky, M., et al. Neuronal and Nonneuronal Influences on Retinal Ganglion Cell Survival, Axonal Regrowth and Connectivity after Axotomy. Annals New York Academy of Sciences 633: 214–228, 1991.
6. Aguayo, A. J. Repair of immature mammalian spinal cord in culture. In: Axonal regrowth in the mammalian spinal cord and peripheral nerve, Abstracts, (022.) International Symposium, Normandy, 1995.
7. Altar, C. A., Boylan, C. B., Jackson, C., et al. Brain-derived neurotrophic factor augments rotational behavior and nigrostriatal dopamine turnover in vivo. P.N.A.S., U.S.A. 89: 11347–11351, 1992.
8. Altar, C. A., Criden, M. R., Lindsay, R. M., et al. Characterization and topography of high affinity [^{125}I] neurotrophin-3 binding to mammalian brain. J. Neuroscience 13: 733–743, 1993.
9. Arenas, E., and Persson, H. Neurotropin-3 prevents the death of adult central noradrenergic neurons in vivo. Nature 367: 368–371, 1994.
10. Asai, T., Wanaka, A., Kato, H., et al. Differential expression of two members of the FGF gene family, FGFR-1 and FGFR-2 mRNA, in the adult rat central nervous system. Mol. Brain. Res. 17: 174–178, 1993.
11. Asipu, A., and Eric Blair, G. Regulation of myeln basic protein-encoding gene transcription in rat oligodendrocytes. Gene 150: 227–234, 1994.
12. Azmitia, E. C., and de Kloet, R. ACTH neuropeptide stimulation of serotonergic neuronal maturation in tissue culture: Modulation of hippocampal cells. Prog. Brain Res. 72: 311–318, 1987.
13. Azmitia, E. C., and Liao, B. Dexamethasone reverses adrenalectomy-induced neuronal de-differentiation in the mid-brain raphe-hippocampus axis. Annals of the New York Academy of Sciences 746: 193–194, 221–222, 1994.
14. Azmitia, E. C. Cell Death and Maturation. In: Lectures in Neuronal Development and Plasticity, NYU, 1995.
15. Balazs, R., and Hack, N. Trophic effects of excitatory amino acids in the developing nervous system. In: Excitatory amino acids and neuronal plasticity, edited by Y. Ben-Yari, pp. 221–228. Plenum Press, New York; 1990.
16. Bandtlow, C., Zachleder, T., and Schwab, M. E. Oligodendrocytes arrest neurite growth by contact inhibition. J. Neurosci. 101(12): 3837–3848, 1990.
17. Bandtlow, C. E., Schmidt, M. F., Hassinger, T. D., et al. Role of intracellular calcium in NI-35 evoked collapse of neuronal growth cones. Science 259: 80–85, 1993.
18. Barbacid, M. The trk family of neurotrophin receptors. J. Neurobiol. 25: 1386–1403, 1994.
19. Bastmeyer, M., Beckmann, M., Schwab, M. E., et al. Growth of Regenerating Goldfish Axons is Inhibited by Rat Oligodendrocytes and CNS Myelin but Not By Goldfish Optic Nerve Tract Oligodendrocytelike Cells and Fish CNS Myelin. J. Neurosci. 11: 626–650, 1991.
20. Bazan, J. F. Neuropoetic cytokines in the hematopoetic fold. Neuron 7: 197–208, 1991.
21. Benedetti, M., Levi, A., and Chao, M. V. Differential expression of nerve growth factor receptors leads to altered binding affinity and neurotrophin responsiveness. P.N.A.S., USA. 90: 7859–7863, 1993.
22. Berkemeier, L. R., Winslow, J. W., Kaplan, D. R., et al. Neurotrophin-5; and novel neurotrophic factor that activates both trk and trkB. Neuron 7: 857–866, 1991.
23. Bjorklund, A. Dopaminergic transplants in experimental parkinsonism: cellular mechanisms of graft-

induced functional recovery. Current Opinions Neurobiology *2:* 683–689, 1992.

24. Bjorklund, A. Long distance axonal growth in the adult nervous system. J. Neurology *241:* S33–S35, 1994.

25. Blaugrund, E., Lavie, V., Cohen, I., *et al.* Axonal regeneration is associated with glial migration: comparison between the injured optic nerves of fish and rats. J. Comp. Neurology. *330:* 105–112, 1993.

26. Blottner, D., and Baumgarten, H. G. Neurotrophy and regeneration in vivo. Acta Anatomica, *150:* 235–245, 1994.

27. Bergman, B. S., and Bernstein-Goral, H. Both regenerating and late-developing pathways contribute to transplant-induced anatomical plasticity after spinal cord lesions at birth. Experimental Neurology *112:* 49–55, 1991.

28. Bregman, B. S., and McAtee, M. Neural tissue transplantation to study development and regeneration. Neuroprotocols *3:* 15–23, 1993.

29. Bregman, B. S., and Kunkel-Bagden, E. Potential Mechanisms Underlying Transplant Mediated Recovery of Function After Spinal Cord Injury. In: *Recent Advances: Neural Transplantation. CNS Neuronal Injury, and Regeneration,* pp. 81–102. CRC Press, Boca Raton, 1994.

30. Bregman, B. S. Repair of immature mammalian spinal cord in culture. In: Axonal regrowth in the mammalian spinal cord and peripheral nerve, Abstracts, (02.) International Symposium, Normandy, 1995.

31. Brittis, P. A., Canning, D. R., and Silver, J. Chondroitan sulfate as a regulator of neuronal patterning in the retina. Science *255:* 733–736, 1992.

32. Brunelli, J. P., and Pall, M. L. Lamda/Plasmid vector construction by in vivo cre-lox-mediated recombination. Biotechniques *16(6):* 1061–64, 1994.

33. Bunge, M. P. Transplantation of purified populations of Schwann cells into lesioned adult rat spinal cord. J. Neurol. *241:* S36–S39, 1994.

34. Bunge, R. P., and Johnson, M. I. Primary Cell Cultures of Peripheral and Central Neurons and Glia. In: *Protocols for Neural Cell Culture,* pp. 13–38. Humana Press, New Jersey, 1994.

35. Bunge, R. P. The role of the Schwann cell in trophic support and regeneration. J. Neurol. *241:* S19–S21, 1994.

36. Burgess, W. H., Dionne, C. A., Kaplow, J., *et al.* Characterization and cDNA cloning of phospholipase C-gamma, a major substrate for heparin-binding growth factor 1 (acidic FGF)-activated tyrosine kinase. Mol. Cell. Biol. *10:* 4770–4777, 1990.

37. Cajal, R. S. Degeneration and Regeneration of the Nervous System. Trans. by May, R. M. Oxford Univ. Press, 1928.

38. Cambray-Deakin, M. A., Foster, A. C., and Burgoyne, R. D. The expression of excitatory amino acid binding sites during neuritogenesis in the developing rat cerebellum. Dev. Brain Res. *54:* 265–271, 1990.

39. Campagnoni, A. T., Kashima, T., Tiu, S. N., *et al.* Expression of Oligodendrocyte-associated genes in cell lines derived from human gliomas and neuroblastomas. Cancer Research *53:* 170–175, 1993.

40. Caramn-Krzan, M., Vige, X., and Wise, B. C. Regulation by interleukins of nerve growth factor secretion and nerve growth factor mRNA expression in rat primary astroglial cultures. J. Neurochemistry *56:* 636–643, 1991.

41. Carey, D. J., Stahl, R. C., Asundi, V. K., *et al.* Processing and subcellular distribution of the Schwann cell lipid-anchored heparan sulfate proteoglycan and identification as glypican. Exp. Cell Res. *208:* 10–18, 1993.

42. Carroll, P., Sendtner, M., Meyer, M., *et al.* Rat CNTF: gene structure and regulation of mRNA in glial cell cultures. Glia *9:* 176–187, 1993.

43. Chandross, K. J., Chanson, M., Spray, D. C., *et al.* Transforming Growth Factor-B1 and forskolin modulate gap junctional communication and cellular phenotype of cultured Schwann cells. J. Neurosci. *15(1):* 262–273, 1995.

44. Chao, M. V. The p75 neurotrophin receptor. J. Neurobio. *25:* 1373–1385, 1994.

45. Chao, M. V., and Hempstead, B. L. p75 and trk: a two receptor system. J. Dev. Neurosci. (1995) In press.

46. Cohen, A., Bray, G. M., and Aguayo, A. J. Neurotrophin-4/5 (NT-4/5) increases adult rat retinal ganglion survival and outgrowth. J. Neurobiology, *25(8):* 953–959, 1994.

47. Cohen-Cory, S., Dreyfus, C. F., and Black, I. B. NGF and excitatory neurotransmitters regulate survival and morphogenesis of cultured cerebellar Purkinje cells. J. Neurosci. *11:* 462–471, 1991.

48. Colamarino, S. A., and Tessier-Lavigne, M. The axonal chemoattractant netrin-1 is also a chemorepellent for trochlear motor axons. Cell, *81:* 621–629, 1995.

49. Colello, R. J., Kapfhammer, J., and Schwab, M. E. A Role for Oligodendrocytes in the Stabilization of Optic Nerve Axon Numbers. Soc. Neurosci. Abstr. *17:* 211, 1991.

50. Conner, J. M., Fass-Holmes, B., and Varon, S. Changes in nerve growth factor immunoreactivity following entorhinal cortex lesions-possible molecular mechanism regulating cholinergic sprouting. J. Comparative Neurology *345:* 408–418, 1994.

51. Croll, S. D., Wiegand, S. J., Anderson, K. D., *et al.* Neuropeptide regulation by BDNF and NGF in adult rat forebrain. Society for Neuroscience Abstracts *19:* 662, 1993.

52. Crowley, C., Spencer, S. D., Nishimura, M. C., *et al.* Mice lacking nerve growth factor display perinatal loss of sensory and sympathetic neurons yet develop basal forebrain cholinergic neurons. Cell *78:* 1001–1011, 1994.

53. Crutcher, K. A. Tissue Sections from the Mature Rat Brain and Spinal Cord as Substrates for Neurite Outgrowth In Vitro: Extensive Growth on Gray but Little Growth on White Matter. Experimental Neurology *104:* 39–54, 1989.

54. D'arcangelo, G., Paradiso, K., Shepherd, D., *et al.* Neuronal growth factor regulation of two different sodium channel types through distinct signal transduction pathways. J. Cell Biol. *122:* 915–921, 1993.

55. Davis, S., Aldrich, T. H., Stahl, N., *et al.* LIFR-Beta and gp130 as heterodimerizing signal transducers of the tripartite CNTF receptor. Science *260:* 1805–1808, 1993.

56. DiStefano, P. S., Friedman, B., Radziejewski, C., *et al.* The neurotrophins BDNF, NT-3, and NGF display distinct patterns of retrograde axonal transport in peripheral and central neurons. Neuron *8:* 983–993, 1992.

57. Dugich-Djordjevic, M. M., Tocco, G., Willoughby, D. A., *et al.* BDNF mRNA expression in the developing rat brain following kainic acid induced seizure activity. Neuron *8:* 1127–1138, 1992.

58. Ebendal, T., Lonnerberg, P., Pei, G., *et al.* Engineering cells to secrete growth factors. J. Neurology *241:* S5–S7, 1992.

59. Eckenstein, F. P. Fibroblast growth factors in the nervous system. J. Neurobiol. *25:* 1467–1480, 1994.

60. Egan, S. E., and Weinberg, R. A. The pathway to signal achievement. Nature *365:* 781–783, 1993.

61. Falls, D. L., Rosen, K. M., Corfas, G., *et al.* ARIA, a protein that stimulates acetylcholine receptor synthesis, is a member of the neu ligand family. Cell *72:* 801–815, 1993.

62. Fawcett, J. W., Houdson, E., Smith-Thomas, L., *et al.* The Growth of Axons in Three-Dimensional Astrocyte Cultures. Dev. Biology. *135:* 449–458, 1989.

63. Fawcett, J. Astrocytes and axon regeneration in the central nervous system. J. Neurol. *241:* S25–S28, 1994.

64. Feltri, M. L., Scherer, S. S., Nemni, R., *et al.* Beta 4 integrin expression in myelinating Schwann cells is polarized, developmentally regulated and axonally dependent. Development *120:* 1267–1301, 1994.

65. Felts, P. A., and Smith, K. J. Conduction properties of central nerve fibers remyelinated by Schwann cells. Brain Res. *574:* 178–192, 1992.

66. Fernandez-Sanchez, M. T., and Novelli, A. Neurotrophins and excitotoxicity. Science *270:* 2019, 1995.

67. Fields, R. D., Neale, E. A., and Nelson, P. G. Effects of patterned electrical activity on neurite outgrowth from mouse sensory neurons. J. Neurosci. *10:* 2950–2964, 1990.

68. Franklin, R. J. M., Crang, A. J., and Blakemore, W. F. The role of Astrocytes in the remyelination of glia-free areas of demyelination. Adv. In Neurology *59:* 125–133, 1993.

69. Frenz, M. Y., Bhatt, P. M. H., Jani, N. D., *et al.* In: Trophic Support after Paralysis, edited by H. C. Bhatt and M. H. Bhatt, pp. 102–111. Dacron Press, New York, 1989.

70. Frisen, J., Verge, V. M., Cullheim, S., *et al.* Increased levels of glial mRNA and trkB protein-like immunoreactivity in the rat and cat spinal cord. P.N.A.S., U.S.A. *89:* 11282–11286, 1992.

71. Frisen, J., Verge, V. M., Fried, K., *et al.* Characterization of glia trkB receptors: differential response to injury in the central and peripheral nervous system. P.N.A.S., U.S.A. *90:* 4971–4975, 1993.

72. Fuss, B., Pott, U., Fischer, P., *et al.* Identification of a cDNA clone specific for the oligodendrocyte-derived repulsive extracellular matrix molecule J1-160/180. J. Neurosci. Res. *29(3):* 299–307, 1991.

73. Gage, F. H., Tuszynski, M. H., Chen, K. S., *et al.* Nerve growth factor function in the central nervous system. Current Topics in Microbiology and Immunology *165:* 71–93, 1991.

74. Geunard, V., Aebischer, P., and Bunge, R. P. The astrocyte inhibition of peripheral nerve regeneration is reversed by Schwann cells. Exp. Neurology *126:* 44–60, 1994.

75. Goodearl, A. D. J., Davis, J. B., Mistry, K., *et al.* 54.

76. Gow, A., Friedrich, V. L., and Lazzarini, R. A. Myelin Basic Protein gene contains separate enhancers for oligodendrocyte and Schwann cell expression. J. Cell Biology *119:* 605–616, 1992.

77. Groves, A. K., Barnett, S. C., and Franklin, R. J. M. Repair of demyelinated lesions by transplantation of purified O-2A progenitor cells. Nature *362:* 453–455, 1994.

78. Gu, H., Marth, J. D., Orban, P. C., *et al.* Deletion of a DNA polymerase B segment in T cells using cell type specific gene targeting. Science *265:* 103–106, 1994.

79. Guest, J. D., and Bunge, R. P. Functional studies of cultured human Schwann cells transplanted to the nude rat spinal cord. In: Axonal Regrowth in the Mammalian Spinal Cord and Peripheral Nerve Abstr. IRME, Normandy France, April 1995.

80. Hagg, T., Quon, D., Higaki, J., *et al.* CNTF prevents neuronal degeneration and promotes low affinity NGF receptor expression in the adult rat CNS. Neuron *8:* 145–158, 1992.

81. Hagg, T., and Varon, S. CNTF prevents degeneration of adult rat substantia nigra dopaminergic neurons in vivo. P.N.A.S., U.S.A. *90:* 6315–6319, 1993.

82. Hagg, T., and Varon, S. Neurotropism of nerve growth factor for adult rat septal cholinergic axons in vivo. J. Experimental Neurology *119:* 37–45, 1993.

83. Hallbook, F., Ibanez, C. F., and Persson, F. Evolutionary studies of the nerve growth factor family reveal a novel member abundantly expressed in Xenopus ovary. Neuron *6:* 845–858, 1991.

84. Hamburger, V. The history of the discovery of the nerve growth factor. J. Neurobiology *24:* 893–897, 1993.

85. Hasan, N., Koob, M., and Szybalski, W. Escherichia coli genome targeting, I. Cre-lox-mediated in vitro generation of ori- plasmids and their in vivo chromosomal integration and retrieval. Gene *150:* 51–56, 1994.

86. Hefti, F. Neurotrophic factor therapy for nervous system degenerative diseases. J. Neurobiol. *25:* 1418–1435, 1994.

87. Hyman, C., Hoffer, M., Barde, Y-A., *et al.* BDNF is a neurotrophic factor for dopaminergic neurons of the substantia nigra. Nature *350:* 230–232, 1991.

88. Hyman, C., Juhasz, M., Jackson, C., *et al.* Overlapping and distinct actions of neurotrophins BDNF, NT-3, and NT-4/5 on cultured dopaminergic and GABAergic neurons of the ventral mesencephalon. J. Neuroscience *14(1):* 335–347, 1994.

89. Ibanez, C. F., Ebendal, T., Barbany, G., *et al.* Disruption of the low affinity receptor-binding site in NGF allows neuronal survival and differentiation by binding to the trk gene product. Cell *69:* 329–341, 1992.

90. Ibanez, C. F., Ebendal, T., Barbany, G., *et al.* An extended surface of binding to Trk tyrosine kinase receptors in NGF and BDNF allows the engineering of a multifunctional pan-neurotrophin. EMBO. J. *12:* 2281–2293, 1993.

91. Ip, N. Y., Ibanez, C. F., Nye, S. H., *et al.* Mammalian neurotrophin-4: structure, chromosomal localization, tissue distribution, and receptor specificty. P.N.A.S., U.S.A. *89:* 3060–3064, 1992.

92. Ip, N. Y., Li, Y., Yancopoulos, G. D., *et al.* Cultured hippocampal neurons show responses to BDNF, NT-3, and NT-4, but not NGF. J. Neuroscience *13(8):* 3394–3405, 1993.

93. Ip, N. Y., Stitt, T. N., Tapley, P., *et al.* The Trk receptor specificities of NGF, BDNF, NT-3 and NT-4/5 in fibroblasts, PC12 cells, and neurons. Neuron *10:* 137–149, 1993.

94. Ip, N. Y., Stitt, T. N., Tapley, P., *et al.* Similarities and differences in the way neurotrophins interact with the trk receptors in neuronal and nonneuronal cells. Neuron *10:* 137–149, 1993.

95. Ip, N. Y., Weigand, S. J., Morse, J., *et al.* Injury-induced regulation of CNTF mRNA in the adult rat brain. Eur. J. Neurosci. *5:* 25–33, 1993.

96. Iwashita, Y., Kawaguchi, S., and Murata, M. Restoration of function by replacement of spinal cord segments in the rat. Nature *367:* 167–170, 1994.

97. Jing, S., Tapley, P., and Barbacid, M. Nerve growth factor mediates signal transduction through trk homodimer receptors. Neuron *9:* 1067–1079, 1992.

98. Johnson, D. E., and Williams, L. T. Structural and functional diversity in the FGF receptor multigene family. Adv. Cancer Res. *60:* 1–41, 1993.

99. Kaplan, D. R., Hempstead, B. L., Martin-Zanca, D., *et al.* The trk proto-oncogene product: signal transducing receptor for nerve growth factor. Science *252:* 554–558, 1991.

100. Kaplan, D. R., and Stephens, R. M. Neurotrohpin signal transduction by the trk receptor. J. Neurobiol. *25:* 1404–1417, 1994.

101. Kawaguchi, S. Axonal regeneration in the spinal cord with functional restoration in young rats. In: Axonal Regrowth in the Mammalian Spinal Cord and Peripheral Nerve Abstr. IRME, Normandy France, April 1995.

102. Kiefer, M. C., Stephans, J. C., Crawford, K., *et al.* Ligand affinity cloning and structure of a cell surface heparan sulfate proteoglycan that binds basic FGF. P.N.A.S., U.S.A. *87:* 6985–6989, 1990.

103. Kishimoto, T., Akira, S., and Taga, T. IL-6 and its receptor: a paradigm for cytokines. Science *258:* 593–597, 1992.

104. Klagsbrun, M., and Baird, A. A dual receptor system is required for basic FGF activity. Cell *67:* 229–231, 1991.

105. Klein, R., Jing, S., Nanduri, V., *et al.* The trk proto-oncogene encodes a receptor for nerve growth factor. Cell *65:* 189–197, 1991.

106. Klein, R., Nanduri, V., Jing, S., *et al.* The trkB tyrosine protein kinase is a receptor for brain-derived neurotrophic factor and neurotrophin-3. Cell *66:* 395–403, 1991.

107. Klein, R., Lamballe, F., Bryant, S., *et al.* The trkB tyrosine protein kinase is a receptor for neurotrophin-4. Neuron *8:* 947–956, 1992.

108. Kleitman, N., Wood, P., Johnson, M. I., *et al.* Schwann cell surfaces but not extracellular matrix organized by Schwann cells support neurite out-

109. Knusel, B., Beck, K. D., and Winslow, J. W. BDNF administration protects basal forebrain cholinergic but not nigral dopaminergic neurons from degenerative changes after axotomy in the adult brain. J. Neuroscience *12:* 4391–4402, 1992.

110. Korsching, S. The neurotrophic factor concept: a re-examination. J. Neuroscience *13:* 2739–2748, 1993.

111. Kromer, L. F., and Cornbrooks, C. J. Transplants of Schwann cell cultures promote axonal regeneration in the adult mammalian brain. P.N.A.S., U.S.A. *82:* 6330–6334, 1985.

112. Kunkel-Bagden, E., Dai, H. N., and Bregman, B. S. Recovery of function after spinal cord hemisection in newborn and adult rats: differential effects on reflex and locomotor function. Experimental Neurology *116:* 40, 1993.

113. Lam, A., Fuller, F., Miller, J., *et al.* Sequence and structural organization of the human gene encoding CNTF. Gene *102:* 271–276, 1991.

114. Lamballe, F., Klein, R., and Barbacid, M. TrkC, a new member of the trk family of tyrosine protein kinases, is a receptor for neurotrophin-3. Cell *66:* 967–979, 1991.

115. Lang, D. M., Rubin, B. P., Schwab, M. E., *et al.* CNS Myelin and Oligodendrocytes of the Xenopus spinal cord-not optic nerve-are nonpermissive for axon growth. J. Neurosci. *15(1):* 99–109, 1995.

116. Lavail, M. M., Unoki, K., Yasumura, D., *et al.* Multiple growth factors, cytokines and neurotrophins rescue photoreceptors from the damaging effects of constant light. P.N.A.S. U.S.A. *89:* 11249–11253, 1992.

117. LeRoith, D., Roberts, Jr., C. T., Werner, H., *et al.* Insulin-like growth factor in the brain. In: Neurotrophic Factors, edited by S. E. Loughin and J. H. Fallon, pp. 391–414. Academic Press Inc., San Diego, Ca., 1993.

118. Leslie, F. Neurotransmitters as neurotrophic factors. In: Neurotrophic factors, edited by S. E., Loughlin and J. H. Fallon, pp. 565–598. Academic Press Inc., San Diego, Ca., 1993.

119. Leung, D. W., Parent, A. S., Cachianes, G., *et al.* Cloning, expression during development, and evidence for release of a trophic factor for ciliary ganglion neurons. Neuron *8:* 1045–1053, 1992.

120. Levi, A. D. O., Bunge, R. P., Lofgren, J. A., *et al.* The influence of heregulins on human Schwann cell proliferation. J. Neurosci. *15(2):* 1329–1340, 1995.

121. Li, Y., and Raisman, G. Sprouts from cut corticospinal axons persist in the presence of astrocytic scarring in long-term lesions of the adult rat spinal cord. Exp. Neurol. *134:* 102–111, 1995.

122. Lin, L-F. H., Doherty, D. H., Lile, J. D., *et al.* GDNF-a glial cell line-derived neurotrophic factor for midbrain dopaminergic neurons. Science *260:* 1130–1132, 1993.

123. Lindholm, D. Role of neurotrophins in preventing glutamate induced neuronal cell death. J. Neurology. *241:* S16–S18, 1994.

124. Lindholm, D., Castren, E., Berzaghi, M., *et al.* Activity-dependent and hormonal regulation of neurotro-

phin mRNA levels in the brain-implications for neuronal plasticity. J. Neurobio. *25:* 1362–1372, 1994.

125. Lindsay, R. M., Altar, C. A., Cedarbaum, J. M., *et al.* The therapeutic potential of neurotrophic factors in the treatment of Parkinson's disease. Experimetnal Neurology *124:* 103–118, 1993.

126. Lindsay, R. M. Neurotrophins and receptors. Progress in Brain Research *103:* 3–14, 1994.

127. Lindvall, O., Sawle, G., Widner, H., *et al.* Evidence for long term survival of dopaminergic grafts in progressive Parkinson's disease. Annals Neurology *35:* 172–180, 1994.

128. Lipton, S. A., and Rosenberg, P. A. Excitatory amino acids as a final common pathway for neurological disorders. New England J. Medicine *330:* 613–622, 1993.

129. Lu, X., and Richardson, P. M. Inflammation near the nerve cell body enhances axonal regeneration. J. Neuroscience *11:* 972–978, 1991.

130. Malhotra, S. K., Svensson, M., Aldskogius, H., *et al.* Diversity among reactive astrocytes: proximal reactive astrocytes in lacerated spinal cord preferentially react with monoclonal Ab J1–31. Brain Res. Bull. *30:* 395–404, 1993.

131. Mansour-Robaey, S., Clarke, D. B., Wang, Y. C., *et al.* Effects of ocular injury and administration of brain-derived neurotrophic factor on survival and regrowth of axotomized retinal ganglion cells. P.N.A.S., U.S.A. *91:* 1632–1636, 1994.

132. Marwah, J., Teitelbaum, H., and Prasad, K. N. In: Neural Transplantation, CNS Neuronal Injury, and Regeneration, Recent Advances, 1st ed. CRC Press, Florida, 1994.

133. Marx, J. Helping neurons find their way. Science *268:* 971–973, 1995.

134. Masu, Y., Wolf, E., Holtmann, B., *et al.* Disruption of the CNTF gene results in motor neuron degeneration. Nature *365:* 27–32, 1993.

135. Mattson, M. P., Lee, R. E., Adams, M. E., *et al.* Interactions between entorhinal axons and target hippocampal neurons: a role for glutamate in the development of hippocampal circuitry. Neuron *1:* 865–876, 1988.

136. Mattson, M. P., Kumar, K. N., Wang, H., *et al.* Basic FGF regulates the expression of a functional 71 kDa NMDA receptor protein that mediates calcium influx and neurotoxicity in hippocampal neurons. J. Neurosci. *13:* 4575–4588, 1993.

137. Meiners, S., Marone, M., Rittenhouse, J. L., *et al.* Regulation of astrocytic tenascin by basic FGF. Dev. Biol. *160:* 480–493, 1993.

138. Merlio, J., Ernfors, P., Jaber, M., *et al.* Molecular cloning of rat trkC and distribution of cells expressing messenger RNA for members of the trk family in the rat central nervous system. Neuroscience *51:* 513–532, 1992.

139. Mey, J., and Thanos, S. Intravitreal injections of neurotrophic factors support the survival of axotomized retinal ganglion cells in adult rats in vivo. Brain Research *602:* 304–317, 1993.

140. Morrissey, T. K., Kleitman, N., and Bunge, R. P. Isolation and functional characterization of Schwann cells derived from adult peripheral nerve. J. Neurosci. *11:* 2433–2442, 1991.

141. Morse, J. K., Wiegand, S. J., Anderson, K., *et al.* Brain-derived neurotrophic factor (BDNF) prevents the degeneration of medial septal cholinergic neurons following fimbria transection. J. Neuroscience *13(10):* 4146–4156, 1993.

142. Murakami, M., Hibi, M., Nakagawa, N., *et al.* IL-6 induced homodimerization of gp130 and associated activation of a tyrosine kinase. Science *260:* 1808–1811, 1993.

143. Nawa, H., Bessho, Y., Carnahan, J., *et al.* Regulation of neuropeptide expression in cultured cerebral cortical neurons by brain-derived neurotrophic factor. Neurochemistry *60:* 772–775, 1993.

144. Nicholls, J. G. Repair of immature mammalian spinal cord in culture. In: Axonal regrowth in the mammalian spinal cord and peripheral nerve, Abstracts, 07. International Symposium, Normandy, 1995.

145. Nishi, R., and Breg, D. K. Two components from eye tissue that differentially stimulate the growth and development of ciliary ganglion neurons in cell culture. J. Neurosci. *1:* 505–513, 1981.

146. Obermeier, A., Lammers, R., Wiesmuller, K. H., *et al.* Identification of trk binding sites for SHC and phosphatidylinositol 3'-kinase and formation of multimeric signaling complex. J. Biol. Chem. *268:* 22963–22966, 1993.

147. Okamoto, T., Asano, T., Harada, S., *et al.* Regulation of transmembrane signal transduction of insulin-like growth factor II by competence type growth factors or viral ras p21. J. Bio. Chem. *266:* 1085–1091, 1991.

148. Olson, L., Backman, L., Ebendal, T., *et al.* Role of growth factors in degeneration and regeneration in the central nervous system; clinical experiences with NGF in Parkinson's and Alzheimer's diseases. J. Neurology *241:* S12–S15, 1992.

149. Oppenheim, R. W. Neuronal death, a tradition of dying. J. Neurobiology *23:* 1111–1115, 1992.

150. Otto, D., and Unsicker, K. Basic FGF reverses chemical and morphological deficits in the nigrostriatal system of MPTP-treated mice. J. Neurosci. *10:* 1912–1921, 1990.

151. Oudega, M., Varon, S., and Hagg, T. Regeneration of adult sensory axons into intraspinal peripheral nerve grafts: promoting effects of conditioning lesions, graft degeneration and NGF. Society for Neuroscience Abstracts *19:* 422, 1993.

152. Paino, C. L., and Bunge, M. B. Induction of axon growth into Schwann cell implants grafted into lesioned adult rat spinal cord. Exp. Neurol. *114:* 254–257, 1991.

153. Paino, C. L., Fernandez-Valle, C., Bates, M. L., *et al.* Regrowth of axons in lesioned adult spinal cord. J. Neurocytol. *23:* 433–452, 1994.

154. Patterson, P. H., and Nawa, H. Neuronal differentiation factors/cytokines and synaptic plasticity. Cell. Suppl. 123–137, 1993.

155. Phillips, H. S., Hains, J. M., Armanini, M., *et al.* BDNF mRNA is decreased in the hippocampus of individuals with Alzheimer's disease. Neuron *7:* 695–702, 1991.

156. Rapraeger, A. C., Krufka, A., and Olwin, B. B. Re-

quirement of heparan sulfate for bFGF-mediated fibroblast growth and myoblast differentiation. Science *252:* 1705–1708, 1991.

157. Reier, P. J., Anderson, D. K., Thompson, F. J., *et al.* Neural tissue transplantation and CNS trauma: anatomical and functional repair of the injured spinal cord. J. Neurotrauma *9:* S221–234, 1992.

158. Richardson, P. M. Neurotrophic factors in regeneration. Current Opinions in Neurobiology *1:* 401–406, 1991.

159. Richardson, P. M., and Lu, X. Inflammation and axonal regeneration. J. Neurology *241:* S57–S60, 1994.

160. Risling, M., Fried, K., Linda, H., *et al.* Changes in nerve growth factor receptor-like immunoreactivity in the spinal cord after ventral funiculus lesion in adult cats. J. Neurocytology *21(2):* 79–93, 1992.

161. Risling, M., Fried, K., Hammarberg, H., *et al.* Studies on scar formation and axonal regrowth after spinal cord injury. In: Axonal Regrowth in the Mammalian Spinal Cord and Peripheral Nerve Abstr. IRME, Normandy France, April 1995.

162. Rodriguez-Tebar, A., Dechant, G., Gotz, R., *et al.* Binding of neurotrophin-3 to its neuronal receptors and interactions with nerve growth factor and brain-derived neurotrophic factor. EMBO. *11:* 917–922, 1992.

163. Rosen, O. M. After insulin binds. Science. *237:* 1452–1458, 1987.

164. Rubin, B. P., Dusart, I., and Schwab, M. E. A monoclonal antibody (IN-1) which neutralizes neurite growth inhibitory proteins in the rat CNS recognizes antigens localized in CNS myelin. J. Neurocytology *23:* 209–217, 1994.

165. Rudge, J. S., Alderson, R. F., Pasnikowski, E., *et al.* Expression of ciliary neurotrophic factor and the neurotrophins-nerve growth factor, brain-derived neurotrophic factor and neurotrophin-3-in cultured rat hippocampal astrocytes. European J. Neuroscience *4:* 459–471, 1992.

166. Rudge, R. S., Li, Y., Pasnikowski, E. M., *et al.* Neurotrohpic factor receptors and their signal transduction capabilities in rat astrocytes. European J. Neoriscience *6:* 693–705, 1994.

167. Savio, T., and Schwab, M. E. Lesioned corticospinal tract axons regenerate in myelin-free rat spinal cord. P.N.A.S., U.S.A. *87:* 4130–4133, 1990.

168. Schlessinger, J., and Ullrich, A. Growth factor signaling by receptor tyrosine kinases. Neuron *9:* 383–391, 1992.

169. Schnell, L., Schneider, R., and Kolbeck, R. Neurotrophin-3 enhances sprouting of corticospinal tract during development and after adult spinal cord lesion. Nature *367:* 179–173, 1994.

170. Schwab, M. E., and Thoenen, H. Dissociated neurons regenerate into sciatic but not optic nerve explants in culture irrespective of neurotrophic factors. J. Neurosci. *5:* 2415–23, 1985.

171. Schwab, M. E., and Caroni, P. Oligodendrocytes are non-permissive substrates for neurite growth and fibroblast spreading in vitro. J. Neurosci. *8:* 2381–2393, 1988.

172. Schwab, M. E., and Schnell, L. Antibodies against myelin-associated neurite growth inhibitors combined with trophic factors and bridges improve regeneration of lesioned nerve fibers in spinal cord and optic nerve. Nature *343:* 269–272, 1990.

173. Schwab, M. E., and Schnell, L. Channelling of developing rat corticospinal tract axons by myelin-associated neurite growth inhibitors. J. Neurosci. *18:* 161–169, 1991.

174. Schwab, M. E., Kapfhammer, J. P., and Bandtlow, C. E. Inhibitors of Neurite Outgrowth. Annual Review of Neuroscience *16:* 565–595, 1993.

175. Schwab, P. M. Inhibition of axonal regeneration by myelin and glial scars. In: Axonal Regrowth in the Mammalian Spinal Cord and Peripheral Nerve Abstr. IRME, Normandy France, April 1995.

176. Sendtner, M., Arakawa, Y., Stoeckli, K. A., *et al.* Effect of CNTF on motor neuron survival. J. Cell Sci. Suppl. *15:* 103–109, 1991.

177. Sendtner, M., Carroll, P., Holtmann, B., *et al.* Ciliary neurotrophic factor. J. Neurobiol. *25:* 1436–1453, 1994.

178. Shao, Y., and McCarthy, K. D. Plasticity of astrocytes. Glia *11(2):* 147–155, 1994.

179. Shimizu, I., Oppenheim, R. W., O'Brien, M., *et al.* Anatomical and functional recovery following spinal cord transection in the chick embryo. J. Neurobiol. *21:* 918–937, 1990.

180. Silver, J. Inhibitory molecules in development and regeneration. J. Neurol. *241:* S22–S24, 1994.

181. Skaper, S. D., Negro, A., Dal Toso, R., *et al.* Recombinant human CNTF alters the threshold of hippocampal pyramidal neuron sensitivity to excitotoxin damage: synergistic effects of monosialogangliosides. J. Neurosci. Res. *33:* 330–337, 1992.

182. Soppet, D., Escandon, E., Maragos, J., *et al.* The neurotrophic factors brain-derived neurotrophic factor and neurotrophin-3 are ligands for trkB tyrosine kinase receptor. Cell *65:* 895–903, 1991.

183. Spina, M. B., Squinto, S. P., Miller, J., *et al.* Brain-derived neurotrophic factor protects dopamine neurons against 6-hydroxydopamine and N-methyl-4-phenylpyrimidinium ion toxicity: involvement of the glutathione system. J. Neurochemistry *59:* 99–106, 1992.

184. Stahl, N., Davis, S. V. W., Taga, T., *et al.* Cross-linking of CNTF and LIF to endogenous and reconstructed receptor complexes identifies LIF binding protein as a CNTF receptor component. J. Biol. Chem. *268:* 7628–7631, 1993.

185. Stahl, N., and Yancopoulos, G. D. The tripartite CNTF receptor complex: activation and signaling involves components shared with other cytokines. J. Neurobiol. *25:* 1454–1466, 1994.

186. Stahl, N., Boulton, T. G., Farruggella, T., *et al.* Association and activation of Jak-Tyk kinases by CNTF-LIF-OSM-IL-6 Beta receptor components. Science *263:* 92–95, 1994.

187. Stroobant, P. Purification of multiple forms of glial growth factor. J. Biol. Chem. *268:* 18095–18102, 1993.

188. Takeichi, M. Cadherin cell adhesion receptors as a morphogenetic regulator. Science *251:* 1451–1455, 1991.

189. Tartaglia, L. A., Ayres, T. M., Wong, G. H. W., *et al.*

A novel domain within the 55kd TNF receptor signals cell death. Cell *73:* 213–216, 1993.

190. Taylor, J., Docherty, M., and Gordon-Weeks, P. R. GABAergic growth cones: release of endogenous gamma-aminobutyric acid precedes the expression of synaptic vesicle antigens. J. Neurochem. *54:* 1689–1699, 1990.

191. Thanos, S., Mey, J., and Wild, M. Treatment of the adult retina with microglia-suppressing factors retards axotomy-induced neuronal degradation and enhances axonal regeneration in vivo and in vitro. J. Neuroscience *13:* 455–466, 1993.

192. Thomas, S. M., DeMarco, M., D'Arcangelo, G., *et al.* Ras is essential for nerve growth factor- and phorbyl ester-induced tyrosine phosphorylation of MAP kinases. Cell *68:* 1031–1040, 1992.

193. Tooyama, I., Kawamata, T., Walker, D., *et al.* Loss of basic FGF in substantia nigra neurons in Parkinson's disease. Neurology *43:* 372–376, 1993.

194. Treherne, J. M., Woodwards, S. K. A., Varga, Z. M., *et al.* Restoration of conduction and growth of axons through injured spinal cord of neonatal opossum culture. P.N.A.S., U.S.A. *89:* 431–434, 1992.

195. Tuszynski, M. H., and Gage, F. H. In vivo assay of neuron-specific effects of nerve growth factor. Methods in Enzymology *198:* 35–48, 1991.

196. Ullrich, A., Gray, A., Tarn, A. W., *et al.* Insulin-like growth factor I receptor primary structure: Comparison with insulin receptor suggests structural determinants that define functional specificity. EMBO J. *5:* 2503–2512, 1986.

197. Valenzuela, D., Maisonpierre, P., Glass, D., *et al.* Alternate forms of rat TrkC with different functional capabilities. Neuron *19:* 666, 1993.

198. Van Hoof, C. O. M., De Graan, P. N. E., Oestreicher, A. B., *et al.* B-50 phosphorylation and polyphosphoinositide metabolism in nerve growth cone membranes. J. Neurosci. *8:* 1789–1795, 1988.

199. Vaneslow, J., Schwab, M. E., and Thanos, S. Responses of regenerating rat retinal ganglion cell axons to contacts with central nervous system myelin in vitro. Eur. J. Neurosci. *2:* 121–125, 1990.

200. Varon, S., and Conner, J. M. Nerve growth factor in CNS repair. J. Neurotrauma *11:* 473–486, 1994.

201. Verdi, J., Birren, S., Ibanez, C., *et al.* P75^{LNGFR} regulates Trk signal transduction and NGF-induced neurinal differentiation in MAH cells. Neuron *12:* 733–745, 1994.

202. Volone, C., Angelastro, J. M., and Greene, L. A. Association of protein kinases ERK1 and ERK2 with p75 nerve growth factor receptors. Mol. Biol. Cell *4:* 71–78, 1993.

203. Walker, P. S., Donovan, J. A., Van Ness, B. G., *et al.* Glucose-dependent regulation of glucose transport activity, protein and mRNA in primary culture of rat brain glial cells. J. Bio. Chem. *263:* 15594–15601, 1988.

204. Wanaka, A., Johnson, E. J., and Milbrandt, J. Localization of the FGF receptor mRNA in the adult rat CNS by in situ hybridization. Neuron *5:* 267–281, 1990.

205. Weibel, D., Cadelli, D., and Schwab, M. E. Regeneration of lesioned rat optic nerve fibers is improved after neutralization of myelin-associated neurite growth inhibitors. Brain Research *642:* 259–266, 1994.

206. Welcher, A. A., Suter, U., DeLeon, M., *et al.* Molecular approaches to nerve regeneration. Philosophical Transactions of the Royal Society of London, *331:* 295–301, 1991.

207. Werner, H., Raizada, M. K., Mudd, L. M., *et al.* Regulation of rat brain/Hep-G2 glucose transporter gene expression by insulin and insulin-like growth factor-I in primary cultures of neuronal and glial cells. Endocrinology *125:* 314–320, 1989.

208. Weskamp, G., and Reichardt, L. F. Evidence that biological activity of NGF is mediated through a novel subclass of high affinity receptors. Neuron *6:* 649–663, 1991.

209. Whitaker-Azmitia, P. M., and Azmitia, E. C. Autoregulation of fetal serotonergic neuronal development: Role of high affinity serotonin receptors. Neurosci. Lett. *67:* 307–312, 1986.

210. Whitaker-Azmitia, P. M., Murphy, R., and Azmitia, E. C. Stimulation of astroglial 5-HT1A receptors releases the serotonergic growth factor, protein S-100, and alters astroglial morphology. Brain Rresearch *528:* 155–158, 1990.

211. White, L. A., Eaton, M. J., Castro, M. C., *et al.* Distinct regulatory pathways control neurofilament expression and neurotransmitter synthesis in immortalized serotonergic neurons. J. Neurosci. *14:* 6744–6753, 1994.

212. Wrabetz, L., Shumas, S., Grinspan, J., *et al.* Analysis of the human MBP promoter in primary cultures of oligodendrocytes: positive and negative cis-acting elements in the proximal MBP promoter mediate oligodendroycte-specific expression of MBP. J. Neurosci. Res. *36:* 455–471, 1993.

213. Xu, X. M., Guenard, V., Kleitman, N., *et al.* Axonal growth into Schwann cell-seeded guidance channels grafted into transected adult rat spinal cord. Soc. Neurosci. Abstr. *18:* 1479, 1992.

214. Xu, X. M., Guenard, V., Chen, A., *et al.* Rostral and caudal axonal regeneration into Schwann cell-seeded guidance channels grafted into a gap in the adult rat spinal cord. Soc. Neurosci. Abstr. *19:* 681, 1993.

215. Xu, X. M., Guenard, V., Kleitman, N., *et al.* Methylprednisilone and neurotrophin treated rat/rat syngeneic transplants. J. Comp. Neurol. *351:* 145–160, 1995.

216. Yamamoto, Y., Mizuno, R., Nishimura, T., *et al.* Cloning and expression of myelin-associated oligodendrocytic basic protein. J. Biol. Chem. *269:* 31725–31730, 1994.

217. Yoshida, K., and Gage, F. H. Cooperative regulation of nerve growth factor synthesis and secretion in fibroblasts and astrocytes by fibroblast growth factor and other cytokines. Brain Research *569:* 14–25, 1992.

PART VI

The Genetics and Subcellular Basis of Epilepsy

CHAPTER 20

Molecular Biology and Genetics of Epilepsy Syndromes

MURAT GUNEL, M.D. and DENNIS D. SPENCER, M.D.

Epilepsy syndromes are common neurological disorders that affect 1% to 2% of the population and have a significant impact on the individual and the society (46). Current treatment is palliative; except for surgery in selected cases, there is no available cure. Even though the cellular and molecular mechanisms underlying these syndromes are incompletely understood, ample evidence suggests that genetic as well as environmental factors contribute to the pathogenesis of many of these syndromes (22, 69).

In the first part of this chapter, temporal lobe epilepsy (TLE), the most common form of symptomatic epilepsies, is discussed with particular emphasis on the underlying pathology and pathophysiology. The most common pathology underlying this syndrome, Ammon's horn sclerosis, was identified nearly 170 years ago (14), and since then, first cellular, then molecular studies have revealed several different abnormalities in the brains of individuals suffering from this disorder. However, despite this progress, the basic pathophysiological mechanism underlying TLE is yet unknown.

In the second part, known pathophysiological mechanisms underlying other epilepsy syndromes will be presented. This will be followed by a review of the inherited human epilepsy syndromes, animal models of epilepsy and the use of genetic tools in dissecting the molecular mechanisms underlying these disorders.

TEMPORAL LOBE EPILEPSY (TLE)

TLE is classified by the International League Against Epilepsy (ILAE) as one of the symp-

tomatic epilepsies (20). This designation indicates a focal origin and is an anatomical classification based on the concordance of electrophysiology and ictal behavior. Modern imaging and analysis of tissue resected from patients with medically intractable seizures have modified this simple anatomical classification to include etiological substrates such as mesial temporal sclerosis (MTS), developmental abnormalities, tumors, and vascular lesions. Among these, MTS is the most common substrate; MTS is seen in approximately 50% of the surgical specimens resected from patients suffering from medically intractable temporal lobe seizures (16). Even though the exact number of patients with a developmental abnormality as an etiological substrate is unknown, postmortem studies have identified developmental abnormalities in as many as 40% of epileptic brains (71). Furthermore, developmental abnormalities are seen in 30% to 50% of surgical specimens (44). These abnormalities are especially prevalent in children with severe epilepsy (32). In addition to MTS and developmental abnormalities, intracranial mass lesions such as low-grade gliomas or vascular lesions are found as etiological substrates in another 20% of the MTLE cases (16, 108).

Mesial Temporal Sclerosis (MTS)

In 30% to 50% of all surgical cases, uniform changes affecting the medial temporal lobe structures, including the hippocampus ("Ammon's horn sclerosis"), are observed. These changes include neuronal loss and gliosis, sprouting of neurons and their reorganization into new circuitry, and hyperexcitability of the medial temporal lobe structures. MTS frequently is associated with cerebral injury such as febrile seizure, trauma or meningitis that occurs before age 5. This association between an injury during early childhood, specific EEG ictal and interictal behavior patterns, and hippocampal atrophy evident on MRI occurs in approximately 40% of all epilepsy cases and has been designated the syndrome of medial temporal lobe epilepsy (MTLE) (16, 20, 92).

Even though the molecular pathways underlying MTS have been debated for over 150 years, they are still poorly understood. The pathological changes in temporal lobe structures in patients with epilepsy were first described in 1825 by Bouchet and Cazauveilh. They found gross atrophy and induration of one or both temporal lobes, especially the hippocampus, and sclerosis of the white matter in 9 out of 18 patients with epilepsy (14). Sommer, in 1880, described severe neuron loss in a restricted area of the pyramidal band of the hippocampus and designated it as Ammon's horn sclerosis (105). Sommer considered the hippocampus to be the sensory center (Fuhlcentrum) and speculated that the sensory phenomena experienced before or between the seizures was the result of Ammon's horn pathology (105).

In 1925, Vogt and Spielmeyer separately described selective destruction of various pyramidal neurons in different fields of the hippocampus (109, 124). Vogt explained this on the basis of the "pathoclisis" theory, which stated that physiochemical properties of certain neurons make them susceptible to particular pathological agents (124). Spielmeyer argued that the neuronal loss in the hippocampi of epileptic patients was not attributable to specific vulnerability of these cells but was nonspecific, because this neuronal loss was seen in many different conditions (109). He suggested that ischemia caused the neuronal loss. He argued that the hippocampus was supplied by a long and tortuous end artery that was susceptible to spasm and occlusion that caused hippocampal ischemia. This vascular theory of Spielmeyer's gained more support than the pathoclisis theory at that time and was considered as the cause of hippocampal sclerosis and thus MTLE for many years.

In 1936, Strauder first correlated the clinical phenomena of seizures with pathological changes in the hippocampus (112). Although Strauder revealed a very strong relationship between temporal lobe epilepsy and Ammon's horn sclerosis, he concluded that the hippocampal damage was not the cause of seizures, but rather the consequence of the frequent head trauma so common in epileptics.

The first surgical cases demonstrating Ammon's horn sclerosis were reported in 1951 by Scholz who supported Spielmeyer's vascular theory and suggested that the hippocampal pathological changes resulted from the vascular and anoxic disturbances seen with severe generalized convulsions (96). After this, continued reports of hippocampal sclerosis in either autopsy or surgical specimens were published, but the cause of neuronal loss in epilepsy continued to be controversial. Lindenberg in 1955 and Pia in 1957 proposed that edema resulting from seizure induced venous stasis, compression of arteries against the tentorium, and neuronal loss (64, 85). The role of edema in neuronal loss was also emphasized by Penfield in 1954 and by Gastaut in 1959 (37, 83). Scholz, in an attempt to combine the theories of Spielmeyer and Vogt, suggested that the increased oxygen and energy requirements during seizure activity contributed to neuronal loss (97).

However, it was not until Falconer's careful light histological description of medial temporal lobe neuronal loss and gliosis that the descriptive term MTS was used to describe this pathology. He pointed out that MTS was the single most common finding in his surgical series (47/100 patients undergoing temporal lobectomy for epilepsy). The firm association of this injury pattern and "prolonged convulsions of early childhood" including febrile seizures (33/47 patients) was noted. The higher rate of seizure control when this pathology rather than histologically normal hippocampus (50% vs. 33%) was resected supported this theory (31). Although the relationship of early childhood injury, the development of spontaneous seizures and the underlying ictal and interictal, electrical events are still not understood, Falconer's observations defined the puzzle that basic investigators are still attempting to solve.

Biochemical Changes in TLE

Since these early reports, more recent histochemical analysis of the hippocampi removed from epilepsy patients has yielded important insights into the pathology and pathophysiology of MTLE. These hippocampi, compared to those with medial temporal epileptogenic masses such as low-grade gliomas or autopsy controls, have demonstrated loss of more than 50% of neurons, and proportional increase in gliosis (4, 5, 54). This neuronal loss affected the pyramidal cells in all cornu ammonis (CA) fields, the interneurons in the hilus, and the granule cells in the dentate gyrus (54). Immunohistochemical (IHC) techniques have characterized the depleted pyramidal cells in the CA fields as glutaminergic and the hilar interneurons as a neuropeptide system involving neuropeptide Y (NPY), somatostatin (SOM), and substance P (SP) (57, 58). Although GABAergic interneurons seemed to be relatively preserved (6), this important inhibitory neurotransmitter colocalizes with certain hilar cells that are uniformly depleted.

TIMM staining of mossy fibers has revealed a unique reorganization and new sprouting of neuropeptide neurons containing dynorphin (DYN), NPY, SOM, and SP in the dentate gyrus of epileptic hippocampi (113, 114, 118). Immunohistochemical electron-microscopical studies of these projections revealed abundant new synapses, many of which are in the inner molecular layer and on proximal granule cell apical dendrites (57). The reorganization also affects the neurotransmitter and neuromodulator receptors; receptors for SOM, NPY, vasoactive intestinal polypeptide (VIP), dopamine D2 and kainic acid (KA) are redistributed and upregulated (7, 58). Although this reorganization and sprouting may contribute to hyperexcitability, it may alternatively reflect a response to excess excitation. This new circuitry leaves an unbalanced system favoring excitation. As demonstrated by the in vitro electrophysiological studies of the human sclerotic hippocampal slice, even a low frequency stimulation of the perforant path elicits increased population spikes in the abnormal dentate gyrus (68). More recently, intracellular electrophysiology of the sclerotic granule cells in these hippocampi found them NMDA dependent and hyperexcitable in response to perforant path stimulation (55, 131). These results suggest that both a decrease in inhibitory activity and an NMDA receptor mediated excitatory enhancement are important in the pathophysiology of MTLE.

In vitro, hyperexcitability can also be demonstrated in the glia cultured from medial temporal lobe structures by Ca^{2+} flou-3 imaging with confocal microscopy (41). In addition, microdialysis studies with dialysis membranes attached to depth electrodes in epileptic patients have sampled the human hippocampal extracellular fluid space before, during and after medial temporal lobe ictal events. In the epileptogenic hippocampus, compared to the contralateral side, glutamate levels rose immediately before the ictal event (26). This elevation in glutamate levels peaked at a level sixfold higher than the baseline, and remained elevated for a prolonged period of time (26). On the other hand, GABA levels were relatively stable in the epileptogenic hippocampus compared to a brisk fourfold responsive rise on the opposite side. Initially, the death of GABAergic neurons was thought to result in the loss of GABA-mediated inhibition and this loss of inhibition was held responsible for focal hyperexcitability within the epileptic hippocampus. However, as mentioned above, GABA interneurons seem to be relatively resistant to seizure-induced neuronal cell loss and are relatively preserved in the epileptic hippocampus (6). One explanation which takes this and the microdialysis results into account comes from data supporting malfunction or reversal of the GABA transporter. This malfunction could provide a functional loss of inhibitory response to glutamate release of either neuronal or glial origin. Regardless, much of this data implicates altered release and/or reuptake of many different neurotransmitters in the human epileptic hippocampi.

One important aspect of this hyperexcitability, poorly understood at the molecular level, is its transient and intermittent nature. As both excitatory and inhibitory mechanisms can contribute to hyperexcitability, either could underlie progression to an epileptic attack. Positron emission tomography (PET) studies have revealed hypometabolism of the temporal lobe in patients with TLE; this suggests that epileptogenic brain is hypoactive between seizures (29). Although this phenomenon is also not well understood, it could reflect increased inhibition within the epileptogenic region or interference with energy metabolism. The main interictal abnormality in these epileptogenic regions is the interplay between the hypersynchronous excitatory and inhibitory events evident as the spike-and-wave pattern on the interictal EEG (12). Any mechanism that interferes with the inhibitory component of this complex could lead to persistent depolarization and a low-voltage fast rhythm, the characteristic rhythm seen in the generalized convulsive seizures. Mechanisms that increase the synchronicity of the complex could lead to a repeated spike-and-wave pattern on the EEG, the characteristic pattern seen in an absence seizure. Partial seizures, on the other hand, could show either pattern. Thus, abnormalities in either the excitatory or the inhibitory circuitry can affect the excitability and synchronicity of the neurons and can lead to an epileptic attack. These abnormalities in the circuitry could arise from abnormalities in development, as seen in the neuronal migration disorders, or from plasticity of the developing brain in response to various noxious stimuli.

The dormant basket cell theory and the mossy fiber sprouting theory offer alternative explanations of the imbalance affecting the excitatory and inhibitory systems within the epileptic hippocampus (75, 103, 118). The former holds that the neuronal cell loss following seizures represents excitatory cells in the hilus, removing the excitatory input to the GABAergic basket neurons. The basket neurons are thus rendered functionally inactive resulting in focal hyperexcitability. The latter theory holds that the hyperexcitability is a consequence of pathologic reorganization of the circuitry in the epileptic hippocampus. The self-innervation of the excitatory granule cells creates a recurrent excitatory loop (75, 118). This re-organization may reflect loss of interneurons that normally innervate the dendrites of the granule cells. There is insufficient immunohistochemical and electrophysiologic evidence to prove either theory, and controversies regarding the underlying pathophysiological mechanism(s) persist.

The two mechanistic questions central to the pathophysiology of MTLE are: 1—What are the cellular and molecular mechanisms that underlie the selective neuronal loss? and 2—How do these acute changes induce long term re-organization and excitatory imbalance? Excitotoxicity with massive calcium influx may answer the first question. First introduced in epilepsy by Olney, excitotoxicity appears to be the final common pathway for neuronal injury and cell death in a variety of diseases with diverse pathophysiological mechanisms (77, 78) including epilepsy, stroke, trauma, and neurodegenerative disorders such as Huntington's disease.

EXCITOTOXICITY

Glutamate is the most abundant excitatory neurotransmitter in the brain; the intracellular and extracellular concentrations of glutamate are estimated to be 10 and 0.6 milimols per liter, respectively. Excitotoxic damage occurs when extracellular glutamate concentrations rise to the range of 2 to 5 micromol per liter. Thus, extracellular glutamate concentration needs to be tightly regulated. This is mainly achieved by sodium dependent, high-affinity glutamate uptake systems which are located on both neurons and astrocytes. These glutamate transporters, under normal physiologic conditions, efficiently transport glutamate into cells against a chemical gradient by using energy. Under pathological conditions, however, the transporter can work backwards and increase the extracellular glutamate concentration. This pathologic mechanism is active following the swelling of astrocytes after trauma, ischemia or any insult that results in energy deficiency. The direction of the transporter's function is completely dependent on the energy generated from the sodium gradient maintained by the Na/K ATPase. Any loss of function of this enzyme results in the reversal of transport of the glutamate molecules across the membrane and increase in the amount of extracellular glutamate (reviewed in 18).

Glutamate exerts its effect through different receptor systems, and at least 20 genes are known to encode for subunits of these receptors (48). Different combinations of these subunits result in different functional receptor types. The three main types of glutamate receptors are N-methyl-D-aspartate (NMDA), alpha-amino-3-hydroxy-5-methyl-4-isoxazolepropionate (AMPA) and kainate (KA) receptors. Among these, NMDA receptors seem to be unique in being responsive to both neurotransmitter (glutamate) and voltage. At rest, the NMDA receptors are blocked by magnesium unless the cell is depolarized. Activation of these receptors by glutamate or by depolarization of the membrane results in a direct influx of calcium ions through NMDA receptor coupled calcium channels. The AMPA and kainate receptors, on the other hand, cause influx of Na+ ions following their activation by glutamate. However, influx of these positively charged Na+ ions depolarizes the membrane and thus indirectly activates voltage-gated L-type calcium channels. There are at least four types of voltage-dependent calcium channels: T (transient current), N (neuronal), L (long duration current, large conduction channels) and P (Purkinje type). Among these, the L-type calcium channels appear to be the most important calcium channel that contributes to excitotoxicity. Thus, excessive glutamate appears to cause neuronal injury by excessive activation of calcium channels coupled to the NMDA receptors, and at the same time, by membrane depolarization through AMPA and kainate receptors that results in the activation of the voltage sensitive calcium channels, mainly the L-type. Excessive intracellular calcium then activates certain cytosolic enzyme systems such as protein kinase C, phospholipases, proteases, protein phosphotases and nitric oxide synthase. Activation of these enzyme systems result in production of toxic materials such as oxygen free radicals, arachidonic acid and its metabolites which ultimately cause protein breakdown, lipid peroxidation and membrane disintegration. This process, also, activates immediate-early gene expression and results in long term structural changes. Thus, short term changes may induce long term re-organization.

DIFFERENTIAL GENE EXPRESSION UNDERLYING LONG TERM CHANGES IN MEDIAL TEMPORAL LOBE EPILEPSY

Neuronal gene expression, modulated by neurotrophic factors, neurotransmitters and synaptic activity is critically involved in the development and plasticity of the nervous system. Even though the effects of neurotrophic factors and neurotransmitters and changes in membrane activity last only milliseconds, long-term consequences of these stimulations mediated by new gene expression may occur. The changes in gene expression may lead to alterations in neuronal synaptic density, in the expression and density of neurotransmitter receptors, and even in neuronal sprouting. The genes that are activated following these diverse stimuli are now grouped into two classes: the immediate early genes (IEG) and late response genes. Even though the distinction between these two

classes is not always sharp, IEGs generally regulate genes that control the expression of late response genes that then serve more specific effector functions (100).

First identified in non-neuronal cells, IEGs, which encode transcription factors, control the re-entry of G_0 resting cells into the cell cycle. c-fos and c-myc were among the first IEGs to be identified (40, 53). In general, these IEGs share several common characteristics. Their expression is very tightly controlled. Their basal expression is very low in quiescent cells, but following appropriate extracellular stimuli, their expression is rapidly induced at the transcriptional level, independent of new protein synthesis. The mRNA synthesized usually has a very short half life and the termination of this transcription requires new protein synthesis. Most of these IEGs use Ca^{2+} as a major second messenger system. Many IEG's are active as a homo- or heterodimer. The best known example is c-fos and c-jun, which interact through a conserved dimerization domain referred to as the leucine zipper and bind to a highly conserved DNA domain -TGACTCA-. This sequence was first identified as a phorbol ester-inducible promoter site for a transcription factor termed AP-1 (2), later shown to consist of c-fos and c-jun (13). Other genes that are closely related to c-fos (fos-B, fra-1) and c-jun (jun-B) not only bind to the consensus AP-1 site in vitro, but also dimerize both with themselves and other members of the c-fos and c-jun family. Several other genes (zif/268, nur/77) also have homologies to known transcriptional factors and are induced by extracellular stimuli; most of these genes are not as well characterized as c-fos and c-jun, but are very likely to act as IEGs. Even though these IEG's can be activated by diverse stimuli, different extra-cellular stimuli appear to induce different sets of IEG's. For example, whereas nerve growth factor (NGF) and epidermal growth factor induce one set of IEG's with virtually identical kinetics, membrane depolarization and Ca^{2+} influx activate a different set of IEG's. Each set of IEGs in turn, induces particular downstream late response genes, depending on the cell type. These late response genes, best characterized in NGF treated PC12 cells, include a neural cell adhesion molecule, transin, a metalloprotease, filament proteins such as peripherin and neurofilament subunits NF-L and NF-M, Ca^{2+} binding proteins, and others (99, 100).

Activation of IEG's such as c-fos, fra-1, zif/268, nur/77, jun-B and c-jun has been shown in neurons of the rodent brain following pharmacologically induced generalized seizures (24, 72, 91, 107, 126). In the best characterized example, following generalized seizures, c-fos, expression increases throughout the brain; the most rapid and substantial induction occurs in the dentate gyrus. Interestingly, this induction can be blocked by stopping the seizure activity by diazepam (72) or carbamazepine (24). Induction of these IEG's also occurs following electrical stimulation of the cortex (93) and after kindling (see below) (23).

Of the other IEG's, zif/268 is preferentially activated in the ipsilateral dentate gyrus following electrical stimulation of the perforant path of the hippocampus (19). Interestingly, only high, and not low, frequency stimulation, which induces long term potentiation (LTP), causes a substantial increase in the zif/268 mRNA levels. In this model, induction of both zif/268 and LTP is dependent on activation of NMDA receptors and is inhibited by NMDA antagonists (19). c-fos is also induced by NMDA receptor activation (116); the brain regions that show high levels of c-fos following seizures have high levels of NMDA receptors; LTP induction, however, does not stimulate c-fos expression (19).

The molecular pathways leading to c-fos activation by extra-cellular stimuli have revealed Ca^{2+} influx as the crucial event. This influx in Ca2+ can be achieved by activating either the N-methyl-D-aspartate (NMDA) subtype of the glutamate receptor or the L-type Ca2+ channel through the AMPA/KA receptor (reviewed in 21). If achieved through the L-type Ca2+ channel, the increase in calcium influx activates a multifunctional Ca2+-calmodulin-dependent protein kinase (CaM kinase II) (100), which phosphorylates and thus activates the cAMP response element binding protein (CREB). CREB binds to the calcium/cAMP responsive element (Ca/CRE) which activates the transcription of c-fos. The expression of other IEG's like nur/77, zif/268 and neuropeptide genes such as somatostatin, vasoactive intestinal polypeptide and proenkephalin is activated via this pathway (reviewed in 100). Interestingly, mice lacking the CaM gene (see below)

exhibit hyperexcitability, suggesting that this pathway might have a role in the pathogenesis of hyperexcitability in vivo (17). However, if the increase in Ca2+ influx is obtained through the NMDA receptor pathway, CaM is not activated. The NMDA pathway and the L-type Ca2+ pathway act through distinct DNA regulatory elements (8). These results suggest that these two pathways may induce distinct patterns of gene expression.

The expression pattern of these IEG's ultimately determines the long term structural changes seen in different chronic disease states. Thus, these transcription factors could potentially be the link between recurrent seizures and resultant structural changes. The mechanism of activation of these molecules is not known, but second messenger systems involving calcium have been implicated.

Other genes are also differentially activated in epileptic brain. Differential screening of a hippocampal cDNA library with two probes, one derived from the mRNA isolated from the cortex of control animals and the other one from the cortex of animals treated with metrazol to induce seizures, revealed that, besides c-fos and zif268, 5 novel genes, including a putatively secreted protein named PC3 or T1S21 of unknown function, and tissue-type plasminogen activator (tPA) were differentially expressed in the epileptic tissue (86). Expression of all these genes were induced by seizure activity. Among these, tPA, which is an extracellular serine protease, is induced by kindling.

In kindling, a good experimental model for neuronal plasticity, a stimulus that initially evokes only a brief after-discharge after multiple repetition becomes capable of consistently initiating a generalized seizure. Once seizures are inducible they can be reproduced throughout the animal's life-time. Both kindling and human epilepsy are associated with similar structural changes in the central nervous system. They may also share a common pathophysiological pathway with long term plastic changes, for example, activation of tPA following seizures or after kindling stimuli. tPA may cause structural changes in the nervous system either by affecting the adhesions between neurons, by changing the spatial and temporal relationships between proteases and their inhibitors, or by activating a yet unidentified receptor (86). More recently, tPA has been directly implicated in the pathogenesis of neuronal degeneration. Transgenic mice lacking the tPA gene (tPA-/-) are resistant to neuronal degeneration induced by excitotoxins (121). These mice are also less susceptible to pharmacologically induced seizures than are wild-type mice. Brains of the tPA-/- mice lack obvious abnormalities before or after the seizures. Detailed histological analysis of wild-type and mutant mice reveal that tPA is expressed by microglia in the brain. Activated microglia have previously been implicated in neuronal injury (70), and the NMDA antagonist MK-801 which, in vitro, can prevent the excitotoxic effects of glutamate, has been shown to block microglial activation and transcriptional induction of tPA (86). Thus, microglial activation with resultant toxic affects could be important in the pathogenesis of the neuronal degeneration following seizure activity.

Another molecule induced following seizures is nerve growth factor (34). Induction of growth factors following seizures is interesting as these factors could be responsible for new axonal growth and synaptic reorganization. In rats, following recurrent seizures induced by the electrical stimulation of the dentate gyrus of the hippocampus, expression of nerve growth factor mRNA is increased in the hippocampus. This is followed by increases in the nerve growth factor levels in stratum granulosum, the entorhinal cortex, piriform cortex, amygdala and broad fields of the neocortex, mainly in layers II, III, and VI (34). The expression seen in the hippocampus mainly affected the dentate gyrus granule cells and its temporal pattern closely resembled the expression pattern of c-fos and tPA, reaching a post-ictal maximum in less than 6 hours, and then declining rapidly. This temporal pattern differs greatly from that of other molecules induced in the dentate gyrus following seizures. These molecules include preproenkephalin and preproneuropeptide Y mRNAs which are elevated for a longer time (33, 129). Another change seen following recurrent limbic seizures is a decrease in the abundance of preprodynorphin mRNA (73, 74).

ANIMAL MODELS (TABLE I)

Genetic models of epilepsy have been identified in diverse animal species. It is hoped that specific genes underlying the hyperexcitability in different animal models will be identified.

TABLE 1
Animal Models

a—Ion channels
 i—weaver (wv) mutant
 ii—Shaker
b—Transcription factors
 i—jerky (Jrk)
c—Neurotransmitter metabolism
 i—Mice lacking tissue non-specific alkaline phosphatase
 ii—Editing deficient GluR-B mouse
 iii—lethargic (lh/lh) mouse
 iv—5-HT2c serotonin receptor knock-out mouse
d—Synaptic transmission
 i—synapsin I and II mutant mice
e—Others
 i—El mouse
 ii—calcium/calmodulin kinase II knock-out mouse

The human homologs of these genes may have importance in the pathogenesis of at least some forms of epilepsy. Despite this progress, it is still unknown if any of these animal models use mechanisms analogous to human epileptic syndromes. Noebels, in 1986, described over 17 single locus mutations that result in epilepsy in mice (76). Since then, the molecular bases of several animal models have been delineated and other models that closely resemble human epilepsy syndromes have been identified. In these models, diverse mechanisms underlie the observed hyperexcitability and seizure susceptibility; these range from interference with a neurotransmitter or an ion channel to malfunction of a transcription factor.

Ion Channels

weaver (wv) mutant: The gene responsible for the weaver (wv) mutant in mice has recently been identified (81). In wv mutant, early stages of neuronal differentiation immediately after cessation of cell division, including expression of late neuronal markers, axon extension, and glia-induced neuronal migration, fail. This failure in differentiation results in severe architectonic rearrangements and phenotypically is characterized by seizures. A missense mutation in the conserved transmembrane domain of a brain G protein coupled rectifier K+ channel (GIRK2), has been shown to be responsible for the phenotype (81). This missense mutation, which changes a glycine residue to serine, results in alterations in the channel conductance. As early events in neuronal differentiation are not thought to be regulated by changes in membrane permeability, it is surprising that the observed phenotype is expressed at that level. How mutations in GIRK2 can lead to the severe architectonic rearrangements seen in wv mice is yet unknown.

Shaker: Mutation in the Shaker gene is another example of an ion channel mutation leading to an epileptic phenotype. Deletion in mKv1.1, one of the 16 murine homologs of the Shaker gene, results in a lethal epilepsy phenotype lacking a functional delayed rectifier K+ channel (104).

Transcription Factors

jerky (Jrk): jerky phenotype was incidentally identified as a line of transgenic mice that showed handling-induced seizures after inserting SV40 large T antigen (SV40 TAg) (120) into brain precursor cells. Chronic recordings in these transgenic mice revealed large amplitude interictal-like spikes in the dentate gyrus and spike-and-wave patterns in the neocortex. Fifty percent of the animals that were homozygous for the trait died by age 3 months; all the surviving animals had a seizure disorder. These seizures did not develop to their full state in hemizygotes, indicating genetic heterogeneity. The molecular basis of this model was revealed by identifying the insertional site of the SV40 TAg transgene into the genome. The fact that this transgene did not cause tumors in any of the transgenic animals and that two other transgenic lines created in the same way did not have seizures suggested that the insertional mutagenesis of a cellular gene was responsible for seizures. The gene disrupted by the insertion has been identified, and it encodes a 58kD protein that shows homology with a number of transcription factors (120). How mutations in this gene lead to neuronal hyperexcitability and seizure is not known; however, reduced levels of this protein during crucial stages of development is thought to result in neuronal degeneration or death or alternatively in disturbances in the synthesis of certain molecules such as neurotransmitters and/or channel proteins.

Neurotransmitter Metabolism

Mice lacking tissue non-specific alkaline phosphatase: Mice lacking the tissue non-specific alkaline phosphatase (TNAP) die from seizures at approximately two weeks after birth (127). Defective metabolism of pyridoxal 5′ phosphate (plp) which results in reduced levels of GABA is responsible for these seizures. Lack of TNAP activity results in a 20 fold increase in plp levels. plp, without de-phosphorylation by TNAP, is unable to cross biological membranes and thus cannot act as a cofactor to many enzyme systems including glutamic acid decarboxylase which synthesizes GABA. The mutant seizure phenotype is shown to be reversed by pyridoxal which restores the normal levels of GABA. These mutant mice provide an excellent genetic model of vitamin B6 deficient seizures.

Editing deficient GluR-B mouse: One type of glutamate receptor, the alpha-amino-3-hydroxy-5-methyl-4-isoxazolepropionate (AMPA) receptor, is a ligand-activated cation channel assembled from four related subunits (GluR-A to GluR-D or GluR1 to GluR4). AMPA receptors, unlike NMDA receptors, are impermeable to Ca^{2+} (48). This is due to the GluR-B subunit of the channel, specifically the arginine residue at position 586 (47). Even though this arginine (R) is not encoded at the DNA level, it is post-transcriptionally introduced by site-specific adenosine deamination of the glutamine (Q) residue (106). This process is called Q/R editing. Heterozygous mice engineered to be incompetent in this Q/R editing expressed AMPA receptors with markedly increased calcium permeability, developed seizures, and died by 3 weeks of age (15). Histological examination of the brains of these mice revealed selective neuronal degeneration in the hippocampal CA3 field.

lethargic (lh/lh) mouse: The lh/lh mouse has spontaneous seizures and a single gene-locus defect on chromosome 2 (49). EEG recordings exhibit bilateral synchronous electrographic bursts of 5- to 6-Hz spike-wave complexes (76). This strain is thought to be a valid model of absence seizures. Human absence (petit mal) seizures demonstrate bilateral synchronous, rhythmic 3-Hz spike wave discharges generated by the cerebral cortex and the thalamus. They are thought to be a result of the interplay between low threshold Ca^{2+} currents (T currents) and the $GABA_B$ receptor mediated inputs. T currents can trigger rhythmic firing of thalamic neurons. They are activated from their normal resting state by $GABA_B$ receptor mediated hyperpolarization. Once T currents become active, they trigger rhythmic firing of thalamic neurons. In lh/lh mice, there is enhanced $GABA_B$ receptor mediated synaptic responses that could potentially activate the T currents responsible for seizure activity (49). In these mice, GABA$_B$ receptor agonists exacerbated the seizures, whereas GABA$_B$ receptor antagonists suppressed seizure activity. Thus GABA$_B$ receptor mediated mechanisms may underlie human absence seizures and GABA$_B$ receptor antagonists may hold promise as anti-convulsants for human absence seizures (49).

5-HT2c serotonin receptor knock-out mouse: Mice lacking the 5-HT2c serotonin receptors were generated by introducing a nonsense mutation into the gene (119). Although these animals appeared to have normal central nervous systems, hippocampal long-term potentiation, and sensitivity to thermal and mechanical stimuli, a significant proportion of the mutant mice died prematurely. Continuous video-monitoring of the animals revealed that the mutant animals suffered from recurrent spontaneous seizures, often preceded by repetitive snout grooming progressing to generalized tonic-clonic seizure activity. In addition, infusion of metrazol, a GABA$_A$ antagonist, proved to be more lethal in the mutant mice. These animals had a lower seizure threshold, and a more rapid progression of seizure induction. The relevance of this model to human epilepsy is unknown, but it demonstrates that a variety of different neurotransmitter and/or neuromodulator systems may be important in the pathophysiology of different epilepsy syndromes.

Synaptic Transmission

synapsin I and II mutant mice: Another knock-out mouse model with seizures is the synapsin I and II mutant (90). Synaptic vesicles are coated by these two glycoproteins which make up approximately 10% of the total vesicle protein. These proteins were initially thought to be important in synaptogenesis and basic mechanisms of synaptic vesicle traffic; however, mice mutant for these proteins have no major morbidity other than seizures precipitated by sensory stimuli. The seizure frequency in these mice is directly proportional to the number of mutant alleles, suggesting that these proteins are important for accelerating the synaptic vesicle traffic during repetitive stimulation. The epileptic phenotype of the synapsin knockouts could be due to deficient recruitment of vesicles at the active zone or impaired maturation prior to release. GABAergic interneurons which fire at high frequencies, would be particularly affected by deficient recruitment of vesicles. This would in turn result in the functional loss of the inhibitory system and an imbalance between inhibitory and excitatory systems in favor of the excitatory one. Thus, the hyperexcitable phenotype seen in the synapsin mutants could be due to a loss of the GABAergic system.

Others

El mouse: The El (epilepsy) mouse is considered to be a good model of human complex partial seizures with secondary generalization (115). Seizures in these mice appear to originate from the parietal cortex or the hippocampus and are associated with appropriate EEG changes (50). Clinically, they are characterized by incontinence, loss of equilibrium, excessive salivation and automatisms involving head, limbs and mouth. They respond well to anti-convulsants such as phenytoin and phenobarbital. On pathological examination, these animals reveal extensive gliosis in the hippocampus but no neuronal loss. Seyfried and his colleagues first mapped the major seizure susceptibility locus to mouse chromosome 9 near the predicted location for the ceruloplasmin gene and designated it as the El-1 locus (89). They also mapped a modifying allele on chromosome 2 and called it the El-2 locus (89). Even though partial gene duplication of the 5′ end of the ceruloplasmin gene was thought to be responsible for susceptibility to epilepsy (36), further studies did not confirm this. Thus, the mechanism underlying seizure susceptibility in El mouse is still not known.

Calcium/calmodulin kinase II knock-out mouse: The homozygous mutant mice carrying the null mutation for the gene encoding the alpha-subunit of the Ca2+-calmodulin kinase II exhibit profound hyperexcitability. Administration of a single, normally subconvulsive stimulation pulse to the amygdala results in prolonged, repeated and sometimes fatal seizures (17). Histologic examination of the unstimulated homozygous mouse reveals extensive sprouting of the mossy fibers in the dentate gyrus of the hippocampus compared to that in the heterozygous mouse (17). This animal model seems to reveal the importance of the CaM pathway in vivo (see above).

INHERITED EPILEPSY SYNDROMES IN HUMANS (TABLE II)

In certain human epileptic syndromes, there is ample evidence to suggest the contribution of genetic factors to the pathophysiology of seizures. Sibling risk of epilepsy is between 2 and 5%, and up to 20–30% if those with EEG abnormalities are included (102). The overall incidence of seizures among the children of patients with epilepsy is about 6% (102). Until recently little progress has been made in mapping specific loci that contribute to the propensity of an individual to develop seizures. This slow progress is in part due to the complex inheritance pattern of epileptic syndromes; they do not fit a simple Mendelian pattern. This could reflect the need for specific environmental factors or modifying genes for the phenotypic expression of these syndromes. It is very likely that both genetic and non-genetic factors are important and that there is more than one modifying allele for each of these syndromes. There are only a few syndromes in which the mode of inheritance has been determined and the relevant chromosomal loci mapped by positional cloning techniques.

In recent years, positional cloning techniques have revealed important disease genes in disorders that are known to be transmitted as simple Mendelian traits. These include cystic fibrosis, neurofibromatosis, Duchenne muscular dystrophy, and amytrophic lateral sclerosis. In positional cloning, the chromosomal location of a disease gene is determined by linkage analysis based on the fact that spatially proximate genes are inherited together at a higher frequency than distant ones. The co-segregation of a disease gene with various polymorphic markers is assessed in families afflicted with the disease. The probability that the observed inheritance of a polymorphic marker and the disease locus could occur by chance alone is calculated. The calculation is then repeated assuming a particular degree of linkage between a polymorphic marker and the disease locus and the ratio of these two probabilities are calculated. This final ratio, called the logarithm of odds (lod) score, gives the likelihood of linkage of each marker to the disease gene and localizes the gene to a particular chromosomal region. The same principle is then applied to markers within that chromosomal region in order to clone the disease gene. By collecting a sufficiently large number of families, strong evidence of genetic linkage can be found despite confounding factors such as genetic heterogeneity, incomplete penetrance and multifactorial determination. If candidate genes are known to be within a small linked region, mutational analysis techniques can be used to identify the disease gene. These techniques include genomic southern blots or restriction fragment length polymorphism (RFLP) assays if deletions or any other chromosomal rearrangements are suspected and single strand conformational polymorphism (SSCP) or heteroduplex analysis if mis-sense or non-sense point mutations are suspected. If, however, no known genes are known to lie in that chromosomal region, positional cloning is further pursued by defining the narrowest region in which the disease gene might lie. This region is then physically mapped and screened for the presence of expressed sequences by molecular biological techniques such as direct cDNA selection, exon trapping or direct sequencing. When new genes are identified and cloned by these approaches, and if these genes are expressed in the appropriate tissue(s), mutational analysis is performed. When the disease gene is successfully isolated, a large population of patients is screened in an attempt to define the proportion of genetic cases within the af-

TABLE 2
Inherited Epilepsy Syndromes in Humans

---

a—Idiopathic generalized epilepsy syndromes
    i—Juvenile myoclonus epilepsy (Herpin-Janz
        syndrome) 6p
    ii—Benign neonatal epilepsy EBN1-20q (?CHRNA4),
        EBN2-8q
b—Idiopathic partial epilepsy syndromes
    i—Nocturnal frontal lobe epilepsy 20q (ADNFLE)
    ii—Partial epilepsy with auditory symptoms 10q
**c—Single gene disorders with epilepsy as a major
feature**
    i—Cerebral cavernous malformation (CCM)
    ii—Neuronal migration disorders
    Tuberous sclerosis (TCS2)
    Lissencephaly, Miller-Dieker type (LIS1 gene)
    X-linked periventricular heterotopia
    iii—Progressive myoclonus epilepsy syndromes
    Unverricht-Lundborg type (EPM1)
    Myoclonic epilepsy with ragged red fibers
      (MERRF) Neuronal ceroid lipofuscinosis
    Lafora's disease Sialidosis (neuraminidase
      deficiency)
    iv—Northern epilepsy syndrome 8p

fected population and the spectrum of mutations that effect the disease gene.

For most of the human epilepsy syndromes inherited as a simple Mendelian traits, relevant chromosomal locations have been mapped by linkage. However, for most of the remaining epilepsy syndromes, the genetic influence in pathogenesis appears to be much more complicated. For example, evidence suggests that genetic factors play an important role in temporal lobe epilepsy (TLE). As mentioned above, medial temporal lobe sclerosis, the most common etiologic substrate underlying temporal lobe epilepsy, frequently is associated with an injury, most commonly a febrile seizure under age 5. Febrile seizures, like other causes of secondary seizures, such as head trauma and CNS infection, are natural reactions of a normal brain to transient noxious stimuli. However, normal brains, because of variations in the individual's genetic endowment and diverse environmental conditions, have different predisposition to secondary or reactive seizures when exposed to such noxious stimuli. For example, 2% to 5% of all North American children suffer from febrile seizures during early childhood (52); however, only a few percent of these become epileptics and suffer from recurrent seizures during adolescence. A history of febrile seizures is especially prevalent in temporal lobe epilepsy patients with hippocampal atrophy (56). All this data suggests that the subgroup of patients who continue to suffer from TLE following a febrile seizure during childhood have a genetic predisposition to develop epilepsy. Furthermore, a genetic predisposition for having a febrile seizure has been described; a sibling of a patient with a febrile seizure is more likely to suffer from a febrile seizure compared to the normal population (52, 122). The genetic components contributing to the pathogenesis of these syndromes are yet to be defined.

The genetic predisposition to develop TLE could also be due to a structural defect. With highly sophisticated imaging techniques and careful histological examination of surgical specimens from TLE patients, minor neuronal migrational disorders, so called microdysgenesis, are being discovered. Microdysgenesis usually co-exists with hippocampal sclerosis. The pathological substrate underlying epilepsy in patients who have the dual pathology of MTS and migrational disorder, remains controversial.

One possible explanation is that this minor migrational abnormality is the underlying defect that renders TLE patients vulnerable to otherwise benign insults such as febrile seizures or head trauma during a critical developmental period during childhood. Indeed, one study described a bilaminar pattern of the hippocampus in patients with hippocampal sclerosis, suggesting that such a migrational abnormality could be the underlying defect (46). If such a benign insult occurs during a critical period, most likely before age 5, it could possibly render individuals with minor migrational disorders susceptible to recurrent seizures. In TLE patients, epileptic seizures appear years after the initial insult; this latent period may be required for the plastic changes that render the brain hyperexcitable and subsequently epileptic to occur.

The human epilepsy syndromes inherited as a simple Mendelian trait can be classified into three different categories: Idiopathic generalized epilepsy syndromes, idiopathic partial epilepsy syndromes, and single-gene disorders with symptomatic epilepsy as a major feature.

a—idiopathic generalized epilepsy syndromes: The three epilepsy syndromes in this category include the two forms of benign familial neonatal convulsions that have been mapped to specific chromosomal sites on 20q (BFNC1) and 8q (BFNC2) and juvenile myoclonic epilepsy (EJM1), which has been mapped to chromosome 6 in the HLA region, although one study has found evidence against this localization.

juvenile myoclonus epilepsy (Herpin-Janz syndrome) 6p: This is a common idiopathic generalized epilepsy characterized by mild myoclonic seizures. Onset is usually between 13 to 15 years of age. Seizures mainly affect the upper extremities and most commonly occur during awakening. The majority of these patients also suffer from generalized tonic-clonic seizures. This disease is not progressive and usually responds well to treatment. Even though there is substantial evidence of a genetic component to this disorder, the mode of inheritance is uncertain and different studies have suggested autosomal dominant, autosomal recessive, two-locus and polygenic inheritance. Linkage was first reported to the HLA region of chromosome 6p assuming an autosomal dominant inheritance with 90% penetrance (39). These results were later confirmed by Weissbecker (128) and by Durner (27). However, a more recent study of 25 families excluded this region (130). The conflicting results of these studies either reflect genetic heterogeneity or suggest that the phenotypic assignments of one of the studies were wrong.

benign neonatal epilepsy EBN1-20q (CHRNA4), EBN2-8q: This rare form of epilepsy is characterized by frequent generalized or focal and apneic seizures. The onset is between two days and three months after birth. The infants are otherwise healthy; development proceeds normally and the outcome is usually good. The inheritance of this disorder is autosomal dominant and a responsible gene has been mapped to the long arm of chromosome 20 by linkage analysis in a large family with 19 affected members (62). Some additional families confirmed this localization whereas others excluded chromosome 20q and showed linkage to 8q (63, 67). Recently, the alpha-4 subunit of the neuronal nicotinic acetylcholine receptor (CHRNA4) has been localized to 20q (111) and mutations in this gene have been identified in one of the families that has linkage to 20q (10). Mutations in CHRNA4, therefore, are responsible for benign neonatal epilepsy. This represents the first example of identification of the mutation underlying an idiopathic human epilepsy syndrome.

b—idiopathic partial epilepsy syndromes: Most partial or focal epilepsy syndromes in which seizure activity originates from a specific brain region are assumed to be nongenetic. However, relatives of probands with partial seizures have an increased risk of epilepsy compared to the general population; this suggests a possible genetic contribution to these syndromes.

nocturnal frontal lobe epilepsy 20q (AD-NFLE): Autosomal dominant nocturnal frontal lobe epilepsy (ADNFLE) was recently described in five families (94, 95). This syndrome is characterized by the focal frontal lobe origin of seizures and their almost exclusive occurrence during sleep. Another characteristic of the syndrome is the variable expression in the same family with some individuals suffering from mild seizures diagnosed as nightmares or other sleep disorders (94, 95). The disease locus has been localized to chromosome 20q13.2 by study of a large Australian family with 27 affected

individuals spanning 6 generations (84). In some families, the gene for benign familial neonatal convulsions (BFNC, EBN1 locus) localizes to this same region (63, 67). A normal low voltage variant of the human electroencephalogram (EEGV1) also maps to this same region; all three disorders give zero recombination fractions with the same marker: D20S19 (110, 111). As mentioned above, neuronal nicotinic acetylcholine receptor alpha-4 subunit (CHRNA4) maps to the same area and a stop codon affecting this gene has been shown to co-segregate in individuals affected with benign familial neonatal convulsions (10). It remains to be seen whether mutations of the same gene are responsible for nocturnal frontal lobe epilepsy or EEGV1.

partial epilepsy with auditory symptoms 10q: Ottman and colleagues (80) have recently described a family with 17 individuals affected by seizures. They identified 11 individuals over 3 generations as suffering from a similar form of non-specific auditory partial epilepsy after excluding three individuals who had acute seizures and another three individuals who had epilepsy due to other CNS diseases. They found linkage to markers located on the long arm of chromosome 10 (10q22-q24). They have localized the disease to a 10 centimorgan region (approximately 10 million base pairs in the human genome). In this region there are more than 50 known genes, including genes for two neurotransmitter receptors (beta-1 and alpha-2A adrenergic receptors) and genes involved in the metabolism of glutamate or calcium/calmodulin-dependent protein kinase gamma. Further investigation is required to see if any of these genes or another, yet unknown gene, is responsible for the susceptibility to seizures in this family.

c—Single Gene Disorders with Epilepsy as a Major Feature

i—Cerebral cavernous malformation (CCM): Cerebral cavernous malformation (CCM) is a disease of the brain characterized by hemorrhagic lesions comprised of cavernous vascular spaces without intervening brain parenchyma. The thin-walled cavernous channels contain blood at various stages of organization, are lined by endothelium, and lack mature vessel wall elements. CCM is a relatively common disease; lesions are found by magnetic resonance imaging (MRI) of the brain or at autopsy in approximately 0.5% of the population; symptomatic disease is considerably less common. Symptomatic subjects typically present between ages 20 and 40 years with seizure, brain hemorrhage, focal neurological deficits or headaches. Diagnosis is usually made by MRI of the brain which reveals a characteristic image of heterogeneous signal intensity surrounded by a dark ring attributable to hemosiderin deposition.

As the majority of CCM lesions are supratentorial and lobar, it is not surprising that seizures are the most common presenting symptom, occurring in 38% to 100% of cases (3). All seizure types have been observed, including simple seizures in 27% to 31% of cases, complex partial seizures in 6% to 45% of cases, and generalized seizures in 27% to 63%. Furthermore, CCM accounts for many cases of medically intractable epilepsy; in one series of 27 vascular malformations associated with intractable epilepsy, 75% were CCM (3).

The pathophysiology of seizures in CCM is postulated to involve irritation and compression secondary to mass effect, multiple local hemorrhages with exposure of surrounding brain to blood breakdown products, particularly iron, and the subsequent local gliotic reaction. Calcification, temporal lobe location, and extensive hemosiderin deposition are frequently associated with a clinical presentation of epilepsy.

Genetic predisposition is important in the pathophysiology of CCM, and many familial cases of CCM have been reported in the literature. By using linkage analysis, a gene responsible for CCM (CCM1) has recently been localized to chromosome 7q (25, 42). Familial CCM is particularly prevalent among Hispanic Americans of Mexican descent, with over 50% of affected patients having one or more relatives with CCM (88). By using linkage disequilibrium, this increased prevalence among Hispanic Americans has been ascribed to a founder effect; virtually all familial and apparently sporadic cases have inherited the identical mutation from a common ancestor, proving that among Hispanic Americans the disease is genetic in close to 100% of cases (43). The apparently sporadic cases have been explained by incomplete penetrance of the symptomatic disease (43).

The CCM-1 gene has been mapped to a narrow interval on 7q (43, 51) and further work is currently underway to clone the CCM-1 gene that is responsible for cavernous malformations.

ii—Neuronal migration disorders: Any event, whether congenital or acquired, that interferes with developmental processes such as neurogenesis, neural migration or differentiation and synapse formation, can result in seizure disorders. Neuronal migration disorders such as agyria (lissencephaly), macrogyria (pachygyria), polymicrogyria, schizencephaly and other heterotopias of the gray matter (9) involve developmental structural anomalies such as cytoarchitectonic disorganization with aberrant columnar and laminar neuronal arrangement.

Two genes involved in human migrational disorders, TCS2, responsible for most of the tuberous sclerosis cases and LIS1, the gene for lissencephaly of the Miller-Dieker type, have been cloned and the gene for another syndrome, periventricular heterotopia, has been localized to chromosome X (28, 30, 87). Tuberous sclerosis is characterized by development of hamartomas in many tissues and organs. Clinical presentation varies according to organ involvement but includes seizures in cases with brain involvement. The TCS2 gene responsible for tuberous sclerosis resides on chromosome 16 and has recently been cloned. It encodes tuberin, a protein homologous to the GTPase activating protein, GAP3, which is expressed in both the developing and the adult cortex (30).

Lissencephaly is a neuronal migration disorder characterized by lack of the sulci-gyri pattern (agyria-pachygyria) of normal cerebral cortex. Isolated forms of the disorder and those associated with the dysmorphic facial features of Miller-Dieker syndrome have been described. A gene located on chromosome 17p13.3, LIS1 is responsible for more than 90% of Miller-Dieker syndrome and about 15% of the isolated cases of lissencephaly (59). Recently, LIS1 gene has been cloned and shown to encode a protein with significant homology to β-subunits of the heterotrimeric G proteins (87). LIS-1 gene is the human homolog of the 45K subunit of intracellular platelet-activating factor (PAF) acetylhydrolase, which is involved in inactivating PAF. Thus, the LIS-1 gene is involved in a signaling pathway activated by the platelet activating factor (45). Perhaps PAF is involved in the signaling pathway that initiates or continues migration or, in the ability of neurons to respond to this signal and abnormalities in the response to PAF may underlie the migrational disorder seen in lissencephaly. Elucidation of the function of LIS2 and TSC2 gene products will likely reveal previously unidentified signaling pathways operant in the developing and adult brain.

iii—progressive myoclonus epilepsy syndromes: The progressive myoclonus epilepsies are a heterogeneous group of disorders that include at least five diseases: Unverricht-Lundborg type (EPM1), Lafora's disease, myoclonic epilepsy with ragged red fibers (MERRF), neuronal ceroid lipofuscinosis and sialidosis. All of these diseases are characterized by myoclonus, epileptic seizures and progressive neurological deterioration including ataxia and dementia.

Unverricht-Lundborg type 1 (EPM1) myoclonic epilepsy displays autosomal recessive inheritance, and is mainly seen in Finland and in the Mediterranean region (11, 66, 123). Clinically, the onset is usually between 8 and 15 years of age. The course of the disease is progressive and mild mental deterioration, ataxia and dysarthria may evolve. The locus responsible for this disease, EPM1, has been mapped to chromosome 21q22.3 region (61). Recently, a direct cDNA selection technique revealed a gene with partial homologies to a group of transmembrane proteins that includes sodium channel proteins. Initially this gene was thought to be a good candidate for the disease but further work revealed very surprising results. The gene coding cystatin B, a member of a superfamily of cysteine protease inhibitors whose function is to inactivate proteases that leak out of the lysosome, was found to be in the region (82). Levels of mRNA encoding this gene are significantly decreased in affected subjects either due to a splice site mutation or a stop codon mutation. This strongly suggests that mutations in cystatin B are responsible for EPM1 (82). These findings are unexpected as cystatin B is a component in no known biological pathway involved in epilepsy. Cystatin B is ubiquitously expressed in every cell in the body. It is completely unclear how mutations in this gene affect only the brain and cause an epileptic syndrome. Mutations in another member of this family of protease inhibitors, cystatin C, is responsible for cerebral amyloid angiopathy which is clinically and pathologically dissimilar to EPM1 (1, 38). This finding opens a new

chapter in epilepsy research and it remains to be seen whether mutations in this family of genes will prove to be responsible for any other progressive myoclonic epilepsy syndrome.

The relevance of mitochondrial disorders to epilepsy was demonstrated by the discovery of a point mutation in mitochondrial tRNA for lysine (tRNAlys) which causes myoclonic epilepsy and ragged red fiber disease (MERRF) (101, 125). Since mitochondrial DNA is solely maternally transmitted, diseases like MERRF are inherited only from the mother. The clinical expression of MERRF varies widely among individuals and depends on the percentage of mutated mitochondrial DNA and the age of the patient. The mitochondrial DNA damage is manifested in dysfunction of the oxidative phosphorylation system. The pathophysiology underling MERRF is not completely understood; however, the mutation in tRNAlys is thought to interfere with the synthesis of higher molecular weight peptides and result in a combined complex I and IV defect in oxidative phosphorylation (125). Oxidative phosphorylation is quantified by measuring the anaerobic threshold in affected individuals as an indicator of the skeletal muscle oxidative work capacity. This index correlates very well with the clinical severity of the disease. However, the mechanism by which this defect in oxidative phosphorylation engenders myoclonic epilepsy is not yet known.

Ceroid lipofuscinosis is a heterogeneous group of inherited neurodegenerative syndromes characterized by the accumulation of a lipopigment in neural tissues. The underlying enzymatic defect is not known. Three subtypes have been described: infantile (Haltia-Santavuori disease, locus CLN1), late infantile (Jansky-Bielschowsky disease, locus CLN2), and juvenile (Spielmeyr-Sjogren-Bogt or Batten disease, locus CLN3).

The infantile type, which mainly affects the Finnish population, is characterized by onset at 8 to 20 months of age, hypotonia, seizures, visual failure, ataxia and choreoathetosis. The EEG is usually iso-electric by three years of age. Linkage to chromosome 1 and finer mapping was achieved by using linkage disequilibrium in 26 Finnish families. Work is currently under way to clone the gene.

The juvenile type is characterized by visual failure followed by progressive intellectual deterioration and seizures. Onset is usually between 6 to 10 years of age. Linkage analysis in 26 families revealed that the CLN3 locus is on chromosome 16 (35). Further analysis localized the gene to a 1 cM region on chromosome 16p12.

The late infantile type is characterized by progressive dementia and seizures beginning by age 2 to 4 years. CLN1 and CLN3 regions on chromosome 1p and 16p have been excluded as the location and linkage to any other chromosome has not yet been reported.

In Lafora's disease, clinical onset is usually around 15 years of age. Grand mal seizures and/or myoclonus are followed by rapid and severe mental deterioration. Survival is usually less than 10 years after the onset. Through linkage studies, the locus responsible for the Unverricht-Lundborg type on chromosome 21q22.3 was excluded (60). Later, Serratosa and others (98) by using linkage analysis in 9 families and homozygosity mapping in 4 consanguineous families assigned the gene responsible for Lafora's disease to 6q23-q25, a 2.5-cM region surrounding D6S403. The gene is yet unknown.

Sialidosis is a lysosomal storage disease that usually presents with progressive debilitating myoclonic seizures in childhood. Affected individuals usually have normal intelligence. The gene has been localized to chromosome 6p21.3 (65, 79).

iv—Northern epilepsy syndrome 8p: An autosomal recessive form of progressive epilepsy with mental retardation known as Northern epilepsy has been reported among the population of northern Finland. Patients with this syndrome are normal at birth and develop normally. Seizures begin at the age of 5 to 10 years (mean, 6.7 years) (generalized tonic-clonic). The frequency of seizures increases until puberty, and then decreases, such that after 35 years of age, many patients are seizure-free. Tahvanainen and others (117) assigned the EPMR gene to the telomeric region of 8p (8pter-p22 region) by linkage analysis. Further analysis of haplotypes in this interval showed that a single founding mutation affected almost all of the diseased individuals. The responsible gene remains unknown.

CONCLUSIONS

Recent years have witnessed rapid progress in understanding molecular mechanisms under-

lying different epilepsy syndromes. Approaches in very diverse fields, from cellular electrophysiology to molecular genetics, have yielded complementary and invaluable information regarding the pathophysiology of the different epilepsy syndromes. This emphasizes that a variety of epileptogenic substrates may be created by the combination of genetic predisposition, acquired injury and developmental abnormalities interacting with specific CNS regions that are prone to excitability. Knowledge regarding certain subtypes of the symptomatic epilepsies has reached the critical point at which basic mechanisms will soon be better understood. Molecular genetic work in animals has already identified genes that are responsible for certain epileptic syndromes. The human homologs of most of these genes are known and work is currently underway to elucidate the role, if any, of these genes in human epileptogenic pathology. Together, these approaches should lead to novel gene therapies or more rational pharmacological therapies based on pathophysiological mechanisms. This approach may not only cure but also prevent different epileptic syndromes.

REFERENCES

1. Abrahamson, M., Islam, M. Q., Szpirer, J., Szpirer, C., and Levan, G. The human cystatin C gene (CST3), mutated in hereditary cystatin C amyloid angiopathy, is located on chromosome 20. Hum. Genet. *82:*223–226, 1989.
2. Angel, P., Imagawa, M., Chiu, R., Stein, B., Imbra, R. J., Rahmsdorf, H. J., Jonat, C., Herrlich, P., and Karin, M. Phorbol ester-inducible genes contain a common cis element recognized by a TPA-modulated trans-acting factor. Cell *49:*729–739, 1987.
3. Awad, I., and Robinson, J. Cavernous malformation and epilepsy, in Awad, I. A., Barrow, D. L. (eds.): *Cavernous Malformations.* Park Ridge, AANS, 1993:49–63.
4. Babb, T. L., Lieb, J. P., Brown, W. J., Pretorius, J., and Crandall, P. H. Distribution of Pyramidal Cell Density and Hyperexcitability in the Epileptic Human Hippocampal Formation. Epilepsia *25:*721–728, 1984.
5. Babb, T. L., Brown, W. J., Pretorius, J., Davenport, C., Lieb, J. P., and Crandall, P. H. Temporal lobe volumetric cell densities in temporal lobe epilepsy. Epilepsia *25:*729–740, 1984.
6. Babb, T. L., Pretorius, J. K., Kupfer, W. R., and Crandall, P. H. Glutamate decarboxylase-immunoreactive neurons are preserved in human epileptic hippocampus. J. Neurosci. *9:*2562–2574, 1989.
7. Babb, T. L., Pretorius, J. K., Kupfer, W. R., Mathern, G. W., Crandall, P. H., and Levesque, M. F. Aberrant synaptic reorganization in human epileptic hip-

pocampus: evidence for feedforward excitation. Dendron *1:*7–25, 1992.

8. Bading, H., Ginty, D. D., and Greenberg, M. E. Regulation of gene expression in hippocampal neurons by distinct calcium signaling pathways. Science *260:*181–186, 1993.

9. Barth, P. Disorders of neuronal migration. Can. J. Neurol. Sci. *14:*1–16, 1987.

10. Beck, C., Moulard, B., Steinlein, O., Guipponi, M., Vallee, L., Montpied, P., Baldy-Moulnier, M., and Malafosse, A. A nonsense mutation in the alpha-4 subunit of the nicotinic acetylcholine receptor (CHRNA4) cosegregates with 20q-linked benign neonatal familial convulsions (EBN1). Neurobiol. Dis. *1:*95–99, 1994.

11. Berkovic, S. F., Andermann, F., Carpenter, S., and Wolfe, L. S. Progressive myoclonus epilepsies: specific causes and diagnosis. N. Eng. J. Med. *315:* 296–305, 1986.

12. Bloom, F. E., and Engel, J., Jr. Aberrant genetic expression and opportunities for epilepsy research in Engel, J., Jr., Wasterlain, C., Cavalheiro, E. A., Heinemann, U., Avanzini, G. (eds): *Molecular Neurobiology of Epilepsy (Epilepsy Res. Suppl. 9).* Elsevier Science Publishers, 1992.

13. Bohmann, D., Bos, T. J., Admon, A., Nishimura, T., Vogt, P. K., and Tjian, R. Human proto-oncogene c-jun encodes a DNA binding protein with structural and functional properties of transcription factor AP-1. Science *238:*1386–1392, 1987.

14. Bouchet, C., and Cazauvielh, C. De l'epilepsie sideree dans ses rapports avec l'alienation mentale. Recherche sur la nature et le siege de ces deux maladies; memoire qui a remporte le prix au concours etabli par M. Esquirol. Arch. Gen. Med. *9:*510–542, 1825.

15. Brusa, R., Zimmermann, F., Koh, D. S., Feldmeyer, D., Gass, P., Seeburg, P. H., and Sprengel, R. Early-onset epilepsy and postnatal lethality associated with an editing-deficient GluR-B allele in mice. Science *270:*1677–1680, 1995.

16. Bruton, C. J. *The neuropathology of temporal lobe epilepsy.* New York, Oxford UP, 1988.

17. Butler, L. S., Silva, A. J., Abeliovich, A., Watanabe, Y., Tonegawa, S., and McNamara, J. O. Limbic epilepsy in transgenic mice carrying a Ca2+/calmodulin-dependent kinase II alpha-subunit mutation. Proc. Nat. Acad. Sci. *92:*6852–6855, 1995.

18. Choi, D. W., and Rothman, S. M. The role of glutamate neurotoxicity in hypoxic-ischemic neuronal death. Annu. Rev. Neurosci. *13:*171–182, 1990.

19. Cole, A. J., Saffen, D. W., Baraban, J. M., and Worley, P. F. Rapid increase of an immediate early gene messenger RNA in hippocampal neurons by synaptic NMDA receptor activation. Nature *340:*474–476, 1989.

20. Commission on Classification and Terminology of the International League Against Epilepsy. Proposal for revised classification of epilepsies and epilepsy syndromes. Epilepsia *30:*389–399, 1989.

21. Curran, T., and Morgan, J. I. Memories of fos. Bioessays *7:*255–258, 1987.

22. Delgado-Escueta, A. V., Serratosa, J. M., Liu, A., Weissbecker, K., Medina, M. T., Gee, M., Treiman, L. J., and Sparkes, R. S. Progress in mapping human epilepsy genes. Epilepsia *35* Suppl. 1:S29–40, 1994.

23. Dragunow, M., and Robertson, H. A. Kindling stimulation induces c-fos protein(s) in granule cells of the rat dentate gyrus. Nature *329:*441–442, 1987.

24. Dragunow, M., and Robertson, H. A. Seizure-inducible c-fos protein(s) in mammalian neurons. Trends Pharmacol. Sci. *9:*5–6, 1988.

25. Dubovsky, J., Zabramski, J. M., Kurth, J., Spetzler, R. F., Rich, S. S., Orr, H. T., and Weber, J. L. A gene responsible for cavernous malformations of the brain maps to chromosome 7q. Hum. Mol. Genet. *4:*453–458, 1995.

26. During, M. J., and Spencer, D. D. Extracellular hippocampal glutamate and spontaneous seizure in the conscious human brain. Lancet *341:*1607–1610, 1993.

27. Durner, M., Sander, T., Greenberg, D. A., Johnson, K., Beck-Mannagetta, G., and Janz, D. Localization of idiopathic generalized epilepsy on chromosome 6p infamilies of juvenile myoclonic epilepsy patients. Neurol. *41:*1651–1655, 1991.

28. Eksioglu, Y. Z., Scheffer, I. E., Cardenas, P., Knoll, J., DiMario, F., Ramsby, G., Berg, M., Kamuro, K., Berkovic, S. F., Duyk, G. M., Parisi, J., Huttenlocher, P. R., and Walsh, C. A. Periventricular heterotopia: an X-linked dominant epilepsy locus causing aberrant cerebral cortical development. Neuron. *16:*77–87, 1996.

29. Engel, J., Jr., Brown, W. J., Kuhl, D. E., Phelps, M. E., Mazziotta, J. C., and Crandall, P. H. Pathological findings underlying focal temporal lobe hypometabolism in partial epilepsy. Ann. Neurol. *12:* 518–28, 1982.

30. The European Chromosome 16 Tuberous Sclerosis Consortium: Identification and characterization of the tuberous sclerosis gene on chromosome 16. Cell *5:*1305–1315, 1993.

31. Falconer, M. A., and Taylor, D. C. Surgical treatment of drug-resistant epilepsy due to mesial temporal sclerosis. Etiology and significance. Arch. Neurol. *19:*353–361, 1968.

32. Farrell, M. A., DeRosa, M. J., Curran, J. G., Lenard Secor, D., Cornford, M. E., Comair, Y. G., Peacock, W. J., Shields, W. D., and Vinters, H. V. Neuropathologic findings in cortical resections (including hemispherectomies) performed for the treatment of intractable childhood epilepsy. Acta Neuropath. *83:*246–259, 1992.

33. Gall, C. M. Localization and seizure-induced alterations of opioid peptides and CCK in the hippocampus. NIDA Research Monograph. *82:*12–32, 1988.

34. Gall, C. M., and Isackson, P. J. Limbic seizures increase neuronal production of messenger RNA for nerve growth factor. Science *245:*758–761, 1989.

35. Gardiner, M., Sandford, A., Deadman, M., Poulton, J., Cookson, W., Reeders, S., Jokiaho, I., Peltonen, L., Eiberg, H., and Julier, C. Batten disease (Spielmeyer-Vogt disease, juvenile onset neuronal ceroid-lipofuscinosis) gene (CLN3) maps to human chromosome 16. Genomics *8:*387–390, 1990.

36. Garey, C. E., Schwarzman, A. I., Rise, M. I., and Seyfried, T. N. Ceruloplasmin gene defect associ-

ated with epilepsy in EL mice. Nat. Genet. *6:*426–431, 1994.

37. Gastaut, H., Toga, M., Roger, J., and Gibson, W. C. A correlation of clinical, electroencephalographic and anatomical findings in nine autopsied cases of "temporal lobe epilepsy." Epilepsia *1:*56–59, 1959.

38. Ghiso, J., Jensson, O., and Frangione, B. Amyloid fibrils in hereditary cerebral hemorrhage with amyloidosis of Icelandic type is a variant of gamma-trace basic protein (cystatin C). Proc. Nat. Acad. Sci. *83:*2974–2978, 1986.

39. Greenberg, D. A., Delgado-Escueta, A. V., Widelitz, H., Sparkes, R. S., Treiman, L., Maldonado, H. M., Park, M. S., and Terasaki, P. I. Juvenile myoclonic epilepsy (JME) may be linked to the BF and HLA loci on human chromosome 6. Am. J. Med. Genet. *31:*185–192, 1988.

40. Greenberg, M. E., and Ziff, E. B. Stimulation of 3T3 cells induces transcription of the c-fos proto-oncogene. Nature *311:*433–438, 1984.

41. Günel, M., Thomas, P. G., Cornell-Bell, A. H., Brines, M. L., Spencer, D. D., and de Lanerolle, N. C. Human glia cultured from epileptogenic foci demonstrate increased basal and glutamate induced calcium fluxes. Epilepsia *1991:*32S3:66.

42. Günel, M., Awad, I. A., Anson, J., and Lifton, R. P. Mapping a gene causing cerebral cavernous malformation to 7q11.2-q21. Proc. Nat. Acad. Sci. *92:*6620–6624, 1995.

43. Günel, M., Awad, I. A., Finberg, K., Anson, J., Steinberg, G. K., Batjer, H. H., Giannotta, S. L., Nelson-Williams, C., and Lifton, R. P. A founder mutation as a cause of cerebral cavernous malformation in Hispanic Americans. N. Engl. J. Med. *334:*946–951, 1996.

44. Hardiman, O., Burke, T., Phillips, J., Murphy, S., O'Moore, B., Staunton, H., and Farrell, M. A. Microdysgenesis in resected temporal neocortex: incidence and clinical significance in focal epilepsy. Neurology *38:*1041–1047, 1988.

45. Hattori, M., Adachi, H., Tsujimoto, M., Arai, H., and Inoue, K. Miller-Dieker lissencephaly gene encodes a subunit of brain platelet-activating factor acetylhydrolase. Nature *370:*216–218, 1994.

46. Hauser, W. A., and Hesdorffer, D. C. *Epilepsy: frequency, causes and consequences.* New York, Demos, 1990.

47. Hollmann, M., Hartley, M., and Heinemann, S. Ca2+ permeability of KA-AMPA-gated glutamate receptor channels depends on subunit composition. Science *252:*851–853, 1991.

48. Hollmann, M., and Heinemann, S. Cloned glutamate receptors. Annu. Rev. Neurosci. *17:*31–108, 1994.

49. Hosford, D. A., Clark, S., Cao, Z., Wilson, W. A., Jr., Lin, F. H., Morrisett, R. A., and Huin, A. The role of GABA$_B$ receptor activation in absence seizures of lethargic (lh/lh) mice. Science *257:*398–401, 1992.

50. Ishida, N., Kasamo, K., Nakamoto, Y., and Suzuki, J. Epileptic seizure of El mouse initiates at the parietal cortex: depth EEG observation in freely moving condition using buffer amplifier. Brain Res. *608:*52–57, 1993.

51. Johnson, E. W., Iyer, L. M., Rich, S. S., Orr, H. T., Gil-Nagel, A., Kurth, J. H., Zabramski, J. M., Marchuk, D. A., Weissenbach, J., Clericuzio, C. L., Davis, L. E., Hart, B. L., Gusella, J. F., Kosofsky, B. E., Louis, D. N., Morrison, L. A., Green, E. D., and Weber, J. L. Refined localization of the cerebral cavernous malformation gene (CCM1) to a 4 cM interval of chromosome 7q contained in a well-defined YAC contig. Genome Res. *5:*368–380, 1995.

52. Johnson, W. G., Kugler, S. L., Stenroos, E. S., Meulener, M. C., Rangwalla, I., Johnson, T. W., and Mandelbaum, D. E. Pedigree analysis in families with febrile seizures. Am. J. Med. Genet. *61:*345–352, 1996.

53. Kelly, K., Cochran, B. H., Stiles, C. D., and Leder, P. Cell-specific regulation of the c-myc gene by lymphocyte mitogens and platelet-derived growth factor. Cell *35:*603–610, 1983.

54. Kim, J. H., Guimaraes, P. O., Shen, M. Y., Masukawa, L. M., and Spencer, D. D. Hippocampal neuronal density in temporal lobe epilepsy with and without gliomas. Acta Neuropathol. *80:*41–45, 1990.

55. Knowles, W. D., Awad, I. A., and Nayel, M. H. Differences of in vitro electrophysiology of hippocampal neurons from epileptic patients with mesiotemporal sclerosis versus structural lesions. Epilepsia *33:*601–609, 1992.

56. Kuks, J. B., Cook, M. J., Fish, D. R., Stevens, J. M., and Shorvon, S. D. Hippocampal sclerosis in epilepsy and childhood febrile seizures. Lancet *342:*1391–1394, 1993.

57. de Lanerolle, N. C., Kim, J. H., Robbins, R. J., and Spencer, D. D. Hippocampal interneuron loss and plasticity in human temporal lobe epilepsy. Brain Res. *495:*387–395, 1989.

58. de Lanerolle, N. C., Brines, M. L., Williamson, A., Kim, J. H., and Spencer, D. D. Neurotransmitters and their receptors in human temporal lobe epilepsy in Ribak, C., Gall, C., Mody, I. (eds.): *The Dentate Gyrus and its Role in Seizures*, Epilepsy Res. Suppl. 7, New York, Elsevier, 1992.

59. Ledbetter, S. A., Kuwano, A., Dobyns, W. B., and Ledbetter, D. H. Microdeletions of chromosome 17p13 as a cause of isolated lissencephaly. Am. J. Med. Genet. *50:*182–189, 1992.

60. Lehesjoki, A.-E., Koskiniemi, M., Pandolfo, M., Antonelli, A., Kyllerman, M., Wahlstrom, J., Nergardh, A., Burmeister, M., Sistonen, P., Norio, R., and de la Chapelle, A. Linkage studies in progressive myoclonus epilepsy: Unverricht-Lundborg and Lafora's diseases. Neurology *42:*1545–1550, 1992.

61. Lehesjoki, A.-E., Koskiniemi, M., Norio, R., Tirrito, S., Sistonen, P., Lander, E., and de la Chapelle, A. Localization of the EPM1 gene for progressive myoclonus epilepsy on chromosome 21: linkage disequilibrium allows high resolution mapping. Hum. Molec. Genet. *2:*1229–1234, 1993.

62. Leppert, M., Anderson, V. E., Quattlebaum, T., Stauffer, D., O'Connell, P., Nakamura, Y., Lalouel, J.-M., and White, R. Benign familial neonatal convulsions linked to genetic markers on chromosome 20. Nature *337:*647–648, 1989.

63. Lewis, T. B., Leach, R. J., Ward, K., O'Connell, P., and Ryan, S. G. Genetic heterogeneity in benign familial neonatal convulsions: identification of a new locus on chromosome 8q. Am. J. Hum. Genet. *53:*670–675, 1993.

64. Lindenberg, R. Compression of brain arteries as pathogenetic factor for tissue necroses and their areas of predilection. J. Neuropath. Exp. Neurol. *14:*223, 1955.

65. Lowden, J. A., and O'Brien, J. S. Sialidosis: a review of human neuraminidase deficiency. Am. J. Hum. Genet. *31:*1–18, 1979.

66. Lundborg, H. B. *Medizinisch-biologische Familienforschungen innerhalb eines 2232 koepfigen Bauerngeschlechtes in Schweden.* Jena, Fischer (pub), 1913.

67. Malafosse, A., Leboyer, M., Dulac, O., Navelet, Y., Plouin, P., Beck, C., Laklou, H., Mouchnino, G., Grandscene, P., Vallee, L., Guilloud-Bataille, M., Samolyk, D., Baldy-Moulinier, M., Feingold, J., and Mallet, J. Confirmation of linkage of benign familial neonatal convulsions to D20S19 and D20S20. Hum. Genet. *89:*54–58, 1992.

68. Masukawa, L. M., Higashima, M., Kim, J. H., and Spencer, D. D. Epileptiform discharges evoked in hippocampal brain slices from epileptic patients. Brain Res. *493:*168–174, 1989.

69. McNamara, J. O. Cellular and molecular basis of epilepsy. J. Neuroscience *14:*3413–3425, 1994.

70. Meda, L., Cassatella, M. A., Szendrei, G. I., Otvos, L., Baron, P., Villalba, M., Ferrari, D., and Rossi, F. Activation of microglial cells by beta-amyloid protein and interferon-gamma. Nature *374:*647–650, 1995.

71. Meencke, H. J., and Janz, D. Neuropathological findings in primary generalized epilepsy: a study of eight cases. Epilepsia *25:*8–21, 1984.

72. Morgan, J. I., Cohen, D. R., Hempstead, J. L., and Curran, T. Mapping patterns of c-fos expression in the central nervous system after seizure. Science *237:*192–197, 1987.

73. Morris, B. J., Moneta, M. E., ten Bruggencate, G., and Hollt, V. Levels of prodynorphin mRNA in rat dentate gyrus are decreased during hippocampal kindling. Neurosci. Letters *80:*298–302, 1987.

74. Morris, B. J., Feasey, K. J., ten Bruggencate, G., Herz, A., and Hollt, V. Electrical stimulation in vivo increases the expression of proenkephalin mRNA and decreases the expression of prodynorphin mRNA in rat hippocampal granule cells. Proc. Nat. Acad. Sci. *85:*3226–3230, 1988.

75. Nadler, J. V., Perry, B. W., and Cotman, C. W. Selective reinnervation of hippocampal area CA1 and the fascia dentata after destruction of CA3-CA4 afferents with kainic acid. Brain Res. *182:*1–9, 1980.

76. Noebels, J. L. Mutational analysis of inherited epilepsies. Adv. Neurol. *44:*97–113, 1986.

77. Olney, J. W. *Excitotoxins, an overview.* In: Excitotoxins (Fuxe, K., Roberts, P., Schwarcz, R., eds.), pp. 82–96. New York: Plenum, 1984.

78. Olney, J. W. Excitatory transmitters and epilepsy-related brain damage. Int. Rev. Neurobiol. *27:*337–362, 1985.

79. Oohira, T., Yoshida, M. C., and Matsuda, I. Additional evidence for the location of the alpha-neuraminidase gene on chromosome 6. Jpn. J. Hum. Genet. *31:*309–310, 1986.

80. Ottman, R., Risch, N., Hauser, W. A., Pedley, T. A., Lee, J. H., Barker-Cummings, C., Lustenberger, A., Nagle, K. J., Lee, K. S., Scheuer, M. L., Neystat, M., Susser, M., and Wilhelmsen, K. C. Localization of a gene for partial epilepsy to chromosome 10q. Nat. Genet. *10:*56–60, 1995.

81. Patil, N., Cox, D. R., Bhat, D., Faham, M., Myers, R. M., and Peterson, A. S. A potassium channel mutation in weaver mice implicates membrane excitability in granule cell differentiation. Nat. Genet. *11:*126–129, 1995.

82. Pennacchio, L. A., Lehesjoki, A.-E., Stone, N. E., Willour, V. L., Virtaneva, K., Miao, J., D'Amato, E., Ramirez, L., Faham, M., Koskiniemi, M., Warrington, J. A., Norio, R., de la Chapelle, A., Cox, D. R., and Myers, R. M. Mutations in the gene encoding cystatin B in progressive myoclonus epilepsy (EPM1). Science *271:*1731–1734, 1996.

83. Penfield, W., and Jackson, H. H. *Epilepsy and functional anatomy of the human brain.* Boston, Little Brown & Co, 1954.

84. Phillips, H. A., Scheffer, I. E., Berkovic, S. F., Hollway, G. E., Sutherland, G. R., and Mulley, J. C. Localization of a gene for autosomal dominant nocturnal frontal lobe epilepsy to chromosome 20q13.2. Nat. Genet. *10:*117–118, 1995.

85. Pia, H. W. Die Schadigungen des Hirnstammes bei den raumfordernden Prozessen des Gehirns. Acta Neurochir. Supp. IV, Springer, Vienna, 1957.

86. Qian, Z., Gilbert, M. E., Colicos, M. A., Kandel, E. R., and Kuhl, D. Tissue-plasminogen activator is induced as an immediate-early gene during seizure, kindling and long-term potentiation. Nature *361:*453–457, 1993.

87. Reiner, O., Carrozzo, R., Shen, Y., Wehnert, M., Faustinella, F., Dobyns, W. B., Caskey, C. T., and Ledbetter, D. H. Isolation of a Miller-Dieker lissencephaly gene containing G protein beta-subunit-like repeats. Nature *364:*717–721, 1993.

88. Rigamonti, D., Hadley, M. N., Drayer, B. P., Johnson, P. C., Hoenig-Rigamonti, K., Knight, J. T., and Spetzler, R. F. Cerebral cavernous malformations. N. Engl. J. Med. *319:*343–347, 1988.

89. Rise, M. L., Frankel, W. N., Coffin, J. M., and Seyfried, T. N. Genes for epilepsy mapped in the mouse. Science *253:*669–73, 1991.

90. Rosahl, T. W., Spillane, D., Missler, M., Herz, J., Selig, D. K., Wolff, J. R., Hammer, R. E., Malenka, R. C., and Sudhof, T. C. Essential functions of synapsins I and II in synaptic vesicle regulation. Nature *375:*488–493, 1995.

91. Saffen, D. W., Cole, A. J., Worley, P. F., Christy, B. A., Ryder, K., and Baraban, J. M. Convulsant-induced increase in transcription factor messenger RNAs in rat brain. Proc. Nat. Acad. Sci. *85:*7795–7799, 1988.

92. Sagar, H. J., and Oxbury, J. M. Hippocampal neuron loss in temporal lobe epilepsy: correlation with early childhood convulsions. Ann. Neurol. *22:*334–340, 1987.

93. Sagar, S. M., Sharp, F. R., and Curran, T. Expression

of c-fos protein in brain: metabolic mapping at the cellular level. Science *240:*1328–1331, 1988.

94. Scheffer, I. E., Hopkins, I. J., Harvey, A. S., and Berkovic, S. F. New autosomal-dominant partial epilepsy syndrome. Pediat. Neurol. *11:*95, 1994, abstract.

95. Scheffer, I. E., Bhatia, K. P., Lopes-Cendes, I., Fish, D. R., Marsden, C. D., Andermann, E., Andermann, F., Desbiens, R., Keene, D., Cendes, F., Manson, J. I., Constantinou, J. E. C., McIntosh, A., and Berkovic, S. F. Autosomal dominant nocturnal frontal epilepsy: a distinctive clinical disorder. Brain *118:*61–73, 1995.

96. Scholz, W. *Die krampdshadigungen des gehirns.* Berlin, Springer-Verlag, 1951.

97. Scholz, W. *Topistic lesions,* in Schade, J. P., Ms-Meheney, W. D. (eds.): Selective vulnerability of brain in hypoxaemia. Blackwell Sci. Publ., 1963, pp. 257–267.

98. Serratosa, J. M., Delgado-Escueta, A. V., Posada, I., Shih, S., Drury, I., Berciano, J., Zabala, J. A., Antunez, M. C., and Sparkes, R. S. The gene for progressive myoclonus epilepsy of the Lafora type maps to chromosome 6q. Hum. Molec. Genet. *4:*1657–1663, 1995.

99. Sheng, M., Dougan, S. T., McFadden, G., and Greenberg, M. E. Calcium and growth factor pathways of c-fos transcriptional activation require distinct upstream regulatory sequences. Mol. Cell Biol. *8:*2787–2796, 1988.

100. Sheng, M., and Greenberg, M. The regulation and function of c-fos and other immediate early genes in the nervous system. Neuron. *4:*477–485, 1990.

101. Shoffner, J. M., Lott, M. T., Lezza, A. M. S., Seibel, P., Ballinger, S. W., and Wallace, D. C. Myoclonic epilepsy and ragged-red fiber disease (MERRF) is associated with a mitochondrial DNA tRNA-lys mutation. Cell *61:*931–937, 1990.

102. Shorvon, S. The classic genetics of the epilepsies, in Hopkins, A., Shorvon, S., Cascino, G. (eds.): Epilepsy (2nd edition) Chapman & Hall, London, 1995.

103. Sloviter, R. S. Feedforward and feedback inhibition of hippocampal principal cell activity evoked by perforant path stimulation: GABA-mediated mechanisms that regulate excitability in vivo. Hippocampus. *1:*31–40, 1991.

104. Smart, S. L., Messing, A., Chiu, S. Y., Schwartzkroin, P., and Tempel, B. Mice lacking the delayed rectifier potassium channel mKv1.1. Soc. Neuroscience *21:*1824 (718.3, abstr.).

105. Sommer, W. Erkrankung des ammonshorn als aetiologisches moment der epilepsie. Arch. Psychiatr. Nervenkr. *10:*631–675, 1880.

106. Sommer, B., Kohler, M., Sprengel, R., and Seeburg, P. H. RNA editing in brain controls a determinant of ion flow in glutamate-gated channels. Cell *67:*11–19, 1991.

107. Sonnenberg, J. L., Macgregor-Leon, P. F., Curran, T., and Morgan, J. I. Dynamic alterations occur in the levels and composition of transcription factor AP-1 complexes after seizure. Neuron. *3:*359–365, 1989.

108. Spencer, D. D., Spencer, S. S., Mattson, R. H., and Williamson, P. D. Intracerebral masses in patients with intractable partial epilepsy. Neurology *34:*432–436, 1984.

109. Spielmeyer, W. Zur Pathogenese ortlich electiver Gehirnveranderungen. Ztschr. Neurol. Psychiatr. *99:*756–776, 1925.

110. Steinlein, O., Fischer, C., Keil, R., Smigrodzki, R., and Vogel, F. D20S19, linked to low voltage EEG, benign neonatal convulsions, and Fanconi anaemia, maps to a region of enhanced recombination and is localized between CpG islands. Hum. Molec. Genet. *1:*325–329, 1992.

111. Steinlein, O., Anokhin, A., Yping, M., Schalt, E., and Vogel, F. Localization of a gene for the human low-voltage EEG on 20q and genetic heterogeneity. Genomics *12:*69–73, 1992.

112. Strauder, K. H. Epilepsie und schlafenlappen. Arch. Psychiat. Nervenkr. *104:*181–211, 1936.

113. Sutula, T., He, X. X., Cavazos, J., and Scott, G. Synaptic reorganization in the hippocampus induced by abnormal functional activity. Science *239:*1147–1150, 1988.

114. Sutula, T., Cascino, G., Cavazos, J., Parada, I., and Ramirez, L. Mossy fiber synaptic reorganization in the epileptic human temporal lobe. Ann. Neurol. *26:*321–330, 1989.

115. Suzuki, J., and Nakamoto, Y. Seizure patterns and electroencephalograms of El mouse. Electro. Clin. Neurophys. *43*(3):299–311, 1977.

116. Szekely, A. M., Barbaccia, M. L., Alho, H., and Costa, E. In primary cultures of cerebellar granule cells the activation of N-methyl-D-aspartate-sensitive glutamate receptors induces c-fos mRNA expression. Mol. Pharmacol. *35:*401–408, 1989.

117. Tahvanainen, E., Ranta, S., Hirvasniemi, A., Karila, E., Leisti, J., Sistonen, P., Weissenbach, J., Lehesjoki, A.-E., and de la Chapelle, A. The gene for a recessively inherited human childhood progressive epilepsy with mental retardation maps to the distal short arm of chromosome 8. Proc. Nat. Acad. Sci. *91:*7267–7270, 1994.

118. Tauck, D. L., and Nadler, J. V. Evidence of functional mossy fiber sprouting in hippocampal formation of kainic acid-treated rats. J. Neuroscience *5:*1016–1022, 1985.

119. Tecott, L. H., Sun, L. M., Akana, S. F., Strack, A. M., Lowenstein, D. H., Dallman, M. F., and Julius, D. Eating disorder and epilepsy in mice lacking 5-HT2c serotonin receptors. Nature *374:*542–546, 1995.

120. Toth, M., Grimsby, J., Buzsaki, G., and Donovan, G. P. Epileptic seizures caused by inactivation of a novel gene, jerky, related to centromere binding protein-B in transgenic mice. Nat. Genet. *12:*110, 1996.

121. Tsirka, S. E., Gualandris, A., Amaral, D. G., and Strickland, S. Excitotoxin-induced neuronal degeneration and seizure are mediated by tissue plasminogen activator. Nature *377:*340–344, 1995.

122. Tsuboi, T., and Endo, S. Genetic studies of febrile convulsions: analysis of twin and family data. Epilepsy Res. Suppl. *4:*119–28, 1991.

123. Unverricht, H. Die Myoclonie. Berlin, Franz Deuticke, 1891.

124. Vogt, O. Der begriff der pathoklise. J. Psychol. Neurol. (Leipzig) *31:*245–255, 1925.
125. Wallace, D. C., Zheng, X., Lott, M. T., Shoffner, J. M., Hodge, J. A., Kelley, R. I., Epstein, C. M., and Hopkins, L. C. Familial mitochondrial encephalomyopathy (MERRF): genetic, pathophysiological, and biochemical characterization of a mitochondrial DNA disease. Cell *55:*601–610, 1988.
126. Watson, M. A., and Milbrandt, J. The NGFI-B gene, a transcriptionally inducible member of the steroid receptor gene superfamily: genomic structure and expression in rat brain after seizure induction. Mol. Cell Biol. *9:*4213–4219, 1989.
127. Waymire, K. G., Mahuren, J. D., Jaje, J. M., Guilarte, T. R., Coburn, S. P., and MacGregor, G. R. Mice lacking tissue non-specific alkaline phosphatase die from seizures due to defective metabolism of vitamin B-6. Nat. Genet. *11:*45–51, 1995.
128. Weissbecker, K. A., Durner, M., Janz, D., Scaramelli, A., Sparkes, R. S., and Spence, M. A. Confirmation of linkage between juvenile myoclonic epilepsy locus and the HLA region of chromosome 6. Am. J. Med. Genet. *38:*32–6, 1991.
129. White, J. D., and Gall, C. M. Differential regulation of neuropeptide and proto-oncogene mRNA content in the hippocampus following recurrent seizures. Brain Res. *427:*21–9, 1987.
130. Whitehouse, W. P., Rees, M., Curtis, D., Sundqvist, A., Parker, K., Chung, E., Baralle, D., and Gardiner, R. M. Linkage analysis of idiopathic generalized epilepsy (IGE) and marker loci on chromosome 6p in families of patients with juvenile myoclonic epilepsy: no evidence for an epilepsy locus in the HLA region. Am. J. Hum. Genet. *53:*652–62, 1993.
131. Williamson, A., McCormick, C. A., Shepard, C. M., *et al.* Intracellular recordings from epileptic human dentate granule cells show evidence of hyperexcitability. Epilepsia *31:*625, 1990.

PART VII

Cellular and Subcellular Mechanisms of Pain

CHAPTER 21

Molecular Biology of Pain

LUC JASMIN, M.D., Ph.D. and ADAM R. BURKEY, B.A.

INTRODUCTION

Molecular techniques have expanded our knowledge of the mechanisms of pain, not by posing new questions but by allowing a novel approach to old ones: Some of the most pressing questions in pain research have been: what are the mediators of pain? Are there anatomical substrates in the cerebral cortex which are unique to pain? What are the mechanisms governing endogenous and exogenous pain inhibition? Are there irreversible structural and functional events that underlie chronic pain? Until quite recently, pain has been considered a symptom and not a disease. Molecular techniques may allow us to define genetic events peculiar to chronic pain that identify it as a disease. That is, the signs and symptoms of pain could be linked to changes in genomic expression that progress autonomously of the precipitating disease. Pain could also result from an abnormal pattern of constitutive gene expression (23). As we shall see, changes in gene expression have been identified following thermal, mechanical, chemical, and inflammatory stimuli. Genetic events have also been associated with drug treatment of pain, such as with opiates (below). When these changes are understood better, therapeutic strategies can be devised to target the fundamental pathophysiology underlying the clinical presentation.

For the purpose of clarification, several terms prevalent in the literature, such as pain and nociception, will be defined. *Nociception* is the perception of a stimulus that threatens the integrity of body tissues. This perception can be physiological, in proportion to the nature and intensity of the stimulus, or pathological, such as is seen in *hyperalgesia* (excessive response to a nociceptive stimulus) or as in *allodynia* (nociceptive response to a non-nociceptive stimulus). Nociception is a unique category of sensation in that it is mediated by specific receptors and nerve fibers (C and A∂ fibers) and central afferent pathways (13, 14). These central pathways form the afferent portion of defensive reflexes organized at the spinal and brainstem levels. The nociceptive message is also relayed to the cerebral cortex, and here, reaching consciousness, a nociceptive stimulus may be perceived as pain.

Pain is the result of a complex series of events that culminates in the cerebral cortex. It often follows a nociceptive stimulus, but it can appear independently of such a stimulus, as in central pain. The experience of pain encompasses not only the nociceptive sensation but also the alteration of mood, thought, and social behavior of the individual. One, therefore, cannot strictly apply the term pain to animals because they cannot verify in speech the presence of these inner phenomena. In accordance with the concepts of pain and nociception, the treatment of pain can produce either analgesia or antinociception, respectively. *Analgesia* is the absence of pain, and *antinociception* is the absence or decreased perception of a nociceptive stimulus. These two phenomena can often be dissociated. For example, an interruption of thalamo-cortical connections will be analgesic, but not antinociceptive; the patients report feeling the pain, but they are not bothered by it. Finally, one must distinguish between exogenous pain inhibition, such as is experienced after morphine administration, and endogenous pain inhibition, such as is seen with the placebo effect. Significantly, both can be reversed by the opiate receptor antagonist naloxone (40), which underscores the importance of the anatomic substrates that either act or are acted upon by opioid compounds to inhibit pain.

c-fos AND OTHER PROTO-ONCOGENES

The advent of proto-oncogene research has allowed major advancements in the study of pain. Oncogenes were originally identified in oncogenic viruses, and later similar genes found in the normal DNA sequence of eukaryotic cells were called proto-oncogenes (17). Proto-oncogenes have widely divergent functions. Several of the proto-oncogene-encoded proteins are involved in neuronal stimulus-transcription coupling (19). Some are extracellular messengers, others are receptors, such as *trkA*, the nerve growth factor (NGF) receptor, and others are involved in intracellular signaling, such as the immediate early genes (IEG) *c-fos* and *c-jun* whose protein products mediate the induction of a variety of genes.

c-fos was described initially as the gene responsible for tumor induction by the FBJ murine osteosarcoma virus (21). *c-fos* was later found in normal eukaryotic cells where it is transcribed as Fos, a DNA-binding protein. After forming a complex with Jun, a process known as dimerization, Fos will migrate to the cell's nucleus and bind to a specific sequence of DNA called an AP-1 binding site. By binding to the AP-1 site, the Fos-Jun dimer induces transcription of late response genes. The protein products of the late response genes are involved in functional (signaling) and perhaps structural (cytoskeletal) changes that occur in neurons as an adaptation to the new conditions. Thus Fos, Jun and other IEGs are part of a cascade of signaling events along which external conditions, physiological or pathological, lead to long lasting changes in the nervous system (50, 58). *c-fos* is expressed at low levels in mature, non-dividing and unstimulated cells. Many neurons when synaptically stimulated will produce large amounts of newly synthesized Fos. This increase is rapid because it is effected by factors already present in the cytoplasm.

In pain research, Fos has been used extensively to monitor the trans-synaptic responses of spinal neurons to nociceptive stimuli. It is used as an index of activity in quantifying the effect of a treatment on large populations of nociresponsive neurons. After a given stimulus, an increase in Fos protein occurs in regions of the central nervous system functionally associated with the transmission of that stimulus. The increased production of Fos after stimulation is detected easily by screening brain or spinal cord sections with a specific antiserum. Treatment of tissue from an unstimulated animal will reveal little Fos-like immunoreactivity (FLI). Nociceptive stimulation will produce FLI in spinal areas where nociresponsive neurons are known to be concentrated: laminae I-IIo, V, and X (48). When only C-fibers are stimulated, as by a cutaneous injection of capsaicin, FLI increases almost exclusively in the superficial dorsal horn (laminae I and IIo) where the vast majority of these fibers terminate (Fig. 1A). A stimulus such as tooth extraction which activates both C and A∂ fibers, is followed by an increase of Fos in all nociceptive areas of the dorsal horn (Fig. 1B). Importantly, an innocuous stimulus, such as walking on a rotorod, will cause increased FLI only in non-nociceptive areas of the central nervous system, such as in laminae VIII and IX where motoneurons are located (36). This study and others have established that Fos is a marker of neuronal responsiveness in the particular system(s) that has been activated by a given stimulus.

When pain behavior and *c-fos* expression are monitored in an animal, both are found to increase in proportion to the stimulus intensity. When antinociceptive treatment is given prior to the nociceptive stimulus, one observes an inhibition of the increase in FLI in proportion to the decrease in pain behavior (31). Thus, FLI can be used to quantify the response to a treatment. Because of the intrinsic variability of labeling intensity, this method does not quantify gradations of activity; that is, a darkly labeled neuron is not necessarily more active than a more lightly labeled one. Thus, Fos functions as a marker of the activity of specific neuronal populations but does not indicate the degree of activity within that population.

NEUROTRANSMITTERS AND THEIR RECEPTORS

During the past three decades, an effort has been made to define the neurotransmitters involved in nociception. Those first to be recognized included the neurotransmitters involved with primary afferent transmission of noxious stimuli in the spinal and trigeminal dorsal horns. The amino acids glutamate and aspartate and several neuropeptides, including substance P

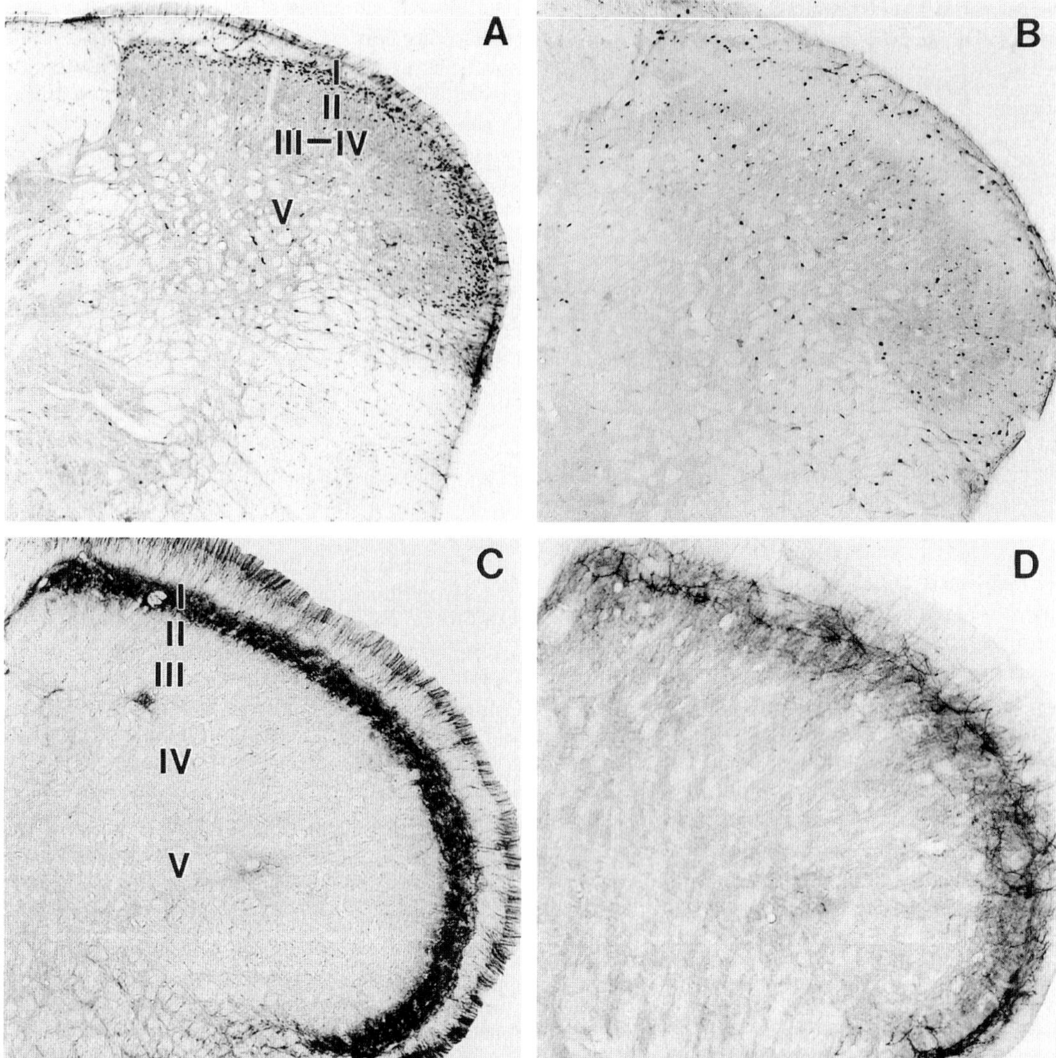

Figure 1. Four transverse hemisections of the caudal medulla at the level of the trigeminal nucleus caudalis, the medullary equivalent of the spinal dorsal horn. Trigeminal nerve nociceptive afferent from the ipsilateral face and oral cavity terminate mainly in laminae I and V. Sections *A* and *B* are slightly more caudal than *C* and *D*. Sections *A* and *B* have been immunoreacted for the Fos antigen after stimulation of ipsilateral trigeminal nociceptive afferents with subcutaneous injection of capsaicin (*A*) and tooth extraction (*B*). Note how capsaicin stimulation activates lamina I neurons only, where unmyelinated C-nociceptive fibers terminate, while tooth extraction also stimulates neurons in other layers, some of which are responding to the activation of small myelinated A∂-nociceptive fibers. Fos immunoreactivity in lamina III and IV would result from activation of non-nociceptive mechanoreceptors. Section *C* and *D* have been immunoreacted for the mu-opioid receptor antigen and the NK1 receptor antigen, respectively. Lamina V NK1 immunoreactive neurons are not seen on these sections. Note that both these receptors are located in superficial layers of nucleus caudalis. Magnification = 12×.

and calcitonin gene-related peptide (CGRP), are among the most significant. Some of these neuropeptides are also released into the peripheral tissues by axonal terminations where they cause hyperalgesia. For example, when substance P is released into the periphery by primary afferents, it will sensitize nociceptors, induce vasodilatation, and cause mast cells to release histamine. Primary afferents often contain more than one neurotransmitter, usually an amino-acid and one or more neuropeptides (11). Thus, the complexity of nociception is reflected in the diversity of neurochemical events that occur at the level of primary afferent transmission. Furthermore, many other neuromodulators influence nociception in the dorsal horn. These include mediators of descending pain inhibition (see below) such as serotonin (5-HT), noradrenaline, acetylcholine, and the endogenous opioids.

Radioligand binding, *in situ* hybridization, and immunocytochemical methods facilitate study of neurotransmitter receptors. The amino acid sequence of some of these receptors, such as the neurokinin-1 receptor (NK1, the substance P receptor) and the μ-opioid receptor (the primary morphine receptor), has been determined by DNA cloning. Raising antibodies against the presumed peptide sequence specific for each of these receptors (4, 62) permits immunohistochemical mapping of their anatomical distribution (Fig. 1 C and D). In discriminating the subcellular distribution of receptors, this is superior to radioligand binding and *in situ* hybridization.

Immunohistochemical techniques have shown that NK1 immunoreactive receptors (3) (Fig. 1D) are found only on neurons and are scattered broadly over 70% of the membrane surfaces of cell bodies and dendrites. Initially most of these receptors were thought to be nonfunctional and merely in transit from the cell body to the distal dendrites. If these receptors were functional, however, either the number of presynaptic terminals containing substance P had previously been underestimated or substance P could be reaching the NK1 receptor by a route other than presynaptic release. In fact, in most instances, there is no visible synaptic specialization apposed to the NK1 receptor. This excludes the involvement of any other neurotransmitter. Double labeling electron microscopy has confirmed disparity between substance P releasing sites and NK1 receptors (44). Approximately 85% of substance P vesicles adjacent to the membrane were not apposed by post-synaptic NK1 receptor sites. Furthermore, when glutamate and substance P colocalize in a pre-synaptic terminal, glutamate is released at the synaptic density while substance P is released from sites outside the synaptic specialization. Thus, substance P must diffuse a considerable distance from its release site to reach its receptor. This type of non-synaptic transmission has been referred to as *volume transmission*. The laminar distribution of NK1 immunoreactivity in the spinal cord is similar to the previously determined distribution of radiolabeled substance P binding sites. This suggests that the NK1 receptor and the substance P binding site are the same. NK1 immunoreactive sites do in fact bind ligand and are not simply nonfunctional isoforms of the receptor.

Substance P released in the superficial dorsal horn derives mostly from the C-primary afferent terminals (27). Peptides released in the superficial dorsal horn under certain conditions diffuse far from their release site in the dorsal horn (28). This occurs only when the activity of the extracellular endopeptidases is low. Since the activity of these enzymes is normally high, substance P should not reach most NK1 receptors on neurons of deeper laminae of the dorsal horn. For example, selective stimulation of C-fibers with capsaicin, presumed responsible for most of the release of substance P, is followed by increased *c-fos* expression in the superficial dorsal horn only (Fig. 1A). The neurons of the deeper laminae, however, have NK1-bearing dendrites extending into the superficial dorsal horn and, therefore, could be activated even when substance P from primary afferents does not diffuse far from the release site. It remains to be determined under which physiological and pathological conditions this activation leads to significant neuronal depolarization. Also unknown is under which conditions substance P reaches the deeper layers of the dorsal horn and how it affects nociceptive transmission.

Finally, the immunocytochemical detection of NK1 receptor demonstrated that, after binding to substance P, the NK1 receptors are rapidly internalized (45). This ligand-induced endocytosis has been proposed previously for G-protein-linked receptors (46, 68) and could serve to regulate neuronal responses to neuropeptide stimulation. Importantly, the receptors would then be recycled back to the membrane surface. Future studies will focus on the molecular mechanisms governing this ligand-induced endocytosis, which may provide insights into the plastic changes that occur in the CNS with chronic pain.

THE EFFECTS OF MORPHINE ON THE CEREBRAL CORTEX

Morphine and other opiates such as methadone are commonly used for cancer pain, where the benefits largely outweigh the side effects. They are also used for chronic non-malignant pain such as that of failed back syndrome refractory to other therapies. Morphine acts diffusely on many neural systems in the cerebral cortex. If this cortical effect predominates in the analgesia produced by systemic opioids, then antinociception should be produced by a purely local action of morphine on the cortex. Morphine applied to the cortex induces analgesia by engendering descending inhibitory activity. Some of the molecular changes induced by morphine in individual neurons termed "drug induced plasticity," are reviewed below (52).

Localized Effects of Morphine in the Cortex

Most studies of the cortical action of morphine have emphasized its psychotropic rather than its antinociceptive effects. Morphine induction of deep analgesia localizes to a discrete region of perirhinal cortex (64). Immunostaining with antiserum against the peptide sequence of the cloned mu-opioid receptor (4) has demonstrated a discrete area of increased reactivity. Application of morphine to this area produces antinociception at much lower doses than are required in other areas that produce morphine induced nociception.

In theory, morphine reaching the cerebral cortex could mediate antinociception through one of two neural mechanisms. Morphine's effect could result entirely from local effects such as inhibition of nociceptive afferents and their post-synaptic target in the cortex. Alternatively, morphine in the cortex could activate the brainstem descending pain inhibitory system (9). This is likely the case in morphine analgesia mediated by intracortical structures. Morphine and other opioid agonists injected in brainstem areas involved in descending inhibition, such as the cerebral ventricles, the periaqueductal gray matter (PAG), or the rostral ventral medulla (RVM), produce strong antinociception with a concomitant inhibition of nociceptive neurons in the dorsal horn (2, 5, 24, 30, 37). Furthermore, the analgesic effect of systemic morphine is abolished by lesions of brainstem nuclei and tracts associated with descending pain inhibition. That is, morphine analgesia is reversed by lesions in the PAG (26), the nucleus raphe magnus (18), the locus coeruleus (33), or the dorso-lateral funiculus (10), through which most of the brainstem descending pathways pass (8).

Descending inhibition is a potent way of inhibiting pain at its origin since many divergent spinal pathways transmit nociceptive information to various supraspinal neural systems. Each aspect of the pain response—discriminative, affective, and cognitive—would be simultaneously suppressed by inhibition of spinal nociceptive neurons. Little data exists to support cortically mediated activation of the descending pain inhibitory system. Two studies in which electrical stimulation of the primary sensory cortex was found to inhibit the firing of spinal and trigeminal nociceptive neurons provide only indirect evidence for cortical activation (56, 67).

To verify that morphine in the cortex activates a descending inhibitory system, the antinociceptive effect of morphine in the perirhinal cortex was correlated with the activity of spinal nociceptive neurons using FLI. The formalin test, a moderately intense stimulus that mimics many aspects of clinical chronic pain was used as a nociceptive stimulus. Nociceptive behavior induced by formalin is quantified over 1 hour to allow statistical comparisons between treatment groups. Following morphine injection into the perirhinal cortex, animals displayed strong behavioral antinociception and had a highly significant reduction in the number of FLI neurons in nociceptive areas of the lumbar spinal cord. This parallel inhibition of behavior and spinal *c-fos* expression indicates that the reduced activity of spinal nociceptive neurons is associated with the antinociception. This antinociception is attributed to an activation of a descending inhibitory system. It is not attributable to diffusion of morphine to the spinal cord or other brain areas since injections in cortical areas surrounding the perirhinal cortex had no effect.

These results demonstrate that morphine acting on a defined region of the cerebral cortex can activate the descending pain inhibitory system. Since some of the Fos-expressing neurons project to supraspinal relay nuclei (36, 48), inhibition of these neurons would block the ascending nociceptive message. Blockade of ascending nociceptive transmission from the spinal cord is thus a dominant feature of cortically induced analgesia.

Drug-Induced Plasticity

Opioid and NK1 receptors, like many other neurotransmitter receptors, are linked to second messenger systems. These receptors are coupled to G-proteins that mediate the intracellular effects of receptor-ligand binding. The role of the mu-opioid receptor in addiction and of the NK1 receptor in pain modulation are being studied. Morphine binding to mu-opioid receptors decreases neuronal firing. Investigations of the intracellular mechanisms through which this inhibition occurs have shown that (51) following the binding of morphine to the mu-opioid receptor, membrane ion channels open to influx of K^+ ions and efflux of Na^+ ions that hyperpolarize the cell. This change in membrane ion gating is mediated by a cascade of second messengers—G. proteins, cyclic AMP (cAMP), CREB (cAMP response element binding) proteins, and protein kinases. CREB factors are proteins that, when phosphorylated, migrate to the nucleus and induce transcription of genes such as *c-fos* and *c-jun*. The protein products of *c-fos* and other immediate early genes regulate the transcription of other genes, late genes such as the tyrosine hydroxylase gene (32) and neurofilament genes (12). The early changes in cellular physiology that follow morphine-induced gene transcription may be responsible for tolerance and dependence. Behavioral tolerance is observed within 4 hours of continuous morphine administration (38). This prompt activation of long term adaptive mechanisms is largely intracellular since the number of opiate binding sites and ion channels are unchanged in tolerant animals. An alteration in mu-receptor signal transduction, however, has been reported in tolerant animals (15). This involves an increase in adenylate cyclase activity that produces an increase in CREB-like proteins that persists at least as long as opiates are available to bind the receptors. Hours after morphine administration has ended, signal transduction returns to normal. Following opiate withdrawal, however, other alterations in gene expression are found in various areas of the brain (20, 35). The mechanisms and consequences of gene induction at the molecular level during withdrawal are currently unknown.

NERVE GROWTH FACTOR AND IMMUNE SYSTEM CYTOKINES IN PAIN AND NOCICEPTION

Pain is not restricted to the nervous system. It is affected by changes in other tissues and systems such as the immune system. Just as the nervous system modulates immunity (for review see Ref. 59), and the immune system influences nociception, especially in the setting of inflammation. Nerve growth factor (NGF), interleukin-1β (Il-1β), and tumor necrosis factor-alpha (*TNF*), whether applied peripherally or centrally, all decrease the nociceptive threshold (hyperalgesia). These cytokines are important not only to inflammation but also to the genesis of pain.

Molecular neuroscience has clarified some of the complex interrelationships between these mediators of response in the nervous and immune systems. NGF, for instance, potently degranulates mast cells to cause hyperalgesia. Some of these mediators influence each other directly: Il-1β can modulate NGF transcription and release (29), and TNF can activate the low-affinity NGF receptor, p75. The functional implications of these relationships are only now being elucidated. The effects of these mediators on nociception and their intracellular second messenger systems and their alteration of gene transcription are discussed below.

NGF-ASSOCIATED HYPERALGESIA

Exogenous NGF-Induced Hyperalgesia

A single dose of systemically administered NGF produces both mechanical and thermal hyperalgesia without allodynia in rats (41). Although no electrophysiological changes are detected in the primary afferent neuron responses, both types of hyperalgesia persist for 3 to 4 days. Both are therefore believed to be centrally maintained. In most other respects, however, these two phenomena differ. First, the NGF-induced thermal hyperalgesia can be attenuated by continuous systemic infusion of the non-competitive NMDA antagonist MK-801, but this drug does not affect mechanical hyperalgesia. Furthermore, thermal hyperalgesia begins within 15 minutes, is fully developed within 50 minutes, and is blocked by pretreatment with 5-HT antagonists or compounds that degranulate mast cells (44). Conversely, mechanical hyperalgesia begins at approximately 6.5 hours, is fully developed at 24 hours, and is not reversed by such pretreatment. Thus, the sensitization of primary afferents by serotonin appears to mediate thermal hyperalgesia in response to NGF. Several hypotheses regarding the etiology of the mechanical hyperalgesia have been proposed. The 6 to 7 hour-latency of mechanical hyperalgesia allows time for new transcription synthesis and fast-axonal transport neuropeptides such as substance P. A novel enhancement, *e.g.*, 'wind-up', of Aβ fiber activity has been detected after a single dose of systemic NGF (1 μg/kg; i.p.). This effect is blocked by an NK-1 receptor antagonist (61). It is uncertain whether this activation of Aβ fibers, which are not normally involved in nociception, underlies the mechanical hyperalgesia and whether this involvement results from alterations in the phenotype of large dorsal root ganglion neurons that might, be induced to express substance P.

Inflammation-Associated NGF Hyperalgesia

Hyperalgesia has been associated with conditions that alter local NGF levels. Transgenic mice, which overexpress NGF in their skin, display mechanical hyperalgesia but NGF knockout mice demonstrate hypoalgesia (22). Chronic inflammation, in which NGF levels are elevated locally, has provided a clinically relevant animal model of pain. An intraplantar inoculation of complete Freund's adjuvant (CFA) creates a model for inflammatory monoarthritis, in which an inflammatory response persists for at least 2 weeks. Anti-NGF antibodies given systemically on the fifth day after onset of inflammation increase thermal response thresholds within 3 hours and mechanical thresholds within 24 hours after administration. This suggests that NGF contributes to hyperalgesia throughout the course of the inflammation. These antibodies do not influence local erythema or edema. They do, however, reduce the expression of *c-fos* in the superficial and deep dorsal horn. Anti-NGF compounds might have therapeutic benefit as analgesics for inflammatory conditions (65).

TNF AND II-β-ASSOCIATED HYPERALGESIA

Central Effects

Il-1β is a proinflammatory cytokine produced primarily by activated macrophages and released at sites of inflammation to act on a variety of target cells, including T and B lymphocytes, neutrophils, epithelial cells, and fibroblasts. Following intracerebroventricular (i.c.v.) injection of this cytokine, hyperalgesia has been reported by some authors but not confirmed by others (1, 53). The issue is complicated by the fact that the induced nociception could be mediated through NGF. Cells that express Il-1β also synthesize NGF mRNA, such that Il-1β may regulate NGF transcription (6). Such regulation occurs in peripheral sensory neurons (43) and in astrocytes, where Il-1β acts synergistically with TNF to promote NGF transcription (29). I.c.v. administration of TNF-alpha increases nociceptive thresholds. The concurrent *decrease* in spontaneous locomotor activity (16) can confound the evaluation of nociceptive thresholds in animals. This antinociceptive effect is completely antagonized by anti-Il-1 antibodies but not by opioid antagonists or antisera to endogenous opioids.

Peripheral Effects

Peripheral injection of both TNF and Il-1β causes hyperalgesia. Intraplantar TNF produces ipsilateral thermal hyperalgesia while Il-1β produces both ipsi- and contralateral thermal hyperalgesia (54). The occurrence of contralateral hyperalgesia suggests it is likely attributable to changes in the spinal cord. Furthermore, bradykinin, a substance involved in both hyperalgesia and inflammation, administered 48 hours after cytokine administration worsened hyperalgesia induced by Il-1β but not that caused by TNF. This suggests that Il-1β induces expression of B1 receptors on primary afferents. Il-1β also produces antinociception locally by precipitating release of endogenous opioids from activated T-cells (60).

MOLECULES, RECEPTORS AND SIGNAL TRANSDUCTION

The central and peripheral changes that lead to nociception ultimately derive from extracellular binding of NGF, TNF and Il-1β to recep-

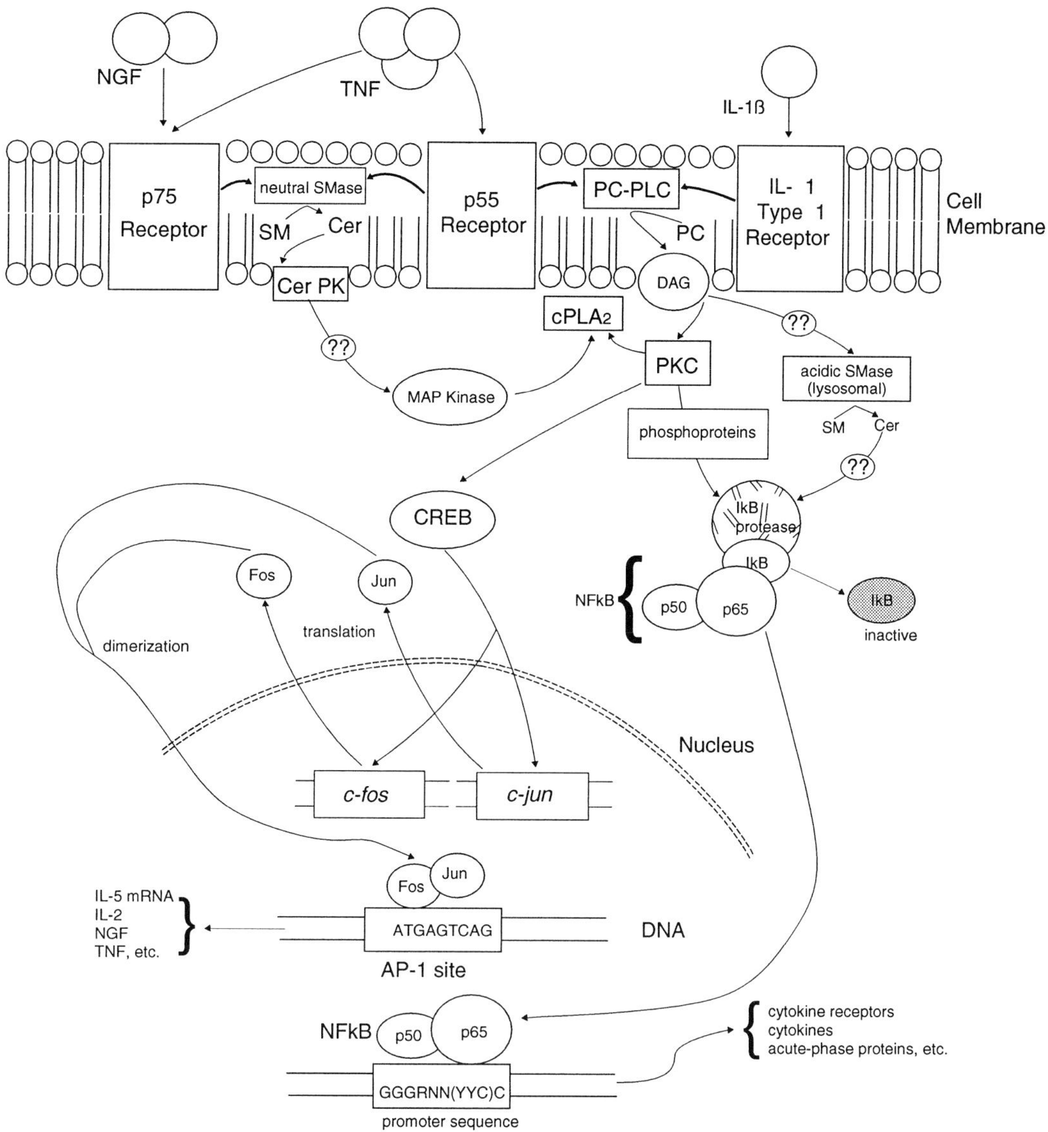

Figure 2. Model for transduction pathways of neural and immune cytokines related to the generation of hyperalgesia. This schematic summarizes the transduction pathways involved in intracellular signaling by receptors for NGF, TNF, and Il-1β. All three receptors activate neutral sphingomyelinase (SMase; Il-1 receptor activation not shown), the enzyme that cleaves sphingomyelin to produce ceramide (Cer). This molecule stimulates its own kinase, ceramide-activated protein kinase (Cer PK), which utilizes mitogen-activated protein (MAP) kinase to activate cytosolic phospholipase A$_2$ (cPLA$_2$). This enzyme releases arachidonic acid from lipids in the plasma membrane that can be metabolized to prostaglandins, molecules known to sensitize sensory neurons to painful stimuli (not shown). Diacylglycerol (DAG), created by the cleavage of phosphatidylcholine (PC) in response to p55 or Il-1 receptor binding, will stimulate both protein kinase C (PKC) and acidic Smase. PKC leads to the transcription and translation of gene regulatory proteins, Fos and Jun, and the activation of nuclear factor kappa B (NFkB). These factors then translocate to the nucleus to act on promoters of inducible genes. Particularly, the transcription of genes for cytokines and cytokine receptors, including TNF and NGF, is increased such that the response of neural and immune cells will increase. IkB: inhibitory subunit of kB; CREB: cAMP response element binding protein.

tors that activate with intracellular signaling pathways. A common enzyme, neutral sphingomyelinase (SMase), is a component of each pathway. NGF is known to bind to two receptors with different affinities, a high-affinity receptor tyrosine kinase, trkA, and a low-affinity receptor, p75, which belongs to the TNF/Fas superfamily of receptors. TNF binds the p75 receptor and its own p55 receptor. Although there is little homology between the two receptors overall, they do have similar sequences of three to four structural repeats. These contain a highly conserved pattern of cysteine residues involved in ligand binding (7, 63, 63). Two receptors are known to bind Il-1β *in vivo*, Il-1R types I and II. Type I, receptors transmit the Il-1 signal. Type II receptors may only competitively modulate Type I receptors. They bind neither TNF nor NGF.

The pathways activated by these ligands have similar signaling cascades (see Fig. 2). Il-1β and TNF induce protein kinases such as MAP kinase and ceramide-activated kinase. They also induce a transcription activator called nuclear factor kappa B (NF-kB) that regulates gene induction. Protein kinase C is also activated in the diacylglycerol (DAG) pathway. The production of DAG following protein kinase C activation also occurs after NGF binds its trkA high-affinity receptor. The role of PKC in Il-1/TNF signaling may be activation of the nuclear transcription factor AP-1 and thus the transcription of the genes it regulates.

Il-1β, TNF and NGF each activate the sphingomyelin pathway. The regulatory role of sphingolipid metabolites (34) was suggested by the finding that activation of a neutral sphingomyelinase (SMase) by cytokines increases intracellular ceramide (19). It is uncertain whether acid SMase mediates sphingomyelin turnover (39). It may activate NF-kB (55). Possible downstream targets of ceramide include a pro-line-directed protein kinase and a Ser/Thr protein phosphatase. Thus, ceramide likely regulates both protein transcription and intracellular phosphorylation/dephosphorylation balance.

IMPLICATIONS FOR PAIN RESEARCH

Mediators of both the immune system and the nervous system contribute to hyperalgesia. These mediators influence not only nociception, but also cell survival, proliferation and re-

growth. Both NGF and Il-1β are expressed in the CNS and often occur together. NGF induces specific histologic changes in the primary afferent nociceptors. SP and CGRP mRNAs increase after either the application of NGF or 5 days of CFA-induced inflammation (25). The mechanism connecting NGF induced signals to the expression of these neuropeptides is currently unknown. Future study of these and other intracellular alterations associated with nociception should reveal the neurophysiologic biochemical and genetic bases of chronic pain syndromes.

REFERENCES

1. Adams, J. U., Bussiere, J. L., Geller, E. B., and Adler, M. W. Pyrogenic doses of intracerebroventricular interleukin-1 did not induce analgesia in the rat hotplate or cold-water tail-flick tests. Life Sci. *53:*1401–1409, 1993.
2. Akaike, A., Shibata, T., Satoh, M., and Takagi, H. Analgesia induced by microinjection of morphine into and electrical stimulation of the nucleus reticularis paragigantocellularis of rat medulla oblongata. Neuropharmacology **17:**775–778, 1978.
3. Allen, C. J., Ghilardi, J. R., Rogers, S. D., *et al.* Antibodies to the C-terminus of the NK-1 (substance P) receptor stain a specific and discrete population of neurons in the cerebral cortex and striatum. In: *Society for Neuroscience 23rd Annual Meeting in Washington, D.C.,* 723 (298.5), 1993.
4. Arvidsson, U., Riedl, M., Chakrabarti, S., *et al.* Distribution and targeting of a mu-opioid receptor (MOR1) in brain and spinal cord. J. Neurosci. **15:** 3328–3341, 1995.
5. Azami, J., Llewelyn, M. D., and Roberts, M. H. T. The contribution of nucleus paragigantocellularis and nucleus raphe magnus to the analgesia produced by systemically administered morphine, investigated with the microinjection technique. Pain *12:*229–246, 1982.
6. Bandtlow, C. E., Meyer, M., Lindholm, D., *et al.* Regional and cellular codistribution of interleukin 1 beta and nerve growth factor mRNA in the adult rat brain: possible relationship to the regulation of the nerve growth factor synthesis. J. Cell. Biol. **111:** 1701–1711, 1991.
7. Banner, D. W., D'Arcy, A., Janes, W., *et al.* Crystal structure of the soluble human 55kd TNF receptor-human TNF (alpha) complex: implications for TNF receptor activation. Cell *73:*431–445, 1993.
8. Basbaum, A. I., and Fields, H. L. The dorsolateral funiculus of the spinal cord: a major route for descending brainstem control. Neurosci. Abst. *3:*499, 1977.
9. Basbaum, A. I., and Fields, H. L. Endogenous pain control mechanisms: review and hypothesis. Ann. Neurol. *4:*451–462, 1978.
10. Basbaum, A. I., Marley, N., O'Keefe, J., and Clanton, C. H. Reversal of morphine and stimulus produced analgesia by subtotal spinal cord lesions. Pain *3:*43–56, 1977.
11. Battaglia, G., and Rustioni, A. Coexistence of gluta-

mate and substance P in dorsal root ganglion neurons of the rat and monkey. J. Comp. Neurol. *277:*302–312, 1988.

12. Beitner-Johnson, D., Guitart, X., and Nestler, E. J. Neurofilament proteins and the mesolimbic dopamine system: Common regulation by chronic morphine and chronic cocaine in the rat ventral tegmental area. J. Neurosci. *12:*2165–2176, 1992.

13. Bernard, J. F., and Besson, J. M. Ascending pain pathways with special reference to the spino(trigeminal)-ponto-amygdaloid tract. In: *Toward the use of noradrenergic agonists for the Treatment of Pain,* edited by J. M. Besson and G. Guilbaud, pp 1–25. Amsterdam, Elsevier, 1992.

14. Besson, J. M., and Chaouch, A. Peripheral and spinal mechanisms of nociception. Physiol. Rev. *67:*67–186, 1987.

15. Bhargava, H. N., and Gulati, A. Down-regulation of brain and spinal cord mu-opiate receptors in morphine tolerant-dependent rats. Eur. J. Pharmacol. 190 (3 1990):305–311.

16. Bianchi, M., Sacerdote, P., Castagnoli, P., *et al.* Central effects of tumor necrosis factor alpha and interleukin-1 alpha on nociceptive thresholds and spontaneous locomotor activity. Neurosci. Lett. *148:*76–80, 1992.

17. Bishop, J. M. Virol oncogenes. Cell *42:*23–38, 1985.

18. Chance, W. T., Krynock, G. M., and Rosecrans, J. A. Effects of medial raphe and raphe magnus lesions on the analgesic activity of morphine and methadone. Psychopharmacology *56:*133–137, 1978.

19. Chatterjee, S. Neutral sphingomyelinase action stimulates signal transduction of tumor necrosis factor-alpha in the synthesis of cholesteryl esters in human fibroblasts. J. Biol. Chem. *269:*879–882, 1994.

20. Chieng, B., Keay, K. A., and Christie, M. J. Increased fos-like immunoreactivity in the periaqueductal gray of anaesthetized rats during opiate withdrawal. Neurosci. Lett. *183:*79–82, 1995.

21. Curran, T., and Teich, N. M. Candidate products of the FBJ murine osteosarcoma virus oncogene. J. Virol. *42:*114–122, 1982.

22. Davis, B. M., Lewin, G. R., Mendell, L. M., *et al.* Altered expression of nerve growth factor in the skin of transgenic mice leads to changes in response to mechanical stimuli. Neuroscience *56:*789–792, 1993.

23. Devor, M., and Raber, P. Heritability of symptoms in an experimental model of neuropathic pain. Pain *42:*51–67, 1990.

24. Dickenson, A. H., Oliveras, J. L., and Besson, J. M. Role of the nucleus raphe magnus in opiate analgesia as studied by the microinjection technique in the rat. Brain Res. *170:*95–111, 1979.

25. Donnerer, J., Schuligoi, R., and Stein, C. Increased content and transport of substance P and calcitonin gene-related peptide in sensory nerves innervating inflamed tissue: Evidence for a regulatory function of nerve growth factor in vivo. Neuroscience *49:*693–698, 1992.

26. Dostrovsky, J. O., and Deakin, J. F. W. Periaqueductal gray lesions reduce morphine analgesia in the rat. Neurosci. Lett. *4:*99–103, 1977.

27. Duggan, A. W., Hope, P. J., Jarrott, H. G., *et al.* Release, spread and persistence of immunoreactive neu-

rokinin A in the dorsal horn of the cat following noxious cutaneous stimulation. Studies with antibody microprobes. Neuroscience *35:*195–202, 1990.

28. Duggan, A. W., Morton, C. R., Zhao, Z. Q., and Hendry, I. A. Noxious heating of the skin releases immunoreactive substance P in the substantia gelatinosa of the cat: a study with antibody microprobes. Brain Res. *403:*345–349, 1987.

29. Gadient, R. A., Cron, K. C., Otten, U. Interleukin-1 beta and tumor necrosis factor-alpha synergistically stimulate nerve growth factor (NGF) release from cultured rat astrocytes. Neurosci. Lett. *117:*335–340, 1990.

30. Gebhart, G. F. Opiate and opioid peptide effects on brain stem neurons: Relevance to nociception and antinociceptive mechanisms. Pain *12:*93–140, 1982.

31. Gogas, K. R., Presley, R. W., Levine, J. D., and Basbaum, A. I. The antinociceptive action of supraspinal opioids results from an increase in descending inhibitory control: Correlation of nociceptive behavior and c-fos expression. Neuroscience *42:*617–628, 1991.

32. Guitart, X., and Nestler, E. J. Identification of morphine- and cyclic AMP-regulated phosphoproteins (MARPPs) in the locus coeruleus and other regions of rat brain: regulation by acute and chronic morphine. J. Neurosci. *9:*4371–4387, 1989.

33. Hammond, D. L., and Proudfit, H. K. Effects of locus coeruleus lesions on morphine-induced antinociception. Brain Res. *188:*79–91, 1980.

34. Hannun, Y. A. The sphingomyelin cycle and the second messenger function of ceramide. J. Biol. Chem. **269:** 3125–3128, 1994.

35. Hayward, M. D., Duman, R. S., and Nestler, E. J. Induction of the c-fos proto-oncogene during opiate withdrawal in the locus coeruleus and other regions of rat brain. Brain Res. *525:*256–266, 1990.

36. Jasmin, L., Gogas, K. R., Ahlgren, S. C., *et al.* Walking evokes a distinctive pattern of Fos-like immunoreactivity in the caudal brainstem and spinal cord of the rat. Neuroscience *58:*275–286, 1994.

37. Jensen, T. S., and Yaksh, T. L. I. Comparison of antinociceptive action of morphine in the periaqueductal gray, medial and paramedial medulla in rat. Brain Res. *363:*99–113, 1986.

38. Kissin, I., Brown, P. T., Robinson, C. A., and Bradley, E. L. Jr. Acute tolerance in morphine analgesia: continuous infusion and single injection in rats. Anesthesiology *74:*166–171, 1991.

39. Kuno, K., and Matsushima, K. The IL-1 receptor signaling pathway. J. Leukocyte Biol. *56:*542–547, 1994.

40. Levine, J. D., Gordon, N. C., and Fields, H. L. Naloxone dose dependently produces analgesia and hyperalgesia in postoperative pain. Nature *278:*740–741, 1979.

41. Lewin, G. R., Ritter, A. M., and Mendell, L. M. Nerve growth factor-induced hyperalgesia in the neonatal and adult rat. J. Neurosci. *13:*2136–2148, 1993.

42. Lewin, G. R., Rueff, A., and Mendell, L. M. Peripheral and central mechanisms of NGF-induced hyperalgesia. Eur. J. Neurosci. *6:*1903–1912, 1994.

43. Lindholm, D., Heumann, R., Meyer, M., and Thoenen, H. Interleukin-1 regulates synthesis of nerve growth

factor in non-neuronal cells of rat sciatic nerve. Nature *330:*658–659, 1987.

44. Liu, H., Brown, J. L., Jasmin, L., Maggio, J. E., *et al.* Synaptic relationship between substance P and the substance P receptor: Light and electron microscopic characterization of the mismatch between neuropeptides and their receptors. Proc. Natl. Acad. Sci. USA *91:*1009–1013, 1994.

45. Mantyh, P. W., DeMaster, E., Malhotra, A., *et al.* Receptor endocytosis and dendrite reshaping in spinal neurons after somatosensory stimulation. Science *268:*1629–1632, 1995.

46. Mazella, J., Leonard, K., Chabry, J., *et al.* Binding and internalization of iodinated neurotensin in neuronal cultures from embryonic mouse brain. Brain Res. *564:*249–255, 1991.

47. McDonald, N. Q., and Hendrickson, W. A. A structural superfamily of growth factors containing a cystine knot motif. Cell *73:*421–424, 1993.

48. Menétrey, D., Gannon, A., Levine, J. D., and Basbaum, A. I. Expression of c-fos protein in interneurons and projection neurons of the rat spinal cord in response to noxious somatic, articular, and visceral stimulation. J. Comp. Neurol. *285:*177–195, 1989.

49. Morgan, J. I. Proto-Oncogene Expression in the Nervous System. Discussion neurosci. *7:*11–50, 1991.

50. Morgan, J. I., and Curran, T. Stimulus-transcription coupling in neurons: role of cellular immediate-early genes. TINS *12:*459–462, 1989.

51. Nestler, E. J. Molecular mechanisms of drug addiction. J. Neurosci. *12:*2439–2450, 1992.

52. Nestler, E. J. Molecular basis of addictive states. Neuroscientist *1:*212–220, 1995.

53. Oka, T., Aou, S., and Hori, T. Intracerebroventricular injection of interleukin-1 beta induces hyperalgesia in rats. Brain Res. *624:*61–68, 1993.

54. Perkins, M. N., and Kelly, D. Interleukin-1 beta induced-desArg9bradykinin-mediated thermal hyperalgesia in the rat. Neuropharmacology *33:*657–660, 1994.

55. Schutze, S., Machleidt, T., and Kronke, M. The role of diacylglycerol and ceramide in tumor necrosis factor and interleukin-1 signal transduction. J. Leukocyte Biol. *56:*533–541, 1994.

56. Sessle, B. J., Hu, J. W., Dubner, R., and Lucier, G. E. Functional properties of neurons in cat trigeminal subnucleus caudalis (medullary dorsal horn). II. Modulation of responses to noxious and non noxious stimuli by periaqueductal gray, nucleus raphe magnus, cerebral cortex, and afferent influences, and

effects of naloxone. J. Neurophysiol. **45:**193–207, 1981.

57. Shen, K. F., and Crain, S. M. Nerve growth factor rapidly prolongs the action potential of mature sensory ganglion neurons in culture, and this effect requires activation of Gs-coupled excitatory kappa-opioid receptors on these cells. J. Neurosci. *14:*5570–5579, 1994.

58. Sheng, M., and Greenberg, M. E. The regulation and function of c-fos and other immediate early genes in the nervous system. Neuron *4:*477–485, 1990.

59. Stanisz, A. M. Neuronal factors modulating immunity. Neuroimmunomodulation *1:*217–230, 1994.

60. Stein, C. Mechanisms of disease: the control of pain in peripheral tissue by opioids. N. Engl. J. Med. *332:*1685–1690, 1995.

61. Thompson, S. W. N., Dray, A., McCarson, K. E., *et al.* Nerve growth factor induces mechanical allodynia associated with novel A fibre-evoked spinal reflex activity and enhanced neurokinin-1 receptor activation in the rat. Pain *62:*219–231, 1995.

62. Vigna, S. R., Bowden, J. J., McDonald, D. M., *et al.* Characterization of antibodies to the rat substance P (NK-1) receptor and to a chimeric substance P receptor expressed in mammalian cells. J. Neurosci. *14:*834–845, 1994.

63. Welcher, A. A., Bitler, C. M., Radeke, M. J., and Shooter, E. M. Nerve growth factor binding domain of the nerve growth factor receptor. Proc. Natl. Acad. Sci. USA *88:*159–163, 1991.

64. Wenniger, J., Proctor, M., Gale, K., and Jasmin, L. The analgesic effect of morphine in the piriform cortex (PC) may be mediated through the descending inhibitory control as evidence by correlation of nociceptive behavior and c-fos expression in the formalin test. Neuroscience Abstract *318:*18, 1994.

65. Woolf, C. J., Safieh-Garabedian, B., Ma, Q-P., *et al.* Nerve growth factor contributes to the generation of inflammatory sensory hypersensitivity. Neuroscience *62:*327–331, 1994.

66. Yan, H., and Chao, M. V. Disruption of cysteine rich repeats of the NGF receptor leads to loss of ligand binding. J. Biol. Chem. *266:*12099–12104, 1991.

67. Yezierski, R. P., Gerhart, K. D., Schrock, B. J., and Willis, W. D. A further examination of effects of cortical stimulation on primate spinothalamic tract cells. J. Neurophysiol. *49:*424–441, 1983.

68. Yu, S. S., Lefkowitz, R. J., and Hausdorff, W. P. Beta-adrenergic receptor sequestration. A potential mechanism of receptor resensitization. J. Biol. Chem. *268:*337–341, 1993.

PART VIII

The Molecular Basis of Deficiency Diseases

CHAPTER 22

Gene Therapy for Neurodegenerative Diseases

MARTIN A. EGLITIS, Ph.D

INTRODUCTION

As gene transfer technology has evolved, its applicability to a wide range of diseases has become apparent. Attribution of many neurologic diseases to single gene defects has made these diseases attractive candidates for gene therapy. This chapter will review the progress in developing gene therapies for lysosomal storage diseases, muscular dystrophy, and Parkinson disease.

Storage Diseases

Gaucher Disease (Glucocerebrosidase deficiency)

Gaucher Disease (GD) is the most common storage disease (17). It is caused by excessive accumulation of glucocerebroside that results from a deficiency of glucocerebrosidase enzyme (EC 3.2.1.43). Neurological symptoms occur in two of the three clinical phenotypes. Enzyme replacement has been beneficial to patients suffering from type 1 GD, which lacks neurological symptoms; gene replacement is likely to be similarly helpful for patients with types 2 and 3 in which neurological manifestations occur.

The cells accumulating glucocerebroside are monocyte/macrophage progenitors in the bone marrow. In fact, bone marrow transplantation has therapeutic benefit in type 1 GD (17). However, the morbidity and mortality of marrow transplantation have encouraged the development of other therapeutic approaches. Enzyme supplementation reverses manifestations of type 1 GD (see references cited in (17)). The blood brain barrier precludes enzymatic correction of the neurologic manifestations of types 2 and 3;

other strategies, such as gene therapy, are needed for the brain.

The success of bone marrow transplantation in treating type 1 GD. Prompted selection of hematopoietic cells as the target cells for gene transfer. Retroviral-mediated transfer of human glucocerebrosidase into mouse bone marrow cells in vivo was first accomplished in 1989 (24). Marrow cells of a patient with GD were harvested and transduced *in vitro* by retroviral vectors carrying the human glucocerebrosidase cDNA. Fourteen days after reinfusion, colonies of transplanted marrow cells (producing glucocerebrosidase) were found in the spleen. Long-term gene expression in mouse hematopoietic cells after bone marrow transplantation was confirmed *in vitro* (88) and *in vivo* (25, 116). Detection of human glucocerebrosidase in macrophages forming colonies in the spleens of secondary bone marrow recipient suggests that the glucocerebrosidase gene was successfully introduced into hematopoietic stem cells (116) and was being expressed in the appropriate target cells (23, 91). That physiologically relevant levels of expression of the glucocerebrosidase gene are achieved was demonstrated in an *in vitro* culture system. A normal level of glucocerebrosidase mRNA, total protein, and actual enzymatic activity was found in treated bone marrow cells of a 5-year-old GD patient *in vitro* (89). Although both the *in vitro* and *in vivo* studies confirmed that the appropriate target cells were susceptible to retroviral mediated gene transfer of the glucocerebrosidase gene, it was unclear if any of these cells could cross the blood-brain barrier. *In situ* hybridization has subsequently shown that cells bearing the human glucocerebrosidase gene enter the brain

(71). Cells expressing human glucocerebrosidase were found in the brains of mice infused with retrovirally transduced bone marrow cells, but they were few in number. Double-labeling analysis identified the cells expressing glucocerebrosidase as microglia; up to 20% of microglia appeared to arise from the genetically altered bone marrow cells (71). This discrepancy between the high proportion of cells containing the therapeutic gene and the few expressing it highlights one significant problem in using retroviral vectors. Silencing of the vector promoter in brain microglia may account for this discrepancy.

Ex vivo transfer of a human glucocerebrosidase cDNA into primate hematopoietic cells and *in vivo* expression of the gene have been shown (129). The retroviral vector used was detected in one animal over a year after transplantation. Interestingly, amphotropic vectors transferred the gene more efficiently into lymphocytes (0.3%–14% transduction rate) than into granulocytes (0.1%–0.5%). Cells of the monocyte/macrophage lineage were not evaluated, and the distribution within the brain of cells expressing the therapeutic gene was not mapped. Nonetheless, these studies demonstrate that retroviral transfer of the glucocerebrosidase gene is possible in primates and, in conjunction with verification of the susceptibility of human hematopoietic cells to retroviral vector transduction (9, 87, 128), herald use of this technique for GD. Although a clinical experimental protocol has been approved by the NIH RAC (D. Kohn, personal communication), the duration of retroviral mediated expression and means of delivering genetically engineered cells to the CNS need further study.

Adeno associated virus (AAV) is also being evaluated for a vector in gene transfer in GD. Fibroblasts derived from a patient with GD sustained expression of glucocerebrosidase in AAV mediated in vitro transfer of the glucocerebrosidase gene producer (115). Whether AAV can deliver glucocerebrosidase to monocytes/macrophages is unknown. A direct comparison of the efficiency of gene transfer mediated by AVV and by retrovirus is needed.

Mucopolysaccharidosis Deficiencies

The mucopolysaccharidoses (MPSs) are a group of lysosomal storage diseases characterized by excessive excretion of amounts of glycosaminoglycans. Glycosaminoglycan accumulation in various organs causes their failure. Serious neurological problems, especially mental retardation are prominent. Seven types of MPS, each due to a deficiency of a different and specific enzyme, have been described. All of the MPSs are potentially treated by enzyme replacement; in fact, cells derived from a patient with one type of MPS therapeutically complement the defect of cells derived from a patient with another type of MPS (45).

Permanent cure of the disease requires continued supply of the enzyme. Bone marrow transplantation has some clinical benefit for MPS type I (1). The potential usefulness of gene replacement has been demonstrated for three different MPSs. The enzymatic deficiency of MPS type I (Hurler Syndrome) has been corrected in vitro using retroviral vectors (5). Retroviral vectors containing a full-length cDNA for the missing enzyme, a-L-iduronidase (EC 3.2.1.76), were constructed and used to transduce fibroblasts derived from patients with MPSI. The observed reduction of glycosaminoglycan accumulation in the cells suggested that the enzyme defect had been corrected. However, over-expression of a-L-iduronidase was counterproductive. This emphasizes that vector design must permit tight control of enzyme expression before gene therapy for MPS type I is undertaken. This is also evident from studies of MPS type VI (Maroteaux-Lamy Syndrome). Retroviral mediated transfer of cDNA of the deficient gene, N-acetylgalactosamine-4-sulphatase, (EC 3.1.6.1) into fibroblasts from a patient with MPS type VI corrected the enzymatic defect but did not increase glycosaminoglycan turnover (6). Concomitant reduction in the activities of other lysosomal sulphatases is one possible explanation. These observations suggest that therapeutic efficacy requires restoration of not just one enzymatic activity, but rather the normal balance among the activities of multiple interrelated lysosomal enzymes.

MPS type II (Hunter Syndrome) has also been evaluated for possible treatment by gene therapy. Transfection of iduronate-2-sulfatase (EC 3.1.6.13) into lymphoblastoid cells from patients with Hunter syndrome by a retroviral vector increased enzyme activity levels up to 70 fold and restored glycosaminoglycan levels to normal (18). This indicates both that MPS type II may be amenable to gene therapy and that regulation of enzyme levels may not need to be as precise in this disease.

Gene replacement for MPS has been evaluated more extensively for Type VII, Sly Syndrome, than for other types. The biochemistry of b-glucuronidase (EC3.2.1.31), the enzyme deficient in the disease, has been well characterized, and a mouse model of the disease is available (15). Replacement of the defective gene ameliorated clinical symptoms in a transgenic MPSVII mouse (72).

HSV vectors have been used to deliver b-glucuronidase to the brains of MPSVII mice (122). Mice inoculated through the eye with 2×105 pfu demonstrated β-glucuronidase activity in the trigeminal ganglion and brainstem as long as 18 weeks after inoculation. While promising, the HSV vector system is currently limited by the number of cells transduced. Transduction may be limited by decline in activity of the endogenous latency-associated promoter linked to the β-glucuronidase cDNA (35). Also, by exclusively targeting the CNS, this strategy does not address the systemic manifestation of MPS type VII.

Transplanting bone marrow cells into which the β-glucuronidase gene has been transfected into β-glucuronidase deficient transgenic mice partially reverses the MPS type VII phenotype (78, 124). Although enzymatic activity remains low in various tissues, gene transfer into hematopoietic stem cells is manifest by persistence of activity in hematopoietic cells of secondary transplant recipients (124). Furthermore, despite low enzyme activity, glycosaminoglycan levels were significantly reduced in both the liver and spleen (78, 124). Glycosaminoglycan levels did not decline in the kidney or retina, as they did when MPS VII mice received transplants of normal bone marrow (14). Higher levels of β-glucuronidase activity are required to produce therapeutic benefit in all target organs. Vectors capable of generating higher levels of β-glucuronidase have been recently described (123); however, it is unknown whether transplanting cells that produce greater amounts of enzyme will result in greater transfer of enzyme to target organs. In particular, the inability of b-glucuronidase to cross the blood-brain-barrier remains an obstacle treatment of CNS manifestations.

An alternative means of restoring β-glucuronidase activity (85), uses autologous skin fibroblasts transduced *in vitro* by a retroviral vector carrying the human b-glucuronidase gene. These modified fibroblasts are embedded in a collagen/PTFE support and implanted into the peritoneum of MPS VII mice. By four days after implantation, excretion of glycosaminoglycan in the urine dropped by approximately half to two or three times normal. This reduction was maintained for almost four months. Furthermore, there was partial reversal of the pathologic alterations of lysosomal storage in the spleen and liver, the two organs exhibiting the highest level of acquired human β-glucuronidase activity. Although many features of the MPS VII phenotype did not return to normal, the treatment slowed progression of the disease. In similar studies using a healthy dog model (84), the implanted cells survived for almost one year, and hepatic levels of human β-glucuronidase activity were similar to those observed in the treated transgenic mice.

Metachromatic Leukodystrophy

Metachromatic leukodystrophy (MLD) is a recessive autosomal storage disorder caused by a deficiency of arylsulphatase A (EC 3.1.6.8). The accumulation of cerebroside sulfate leads to severe neurological problems and early death. Retroviral (97) and AAV (115) vectors carrying human arylsulphatase A cDNA reverse the enzyme deficiency in fibroblasts derived from patients with MLD. The retroviral vector elevated arylsulfatase activity to 10 times that of normal cells (97), and the AAV vector elevated it up to 50 times normal (123). With both vectors, treated cells appeared normal. These preliminary experiments suggest that MLD may also be amenable to gene therapy. Cells derived from patients with a rare form of MLD caused by a deficiency of the sphingolipid activator protein (SAP-1, prosaposin) have also been successfully treated *in vitro* using a retroviral vector carrying the SAP-1 cDNA (95).

Niemann-Pick's Disease (Sphingomyelinosis)

The cloning of the cDNA encoding acid sphingomyelinase (EC 3.1.4.12), the enzyme responsible for Niemann-Pick Disease (NPD) (100), permits testing of the ability of gene transfer to reverse the metabolic defect. A retroviral vector carrying the cDNA for acid sphingomyelinase (106) reduces accumulation of sphingomyelin in fibroblast of patients with NPD. The ability to select cells expressing acid sphingomyelinase (37) may allow selection of transduced bone marrow stem cells for gene therapy.

Other Storage Diseases

A number of other lysosomal storage diseases are potential candidates for treatment by gene therapy. In some cases, cell transplantation corrects the metabolic defect in animal models. For example, bone marrow transplantation halts progressive neurological deterioration in a cat model of a-mannosidosis (114). Dogs with fucosidosis have increased enzyme activity in various tissues after bone marrow transplantation, but disease progression is unaltered (108). Retroviral transfer of a-L-fucosidase (EC 3.2.1.51) cDNA into fibroblasts from both dogs and patients suffering from fucosidosis increases (90) enzyme activity to levels sufficient to correct the metabolic defect. Transplantation of such genetically altered autologous cells may be an effective way to treat fucosidosis. However, given the lack of efficacy of bone marrow transplantation in the adult dog model, cell transplantation may need to occur very early in life to produce clinical benefit.

In vitro tests of retroviral-mediated gene transfer have been successful for both maple syrup urine disease (MSUD) and adrenoleukodystrophy. Patients suffering from MSUD are deficient in mitochondrial branched-chain a-oxo acid dehydrogenase complex, which consists of three catalytic components. A retroviral vector containing the cDNA for one component restored enzymatic activity into fibroblasts of patients with MSUD (69). Similarly, retroviral vectors carrying the cDNA of the gene associated with adrenoleukodystrophy in the oxidation of very-long-chain fatty acids correct the defect found in fibroblasts obtained from a patient with the disease (20).

Thus, genetically altering autologous cells *ex vivo* and reimplanting them is a promising therapeutic strategy for a variety of lysosomal storage diseases. However, because neuronal damage, once sustained, is frequently irreversible, the treatment needs to occur very early in life, perhaps even *in utero* (63).

Muscular Dystrophy

Treatment of Duchenne and Becker muscular dystrophy is complicated by the involvement of muscles through the body. The illness is caused by an absence of dystrophin, a protein expressed in all muscle cells. Cure entails successful targeting of all muscles. Proposed treatments involve cell therapy or gene therapy. Cell therapy is the implantation of normal donor cells containing a normal dystrophin gene. Cell therapy of Duchenne's muscular dystrophy has been tested in humans, but the results have, at best, been equivocal (see (83) for a recent review). Gene therapy has the potential advantage that a muscle specific vector could be designed to deliver the dystrophin gene to muscles throughout the body.

Three types of vectors have been tested for their delivery of dystrophin cDNA into muscles: plasmids, retroviral vectors, and adenoviral vectors. Gene transfer by plasmid has been shown in skeletal muscle (126), cardiac muscle (75), and the diaphragm (2, 33). Injection of plasmid containing human dytrophin linked to the LTR promotor of Rous sarcoma virus into the muscles of mdx mice, a model for muscular dystrophy, resulted in expression of human dystrophin. Only about 1% of the fibers in the target muscle (the rectus femoris) expressed the cDNA 7 days after injection. Preinjection of muscles with a volume of hypertonic sucrose equal to the volume of DNA injected reduced the variability and doubles the efficiency of plasmid-mediated gene transfer. The choice of promoter for the plasmid greatly affects both the magnitude and the persistence of gene expression in muscle. Expression of a luciferase cDNA linked to the SV40 early promoter declines to control levels two weeks after injection. In contrast, a similar plasmid using the Rous sarcoma virus promoter effects gene expression that persists 60 days after injection. Other investigators found a different temporal pattern of gene expression from a similar plasmid: a peak of activity at 1 month and then an abrupt decline (29, 34). A different plasmid containing a chloramphenicol acetyl transferase reporter gene under the transcriptional control of the HSV thymidine kinase gene promoter produced peak activity after only 7 days. Regenerating muscle is more susceptible to plasmid-mediated gene transfer than normal adult muscle (29, 113, 117). In normal adult muscle induced to regenerate by the myotoxic local anesthetic bupivicaine, gene expression is up to 80 times higher than an uninjured muscle. Mdx mice, which regenerate muscle in response to their disease, are more susceptible than normal mice to plasmid-based gene transfer (117). Gene expression did not increase when mdx mice were pretreated with bipivacaine to increase regeneration (117). Furthermore, injuring dystrophic muscles is unwise because of the reduced regenerative capacity in muscular dystrophy.

The chronic muscle regeneration observed in the mdx mouse suggested that such cells may also be susceptible to retroviral-mediated gene transfer, which requires cell division for gene expression to occur. Retroviral transfer of the human dystrophin cDNA into muscle cells of 7–8 week old mdx mice has been accomplished (39). The limited capacity of retroviral vectors necessitated using a truncated dystrophin cDNA from a mild Becker genotype. Two weeks after injection of the retroviral vector, numerous muscle fibers expressed human dystrophin. Furthermore, 4% of fibers in the quadriceps muscle were positive nine months after a single injection of retroviral vector. The large size of even the truncated Becker-type dystrophin cDNA probably reduces the maximum attainable titer of the retroviral vectors carrying this cDNA and the efficiency of gene transfer into muscle. Further truncation of the dystrophin gene (94) may improve results.

An adenovirus vector transduces various tissues after intravenous administration of 2 to 5 day-old mice (104). Animal age significantly affects transduction efficiency because, as the animal gets larger, the limit in vector titer becomes an obstacle in transducing large numbers of cells. The route of administration to 2-day-old rats also influences both the efficiency and tissue distribution transduction (56). Greater than 25% of muscle cells in the diaphragm, intercostal muscles, and heart are positive for the β-galactosidase marker when vector is administered via the heart. In contrast, injection into the tail vein labels fewer than 5% of cells in the same muscle groups, although, 12% of muscles in the tail were labelled. Skeletal muscle was most efficiently transduced by direct injection of the adenoviral vector.

A truncated, Becker-type dystrophin cDNA cloned into an adenoviral vector and introduced into the biceps femoris muscle of 5 to 9 day-old mdx mice produced human dystrophin in 20% of muscle fibers 13 weeks after injection of 3×10^9 pfu of vector (96). Reversal of necrotic degeneration and functional improvement were not detected. Physiological improvement did occur (112), following an injection of 7×10^9 pfu into the gastrocnemius muscle of an 8-day old mdx mouse that produced human dystrophin in 64% of muscle fibers. The proportion of centronucleated fibers, an index of repair necessitated by fiber injury, declined from 60% in untreated muscle to 10% in muscle inoculated with the dystrophin vector.

Thus, three different vector systems are able to transfer genes into skeletal muscle. A direct comparison of gene transfer by plasmid, retrovirus, and adenovirus into normal and regenerating muscles of (32) normal C57Bl/6 mice, found that only plasmid and adenovirus vectors can transduce uninjured muscle. Following an injection of cardiotoxin that induces muscle regeneration, all three vectors transduce muscle cells. Plasmid and adenovirus have similar efficiencies, superior to that of the retrovirus, under these conditions. The inefficiency of the retroviral vector reflected the low titer used—only 5×10^4 pfu compared to 5×10^7 pfu of the adenoviral vector. Both viral vectors, but not plasmid DNA, elicited inflammation. Retroviral vectors and plasmid transduced only muscle cells, whereas adenoviral vector also transduced other cell types. These experiments used submaximal titers of adenovirus in adult (6–7 week old) mice; the higher rates of transduction by the adenoviral vector might have been achieved with younger mice and higher titers of adenoviral vector (104). Thus, adenoviral and plasmid vectors appear more promising than retroviral vectors for gene transfer into muscle, but further study of plasmid stability and adenoviral toxicity is needed.

Parkinson Disease

Parkinson Disease (PD) is caused by progressive loss of dopaminergic neurons from the substantia nigra. The proximate cause of this loss is unknown. Animal models replicate the symptoms, if not the etiology, of PD (see (11) for a review). With these models, grafts of dopamine-producing cells improve Parkinsonian symptoms. Cell grafts of either adrenal medulla or fetal brain tissue have been tested clinically but limited tissue availability, histo-incompatability, and controversy over interpretation of results prevent widespread use of this technique. Gene therapy using implants of genetically engineered autologous cells and direct gene transfer is being tested in animal models as alternatives to allografts.

The initial transplantation efforts to increase L-DOPA production in models of PD used transformed cells such as the rat phenochromocytoma cell line PC12 genetically modified to express tyrosine hydroxylase (TH, EC 1.14.16.2) (54, 125). Behavioral improvements occurred, but the transformed cells proved tumorgenic. Reduction of tumorgenicity by modifying PC12 cells to express nerve growth factor prevented both tumor and TH expression (28).

Nontransformed primary cells proved a better alternative. The first report that transplantation of primary fibroblasts modified to produce L-DOPA reduces Parkinsonian motor defects in Fischer rats appeared in 1991 (43). Primary muscle cells transfected with a plasmid encoding TH have also been used to deliver L-DOPA to denervated striatum (59). After muscle cell transplantation, motor function, as measured by apomorphine-induced rotation, became normal. Improvement persisted for up to 4 months, far superior to the 4 and 8 weeks achieved by fibroblasts transduced with L-DOPO containing retroviral vector. Genetic engineering with retroviral vectors has also been used to improve the performance of fetal mesencephalic cell grafts in rats. Because TH activity is increased by phosphorylation, cells were modified to overexpress protein kinase C (131). Although these implanted cells lived no longer, they did form better synaptic contact with cells of the host striatum.

The utility of implanting neurons engineered with retroviral vectors to express TH has been studied in primate models of PD. Neurons modified to express TH under control of a temperature-sensitive promotor of SV40 virus T antigen produced behavioral improvements in two monkeys for 1 month after transplantation and in rats for 2 months (7).

Because most of the cells engineered to express TH lack the aromatic acid decarboxylase required to synthesize dopamine from L-DOPA, L-DOPA must exit these cells and be taken up by neurons that contain the required enzyme. Alternatively, increased levels of dopamine within neurons of the targeted region may not be achieved and some other mechanism accounts for the improvement in Parkinsonian symptoms that follow grafting. Optimization of clinical results will require further understanding of mechanism.

Both HSV (40) and AAV (65) have been used to deliver the TH gene to the striatum of rats treated with 6-hydroxydopamine (6-OHDA); with HSV, both biochemical and behavioral recovery were noted. Behavioral recovery persist up to 1 year after vector inoculation (40). However, 10% of treated animals died shortly after vector inoculation and some tissue necrosis occurred in the region of the injection even in surviving animals. Also, despite the persistence of effect, the number of transduced cells declined with time after treatment. With AAV, no vector-related toxicity was seen, and expression of a lacZ marker gene persisted for four months. However, the number of cells expressing β-galactosidase did decline over time. With a TH vector, behavioral recovery was seen as long as two months after inoculation. It was not determined whether the vector had stably integrated.

Restoration of dopamine levels attends only to the manifestations of neurodegeneration in PD, not to the actual cause of the loss of dopaminergic neurons. The ability of various neuronal growth factors to slow or even reverse this loss of neurons has been tested using a rat fibroblast cell line transduced with retroviral vectors carrying different growth factors gene. Nerve growth factor (NGF) and basic fibroblast growth factor (bFGF) protect striatal neurons from the neurotoxic effects of quinolinic acid (47); however, brain-derived neurotrophic factor (BDNF) does not. Thus, neurotropic agents may constitute an alternative or supplement to the provision of TH or dopamine in treating PD. BDNF also protects neurons from 1-methyl-4-phenylpyridium (MPTP) toxicity in a rat model. However, because rats are relatively insensitive to MPTP, it is unclear whether the neuroprotective effect of fibroblasts expressing BDNF results from BDNF or rat cells injured by MPTP are inherently more capable of recovering from this insult.

Protection from neurotoxicity is not the only potential benefit of delivering neurotrophic factors to PD lesions. Striatal implantation of cells transduced with retroviral vectors directing expression of NGF (27) or bFGF (107) together with fetal brain cells improves implant viability in a 6-OHDA treated rat. With either growth factor, behavioral improvements persist for at least 2 months. Other neurotrophic factors, such as ciliary neurotrophic factor (53), neurotrophin-4/5 (57), or glial-derived neurotrophic factor by maintaining neuronal viability or improving implant survival may also prove useful in PD (76).

Questions remain regarding the clinical relevance of these implant models. In PD, the degeneration of neurons of the substantia nigra has excitatory and degenerative effects on other brain nuclei. Although the striatum is indirectly affected by the neuronal degeneration within the substantia nigra pars compacta, it is not the primary locus of the effect of PD. Implant models demonstrate that cells engineered to secrete growth factors can ameliorate these secondary striatal effects of nigral neurodegeneration; however, the ability to prevent nigral degeneration has not yet been shown.

Genes other than those for neurotrophic factors have been tested for the ability to promote graft survival in lesioned rats. Embryonic mesencephnalic cells derived from transgenic mice engineered to over-express Cu/Zn superoxide dismutase, survive longer in 6-OHDA lesioned rats than do cells from normal embryos (86). This suggests that protection from oxidative stress may also improve survival of the graft, and its therapeutic effect.

Other Neurodegenerative Disorders

One difficulty in developing gene therapy for neurological disorders is the lack of appropriate animal models. Even though lesioning of the substantia nigra does not reproduce the chronic clinical aspects of PD, it at least produces the same focal loss of neurons. Diseases such as Alzheimer disease (AD), in which the brain undergoes a progressive pathological change, are particularly hard to model. The loss of cholinergic neurons in AD is reproduced by surgical lesions of the rat fimbria and formix which induce retrograde degeneration of cholinergic neurons. In one of the earliest experiments of gene transfer to the CNS, grafting a fibroblast cell line transduced with a retroviral vector carrying the cDNA for NGF reduced the degener-

ation of cholinergic neurons in this model (98). Grafting of cells of fibroblast lines transfected with an NGF expression plasmid (105), or primary fibroblasts transduced with a NGF retroviral vector (67), produces similar results. Although grafts of primary fibroblasts are not as neuroprotective as grafts of cell lines, primary fibroblasts have the advantage of not forming tumors. Furthermore, such grafts of primary cells evoke hippocampal reinnervation from the lesioned fimbria and fornix (67). Implants of cultured cells transfected with a neurotrophin-3 expression plasmid are also neuroprotective (8) in a model of neuronal degeneration involving 6-OHDA ablation of noradrenergic neurons of the locus coeruleus.

In analogy with the restoration of dopamine levels in PD by transfer of TH, transfer of choline acetyl transferase (ChAT) to restore the acetylcholine deleted in AD has been studied. Fibroblasts transduced with a retroviral vector directing expression of ChAT release acetylcholine when provided with choline (44). When these cells are implanted into the hippocampus of rats, they continue to secrete acetylcholine in response to local infusions of choline. Similar grafts in a different rat model amelionate behavioral deficits associated with loss of cholinergic neurons. Following ablation of the cholinergic neurons of the nucleus basalis magnocellularis with ibotenic acid, implants of fibroblasts expressing the Drosophila ChAT significantly improve the rats' performance of a spatial navigation task (120). While the actual relationship between ablation of neurons with ibotenic acid and the behavioral deficits seen in rats remains debatable (11, 16), these results suggest that measurable cognitive improvements can be obtained, even with fibroblasts releasing acetylcholine in a non-regulated, tonic manner.

Huntington Disease (HD) is modeled by neuronal damage caused by other neurotoxins. Quinolinic acid, an excitotoxin that acts primarily on the N-methyl-D-aspartate (NMDA) glutamate receptor, produces striatal neuronal damage similar to that seen in (HD). NGF, delivered by cells implanted at the site of lesion, is neuroprotective against the effects of quinolinic acid when delivered by implanted cells at the site of lesion (46, 101). Inhibition of mitochondrial function by systemic treatment with 3-nitropropionic acid also mimics some of the neurodegeneration seen in HD. Implantation of a fibroblast cell line transduced with a retroviral vector directing expression of NGF protects the striatum (48).

Conclusions and Future Perspectives

Lysosomal storage diseases are the first candidates for treatment by gene therapy. Clinical trial is already underway for GD. Other storage diseases in which bone marrow transplantation is beneficial are likely candidates for gene therapy as well. Despite the great promise of gene therapy for treating these diseases, some caveats must be noted. Many of these diseases primarily involve hematopoietically-derived monocytes. Although monocytes occur in many tissues, the ability of genetically altered cells to seed all the appropriate target tissues sufficiently well to produce clinical improvement is unproved. Particularly in the case of the MPSs, correction of the biochemical defect requires appropriate regulation of gene expression. In addition, because neurological deficits are often irreversible, gene therapy needs to be performed very early in the course of the disease, possibly even *in utero*.

Muscular dystrophy presents the challenge of delivering the therapeutic gene to the majority of cells at a large number of sites throughout the body. Currently, no systemic method of gene delivery provides gene transfer sufficient for clinical effect. Because systemic treatment is likely needed, a means of accurately targeting muscle cells is required. Despite these significant technical hurdles, gene therapy affords the best hope for a cure of muscular dystrophy.

The gene therapy of other neurodegenerative diseases, which currently attempts delivery of neurotrophic factors or augmentation of diminished neurotransmitter level, is hampered by poor understanding of disease etiology. The pleiotropic effects of neurotrophic factors confound interpretation of animal experiments. Neuroprotection may arise indirectly by stimulating an intermediate effector cell (eg. astroglia) rather than directly by sustaining degenerating neurons. Improved understanding of the molecular mechanisms of PD, AD, or HD will permit targeting of therapy to etiology rather than symptoms.

Acknowledgments

I am grateful to Michael Brownstein, Beth Hoffman, and Richard Schneiderman for their comments on drafts of this review. I also thank Rebecca Voorthuis and Kate Walshe for help in preparing this article.

REFERENCES

1. On-line Mendelian Inheritance in Man, OMIM (TM) [database online], Baltimore: Johns Hopkins University, MIM Number: *252800, Mucopolysaccharidosis type I. Date last edited: 13 January, 1995.
2. Acsadi, G., Dickson, G., Love, D. R., et al. Human dystrophin expression in mdx mice after intramuscular infection of DNA constructs. Nature *352:*815–818, 1991.
3. Anson, D. S., Bielicki, J., and Hopwood, J. J. Correction of mucopolysaccharidosis type I fibroblasts by retroviral-mediated transfer of the human alpha-L-iduronidase gene. Hum. Gene Ther. *3:*371–379, 1992.
4. Anson, D. S., Muller, V., Bielicki, J., et al. Overexpression of N-acetylgalactosamine-4-sulphatase induces a multiple sulphatase deficiency in mucopolysaccharidosis-type-VI fibroblasts. Biochem. J. *294:*657–662, 1993.
5. Anton, R., Kordower, J. H., Maidment, N. T., et al. Neural-targeted gene therapy for rodent and primate hemiparkinsonism. Exp. Neurol. *127:*207–218, 1994.
6. Arenas, E. and Persson, H. Neurotrophin-3 prevents the death of adult central noradrenergic neurons in vivo. Nature *367:*368–371, 1994.
7. Bahnson, A. B., Nimgaonkar, M., Fei, Y., et al. Transduction of CD34+ enriched cord blood and Gaucher bone marrow cells by a retroviral vector carrying the glucocerebrosidase gene. Gene Ther. *1:*176–184, 1994.
8. Bankiewicz, K., Mandel, R. J., and Sofroniew, M. V. Trophism, transplantation, and animal models of Parkinson's disease. Exp. Neurol. *124:*140–149, 1993.
9. Birkenmeier, E. H., Barker, J. E., Vogler, C. A., et al. Increased life span and correction of metabolic defects in murine mucopolysaccharidosis type VII after syngeneic bone marrow transplantation. Blood. *78:*3081–3092, 1991.
10. Birkenmeier, E. H., Davisson, M. T., Beamer, W. G., et al. Murine mucopolysaccharidosis type VII. Characterization of a mouse with beta-glucuronidase deficiency. J. Clin. Invest. *83:*1258–1256, 1989.
11. Bjorklund, A. and Dunnett, S. B. Acetylcholine revisited. Nature *375:*446, 1995.
12. Brady, R. O., Barton, N. W., and Grabowski, G. A. The role of Neurogenetics in Gaucher Disease. Arch. Neurol. *50:*1212–1224, 1993.
13. Braun, S. E., Aronovich, E. L., Anderson, R. A., et al. Metabolic correction and cross-correction of mucopolysaccharidosis type II (Hunter syndrome) by retroviral-mediated gene transfer and expression of human iduronate-2-sulfatase. Proc. Natl. Acad. Sci. U. S. A. *90:*11830–11834, 1993.
14. Cartier, N., Lopez, J., Moullier, P., et al. Retroviral-mediated gene transfer corrects very-long-chain fatty

acid metabolism in adrenoleukodystrophy fibroblasts. Proc. Natl. Acad. Sci. U. S. A. *92:*1674–1678, 1995.

15. Correll, P. H., Colilla, S., Dave, H. P., et al. High levels of human glucocerebrosidase activity in macrophages of long-term reconstituted mice after retroviral infection of hematopoietic stem cells. Blood. *80:* 331–336, 1992.

16. Correll, P. H., Fink, J. K., Brady, R. O., et al. Production of human glucocerebrosidase in mice after retroviral gene transfer into multipotential hematopoietic progenitor cells. Proc. Natl. Acad. Sci. U. S. A. *86:*8912–8916, 1989.

17. Correll, P. H., Kew, Y., Perry, L. K., et al. Expression of human glucocerebrosidase in long-term reconstituted mice following retroviral-mediated gene transfer into hematopoietic stem cells. Human. Gene. Ther. *1:*277–287, 1990.

18. Cunningham, L. A., Short, M. P., Breakefield, X. O., et al. Nerve growth factor released by transgenic astrocytes enhances the function of adrenal chromaffin cell grafts in a rat model of Parkinson's disease. Brain Res. *658:*219–231, 1994.

19. Cunningham, L. A., Short, M. P., Vielkind, U., et al. Survival and differentiation within the adult mouse striatum of grafted rat pheochromocytoma cells (PC12) genetically modified to express recombinant beta-NGF. Exp. Neurol. *112:*174–182, 1991.

20. Danko, I., Fritz, J. D., Jiao, S., et al. Pharmacological enhancement of in vivo foreign gene expression in muscle. Gene Ther. *1:*114–121, 1994.

21. Davis, H. L., Demeneix, B. A., Quantin, B., et al. Plasmid DNA is superior to viral vectors for direct gene transfer into adult mouse skeletal muscle. Hum. Gene Ther. *4:*733–740, 1993.

22. Davis, H. L. and Jasmin, B. J. Direct gene transfer into mouse diaphragm. FEBS. Lett. *333:*146–150, 1993.

23. Davis, H. L., Whalen, R. G., and Demeneix, B. A. Direct gene transfer into skeletal muscle in vivo: Factors affecting efficiency of transfer and stability of expression. Human. Gene. Ther. *4:*151–159, 1993.

24. Deshmane, S. L., Valyi-Nagy, T., Block, T., et al. An HSV-1 containing the rat b-glucuronidase cDNA inserted within the LAT gene is less efficient that the parental strain at establishing a transcriptionally active state during latency in neurons. Gene Ther. *2:*209–217, 1995.

25. Dinur, T., Schuchman, E. H., Fibach, E., et al. Toward gene therapy for Niemann-Pick Disease (NPD): Separation of retrovirally corrected and noncorrected NPD fibroblasts using a novel fluorescent sphingomyelin. Hum. Gene Ther. *3:*633–639, 1992.

26. Dunckley, M. G., Wells, D. J., Walsh, F. S., et al. Direct retroviral-mediated transfer of a dystrophin minigene into mdx mouse muscle in vivo. Hum. Mol. Genet. *2:*717–723, 1993.

27. During, M. J., Naegele, J. R., O'Malley, K. L., et al. Long-term behavioral recovery in Parkinsonian rats by an HSV vector expressing tyrosine hydroxylase. Science. *266:*1399–1402, 1994.

28. Fisher, L. J., Jinnah, H. A., Kale, L. C., et al. Survival and function of intrastriatally grafted primary fibroblasts genetically modified to produce L-dopa. Neuron. *6:*371–380, 1991.

29. Fisher, L. J., Raymon, H. K., and Gage, F. H. Cells engineered to produce acetylcholine: Therapeutic potential for Alzheimer's disease. Ann. N. Y. Acad. Sci. *695:*278–284, 1993.

30. Fratantoni, J. C., Hall, C. W., and Neufeld, E. F. Hurler and Hunter syndromes: mutual correction of the defect in cultured fibroblasts. Science *162:*570–572, 1968.

31. Frim, D. M., Short, M. P., Rosenberg, W. S., et al. Local protective effects of nerve growth factor-secreting fibroblasts against excitotoxic lesions in the rat striatum. J. Neurosurg. *78:*267–273, 1993.

32. Frim, D. M., Uhler, T. A., Short, M. P., et al. Effects of biologically delivered NGF, BDNF and bFGF on striatal excitotoxic lesions. Neuroreport. *4:*367–370, 1993.

33. Frim, D. M., Wüllner, U., Beal, M. F., et al. Implanted NGF-producing fibroblasts induce catalase and modify ATP levels but do not affect glutamate receptor binding or NMDA receptor expression in the rat striatum. Exp. Neurol. *128:*172–180, 1994.

34. Hagg, T. and Varon, S. Ciliary neurotrophic factor prevents degeneration of adult rat substantia nigra dopaminergic neurons in vivo. Proc. Natl. Acad. Sci. U. S. A. *90:*6315–6319, 1993.

35. Horellou, P., Brundin, P., Kalen, P., et al. In vivo release of DOPA and dopamine from genetically engineered cells grafted to the denervated rat striatum. Neuron. *5:*393–402, 1990.

36. Huard, J., Lochmuller, H., Acsadi, G., et al. The route of administration is a major determinant of the transduction efficiency of rat tissues by adenoviral recombinants. Gene Ther. *2:*107–115, 1995.

37. Hynes, M. A., Poulsen, K., Armanini, M., et al. Neurotrophin-4/5 is a survival factor for embryonic midbrain dopaminergic neurons in enriched cultures. J. Neurosci. Res. *37:*144–154, 1994.

38. Jiao, S., Gurevich, V., and Wolff, J. A. Long-term correction of rat model of Parkinson's disease by gene therapy. Nature *362:*450–453, 1993.

39. Kantoff, P. W., Flake, A. W., Eglitis, M. A., et al. In utero gene transfer and expression: a sheep transplantation model. Blood. *73:*1066–1073, 1989.

40. Kaplitt, M. G., Leone, P., Samulski, R. J., et al. Long-term gene expression and phenotypic correction using adeno-associated virus vectors in the mammalian brain. Nat. Genet. *8:*148–154, 1994.

41. Kawaja, M. D., Rosenberg, M. B., Yoshida, K., et al. Somatic gene transfer of nerve growth factor promotes the survival of axotomized septal neurons and the regeneration of their axons in adult rats. J. Neurosci. *12:*2849–2864, 1992.

42. Koyata, H., Cox, R. P., and Chuang, D. T. Stable correction of maple syrup urine disease in cells from a Mennonite patient by retroviral-mediated gene transfer. Biochem. J. *295:*635–639, 1993.

43. Krall, W. J., Challita, P. M., Perlmutter, L. S., et al. Cells expressing human glucocerebrosidase from a retroviral vector repopulate macrophages and central nervous system microglia after murine bone marrow transplantation. Blood. *83:*2737–2748, 1994.

44. Kyle, J. W., Birkenmeier, E. H., Babette, G., et al. Correction of murine mucopolysaccharidosis VII by

a human b-glucuronidase transgene. Proc. Natl. Acad. Sci. *87:*3914–3918, 1990.

45. Lin, H., Parmacek, M. S., Morle, G., et al. Expression of recombinant genes in myocardium in vivo after direct injection of DNA. Circulation. *82:*2217–2221, 1990.

46. Lin, L. H., Doherty, D. H., Lile, J. D., et al. GDNF: A glial cell line-derived neurotrophic factor for midbrain dopaminergic neurons. Science *260:*1130–1132, 1993.

47. Marechal, V., Naffakh, N., Danos, O., et al. Disappearance of lysosomal storage in spleen and liver of mucopolysaccharidosis VII mice after transplantation of genetically modified bone marrow cells. Blood. *82:*1358–1365, 1993.

48. Morgan, J. E. Cell and gene therapy in Duchenne muscular dystrophy. Hum. Gene Ther. *5:*165–173, 1994.

49. Moullier, P., Bohl, D., Cardoso, J., et al. Long-term delivery of a lysosomal enzyme by genetically modified fibroblasts in dogs. Nature Med. *1:*353–357, 1995.

50. Moullier, P., Bohl, D., Heard, J. M., et al. Correction of lysosomal storage in the liver and spleen of MPS VII mice by implantation of genetically modified skin fibroblasts. Nat. Genet. *4:*154–159, 1993.

51. Nakao, N., Frodl, E. M., Widner, H., et al. Overexpressing Cu/Zn superoxide dismutase enhances survival of transplanted neurons in a rat model of Parkinson's disease. Nature. Med. *1:*226–231, 1995.

52. Nimgaonakar, M. T., Bahnson, A. B., Boggs, S. S., et al. Transuction of mobilized peripheral blood CD34+ cells with the glucocerebrosidase cDNA. Gene Ther. *1:*201–207, 1994.

53. Nolta, J. A., Sender, L. S., Barranger, J. A., et al. Expression of human glucocerebrosidase in murine long-term bone marrow cultures after retroviral vector-mediated transfer. Blood. *75:*787–797, 1990.

54. Nolta, J. A., Yu, X. J., Bahner, I., et al. Retroviral-mediated transfer of the human glucocerebrosidase gene into cultured Gaucher bone marrow. J. Clin. Invest. *90:*342–348, 1992.

55. Occhiodoro, T., Hopwood, J. J., Morris, C. P., et al. Correction of alpha-L-fucosidase deficiency in fucosidosis fibroblasts by retroviral vector-mediated gene transfer. Hum. Gene Ther. *3:*365–369, 1992.

56. Ohashi, T., Boggs, S., Robbins, P., et al. Efficient transfer and sustained high expression of the human glucocerebrosidase gene in mice and their functional macrophages following transplantation of bone marrow transduced by a retroviral vector. Proc. Natl. Acad. Sci. U. S. A. *89:*11332–11336, 1992.

57. Passos-Bueno, M. R., Vainzof, M., Marie, S. K., et al. Half the dystrophin gene is apparently enough for a mild clinical course: confirmation of its potential use for gene therapy. Hum. Mol. Genet. *3:*919–922, 1994.

58. Rafi, M. A., Amini, S., Zhang, X. L., et al. Correction of sulfatide metabolism after transfer of prosaposin cDNA to cultured cells from a patient with SAP-1 deficiency. Am. J. Hum. Genet. *50:*1252–1258, 1992.

59. Ragot, T., Vincent, N., Chafey, P., et al. Efficient adenovirus-mediated transfer of a human minidystro-

phin gene to skeletal muscle of mdx mice. Nature *361:*647–650, 1993.

60. Rommerskirch, W., Fluharty, A. L., Peters, C., et al. Restoration of arylsulphatase A activity in human-metachromaticleucodystrophy fibroblasts via retroviral-vector-mediated gene transfer. Biochem. J. *280:* 459–461, 1991.

61. Rosenberg, M. B., Friedmann, T., Robertson, R. C., et al. Grafting genetically modified cells to the damaged brain: restorative effects of NGF expression. Science *242:*1575–1578, 1988.

62. Schuchman, E. H., Suchi, M., Takahashi, T., et al. Human acid sphingomyelinase. Isolation, nucleotide sequence and expression of the full-length and alternatively spliced cDNAs. J. Biol. Chem. *266:*8531–8539, 1991.

63. Schumacher, J. M., Short, B. T., Hyman, B. T., et al. Intracerebral implantation of nerve growth factor-producing fibroblasts protects striatum against neurotoxic levels of excitatory amino acids. Neurosci. *45:*561–570, 1991.

64. Stratford-Perricaudet, L. D., Makeh, I., Perricaudet, M., et al. Widespread long-term gene transfer to mouse skeletal muscles and heart. J. Clin. Invest. *90:*626–630, 1992.

65. Stromberg, I., Wetmore, C. J., Ebendal, T., et al. Rescue of basal forebrain cholinergic neurons after implantation of genetically modified cells producing recombinant NGF. J. Neurosci. Res. *25:*405–411, 1990.

66. Suchi, M., Dinur, T., Desnick, R. J., et al. Retroviral-mediated transfer of the human acid sphingomyelinase cDNA: correction of the metabolic defect in cultured Niemann-Pick disease cells. Proc. Natl. Acad. Sci. U. S. A. *89:*3227–3231, 1992.

67. Takayama, H., Ray, J., Raymon, H. K., et al. Basic fibroblast growth factor increases dopaminergic graft survival and function in a rat model of Parkinson's disease. Nature Med. *1:*53–58, 1995.

68. Taylor, R. M., Stewart, G. J., Farrow, B. R. H., et al. The effect of bone marrow-derived cells on lysosomal enzyme activity in the brain after marrow engraftment. Transplant. Proc. *21:*3822–3823, 1989.

69. Vincent, N., Ragot, T., Gilgenkrantz, H., et al. Long-term correction of mouse dystrophic degeneration by adenovirus-mediated transfer of a minidystrophin gene. Nature Genet. *5:*130–134, 1993.

70. Vitadello, M., Schiaffino, M. V., Picard, A., et al. Gene transfer in regenerating muscle. Hum. Gene. Ther. *5:*11–18, 1994.

71. Walkley, S. U., Thrall, M. A., Dobrenis, K., et al. Bone marrow transplantation corrects the enzyme defect in neurons of the central nervous system in a lysosmal storage disease. Proc. Natl. Acad. Sci. U. S. A. *91:* 2970–2974, 1994.

72. Wei, J., Wei, F., Samulski, R. J., et al. Expression of the human glucocerebrosidase and arylsulfatase A genes in murine and patient primary fibroblasts transduced by and adeno-associated virus vector. Gene Ther. *1:*261–268, 1994.

73. Weinthal, J., Nolta, J. A., Yu, X. J., et al. Expression of human glucocerebrosidase following retroviral vector-mediated transduction of murine hematopoietic

stem cells. Bone. Marrow. Transplant. *8:*403–412, 1991.

74. Wells, D. J. Improved gene transfer by direct plasmid injection associated with regeneration in mouse skeletal muscle. FEBS Lett. *332:*179–182, 1993.

75. Winkler, J., Suhr, S. T., Gage, F. H., et al. Essential role of neocortical acetylcholine in spatial memory. Nature *375:*484–487, 1995.

76. Wolfe, J. H., Deshmane, S. L., and Fraser, N. W. Herpesvirus vector gene transfer and expression of b-glucuronidase in the central nervous system of MPS VII mice. Nature Genet. *1:*379–384, 1992.

77. Wolfe, J. H., Kyle, J. W., Sands, M. S., et al. High level expression and export of b-glucuronidase from murine mucopolysaccharidosis VII cells corrected by a double-copy retrovirus vector. Gene Ther. *2:*70–78, 1995.

78. Wolfe, J. H., Sands, M. S., Barker, J. E., et al. Reversal of pathology in murine mucopolysaccharidosis type VII by somatic cell gene transfer. Nature. *360:*749–753, 1992.

79. Wolff, J. A., Fisher, L. J., Xu, L., et al. Grafting fibroblasts genetically modified to produce L-dopa in a rat model of Parkinson disease. Proc. Natl. Acad. Sci. U. S. A. *86:*9011–9014, 1989.

80. Wolff, J. A., Malone, R. W., Williams, P., et al. Direct gene transfer into mouse muscle in vivo. Science *247:*1465–1468, 1990.

81. Xu, L., Stahl, S. K., Dave, H. P., et al. Correction of the enzyme deficiency in hematopoietic cells of Gaucher patients using a clinically acceptable retroviral supernatant transduction protocol. Exp. Hematol. *22:*223–230, 1994.

82. Xu, L. C., Karlsson, S., Byrne, E. R., et al. Long-term in vivo expression of the human glucocerebrosidase gene in nonhuman primates after CD34+ hematopoietic cell transduction with cell-free retroviral vector preparations. Proc. Natl. Acad. Sci. U. S. A. *92:*4372–4376, 1995.

83. Zhu, S. M., Kujirai, K., Dollison, A., et al. Implantation of genetically modified mesencephalic fetal cells into the rat striatum. Brain Res. Bull. *29:*81–93, 1992.

Index

Page references followed by *t* or *f* indicate tables or figures, respectively.